S0-AFF-672

Community Health Nursing
Concepts and Practice

THIRD EDITION

Barbara Walton Spradley, R.N., M.N.

Public Health Nursing, School of Public Health,
University of Minnesota, Minneapolis

SCOTT, FORESMAN/LITTLE, BROWN HIGHER EDUCATION
A Division of Scott, Foresman and Company
Glenview, Illinois   London, England

Credit lines for copyrighted materials appearing in this work appear in the Credits section beginning on page 765.

Library of Congress Cataloging-in-Publication Data

Spradley, Barbara Walton.
   Community health nursing: concepts and practice/Barbara Walton Spradley. — 3rd ed.
      p.   cm.
   Includes bibliographical references.
   1. Community health nursing.   2. Public health nursing.   I. Title.
   [DNLM: 1. Community Health Nursing. WY 106 S766c]
   RT98.S68   1990
   610.73'43 — dc20
   DNLM/DLC
   For Library of Congress   89-24272
                                                                                              CIP

ISBN 0-673-39805-6

Copyright © 1990 by Barbara Walton Spradley.

Artwork, illustrations, and other materials supplied by the publisher.
Copyright © 1990 Scott, Foresman and Company.

1 2 3 4 5 6 -KPF- 94 93 92 91 90 89

To Neil
with love and thanks

Contents

3   Community Health Nursing Foundations: Past and Present   64

4   Family Theory   98

5   Culture and Community   130

24 Research in Community Health Nursing   721

25 Political Involvement and Community Health Advocacy   737

Contributing Authors

Dorothy Brockopp, Ph.D., R.N.
Associate Professor
College of Nursing
University of Kentucky
Lexington, Kentucky

Beverly Dorsey, M.P.H., R.N.
Associate Director
Ambulatory Care Services
University of Minnesota Hospital
  and Clinic
Minneapolis, Minnesota

Sara T. Fry, Ph.D., R.N.
Associate Professor
School of Nursing
University of Maryland
Baltimore, Maryland

Michele Hadeka, M.S., R.N.
Associate Professor
School of Nursing
University of Vermont
Burlington, Vermont

Laura N. Harris, B.A.
Associate Staff
Voyageur Outward Bound
Red Lodge, Montana

**Pamela Thul-Immler,
M.P.H., R.N.C.**
Quality Assurance Chair
Ambulatory Nursing
Hennepin County Medical Center
Minneapolis, Minnesota

Terry W. Miller, M.S.N., P.H.N.
Assistant Professor
Department of Nursing
School of Applied Arts
  and Sciences
San Jose State University
San Jose, California

Elaine Richard, M.S., R.N.
Director of Occupational Health
HealthLine
St. Joseph's Hospital
Tampa, Florida

Preface

The third edition of *Community Health Nursing: Concepts and Practice* represents a continuing effort to capture the essence of community health nursing and to clarify its meaning for the student and practitioner. It is written to share enthusiasm for a field whose complex nature demands and fosters creativity, leadership, and innovation. As a basic text, the third edition, like the first two, is designed to give undergraduate nursing students a comprehensive introduction to the field of community health nursing. As a professional resource it is also designed to enlarge the vision and enhance the impact of practicing community health nurses.

In response to the demands of a changing health care scene, this edition incorporates several new topics and expands on many others. As a result, this edition is even more comprehensive and sharply focused on issues of current and future concern to community health nurses. Four entirely new chapters address maternal and infant health, environmental health, quality assurance, and research in community health nursing. The chapter on epidemiology has been rewritten to clarify the meaning and application of that field of public health for community health nurses. In the epidemiology chapter the host-agent-environment model has been incorporated with the broader multiple-causation view to better prepare nurses for understanding the complexity of causal relationships in health and illness. Expanded topic coverage in the third edition includes strengthened integration of systems theory and community health nursing conceptual models, including the Neuman model (Chapter 3); family theory (Chapter 4); poverty, homelessness, and the health of migrant workers (Chapter 5); ethical decision making (Chapter 6); program planning and evaluation (Chapter 8); and teaching-learning theory (Chapter 11). Woven throughout the book is an even stronger emphasis than in previous editions on the nursing of aggregates.

Reviews and feedback from colleagues affirmed that the basic organization and content of the first two editions should be retained, with changes made primarily for reinforcement and updating. Notable organizational changes in the third edition include the following:

1. A strengthened family theory chapter was moved from Part Three, Care of Communities, to Part One, Conceptual Foundations.
2. The chapter on roles and settings for community health nursing practice was moved from Part One to Part Two, Tools for Practice.
3. New chapters on maternal-infant health and environmental health were added to Part Three.
4. Part Four, Expanding the Nurse's Influence, was broadened with new chapters on quality assurance and research in community health nursing.

Each of the book's four major parts provides the reader with a different perspective on community health nursing. Part One introduces the conceptual foundations for this field of nursing practice with an updated discussion of community health in Chapter 1 and coverage of health care organization and financing in Chapter 2. These two chapters set the stage for expanded coverage in Chapter 3 of the theoretical and conceptual bases for community health nursing practice, as well as its nature and scope. Family theory comes next in Chapter 4, giving the nurse a foundation for understanding this basic societal unit. Chapter 5 features a discussion of the cultural dimension, and Chapter 6 explores values and ethical decision making.

Part Two presents important tools for community health nursing practice. Roles and settings for practice are discussed in Chapter 7, application of the nursing process in Chapter 8, epidemiology in Chapter 9, the helping relationship and contracting in Chapter 10, community health education in Chapter 11, and crisis prevention and intervention in Chapter 12.

Part Three, Care of Communities, begins with coverage of community health assessment in Chapter 13 and small-group and population work in Chapter 14. The remaining chapters focus on specific target communities or populations, including families, mothers and infants, children and adolescents, working adults, the environment, the elderly, and the home care population.

Part Four explores the expanding influence of community health nurses through leadership and management of planned change in Chapter 22, quality assurance in Chapter 23, conducting and using community health nursing research in Chapter 24, and political involvement and advocacy in Chapter 25.

Community health nursing, now more than ever, is a challenging, evolving field of nursing practice — one that is on the cutting edge of many innovations in health care delivery. It is, at the same time, a field of nursing that continues to be surrounded by some confusion. *Community Health Nursing: Concepts and Practice* originally was written to clarify the nature and practice of community health nursing. This third edition seeks to further elucidate the conceptual and philosophical foundations influencing the definition of this nursing specialty. In recent years, the nursing community has engaged in considerable discussion and debate over the meaning of community health nursing versus public health nursing. The two terms have been used synonymously in this and other texts as well as in the field. The rationale continues to be that nurses who incorporate public health theory and principles into their practice, who emphasize the care of communities of people, or who take a population-focused view, are true public health practitioners. Confusion enters when community health nursing is defined by where, rather than how, it is practiced. Dramatic increases in ambulatory and home care are creating an escalating demand for nurses to practice in the community; many of these nurses, however, practice basic nursing or other nursing specialties, not community health nursing as we define it here. The challenge for the nurse who wishes to practice community health nursing lies in incorporating public health knowledge and skills with basic nursing knowledge and skills to offer preventive, health-promoting, protective services that benefit population groups. As beginning practitioners nurses may have limited impact on populations, but a population or aggregate orientation must be germane to their practice. At advanced levels of practice, with advanced training in public health, nurses can become specialists in public or community health.

The third edition of this text thus continues to use the terms *community health nurse* and *public health nurse* interchangeably, based on the belief that either label is appropriate so long as it describes a practitioner whose work incorporates public health theory and skills, including a population-focused practice.

ACKNOWLEDGMENTS

Many individuals have contributed to the completion of this third edition. To acknowledge them all would be impossible, given the limitations of space and memory. Many have unwittingly enriched the writing through sharing their experiences and expertise. Others have directly provided ideas, criticism, encouragement, and support. To all I offer my sincere gratitude, and in so doing am reminded once more that no person is an island. Life's successes depend in large measure on our interdependence with other people. Like the public health principle of collaboration, we need teamwork to get a job done, and this text is no exception.

Four individuals, in particular, made substantial new contributions to this third edition. Michele Hadeka wrote the chapter on maternal and infant populations, Laura Harris coauthored the chapter on environmental health, Pamela Thul-Immler contributed the chapter on quality assurance, and Dorothy Brockopp prepared the chapter on research in community health nursing. My thanks go to each of them.

I am grateful to all my faculty colleagues in the School of Public Health for their ideas and encouragement. I especially wish to thank public health nursing faculty colleagues Mila Aroskar, Janet Berkseth, Debra Froberg, Patricia McGovern, Deborah Olson, and Sharon Ostwald, and co-workers in health administration, Lester Block, Bright Dornblaser, G. Kenneth Gordon, George Johnson, Theodor Litman, Michael Resnick, Lee Stauffer, Robert Veninga, and Vernon Weckwerth.

Others have made a variety of contributions to this third edition. First, I wish to thank my graduate students in public health nursing and public health administration who have provided stimulation and support. In particular, I am grateful to Cecelia Erickson, Ann Rogers, Gaye Davies, Barbara Eaton, and Carol Solie. My thanks also go to the many community colleagues who supported and contributed to my efforts: in particular, Esther Tatley, Elaine Saline, Elaine Sime, Mary Lou Christiansen, Gayle Hallin, LaVohn Josten, Mary Jane Madden, and Linda Stein.

I would like to thank the many people who provided their suggestions and assistance as reviewers throughout the revision process. These include Hedy Mechanic of San Diego State University, Charlotte Patrick of Texas Women's University, Janet Philip of Morningside College, Iowa City, and Carol Jacobson of Gonzaga University, Spokane.

I am deeply indebted to Ann West, my Little, Brown editor, whose ideas, patience, and encouragement energized me to complete the writing. Her contribution is immeasurable. I am also grateful to Janet Tilden for her outstanding editorial work, and to the other helpful people at Scott, Foresman/Little, Brown, especially designer Beth Morrison and photo researcher Aileen Maniates.

Finally, I am grateful to the many friends and family members who provided essential encouragement. I especially wish to thank Dale and Ruth Warland, Bob and Karen Veninga, Tom and Joan Correll, Rick and Pam Immler, Janet Hagberg, Janet Braunstein, Alice Stark, Sister Ann Wylder, Lois Yellowthunder, and Susan Zahner for their unfailing friendship. Thanks to my daughters and sons-in-law, Sheryl and Richard Grassie, Debbie and Steve Teynor, and Laura and Todd Harris and to my new Kittlesen family for their encouragement. I continue to be grateful for the love and prayers of my mother, Lois Walton, my sister and brother-in-law, Lindie and Dan Bacon, and my brother and sister-in-law, Tom and Patti Walton. Most importantly, I wish to thank my husband, Neil Kittlesen, for his unflagging support, interest, and encouragement. His contribution has been invaluable.

1 Community Health

Human beings are social creatures. All of us, with rare exceptions, live out our lives in the company of other people. An Eskimo lives in a small, tightly knit community of close relatives; a rural Mexican lives in a small village with hardly more than two hundred members. In complex societies most people find their lives influenced by many overlapping communities such as their professional societies, political parties, neighborhoods, and cities. Even those who try to escape community membership always begin their lives in some type of group and usually continue to depend on groups for material and emotional support. Communities are an essential and permanent feature of human experience.

The communities in which people live and work have a profound influence on their collective health and well-being. It is commonly known, for example, that exposure to tobacco smoke is associated with negative health effects. An increasing number of communities and organizations (hospitals and airlines included) restrict smoking in public places. Such "community" rules protect nonsmokers and promote the potential for reduced heart and lung disease on a community-wide basis. In recent years Kimberly-Clark instituted a screening and exercise program to reduce coronary heart disease among its employees. More than 90% of the salaried employees were screened, and 25% used the company-furnished exercise facilities. Follow-up tests showed "significant reductions in blood pressure and triglyceride levels and increased treadmill capacity" (Knobel, 1983, p. 19). In this instance, collective health was influenced by the community in which these people worked. On a larger scale, a state that opts to increase its highway speed limit to 65 miles per hour is placing its motorists at greater risk of accidents, injuries, and death. Once again, people's health is influenced by the community of which they are a part.

Although many people tend to think of health and illness as individual matters, it has been established that they are also community matters.

Recent experiences in many parts of the nation with acquired immune deficiency syndrome (AIDS) demonstrate the point (Vladiserri, Brandon, and Lyter, 1984). Communities can influence the spread of disease, provide barriers to protect members from health hazards, organize in ways to combat outbreaks of infectious disease, and promote practices that contribute to individual and collective health (Freudenberg, 1987).

NURSING AND COMMUNITY HEALTH

The relationship between community conditions and people's health is the basis for a challenging field of practice — community health. Many different professionals work in community health to form a complex team. The city planner designing an urban renewal project necessarily becomes involved in community health. The social worker counseling on child abuse or the use of chemical substances among adolescents is involved in community health. A physician treating patients affected by a sudden outbreak of hepatitis and seeking to find the source is engaged in community health practice. Prenatal clinics, meals for the elderly, genetic counseling centers, educational programs for the early detection of cancer, and hundreds of other activities are all part of the community health effort.

Professional nurses are an integral part of community health practice. Their roles and activities are so varied that it is impossible to describe the "typical" community health nurse. They work in every conceivable kind of community health agency from state public health departments to community-based advocacy groups. Their duties range from examining infants in a well-baby clinic or teaching elderly stroke victims in their homes to carrying out epidemiologic research or engaging in health policy analysis and decision making. Community health nursing is a specialty area. It combines all the basic elements of professional, clinical nursing with community health practice. This book examines the unique contribution that community health nursing makes to our health care system. Our discussion of the concepts and theories that make community health nursing an important specialty within nursing begins with the broader field of community health, which provides the context as well as essential content for community health nursing practice.

Community health, also known as public health, is sometimes misunderstood. Even many health professionals think of community health in limiting terms such as sanitation, poverty-area clinics, and massive campaigns to prevent infectious disease. Although these are a part of its ever-broadening practice, community health is much more. In order to understand the nature and significance of this field, it is necessary to look more closely at concepts of community and health.

THE CONCEPT OF COMMUNITY

Broadly defined, a community is a collection of people who share some important feature of their lives. More specifically, Green and Anderson define a community as "a social unit in which there is a transaction of a common life among the people making up the unit. As a social group, functioning with norms of behavior and organization of resources, the community regulates both the environment and behavior" (Green and Anderson, 1986, p. 32). Some communities, such as a tiny village in Appalachia, are composed of people who share almost everything. They live in the same location, work at a limited number of jobs, attend the same churches, and make use of the single health clinic and visiting physician or nurse. Other communities, such as Mothers Against Drunk Drivers (MADD), are large, scattered, and composed of people who may share only their interest and involvement in that particular group. Although most communities share many aspects of their experience, the following criteria are useful for identifying three types of communities in relation to community health practice: geography, common interest, and health problem.

GEOGRAPHIC COMMUNITY

A community is often defined by its geographic boundaries. A city, town, or village is a geographic community. Consider the community of Hayward, Wisconsin. Located in northwestern Wisconsin, it is set in the north woods environment, far removed from any urban center, and in a climatic zone characterized by extremely harsh winters. With a population of less than twenty-five hundred, it is considered a rural community. The population has certain identifiable characteristics such as age and sex ratios, and its size fluctuates with the seasons; summers bring hundreds of tourists and seasonal residents. Hayward is a social system as well as a geographic location. The families, schools, hospital, churches, stores, and government institutions are linked in a complex network. This community, like others, has an informal power structure. It has a communication system that includes gossip, the newspaper, the co-op store bulletin board, and the radio station. In one sense, then, a community consists of a collection of people located in a specific place and is made up of institutions organized into a social system.

Local communities such as Hayward vary in size. A few miles south of Hayward lie several other communities, including Northwoods Beach and Round Lake, but these three, along with other towns and isolated farms, form a larger community called Sawyer County. If you worked for a health agency serving only Hayward, that community would be of primary concern; however, if you worked for the Sawyer County Health Department, you would focus on this larger community. A community health nurse employed by the State Health Department in Madison, Wisconsin, would have an interest in Sawyer County and Hayward, but only as one small part of the larger community of Wisconsin.

Frequently, a single part of a city can be treated as a community. In Seattle, for example, the skid row district near the waterfront is a community of many transients. For certain purposes in community health, it is useful to identify a geographic area as a community.

COMMON-INTEREST COMMUNITY

A community can also be identified by a common interest. A collection of people, widely scattered geographically, can have an interest that binds the members together. The members of a church in a large metropolitan area, a group of migrant workers, or the members of a national professional organization can all be treated as communities. Sometimes within a fairly small geographic area, a group of people become a community by promoting their common interest. Disabled individuals scattered throughout a large city may emerge as a community through a common interest in their need for improved wheelchair facilities. The residents in an industrial community may develop a common interest in air or water pollution issues, while others who work but do not live there may not share that interest. The kinds of shared interests that lead to the formation of communities are almost infinitely varied.

HEALTH-PROBLEM-SOLVING COMMUNITY

Frequently in community health practice a community is an area with fluid boundaries within which a problem can be identified and solved. The shape of this community varies with the size of the geographic area affected and the number of resources needed to address a problem. Such a community has been called "a community of solution" (National Commission on Community Health Services, 1967). A water pollution problem may involve several counties whose agencies and personnel must work together to control upstream water supply, industrial waste disposal, and city water treatment. This group of counties forms a community of solution around a health problem. In another instance, several schools may collaborate with law enforcement and health agencies to study patterns of students' drug use and possible preventive approaches. The boundaries of this community of solution form around the schools and agencies involved. Figure 1-1 depicts some communities of solution related to one city.

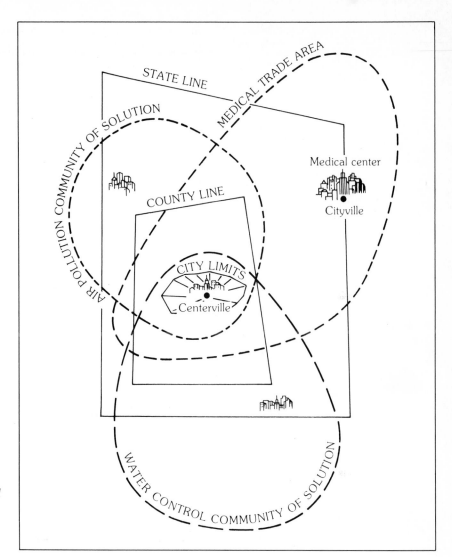

Figure 1-1
A city's communities of solution. State, county, and city boundaries (shown in solid lines) may have little or no bearing on health solution boundaries.

POPULATION OR AGGREGATE CONCEPT

The three types of communities just discussed underscore the meaning of the concept of community: in each instance a collection of people have one or more basic things in common. Having something in common is what makes a group of people into a community. In community health we also use the terms *population* or *aggregate* to refer to a group of people "who share one or more personal or environmental characteristics" (Williams,

1988, p. 296). Like a community, an aggregate may be defined geographically, such as the population of the French Quarter in New Orleans; by common interest or characteristics, such as teenage unwed mothers; or by its shared problem-solving focus, such as Physicians for Social Responsibility. The terms *community* and *aggregate* (or population) share similar definitions and are sometimes used interchangeably. For community health purposes, however, we often consider a population as a subset of some larger community. We may focus intervention, for example, on the population of isolated elderly who are part of the total community of elderly persons residing in a given area.

Community health workers, including the community health nurse, need to be able to define the community targeted for study. That is, who are the people that compose the community? Where are they located and what are their characteristics? A clear delineation of the population must be established before we can assess needs and design interventions (Shamansky and Pesznecker, 1981). We also need to understand the complex nature of communities. What are the characteristics of the people in terms of age, sex, race, and socioeconomic level? How does the community interact with other communities? What is its past history? Is the community undergoing rapid change? Many of these questions, as well as the tools needed to assess a community for health purposes, are discussed in Chapter 13.

THE CONCEPT OF HEALTH

The World Health Organization defines health as "a state of complete physical, mental, and social well-being and not merely the absence of disease or infirmity (WHO, 1986, p. 1)." Our understanding of the concept of health builds on this classic definition. We recognize that health is not just the absence of illness but the presence of a positive capacity to develop one's potential and to lead an energetic, fulfilling, and productive life (Smith, 1983). We value a strong emphasis on well-being or "wellness" as we have come to know it. We are growing to understand health broadly through holistic perspectives that recognize the relationship of health to environment. J. M. Last partially defines health as "a state of equilibrium between humans and the physical, biologic, and social environment..." (Last, 1987, p. 5).

Yet health is an elusive concept. For each person it has acquired dozens of meanings in the course of ordinary conversations. As children, we were encouraged to eat proper foods in order to grow strong and healthy. We later heard of people who "lost" their health. Under the treatment of physicians these people may have "regained" their health. Like barnacles slowly accumulating on the hull of an ocean barge, multiple meanings became attached to the concept of health. Although health is widely accepted as desirable, the exact nature of health is often unclear and ambiguous. In order to clarify the concept for our use in considering community health practice, the distinguishing features of health shall be briefly characterized; then the implications of this concept for the activities of professionals in the field can be examined more fully.

A RELATIVE CONCEPT

Health is a relative, not an absolute, concept. Our language tends to impose on us a black-and-white way of thinking about health. Most people contrast health with illness or disease. A person has either one condition or the other—that is, a person can move from one category to the other, from sick to well again—in an absolute sense. This kind of thinking must be set aside if we are to grasp the nature and significance of community health practice.

Health, according to the concept used in this text, always involves many levels. We are all familiar with degrees of illness. We classify a person with terminal cancer or end-stage renal disease as very ill. Someone else recovering from a cholecystectomy is less ill, yet another person with infectious mononucleosis may be mildly ill. These are degrees or levels of illness. In the same manner we can identify degrees of wellness. From a mildly well person with limited functional activity because of chronic arthritis to a robust 70-year-old person who is fully active and is functioning at an optimal level of wellness, we see variations in degrees of health. Health always involves a continuum—a range of degrees—from optimal health at one end to death or total disability at the other (see Figures 1-2 and 1-3). The health of an in-

Figure 1-2
The wellness-illness continuum. The level (degree) of illness increases as one moves toward total disability or death; the level of wellness increases as one moves toward optimal health. This continuum shows the relative nature of health. At any given time a person can be placed at some point along the continuum.

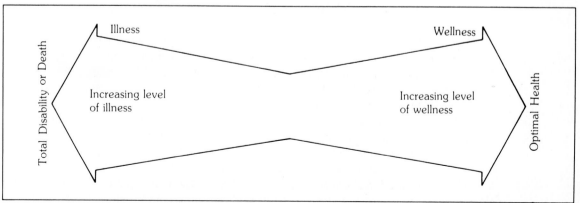

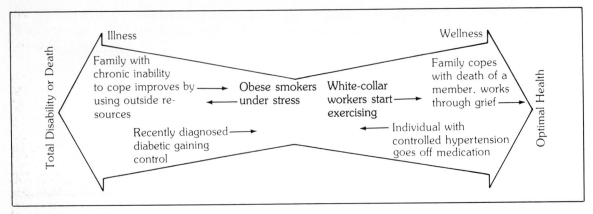

Figure 1-3
Dynamic nature of the wellness-illness continuum. A person's relative health
is usually in a state of flux, either improving or deteriorating. This diagram of
the wellness-illness continuum shows several examples of people in changing
state of health.

dividual, family, group, or community moves back and forth along this continuum throughout life.

By thinking of health relatively, as a matter of degree, we can avoid the
strong tendency to polarize its meaning and thus limit our practice. Traditionally, the majority of health care was focused on treatment of acute and
chronic conditions at the illness end of the continuum. Gradually the emphasis shifted to include attention to the wellness end of the continuum.
Community health practice ranges over the entire continuum; it always
works to improve the degree of health in individuals, families, groups, and
communities. In particular, community health practice emphasizes the promotion and preservation of positive health and the prevention of illness or
disability (Green and Anderson, 1986).

A STATE OF BEING

Health refers to a state of being. Individuals and communities have many
different qualities and characteristics. We might describe a person in such
terms as *energetic, outgoing, enthusiastic, beautiful, caring, loving,* and *intense.* Together, these qualities become the essence of a person's existence;
they describe a state of being. Similarly, a specific geographic community
might be characterized by the terms *congested, deteriorating, unattractive,
dirty,* and *disorganized.* These characteristics suggest diminishing degrees of
vitality. Again, they describe a state of being.

Health, as a set of qualities or a state of being, involves the total person
or the total community. That is, all the dimensions of life affecting everyday
functioning determine an individual's or a community's health. Physical,
psychological, spiritual, and sociocultural experiences influence one's present

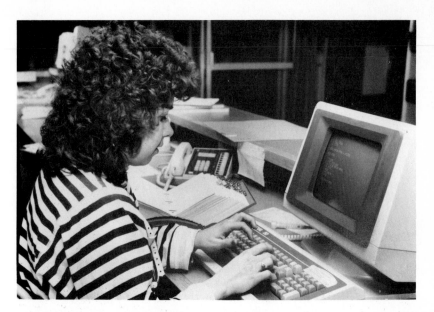

Figure 1-4
Pressured to get her word processing done between interruptions, this secretary is experiencing work stress and an unhealthy life-style that is likely to move her health state to the illness end of the continuum.

condition. Thus, an individual's placement on the wellness-illness continuum can only be known if we consider that person from a holistic perspective (Figure 1-4). Wellness is a relative state of well-being; illness is a relative state of ill-being.

As we consider an aggregate of people in terms of health, it sometimes becomes useful to speak of the "health of a community." With aggregates as well as individuals, health as a state of being does not merely involve the physical condition but includes psychological, spiritual, and sociocultural factors as well.

SUBJECTIVE AND OBJECTIVE DIMENSIONS

Health involves subjective and objective dimensions. Subjectively, a healthy person is one who feels well, who experiences the sensation of a vital, positive state. Healthy people are full of life and vigor, capable of physical and mental productivity. They feel minimal discomfort and displeasure with the world around them. Again, people experience varying degrees of vitality and well-being. The state of feeling well fluctuates. Some mornings we wake up feeling more energetic and enthusiastic than we do on other mornings. How a person feels varies day by day, even hour by hour; nonetheless, it can be a strong indicator of that person's state of health.

Health also involves the objective dimension of ability to function. A healthy individual or community can carry out necessary activities and achieve enriching goals. Unhealthy people not only feel ill but are limited, to some degree, in their ability to carry out daily activities. Indeed, levels of illness or wellness are largely measured in terms of ability to function (Stokes et al., 1982). A person confined to bed is labeled sicker than an ill person managing self-care. A family that meets its members' needs is healthier than one that has poor communication patterns and is unable to provide adequate physical and emotional resources. Degree of functioning is directly related to state of health.

The ability to function can be observed. A man dresses and feeds himself and goes to work. Despite financial exigencies, a family nourishes its members through a supportive emotional climate. A community fails to provide adequate resources and services for its members. These performances, to some degree, can be regarded as indicators of health status. Some community health agencies assess clients' ability to function as a measure of client progress and nursing care effectiveness (Choi et al., 1983).

Underlying performances are the values an individual, family, or community places on actions. Some activities such as walking and taking care of personal needs are functions almost everyone values. Other actions (for example, sports such as running) have more limited appeal. In assessing the health of individuals and communities, the community health nurse can observe their ability to function but must also know their values, which may contrast sharply with those of the professional. We examine more closely the influence of values on health in Chapter 5.

Subjective (feeling well or ill) and objective (function) dimensions together provide us with a clearer picture of people's health. When they feel well and demonstrate functional ability, they are close to the wellness end of the wellness-illness continuum. Even those with a disease such as arthritis or diabetes may feel well and perform well within their capacity. These people can be considered healthy. Figure 1-5 depicts the relationships between the subjective and objective views of health.

HEALTH AND COMMUNITY

Health can be viewed as an important resource, both of individuals and communities. The relationship between health and community has been summarized by Henkel (1970, p. 2):

1. The health and well-being of an individual physically, emotionally, and socially is one of his most important assets.
2. Through judicious use of this asset he will be able to achieve more effectively his goals in life.
3. To develop this asset to the greatest possible level requires the concerted and cooperative efforts of many people.
4. Society as a whole will ultimately benefit from healthy citizens.

The implications of this view of health have far-reaching consequences for persons engaged in health care. No longer can we justify concentrating the majority of our efforts exclusively on healing the sick or even on the prevention of disease. For centuries health work has focused on the illness end of the wellness-illness continuum. We now live in an age when it is not only

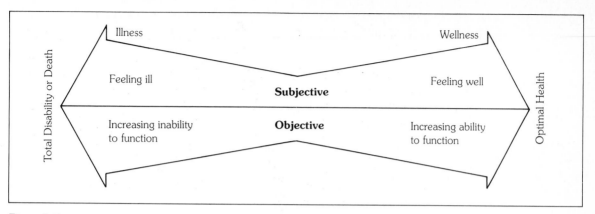

Figure 1-5
Subjective and objective
views of the wellness-illness
continuum.

possible to promote health but our mandate and responsibility to do so (Public Health Service, 1983).

As important as health promotion is the need for health assessment. When one considers health status from the perspective just discussed, its measurement becomes more feasible as well as necessary. Health promotion and health assessment are essential aspects of community health nursing and are discussed in detail in later chapters.

ELEMENTS OF COMMUNITY HEALTH PRACTICE

We have examined the definitions of community and of health. Together, these concepts provide the foundation for understanding community health. In acute care the health of an individual is the primary focus. Community health broadens that focus to concentrate on families, groups, and the community at large. The community becomes the recipient of service, and health becomes the product. Viewed from another perspective, community health is concerned with the interchange between population groups and their total environment, and with the impact of that interchange on collective health.

Just as a whole is greater than the sum of its parts, the health of a community is more than the sum of the health of its individual citizens. A community that achieves high-level wellness is composed of healthy citizens, functioning in an environment that protects and promotes health. Community health, as a field of practice, seeks to provide the organizational structure, resources, and activities needed to accomplish the goal of an optimally healthy community.

What is the difference between community health and public health? Theoretically there is none. Both are organized community efforts aimed at the promotion, protection, and preservation of the public's health. Historically, however, as a field of practice, public health has been associated with official or government efforts. This is in contrast to private health efforts directed toward solving selected health problems. The latter augments the former. Community health practice encompasses both because its focus includes all health agencies and efforts, public or private, concerned with community health. In this text, the term *community health* refers to this broader perspective while recognizing the fundamental concepts and principles of public health as its birthright and foundation for practice.

Winslow's 1920 definition of public health is still timely and forms the basis for our definition of community health in this text. "Public health is the science and art of preventing disease, prolonging life, and promoting health and efficiency through organized community efforts for the sanitation of the environment, the control of communicable infections, the education of the individual in personal hygiene, the organization of medical and nursing services for the early diagnosis and preventive treatment of disease, and the development of the social machinery to insure everyone a standard of living adequate for the maintenance of health, so organizing these benefits as to enable every citizen to realize his birthright of health and longevity" (cited in Hanlon and Pickett, 1984, p. 4).

One of the challenges community health practice faces is to remain responsive to community health needs. As a result, its structure is complex; numerous health services and programs are currently available or will be developed in the future. Examples include health education, family planning, accident prevention, environmental protection, immunization, nutrition, early periodic screening and developmental testing, school programs, mental health, and industry and occupational health.

Community health practice can best be understood by examining six basic elements, which when combined encompass its services and programs: (1) promotion of healthful living, (2) prevention of health problems, (3) treatment of disorders, (4) rehabilitation, (5) evaluation, and (6) research.

PROMOTION OF HEALTHFUL LIVING

Promotion of healthful living is now recognized as one of the most important elements of community health practice. Health promotion programs and activities include many forms of health education, demonstration of healthful practices, and efforts to provide a greater number of health-promoting options. Community health promotion, then, "is any combination of educational, social, and environmental actions conducive to the health of a population..." (Green and Anderson, 1986, p. 5).Wellness programs in business and industry are an example. Health education, although a useful tool, has limited significance alone unless accompanied by desire, opportunity, and resources that encourage more healthful practices (Milio, 1976; Green and Anderson, 1986).

Demonstration of such healthful practices as eating more nutritious foods and exercising more regularly is often performed by individual health workers. In addition, groups and health agencies that support the rights of non-smokers, encourage physical fitness programs for all ages, or demand that food products be properly labeled demonstrate the importance of these practices and create public awareness.

The goal of health promotion is to raise individuals', families', groups', and communities' levels of wellness (Moore and Williamson, 1984). Community health accomplishes this goal through a three-pronged effort: (1) to increase understanding of health, (2) to raise community standards for health, and (3) to assist in developing more positive health practices. More specifically, the U.S. Public Health Service outlined 15 target areas with specific objectives and plans for their implementation (Public Health Service, 1983). They are listed below.

Preventive health services:
　　Family planning
　　Pregnancy and infant care
　　Immunizations
　　Reducing the spread of sexually transmissible diseases
　　Control of high blood pressure
Health protection:
　　Toxic agent control
　　Occupational safety and health
　　Accidental injury control
　　Fluoridation of community water supplies
　　Infectious agent control
Health promotion:
　　Smoking cessation
　　Reduction of alcohol and drug abuse
　　Improved nutrition
　　Exercise and fitness
　　Stress control

Today, this list has expanded to include prevention of the spread of AIDS and provision of preventive health services to the elderly.

It is difficult to provide health-promoting options—that is, opportunities to make more healthful choices—without reexamining and, in many instances, restructuring organizational patterns and policies as well as increasing personal and societal resources. At the local level, many health agencies are offering services at hours more convenient to their clientele and, in some cases, are providing transportation or other means of easier access to service. Furthermore, community residents are forming stronger bonds of partnership with health workers in order to understand and solve their own health problems as well as to assume greater responsibility for achieving positive health for themselves and their communities.

LEVELS OF PREVENTION OF HEALTH PROBLEMS

Prevention of health problems constitutes a major part of community health practice. Prevention means anticipating and averting problems or discovering them as early as possible in order to minimize possible disability and impairment. It is practiced on three levels in community health: (1) primary prevention, (2) secondary prevention, and (3) tertiary prevention (Moore and Williamson, 1984).

Primary prevention obviates the occurrence of a health problem. It keeps it from happening at all: "It precedes disease or dysfunction and is applied to a generally healthy population" (Shamansky and Clausen, 1980, p. 106). For example, a community health nurse who encourages an elderly couple to install safety devices, such as a grab bar by the bathtub or a hand rail on the front steps, is preventing injuries from falls. Local health departments help control and prevent communicable diseases such as rubeola or poliomyelitis by providing regular immunization programs. Primary prevention involves anticipatory planning and action on the part of community health professionals who must project themselves into the future, envision potential needs and problems, and then design programs to counteract them so that they never occur. A nutritionist who instructs a group of overweight women to follow a well-balanced diet during weight loss is preventing the possibility of nutritional deficiency. The concepts of primary prevention and planning for the future are foreign to many social groups who may resist on the basis of conflicting values. The "Parable of the Dangerous Cliff" (Figure 1-6) illustrates such a value conflict.

Secondary prevention seeks to detect and treat existing health problems at the earliest possible stage. Pathology is now involved. Hypertension screening centers, which have been formed in many communities, help identify a high-risk group and encourage early treatment. Another example is breast and testicular self-examination programs. Secondary prevention attempts to discover a health problem at a point when intervention may lead to its control or eradication. This is the reasoning behind water and soil testing for contaminants and hazardous chemicals in community environmental health. It also prompts community health nurses to watch for early signs of child abuse in a family, emotional disturbances in a group of widows, or excessive drinking among adolescents.

Tertiary prevention attempts to reduce the extent and severity of a health problem to its lowest possible level. Rehabilitation of persons following a stroke, postmastectomy exercise programs, and Alcoholics Anonymous support groups are examples. The clients involved have an existing illness or disability whose impact on their lives is lessened through tertiary prevention. In broader community health practice we use tertiary prevention to minimize the effects of an existing unhealthy community condition. An example of such prevention is warning urban residents about rats in the sewer system.

Parable of the Dangerous Cliff

'Twas a dangerous cliff, as they freely confessed,
    Though to walk near its crest was so pleasant;
But over its terrible edge there has slipped
    A duke, and full many a peasant.
The people said something would have to be done
    But their projects did not at all tally.
Some said, "Put a fence around the edge of the cliff";
    Some, "An ambulance down in the valley."
The lament of the crowd was profound and was loud,
    As their hearts overflowed with their pity;
But the cry of the ambulance carried the day
    As it spread through the neighboring city.
A collection was made, to accumulate aid,
    And the dwellers in highway and alley,
Gave dollars or cents.
Not to furnish a fence
But "An ambulance down in the valley."
"For the cliff is all right if you're careful," they said;

"And if folks ever slip and are dropping,
    It isn't the slipping that hurts them so much
As the shock down below when they're stopping."
So for years (we have heard), as these mishaps occurred,
    Quick forth would the rescuers sally,
To pick up the victims who fell from the cliff,
    With the ambulance down in the valley.
Said one, in his plea, "It's a marvel to me
    That you'd give so much greater attention
To repairing results than to curing the cause;
You had much better aim at prevention.
    For the mischief, of course, should be stopped at its source,
Come neighbors and friends, let us rally.
    It is far better sense to rely on a fence
Than an ambulance down in the valley."
"He is wrong in his head," the majority said;
    "He would end all our earnest endeavor.
He's a man who would shirk this responsible work,
    But we will support it forever.

Aren't we picking up all, just as fast as they fall,
    and giving them care liberally?
A superfluous fence is of no consequence,
If the ambulance works in the valley."
The story looks queer as we've written it here,
    But things oft occur that are stranger,
More humane, we assert, than to take care of the hurt,
    Is the plan of removing the danger.
The very best plan is to safeguard the man,
    And attend to the thing rationally;
To build up the fence and try to dispense
    With the ambulance down in the valley.
Better still! Cut down the hill!

—Author Unknown

Figure 1-6
"Parable of the Dangerous Cliff."

Health assessment of individuals, families, and communities is an important part of preventive practice. One must determine health status in order to anticipate problems and select appropriate preventive measures. A community health nurse who discovers that a young mother has herself been a victim of child abuse institutes early treatment for the mother to prevent abuse and foster adequate parenting of her children. If assessment of a community reveals inadequate facilities and activities to meet the future needs of its increasing population of senior citizens, agencies and groups collaborate to plan and develop the needed resources.

Health problems are most effectively prevented by maintaining healthy life-styles and healthy environments. To these ends, community health practice directs many of its efforts to providing safe and satisfying living and working conditions, nutritious food, and clean air and water. This area of practice includes the field of preventive medicine, which is a population-focused, or community-oriented, branch of medical practice that incorporates public health sciences and principles (Last, 1987).

TREATMENT OF DISORDERS

Treatment of disorders, which focuses on illnesses and health problems, is the remedial aspect of community health practice. The first of its three major functions is to provide *direct service* to people with health problems. For example, a family unable to afford the purchase of a wheelchair for a son with multiple sclerosis is provided one through a community agency. If the wife in an older couple is newly diagnosed as diabetic, home visits from a community health nurse, for assistance with diet planning, administration of insulin, and personal care, are arranged. A neighborhood health center forms an educational and support group for people needing to lose weight. Many kinds of community agencies provide direct health care or health-related sevices.

Second, the remedial aspect of community health practice includes indirect service by assisting people with health problems to obtain treatment. In many instances a community agency may not be able to provide needed care and will refer the individuals or groups concerned to a more appropriate resource. A young woman with postpartum bleeding, assisted by the community health nurse, gets an immediate appointment with a physician at the local clinic. A social worker helps a family that is plagued by personal and economic problems to enter a family therapy and counseling program. A number of community agencies provide information and referral services.

Third, treatment of disorders also includes the development of *programs to correct unhealthy conditions*. One community with a high incidence of alcoholism and drug abuse initiated a chemical dependency counseling and treatment center. In another community, the health department developed new regulations for industrial waste disposal as a result of increased pollution of the water supply. Individual community members and health workers also take corrective action to remedy situations such as a case of apparent child abuse, poor nutrition in a school lunch program, or inhumane conditions and treatment in a nursing home.

REHABILITATION

Rehabilitation, the fourth element of community health practice, focuses on reducing disability and, as much as possible, restoring function. People whose handicaps are congenital or acquired through illness or accident such as stroke, heart condition, amputation, or mental illness can be helped to regain some measure of lost function or to develop new compensating skills. For example, a factory worker who lost his leg in an industrial accident received good medical and nursing care, prosthetic fittings, and physical and occupational therapy; he thus retrained to assume an office job.

In community health, the need to reduce disability and restore function applies equally to families, groups, and communities as well as to individuals. (See Figure 1-7.) Many groups form for rehabilitative purposes, such as Alcoholics Anonymous, halfway houses for discharged psychiatric patients, or

Figure 1-7
This retarded young adult, functioning well within her capacity, demonstrates that community health efforts can enable people to achieve a high level of health despite disability.

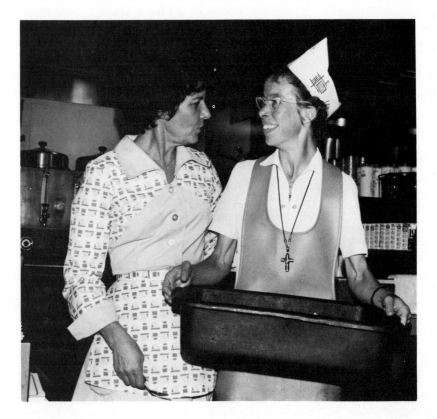

ostomy clubs. Rehabilitation services are often needed and sought by whole communities, as when a ghetto area desires to provide decent, safe playgrounds for its children.

As an element of community health practice, rehabilitation becomes increasingly significant when disease trends and changes in life expectancy are considered. Chronic conditions have replaced acute as the major causes of morbidity; these include such cripplers as cardiovascular disease and cancer, the increased incidence of accidents, and environmentally caused conditions. As a result, the need for long-term care and rehabilitation has increased, stimulated further by a greater proportion of elderly persons in the population.

EVALUATION

Evaluation is the means by which community health practice is analyzed and improved. Evaluation of health and health care should be an integral part of every kind of health service from individual practice to national and international programs. Whether done on the single case or program level, evaluation helps solve problems and provides direction for future health care efforts. Its goals are to determine needs and the success of present activities as well as to develop improved services (Veney and Kaluzny, 1984). In one community, evaluation of mental health services revealed a need for more comprehensive psychiatric emergency care on a 24-hour basis. If a psychiatric crisis occurred during the night, police were the only persons available to help, and jail the only place where the mentally ill could be taken. The deficiency was corrected by providing 24-hour psychiatric emergency service in the community mental health center. A community health nurse, in another instance, developed a contract with a family to whom she was making home visits. The parents wanted to learn how to cope with their adolescent boys. Specific, written objectives and a plan for measuring the outcomes enabled the couple and the nurse to evaluate the successful completion of this helping relationship.

A comprehensive discussion of evaluation is provided in Chapter 8, "The Nursing Process in Community Health."

RESEARCH

Research, a critical element of community health practice, provides a means for solving problems and exploring improved methods of health service. Community health conducts and utilizes scientific investigations at all levels from federal agencies such as the U.S. Public Health Service to state and local groups conducting research. Biostatistics and epidemiology are the primary public health measurement and analytic sciences underlying community health practice. Chapter 9 addresses these sciences in more detail.

Researchers in community health investigate the characteristics and patterns of illness and health. Conditions such as food poisoning, trauma, alcoholism, lung cancer, child abuse, drug dependency, or suicide are studied for possible causes and means of prevention. Health and healthful behavior are analyzed, for example, in nutrition projects and studies of normal human growth and behavior, for better understanding of ways to promote healthful living.

Community health researchers explore ways to improve health care. For example, an experimental program of foster home care for the frail elderly proved to be more beneficial and less costly than nursing home care (Oktay and Volland, 1987). A study of school children in Berkeley, California, demonstrated that after screening, public health nursing follow-up increased dental care utilization (Oda, Fine, and Heilbron, 1986). Other research projects might focus on the effectiveness of drug treatment programs, long-term stroke rehabilitation, or improved treatment approaches to obesity.

Community health researchers also examine the impact of social and environmental factors on health and health services provision. For example, one study of work schedules revealed that people working variable shifts are at much greater risk for health problems (Gordon et al., 1986), while another identified social and psychological as well as environmental factors contributing to the poor health of homeless families (Bassuk, Rubin, and Lauriat, 1986). A growing number of studies center around needs and care of the elderly. Others investigate ways to improve health services planning and policy development through such efforts as studies of community needs and program utilization.

CHARACTERISTICS OF COMMUNITY HEALTH PRACTICE

Several characteristics of community health practice deserve special emphasis. First, community health practice, unlike the individualized focus of acute health care, is *population-focused*. It is concerned with the health status of people in the aggregate, people who, as a group, form a distinct population. These groups or communities, in turn, are multiple and overlapping. Thus, community health must deal with a complex set of interacting physical, psychological, sociocultural, and biological variables that influence human behavior and affect aggregate health (Williams, 1977). Public health, or community health, is fundamentally concerned with the collective good; it focuses on community and on the values of life, health, and security shared by the community (Forster, 1982).

Second, in community health practice the *promotion of health and prevention of illness* are of first-order priority. There is minimal emphasis on curative care. Some corrective actions are always needed, such as cleanup of a toxic waste dump site, stricter enforcement of day care standards, or home care of the ill; however, community health best serves its constituents through preventive and health-promoting actions (Beauchamp, 1984). These include services to mothers and infants, prevention of environmental pollution, school health programs, senior citizens' fitness classes, "workers'-right-to-know" legislation that warns against hazards in the workplace, and numerous other activities.

Third, community health practice uses *aggregate measurement and analysis*. The need to collect and examine data on the entire population under study before making decisions is fundamental to community health practice. Analysis of health states, environmental factors, health-related services, economic patterns, and social policy are among the many foci of community health evaluation and research, described further in Chapter 8.

Finally, community health practice utilizes principles from *management and organization* theory to provide effective administration of health care services. Public health has long been defined as "the protection and improvement of community health by organized community efforts" (U.S. Congress, 1976; Hanlon, 1984). It is the organization and administration of such services that enables practitioners to ultimately address community needs. Chapter 2 elaborates on this subject.

Summary

Community health is much more than environmental programs and large-scale efforts to control communicable disease. To comprehend the nature and significance of community health we must understand the concepts of community and of health.

A community, broadly defined, is a collection of people who share some important feature of their lives. More specifically, it is helpful in community health practice to identify three types of communities: geographic, common-interest, and health-problem-solving. Sometimes a community, such as a city, county, or neighborhood, is formed by geographic boundaries. At other times a community may be identified by its common interest; examples are a religious community, a group of migrant workers, or a gathering of residents concerned about air pollution. A community may also be defined by a pooling of efforts by people and agencies toward solving some health-related problem.

Health is an abstract concept that can be understood more clearly when we recognize its distinguishing features. First, health is a relative, not an absolute, concept. People are not either sick or well in an absolute sense but have levels of illness or wellness. These levels may be plotted along a continuum ranging from optimal health to total disability or death. This is known as the wellness-illness continuum. Thus, a person's state of health is dynamic, varying from day to day and even hour to hour.

Second, health is a state of being. That is, the characteristics of a person, family, or community can be said to describe the essence of their existence.

These characteristics portray people and therefore suggest the presence or absence of vitality. As a state of being, health also involves the total person. All the dimensions of life—physical, psychological, social, and spiritual—affect health.

Third, health has both subjective and objective dimensions. The subjective aspect involves feeling well; the objective aspect refers to the ability to function. How one feels can indicate one's state of health. At the wellness end of the wellness-illness continuum, people feel well; at the illness end, they feel ill. The ability to function, which is observable and often used to measure health status, may be present anywhere along the continuum. Most often, performance diminishes dramatically toward the illness end.

Community health practice is concerned with preserving and promoting the health of the community. It incorporates six basic elements: (1) promotion of healthful living, (2) prevention of health problems, (3) treatment of disorders, (4) rehabilitation, (5) evaluation, and (6) research.

Important characteristics of community health practice include its emphasis on populations, promotion of health and prevention of illness, use of measurement and analysis of aggregates, and effective management and organization of health services.

Study Questions

1. Identify a community of people for whom you have some concern. What makes it a community? What characteristics does this population group share?
2. Place the community you selected on the wellness-illness continuum. What factors influenced your decision?
3. Describe three preventive actions (one primary, one secondary, and one tertiary) that might be taken to move the community you selected closer to optimal wellness.
4. Place yourself on the wellness-illness continuum. What factors influenced your decision?

References

Bassuk, E. L., L. Rubin, and A. S. Lauriat. (1986). Characteristics of sheltered homeless families. *American Journal of Public Health* 76(9): 1097–1101.

Beauchamp, D. (1984). What is public about public health? *Health Affairs* 2(4): 76–87.

Choi, T., L. V. Josten, and M. Christensen. (1983). Health-specific family coping index for non-institutional care. *American Journal of Public Health* 73(11): 1275–77.

Forster, J. (1982). A communitarian ethical model for public health interventions: An alternative to individual behavior change strategies. *Journal of Public Health Policy* 3: 150–63.

Freudenberg, N. (1987). Reassessing communities. *Health/PAC Bulletin* 17(5): 30.

Gordon, N. P., P. D. Clearly, C. E. Parker, and C. A. Czeisler. (1986). The prevalence and health impact of shiftwork. *American Journal of Public Health* 76(10): 1225–28.

Green, L. W., and C. L. Anderson. (1986). *Community Health.* St. Louis: Times Mirror/Mosby.

Hanlon, J. J., and G. E. Pickett. (1984). *Public health: Administration and practice.* 8th ed. St. Louis: Times Mirror/Mosby.

Henkel, B. (1970). *Community Health.* 2nd ed. Boston: Allyn and Bacon.

Knobel, R. J. (1983). Health promotion and disease prevention: Improving health while conserving resources. *Family and Community Health* 5(4): 16–27.

Last, J. M. (1987). *Public health and human ecology.* East Norwalk, Conn.: Appleton and Lange.

Milio, N. (1976). A framework for prevention: Changing health-damaging to health-generating life patterns. *American Journal of Public Health* 66: 435–39.

Moore, P. V., and G. C. Williamson. (1984). Health promotion: Evolution of a concept. Nursing Clinics of North America 19(2): 195–206.

National Commission on Community Health Services. (1967). *Health Is a Community Affair.* Cambridge: Harvard University Press.

Oda, D. S., J. I. Fine, and D. C. Heilbron. (1986). Impact and cost of public health nurse telephone follow-up of school dental referrals. *American Journal of Public Health* 76(11): 1348–49.

Oktay, J. S., and P. J. Volland. (1987). Foster home care for the frail elderly as an alternative to nursing home care: An experimental evaluation. *American Journal of Public Health* 77(12): 1505–10.

Public Health Service. (1983). Public Health Service implementation plans for attaining the objectives for the nation. *Public Health Reports,* September–October 1983 Supplement: 1–177.

Shamansky, S., and C. Clausen. (1980). Levels of prevention: Examination of the concept. *Nursing Outlook* 28: 104–8.

Shamansky, S., and B. Pesznecker (1981). A community is... *Nursing Outlook* 29(3): 182–85.

Smith, J. A. (1983). *The idea of health: Implications for the nursing professional.* New York: Teachers College Press, Columbia University.

Stanhope, M., and J. Lancaster. (1988). *Community health nursing: Process and practice for promoting health.* 2nd ed. St. Louis: C. V. Mosby.

Stokes, III, J., J. J. Noren, and S. Shindell. (1982). Definition of terms and concepts applicable to clinical preventive medicine. *Journal of Community Health* 8: 33–41.

U. S. Congress, House Committee on Interstate and Foreign Commerce, Subcommittee on Health Environment. (1976). *A discursive dictionary of health care,* 94th Congress, 2nd session. Washington, D.C.: U.S. Government Printing Office.

Valdiserri, R. O., W. R. Brandon, and D. W. Lyter. (1984). AIDS surveillance and health education: Use of previously described risk factors to identify high-risk homosexuals. *American Journal of Public Health* 74: 259–60.

Veney, J. E., and A. D. Kaluzny. (1984). *Evaluation and decision making for health services programs.* Englewood Cliffs, N.J.: Prentice-Hall.

Williams, C. A. (1977). Community health nursing—What is it? *Nursing Outlook* 25: 250–54.

Williams, C. A. (1988). Population-focused practice: The basis of specialization in public health nursing. In M. Stanhope and J. Lancaster, *Community Health Nursing: Process and Practice for Promoting Health.* 2nd ed. St. Louis: C. V. Mosby.

World Health Organization: Basic documents. (1986). 36th ed. Geneva: WHO.

Selected Readings

Barsky, A. J. (1988). The paradox of health. *The New England Journal of Medicine* 318(7): 414–18.

Beauchamp, D. (1984). What is public about public health? *Health Affairs* 2(4): 76–87.

Blum, H. (1981). *Planning for health: Generics for the eighties.* 2nd ed. New York: Human Sciences Press.

Dunn, H. (1961). *High-level wellness.* Arlington, Va.: Beatty Press.

Forster, J. (1982). A communitarian ethical model for public health interventions: An alternative to individual behavior change strategies. *Journal of Public Health Policy* 3: 150–63.

Freudenberg, N. (1987). Reassessing communities. *Health/PAC Bulletin* 17(59): 30.

Green, L. W., and C. L. Anderson. (1986). *Community Health.* St. Louis: Times Mirror/Mosby.

Hanlon, J. J., and G. E. Pickett. (1984). *Public Health: Administration and practice.* 8th ed. St. Louis: Times Mirror/Mosby.

Institute of Medicine Committee for the Study of the Future of Public Health. (1988). *The future of public health.* Washington, D.C.: National Academy Press.

Knobel, R. J. (1983). Health promotion and disease prevention: Improving health while conserving resources. *Family and Community Health* 5(4): 16–27.

Last, J. M. (1987). *Public health and human ecology.* East Norwalk, Conn.: Appleton and Lange.

Lauzon, R. (1977). An epidemiological approach to health promotion. *Canadian Journal of Public Health* 68: 311–17.

Leavell, H. R., and E. G. Clark. (1965). *Preventive medicine for the doctor in his community: An epidemiological approach.* 3rd ed. New York: McGraw-Hill.

Milio, N. (1975). *The care of health in communities.* New York: Macmillan.

Milio, N. (1976). A framework for prevention; Changing health-damaging to health-generating life patterns. *American Journal of Public Health* 66: 435–39.

Moore, P. V., and G. C. Williamson. (1984). Health promotion: Evolution of a concept. *Nursing Clinics of North America* 19(2): 195–206.

Public Health Service. (1979). *Healthy people: The Surgeon General's report on health promotion and disease prevention* (DHEW Publication No. PHS 79-55071). Washington, D.C.: U.S. Government Printing Office.

Roemer, R. (1988). The right to health care — Gains and gaps. *American Journal of Public Health* 78(3): 241–47.

Shamansky, S., and C. Clausen. (1980). Levels of prevention: Examination of the concept. *Nursing Outlook* 28: 104–8.

Shamansky, S., and B. Pesznecker. (1981). A community is . . . *Nursing Outlook* 29: 182–85.

Smith, J. A. (1983). *The idea of health: Implications for the Nursing Professional.* New York: Teachers College Press, Columbia University.

Terris, M. (1975). Evolution of public health and preventive medicine in the United States. *American Journal of Public Health* 65: 161–69.

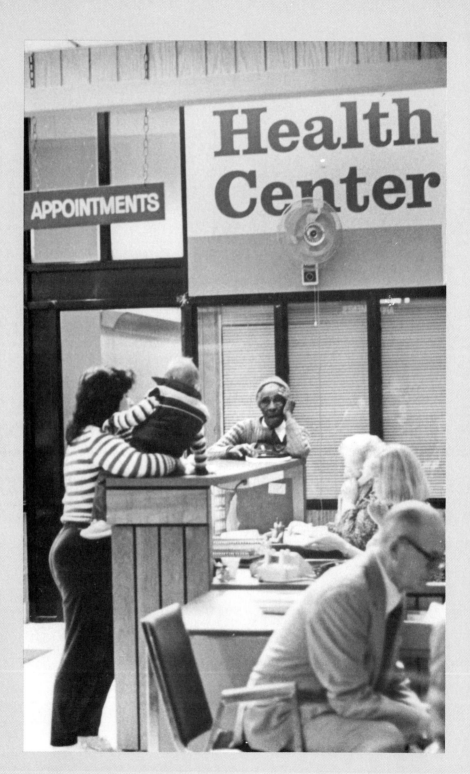

2 Organization and Financing of Community Health Services

Service delivery systems directed at restoring or promoting the public's health have evolved over centuries. The structure, function, and financing of health care systems have changed dramatically over time in response to changing societal needs and demands, scientific advancements, more effective methods of service delivery, new technology, and development of varying approaches to resource acquisition and allocation (Hanlon and Pickett, 1984). We have made considerable progress toward a healthier world society. At the same time we are faced with many problems, particularly those of escalating health care costs, equitable distribution and effectiveness of health services, and assuring the quality of those services (Milio, 1984; Balinsky and Starkman, 1987).

In this chapter we describe the current organization of community health services in the United States and give an overview of historical and legislative events that have influenced health planning and system structure and function. We also discuss the changing picture of health care financing and its incentives and disincentives for enhancing the public's health. More extensive treatment of these important subjects can be found in the selected readings that are listed at the close of the chapter.

HISTORICAL PERSPECTIVES

Health care as we know it today has changed dramatically from previous centuries. Yet there is reason to believe that personal and community hygiene and health care were practiced from the beginning of time. Many primitive tribes appeared to engage in sanitary practices such as burial of excreta, removal of the dead, and isolation of members with certain illnesses along with treatment of the sick using a variety of therapeutic agents administered by a "healer." Whether these activities were purely superstitious or derived from survival needs is unknown. Nonetheless, records show that in Egypt and the Middle East, as early as 3000 B.C., people were building drainage systems and practicing personal cleanliness (Hanlon and Pickett, 1984). The biblical record in Leviticus describes the Hebrew hygienic code, circa 1500 B.C., as a prototype for personal and community sanitation. Even more advanced were the Athenians, circa 1000–400 B.C., who emphasized personal hygiene, diet, and exercise in addition to a sanitary environment, albeit for the benefit of the wealthy. Their successors, the Romans, added many more community health measures such as laws regulating environmental sanitation and nuisances, and construction of paved streets, aqueducts, and a subsurface drainage system.

The Middle Ages (from about A.D. 500 to 1500) marked a distinct change in health beliefs and practices based on the philosophy that to pamper the body was evil. Neglected personal hygiene, improper diets, and accumulation of refuse and body wastes soon led to widespread epidemics and pandemics of disease including cholera and leprosy. Increased trade between Europe and Asia, military conquests, and Christian crusades to the Middle East only furthered the spread of disease. Bubonic plague, known as the Black Death, in the mid-1300s was the most devastating of pandemics, reportedly killing about 43 million people, half the population of the known world (Hanlon and Pickett, 1984). In response to this, the first known quarantine measure was instituted in 1377 at the port of Ragusa (now Dubrovnik in Yugoslavia), where travelers from plague areas were required to wait two months and be free of disease before entry was allowed. Marseilles, in 1383, passed the first quarantine law (Hanlon and Pickett, 1984). During this regressed period in history, health care was scarce, private, and reserved for the wealthy few, and public health problems were minimally and ineffectively addressed.

By the end of the Middle Ages more enlightened European thinkers began to challenge the prevailing beliefs and conditions. They no longer believed that disease was a punishment for sin, although traces of stigma regarding leprosy, tuberculosis, and cancer can be found yet today, and venereal disease is still regarded by some as punishment for immoral conduct. Concepts of human dignity and rights and an emphasis on the search for scientific truth influenced new efforts at reform during the late eighteenth century that continued through the nineteenth century.

Despite these signs of improvement, many serious problems persisted. Hundreds of pauper children died in England's abusive but legally approved workhouses and apprentice slavery system. Most of Europe continued in deplorable conditions of misery and filth. Many householders dumped their refuse out windows or doors into the streets. Stinking rivers and water supplies were seriously contaminated. Numerous diseases including cholera, typhus, typhoid, smallpox, and tuberculosis took a tremendous toll on human life.

Around the turn of the nineteenth century, England became increasingly concerned about social and sanitary reform. The first sanitary legislation, passed in 1837, established vaccination stations in London. One of the most notable reformers, Edwin Chadwick, published his "Report on an Inquiry into the Sanitary Conditions of the Laboring Population of Great Britain" (Hanlon and Pickett, 1984) in 1842. Chadwick, the father of modern public health, believed that disease and poverty were related and could be changed. His efforts resulted in passage of the English Public Health Act and establishment of a General Board of Health for England in 1848 (Lewis, 1952). Conditions improved and scientific study advanced in England and concurrently in France, Germany, Scandinavia, and other European countries. England, however, set the pace for application of research, particularly with reference to public health measures, through steadily improved legislation. British laws subsequently became the pattern for American sanitary ordinances.

HEALTH CARE DEVELOPMENT IN THE UNITED STATES

Early health care in the American colonies consisted of private practice with infrequent governmental action for the public good. Action was usually in the form of isolated local responses to specific dangers or nuisances such as the 1647 regulation to prevent pollution of Boston Harbor or the 1701 Massachusetts law requiring ship quarantine and isolation of smallpox patients. New York City in the late 1700s formed a public health committee to monitor, among other public concerns, water quality, sewer construction, marsh drainage, and burial of the dead.

The U.S. Constitution, adopted in 1789, made no direct reference to public health, nor was the federal government active in health matters. It was the responsibility of each sovereign state to manage its own health affairs. The first federal intervention for health problems was the Marine Hospital Service Act of 1798. It subsidized medical and hospital care for disabled seamen. During the early years a scourge of epidemics, especially yellow fever, smallpox, cholera, typhoid, and typhus, caused many deaths throughout the colonies. Quarantine efforts under local control proved ineffective. Congress, in 1873, finally instituted the national port quarantine system, which was regulated and enforced by the Marine Hospital Service. Epidemics were quickly brought under control, causing society to recognize the benefits of uniform central government policy. Improvements in public health and sanitation generally throughout the states, however, were held back by delayed progress in coping with other competing needs such as police and fire protection.

The Shattuck report, a landmark document, made a tremendous impact on sanitary progress. Lemuel Shattuck, a layman and legislator, chaired a legislative committee that studied health and sanitary problems in the commonwealth of Massachusetts. In 1850, he produced the "Report of the Sanitary Commission of Massachusetts." It described public health concepts and methods upon which much of today's public health practice is based. Among his many recommendations, Shattuck advocated the establishment of state and local boards of health, environmental sanitation, collection and use of vital statistics, systematic study of diseases, control of food and drugs, urban planning, establishment of nurses' training schools (there were none before this time), and preventive medicine. Unfortunately, it was almost 25 years before the recommendations were appreciated and truly implemented. A similar report by John C. Griscom conducted about the same time concluded that illness, premature death, and poverty were directly related. He also recommended sanitary reform (Figure 2-1).

Precursors to an organized health care system in the United States came in the form of official health agencies. Development occurred initially at the local level. Many cities established local boards of health in the late 1700s and early to mid-1800s. Among the earliest were Baltimore, Maryland (1798), Charleston, South Carolina (1815), and Philadelphia (1818). As their efforts expanded from handling public "nuisances" to dealing with epidemics and complex public health problems, local health boards recognized

Figure 2-1
Poverty and environmental conditions have a direct influence on people's health.

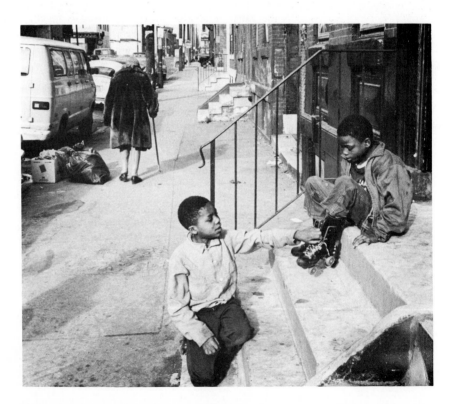

that employment of full-time staff was needed and formed health departments. The first full-time county health departments were established in 1911 in North Carolina and Washington state. Massachusetts formed the nation's first state board of health in 1869 and a few years later the first state department of health. At the national level, the Marine Hospital Service, now broadened in function, became the Public Health and Marine Hospital Service in 1902. Congress gave it a more clearly defined organizational structure and specific functions for its director, the surgeon general. In 1912 it was renamed the U.S. Public Health Service.

Rapidly expanding through the years of World War I and the Great Depression, the U.S. Public Health Service strengthened its research activity based in the National Institutes of Health (founded 1912), added demonstration projects, and initiated greater cooperation with the states. Responding to increasingly complex needs, it added such programs significant to public health as the Children's Bureau (1912), the National Leprosarium at Carville, Louisiana (1917), examination of arriving aliens (1917), the Division of Venereal Diseases (1918), the Food and Drug Administration (1927), and the Narcotics Division (1929), which later became the Division of Mental Hygiene. Title VI of the 1935 Social Security Act promoted stronger federal support of state and local public health services including health manpower training.

As the number of health, welfare, and educational services proliferated, the need for consolidation prompted the creation of the Federal Security Agency in 1939. In 1953 it became the Department of Health, Education and Welfare, now the Department of Health and Human Services. Other significant events included the establishment, during World War II, of the Communicable Disease Center in Atlanta, currently the National Centers for Disease Control, and the development, after World War II, of the National Office of Vital Statistics, now called the National Center for Health Statistics.

The private sector actually responded first to America's health problems and to this day continues to complement and supplement the government's role in provision of health services. Voluntary health agencies began to emerge by the late 1800s. The first of these was the Anti-Tuberculosis Society of Philadelphia formed in 1892 to educate the public and the government about tuberculosis, then causing 10 percent of all deaths. Other agencies followed. The National Society to Prevent Blindness was formed in 1908, the Mental Health Association in 1909, the American Cancer Society in 1913, and several, including the National Easter Seal Society for Crippled Children and Adults and the Planned Parenthood Federation of America in 1921. Also in the late 1800s, organized charities such as the Red Cross, previously denounced for promoting dependent poverty, began to be recognized for their contributions to health and welfare. Philanthropy, too, became respected with the establishment of the Rockefeller Foundation (1913) followed by the Carnegie-Mellon, Kellogg, and other foundations.

Many health-related professional associations over the years have influenced the quality and type of community health services delivery. Among these, the National Organization for Public Health Nursing, formed in 1912, significantly influenced early organization and quality of public health nursing services. It later became the National League for Nursing (1950) and continues to promote quality efforts in community health. The American Public Health Association, founded in 1872, to this day maintains a prominent role in the dissemination of public health information, influence on health policy, and advocacy for the nation's health.

HEALTH CARE ORGANIZATION

The historical record demonstrates that for many centuries people have attempted to address community health needs. Responsibility for these shifted between individuals and governing institutions. Each arm, public and private, offered a unique perspective, different skills, and different resources. Lack of coordination between them, however, and no method for comprehensive planning and delivery of health services left huge gaps in some areas, duplication in others. It has only been within the past 100 years that the two arms have gradually begun to work together to create an emerging system of health care (Roemer, 1984). How does that system work today? What are its strengths and weaknesses? To answer these questions, we will first examine its structure. Why look at structure? Because it becomes the operational base for assessment, diagnosis, planning, implementation, and evaluation of services and because it provides a framework for intersystem and intrasystem communication and coordination.

Health services occur at four levels: local, state, national, and international. Like ever-widening concentric circles, these levels encompass broader and broader populations. The organization of health services at each level can be classified under one of two types, government or private.

GOVERNMENT HEALTH ORGANIZATION

Government health agencies, the tax-supported arm of the community health effort, perform an important function in community health practice. They are the official public health and welfare agencies whose areas of jurisdiction and types of service are dictated by law. They coordinate activities that often can be carried out only by group or community-wide action: for example, proper sewage disposal or the provision of sanitary water systems. Government health agencies develop facilities and programs for special groups, such as native Americans, migrant workers, and military personnel and veterans, whose health care is not the direct responsibility of any one state or locality. Many community health activities require an authoritative legal backing to ensure enforcement (another useful function of official agencies) of control in such areas as environmental pollution, highway safety practices, and harmful use of drugs. Official agencies provide important record-keeping services, which include the collection of vital statistics, research, consultation, and sometimes financial support to other community health groups.

Many different government agencies contribute to the health of a community. Most obvious are the city or county health departments, which provide a variety of direct and indirect health services, including community health nursing. Other tax-supported agencies that sponsor health care or health-related services include welfare departments, departments of public works, public schools and hospitals, police departments, county agricultural services, and local housing authorities.

Local Health Agencies

At the grass-roots level, community health agencies vary considerably from one locality to the next. This is due in part to variations in local needs, size, and priority setting: to differing interpretations of standards; and to the type and stipulations of funding sources. Nonetheless, each local governmental health agency shares some commonly held responsibilities, functions, and structural features.

The primary responsibilities of the local health department are (1) to assess its population's health status and needs, (2) to determine how well those needs are being met, and (3) to take action toward satisfying unmet needs (Hanlon and Pickett, 1984). Local government also plays an important role in "coordinating inputs from the federal and state levels with those from the private sector to produce truly comprehensive health services" (American Public Health Association [APHA], 1975, p. 189). The local health agency is a critical level of health services provision because of its closeness to the ultimate recipients—health care consumers. The American Public Health Association has outlined in an official policy statement the functional areas for which local government should be responsible, either to provide services directly or by arrangement with other providers. Table 2-1 lists these areas (APHA, 1975).

The structure of the local health department varies in complexity with the setting. Rural and small urban agencies need only a simple organization while large metropolitan agencies require more complex organizational structures to support the greater diversity and quantity of work. A local board of health generally holds the legal responsibility for the health of its citizens. Health board members may be appointed by the mayor if the board of health serves a city or by a board of supervisors if the board of health serves a county. In turn, the board of health appoints a health officer, usually a physician with public health training, who employs the remaining

Table 2-1
The Role of Official Local Health Agencies

Community Health Services	Environmental Health Services	Mental Health Services	Personal Health Services	Processes Common to All Services
Communicable disease control	Food protection	Primary prevention of mental disorders	Personal health services, per se	Health data
Chronic disease control	Hazardous substances and product safety	Consultation	Health facilities operations	Agency program planning
Family health	Water supply sanitation	Diagnostic and treatment services	Emergency medical services	Interagency planning
Dental health	Liquid waste control		Home health services	Comprehensive state and regional health planning
Substance abuse	Water pollution control		Employee health programs	Disaster planning
Accident prevention	Swimming pool sanitation and safety		Medical care for inmates of prisons and institutions	Education of the public in health affairs
	Occupational health and safety			Health advocacy
	Radiation control			Continuing education of health personnel
	Air quality management			Involvement of health professionals
	Noise pollution control			Research and development
	Pest control			Community involvement
	Solid waste management			Organization
	Institutional sanitation			Policy direction
	Recreational sanitation			Staffing
	Housing conservation			Financing
	Environmental injury prevention			Relationships with state and federal health authorities

Source: Adapted from A.P.H.A. Position Paper, *American Journal of Public Health* 65: 189–92, 1975.

staff of the health department, including public health nurses, one or more environmental health workers, a health educator, and office personnel. Others, like a nutritionist, statistician, epidemiologist, social worker, physical therapist, veterinarian, or public health dentist, may be added as needs and resources dictate. Figure 2-2 depicts the organization of one local health department serving a population of approximately 270,000.

State Health Agencies

State-level health services, too, vary considerably. Each state, as a sovereign government, establishes its own state health department that, in turn, determines its goals, actions, and administrative structure. The state health department is responsible for providing leadership in and monitoring of public health needs and services in the state. It establishes statewide health policy standards, assists local communities, allocates funds, promotes state-level health planning, conducts and evaluates state-level health programs, pro-

Figure 2-2
Organizational chart of the St. Paul Division of Public Health.

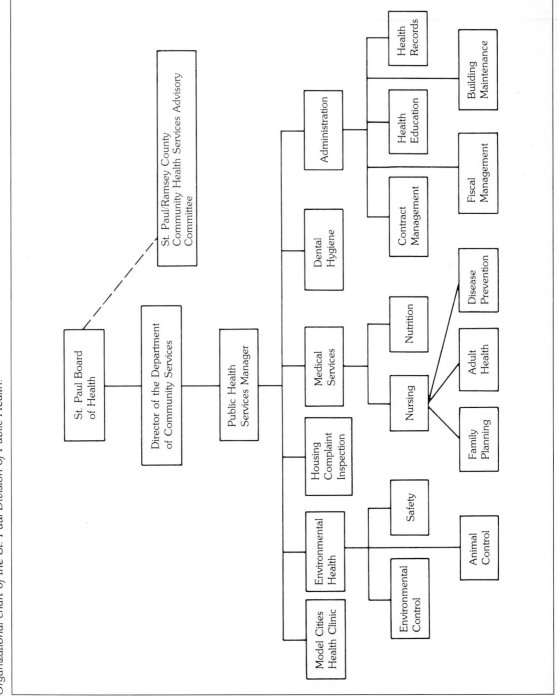

motes cooperation with voluntary health agencies, and collaborates with the federal government for health planning and policy development (Hanlon and Pickett, 1984).

State health department functions have been summarized in the following categories (Hanlon and Pickett, 1984, p. 149):

1. Statewide planning
2. Intergovernmental relations
3. Intrastate agency relations
4. Certain statewide policy determination
5. Standard setting
6. Regulatory functions

Each of the 50 state health departments in the United States has developed its own unique structure. All are overseen by a director of public health, but titles vary. Under the director are a number of divisions or bureaus. Those most commonly found in state health department organizational structures are disease control, local health services (which includes community health nursing), hospital and technical services, laboratory services, state center for health statistics, and medical care. Figure 2-3 shows a state health department organizational chart.

Federal Health Agencies

The federal level of public health organization contains many agencies. Best known is the Public Health Service (PHS), which is concerned with a broad variety of health interests and is directed by the Surgeon General. The PHS encompasses the Centers for Disease Control; the Food and Drug Administration; the National Institutes of Health; the Alcohol, Drug Abuse, and Mental Health Administration; and the Health Resources and Services Administration. Its major functions through these five branches are the administration of grants and contracts. In some instances, as with the Indian Health Service, it provides hospital and clinical services; through the Centers for Disease Control it provides epidemiologic surveillance; and through the Food and Drug Administration it monitors the safety and usefulness of various food and drug products. Figure 2-4 portrays the PHS organizational structure.

At the federal level the primary agencies concerned with health are organized under the Department of Health and Human Services. The PHS is one unit in this department. Formerly it was known as the Department of Health, Education and Welfare, established under President Eisenhower in 1953. In 1979, Education was made a separate cabinet-level department, and the department was renamed Health and Human Services. Figure 2-5 depicts this department's organization.

Figure 2-3
Organizational chart of a state health organization.

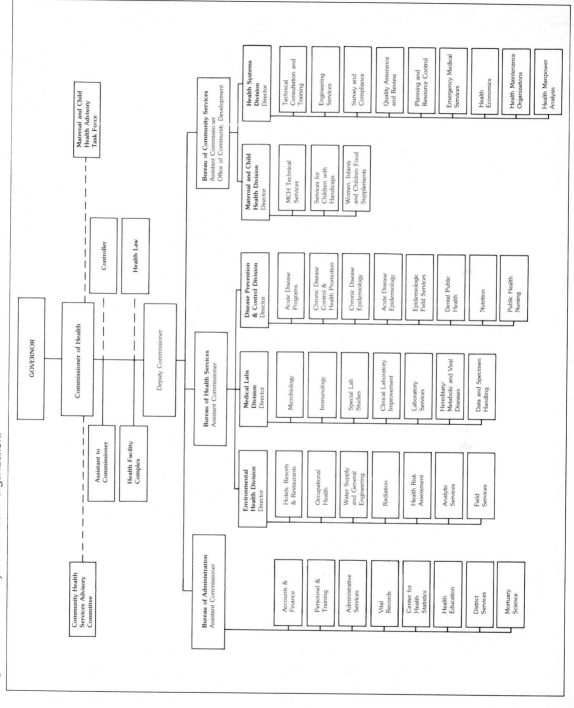

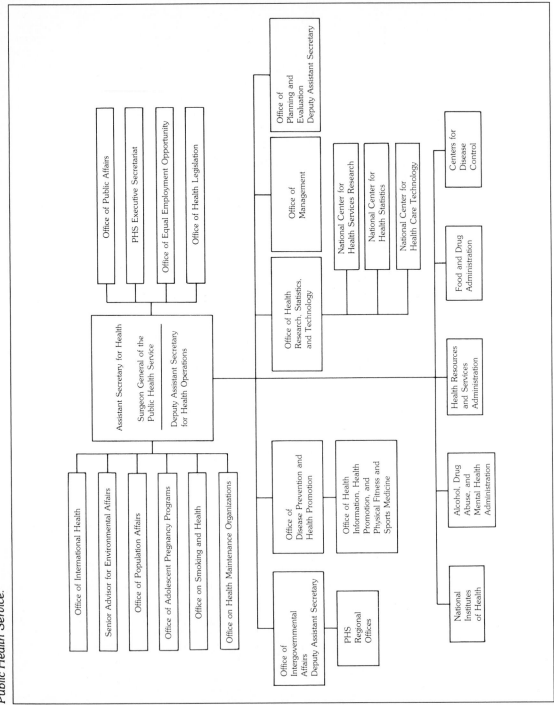

Figure 2-4
Public Health Service.

Figure 2-5
Department of Health and Human Services.

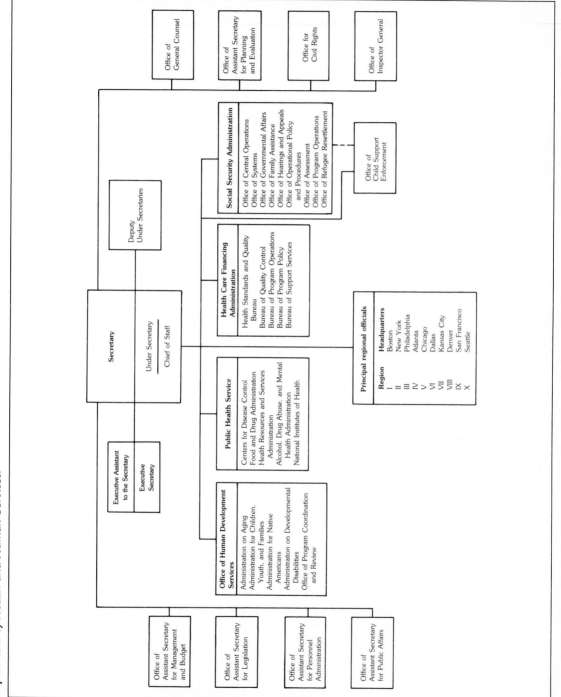

In addition to the PHS, a cluster of federal health agencies deals with special population groups such as the elderly (Administration on Aging), farmers (Agricultural Extension Service), Native Americans (Bureau of Indian Affairs), and the military. Another cluster addresses special programs or problems. Examples are the Bureau of Labor Standards, the Office of Education, the Bureau of Mines, and the Social Security Administration. A final cluster of federal agencies focuses on international health concerns. Two important ones are the Office of International Health, part of the PHS, and the Agency for International Development, part of the Department of State.

INTERNATIONAL HEALTH AGENCIES

The health of other countries cannot be ignored. Besides important humanitarian and moral concerns, there are pragmatic reasons for addressing health issues at the international level. We now live in an age when health, along with politics and economics, has become a global issue. The nations of the world are dependent on one another for goods and services, and as in any set of interdependent systems, a problem in one nation has repercussions on the others. Furthermore, as the constitution of the World Health Organization states, "The health of all peoples is fundamental to the attainment of peace and security" (World Health Organization [WHO], 1986).

International cooperation in health dates back to early concerns for epidemics. In 1851, representatives from 12 countries met in Paris for the First International Sanitary Conference. They later established a more permanent organization, the Office Internationale d'Hygiène Publique in 1907. Epidemics on the American continent prompted representatives from 21 American republics also to meet for the First International Sanitary Conference in Mexico City in 1902. In that same year they formed the International Sanitary Bureau, later renamed the Pan American Health Organization. After World War I, the League of Nations in 1921 formed a health organization with which the Office Internationale d'Hygiène Publique merged.

World Health Organization

The World Health Organization (WHO) was formed in 1948 and assumed the functions of the League of Nation's Health Organization. The Pan American Health Organization remained separate but became WHO's regional office for the Americas. An agency of the United Nations, WHO began its existence with 61 member nations, one of which was the United States. Its membership now numbers 168 (WHO, 1988).

The responsibility or mission of WHO is to serve as "the one directing and coordinating authority on international health work" (Hanlon and Pickett, 1984, p. 79). From its inception, WHO has influenced international thinking with its classic definition of health as "a state of complete physical, mental, and social well-being and not merely the absence of disease or infirmity" (WHO, 1986). WHO's primary function is to help countries improve their health status and services by helping them to help themselves and each other. To accomplish this, it provides member countries with technical services and information from epidemiology and statistics, advisory and consulting services, and demonstration teams.

In addition to its headquarters in Geneva, Switzerland, WHO has six regional offices. The office for the Americas (the Pan American Health Organization) is located in Washington, D.C. Its funding comes from member countries and from the United Nations. It holds an annual World Health Assembly (Figure 2-6) to discuss international health policies and programs (Hanlon and Pickett, 1984).

Pan American Health Organization

The Pan American Health Organization serves as the central coordinating organization for public health in the Western Hemisphere. Founded in 1902, it is the oldest continuously functioning international health organization in the world. As WHO's regional office for the Americas, it disseminates epidemiologic information, provides technical assistance, finances fellowships, and promotes cooperative research and professional education.

Figure 2-6
The World Health Assembly meets annually in Geneva, Switzerland, to discuss international health policies and programs.

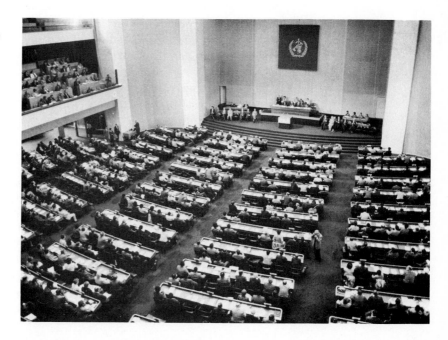

United Nations International Children's Emergency Fund

Organized in 1946, the United Nations Children's Fund, now the United Nations International Children's Emergency Fund (UNICEF), was initially established to assist children of war-torn countries. That focus has broadened. Now it promotes child and mental health and welfare globally through a variety of programs and activities. Some include provision of food and supplies to underdeveloped countries, immunization programs in cooperation with WHO, and promotion of family planning. Its International Children's Center, opened in 1940, has made a significant international impact with its teaching, research, publications, and cooperation on projects related to the health and welfare of children.

PRIVATE SECTOR HEALTH SERVICES

The unofficial arm of the health care delivery system includes many types of services. Voluntary nonprofit health and welfare agencies make up one large group. Privately owned (proprietary) agencies are another, and private professional health care practice forms a third group. They are the non-tax-supported, non-governmental dimension of community health care.

Private health services are complementary and supplementary to government health agencies. They often meet the needs of special groups, such as those with cancer or heart disease; they offer an avenue for private enterprise or philanthropy; they are freer than government agencies to develop innovations in health care; and they have been spurred to development, in part, by impatience or dissatisfaction with government programs. Their financial support comes from voluntary contributions, bequests, or fees.

Proprietary health services are privately owned and managed. They may be nonprofit or for-profit. According to the Institute of Medicine study, 81 percent of nursing homes, 52 percent of psychiatric hospitals, 13 percent of acute care hospitals, and 35 percent of HMOs are for-profit (A Washington Seminar Report, 1987). Many hospitals and nursing homes offer nonprofit services but must generate sufficient revenues to keep ahead of operating costs. Often one or more special services offered by a hospital will generate enough income to cover the drain from more expensive programs or uncompensated care. As more hospitals have merged or become part of larger health conglomerates, the practice has often been to establish a separate for-profit corporation that generates revenues so that the basic organization can retain its nonprofit, tax-exempt status.

Examples of for-profit health services include a wide range of private practices by physicians, nurses, social workers, psychologists, laboratory and X-ray technologists, and many more. With the greater demand for home care services in the 1980s we have also seen a major increase in new for-profit services, such as home care agencies, nursing personnel pools, and durable medical equipment supply companies.

Voluntary health agencies are nonprofit organizations established and administered by private citizens for some specific health-related purpose. Often this purpose is seen as a special need either not addressed or served inadequately by government. An example is visiting nurse associations that were formed to provide care for the sick in their homes. The contribution of the voluntary health agency then becomes complemental to official health services.

Many types of voluntary agencies exist. Most of them have very specialized interests. Some, such as the American Cancer Society and the American Diabetes Association, are concerned with specific diseases. Others, such as the National Society for Autistic Children and the National Council on Aging, focus on the needs of special populations. A third group, such as the American Heart Association and the National Kidney Foundation, is concerned with diseases of specific organs. All of these agencies are funded through private contributions.

Another group of voluntary health agencies includes the many foundations that support health programs, research, and professional education. Examples include the Kellogg Foundation and the Robert Wood Johnson Foundation. Some agencies, like the United Way, exist to fund other voluntary efforts. Still another group includes professional associations that work to improve the public's health through the promotion of standards, research, information, and programs. Examples are the American Public Health Association, the National League for Nursing, the American Nurses Association, and the American Medical Association. These organizations are funded primarily through membership dues.

Hanlon and Pickett, (1984, p. 160) describe the general functions of voluntary agencies as follows:

1. Pioneering—detecting unserved needs or exploring better methods for meeting needs already addressed
2. Demonstration—piloting or subsidizing demonstration projects
3. Education—promoting public knowledge
4. Supplementation of official actions—assisting official agencies with innovative programs not otherwise possible
5. Guarding citizen interest in health—evaluating official programs and assuming a public advocacy role
6. Promotion of health legislation
7. Planning and coordination—promoting collaboration among voluntary services and between voluntary and official agencies
8. Development of well-balanced community health programs seeking to make services relevant and comprehensive

SIGNIFICANT LEGISLATION

During the twentieth century, an ever-widening sense of responsibility for health in the public sector led to passage of an increasing amount of health-related legislation. Some acts are of particular significance to the delivery and financing of community health services.

The Shepard-Towner Act of 1921 provided federal funds for state administration of programs to promote the health and welfare of infants. The act expired in 1929, but it set a pattern for maternal and child health programs that was later revived and strengthened through the successful and far-reaching efforts of the Children's Bureau, housed in the Department of Labor (Hanlon and Pickett, 1984). The Children's Bureau maintained its impact through several administrative changes (moved to the Federal Security Agency in 1946 and to the Department of Health, Education and Welfare in 1953 and became the Office of Child Development) but was phased out in 1972. Since that time federal advocacy for child health per se has considerably weakened.

The Social Security Act of 1935 had tremendous consequences for public health. In addition to its revolutionary welfare insurance and assistance programs, which particularly benefited high-risk mothers and children, Title VI of the act financially assisted states and localities in providing public health services. These funds were and still are allocated on the basis of population, public health problems, economic need, and need for training public health personnel. Many of the grants had to be matched by the states or localities serving to increase their knowledge of and commitment to health programs. The act strengthened local health departments and health programs in nearly all the states (Hanlon and Pickett, 1984).

The Hill-Burton Act (Hospital Survey and Construction Act) of 1946 was an important breakthrough in nationwide health facilities planning. It marked the first real effort to link health planning with population need on a comprehensive basis. The act provided federal funds to states for hospital construction. Allocation of funds, however, was contingent upon the states forming planning councils to survey and document needs for new facilities and other capital expansion. The Hill-Harris Amendments in 1954 shifted the emphasis from purely construction to broader health planning based on needs assessment (Hyman, 1982).

The Heart Disease, Cancer, and Stroke Amendments of 1965 (Pub. L. 89-239) are noteworthy for their establishment of regional medical programs, one of the first real efforts at comprehensive health planning. Fifty-six regions in the United States were designated, each charged with the responsibility to evaluate the overall health needs of its region and cooperate with other regions for program development. Although the amendments were initially categorical in nature (limited to heart disease, cancer, and stroke), amendments in 1970 expanded the focus. The act was important for two additional reasons. It encouraged local participation in health planning, previously done at federal and state levels, and it funded program operations as well as planning.

The Social Security Act Amendments of 1965 produced two pieces of legislation that attempted to address a concern for some type of national health insurance. Title XVIII, Medicare, still provides federal health insurance to persons over 65 years of age on Social Security, to the disabled, and to persons with end-stage renal disease needing dialysis. Part A of this law covers hospitalization. Part B, which is supplementary, pays for physician care and other related health services. Both parts of Medicare are financed by trust funds. Title XIX, Medicaid, is a joint federal-state assistance program; it serves low-income persons and their families as well as the medically indigent (those with high medical expenses). It is administered on a state-by-state basis. These two pieces of legislation have enabled many of the poor and elderly to gain access to high-quality health care (Davis, 1983).

The Comprehensive Health Planning and Public Health Service Amendments Act (Partnership for Health Act) of 1966 (PL. 89-749) promoted further advances in comprehensive health planning. It established comprehensive health planning agencies and attempted to coordinate the many categorical health and research efforts into an integrated system. It emphasized comprehensive health planning and cost containment at local, state, and regional levels. Its goals were improved efficiency and effectiveness of health care. Many problems, including unclear expectations, uncertain funding, and limited authority, prevented full accomplishment of these goals.

The Health Manpower Act of 1968 (PL. 90-490) sought to increase the supply of health personnel by providing federal monies to educational institutions for construction, training, special projects, student loans, and scholarships. The act replaced several previous acts with similar goals but whose efforts were fragmentary in addressing the problem. Among them were the Nurse Training Act (1966) and the Allied Health Professions Personnel Training Act (1966). In 1976, Congress passed the Health Professions Education Assistance Act (PL. 94-484) to effect a better balance between the country's health needs and the supply of available health professionals. One of its major emphases was to address the problem of physician maldistribution between underserved (rural) and overserved (urban) areas through educational incentive programs.

The Occupational Safety and Health Act of 1970 (PL. 91-956) provides protection to workers against personal injury or illness resulting from hazardous working conditions. This and other acts affecting the working population, such as workers' compensation, toxic substance control, access to employee exposure and medical records, and "right-to-know" legislation, are discussed in Chapter 18.

The Professional Standards Review Organization Amendment to the Social Security Act of 1972 (PL. 92-603) had two goals: cost containment and improved quality of care. Professional Standards Review Organization (PSRO) legislation created autonomous organizations, external to hospitals and ambulatory care agencies, to monitor and review objectively the quality of care delivered to Medicare and Medicaid patients. The PSRO review boards, composed mostly of physicians, examined such things as need for care, length of stay, and quality of care against predetermined standards developed locally. Failure to meet standards could mean denial of federal funding. The PSRO concept has created considerable controversy, partly because the two mandated goals, cost containment and quality of care, are potentially incompatible. The federal government's primary emphasis on costs frequently clashed with local concerns for quality. Also, the lack of criteria or standards for review has made it hard to evaluate the program's success. Preliminary studies, however, indicate a substantial cost saving in Medicare expenditures (Hyman, 1982).

The Health Maintenance Organization Act of 1973 (PL. 93-222) added federal support to the concept of prepayment for medical care. Congress authorized funding for feasibility studies, planning, grants, and loans to stimulate growth among qualifying health maintenance organizations (HMOs). In addition, this act requires a business employing 25 or more people to offer an HMO health insurance option, if such an option is available locally.

The National Health Planning and Resource Development Act of 1974 (PL. 93-641) was a major breakthrough in comprehensive health planning. Replacing the Partnership for Health Act, it combined Hill-Burton, comprehensive health planning agencies, and regional medical programs into a single new program. It fostered not only comprehensive heath planning, but regulation and evaluation, and promoted collaborative efforts among regional, state, and federal governments. An important contribution of this act was its emphasis on consumer involvement in health planning. The act was divided into two titles. Title XV, National Health Planning and Development, established national health priorities and assisted the development of area-wide and state planning through health systems agencies and state health planning and development agencies. Title XVI, Health Resources Development, coordinated health facilities planning with health planning, replacing Hill-Burton (Hyman, 1982).

The Social Security Amendments of 1983 (PL. 98-21) became law in response to accelerating health care costs. The act represents a major reform in health care financing from retrospective to prospective payment. Most Medicare-participating hospitals now receive payment from Medicare on the basis of a fixed rate set in advance for each patient by diagnosis. A billing classification system has identified 23 major diagnostic categories and 467 diagnosis-related groups (DRGs) with prospective payment made based on hospital case mix (Joel, 1983; Shaffer, 1983). The fixed payment cannot be increased if hospital costs for care exceed that amount. Conversely, if costs are less than the paid amount, the hospital may keep the difference (Davis, 1983). Thus, a positive incentive was introduced to reduce hospital costs.

HEALTH CARE FINANCING

Behind the financing of health care lies the science of health economics. The field of economics, as a whole, studies and seeks to promote the best use of scarce resources for the greatest good of society. *Health care economics* is the description and analysis of production, distribution, and consumption of health care goods and services. Its goal is to maximize the benefits of using scarce resources for the greatest number of people.

Health care economics encompasses an intricate and complex set of interacting variables. It is concerned with supply and demand: Is the supply of available resources sufficient to meet the demand for use by consumers? It examines costs and benefits, cost effectiveness, and cost efficiency: Are the resources expended achieving the desired outcomes? It looks at the allocation of scarce resources: Where should resources, such as funding and personnel, be applied when there aren't enough to go around? Health economics is a field of study in and of itself. Issues such as cost containment, competition between providers, accessibility of services, and need for accountability have become targets of major concern for the 1980s and 1990s. We can facilitate our understanding of some of these issues and their impact on community health through examination of types of health care financing, trends influencing health care economics, and the effects of financing patterns on community health practice.

TYPES OF HEALTH CARE FINANCING

Financing of health care significantly affects community health practice. It influences the quality of services offered as well as the way those services are utilized. Methods of health care financing fall into three categories: third-party payers, direct consumer payment, and voluntary support.

Third-party payers are so called because they are a third party, or external, to the consumer-provider relationship. Included in this category are four types of payment sources: private insurance companies, independent health plans, government health programs, and claims payment agents (Rapoport, Robertson, and Stewart, 1982).

Private insurance companies market and underwrite policies aimed at decreasing consumer risk of economic loss because of health services utilization. None actually delivers health services. They are composed of three types. First are commercial stock companies that sell health insurance, generally as a sideline. They are private stockholder-owned corporations, such as Aetna, Travelers, and Connecticut General, that sell insurance nationally. Mutual companies are a second type that operates in the national marketplace, but they are owned by their policyholders. Examples are Mutual of

Omaha, Prudential, and Metropolitan Life. The third type, nonprofit insurance plans, include Blue Cross, Blue Shield, and Delta Dental. These operate under special state enabling laws that give them an exclusive franchise to the whole state (or some part of it) and to a specific type of insurance. Blue Cross, for example, in most instances sells only hospital coverage, Blue Shield only medical insurance, and Delta Dental only dental insurance. Because they are nonprofit, they are tax-exempt and at the same time subject to tighter state regulation than the commercial health insurance companies. Combined, the nonprofit and commercial carriers sell 90 percent of the private health insurance in the United States (Rapoport et al., 1982).

Independent health plans underwrite the remaining 10 percent of private health insurance in the nation. These are offered through several hundred smaller organizations such as businesses, unions, consumer cooperatives, and medical groups. HMOs and various company self-insurance plans are included in this category. They may sell only health insurance or, in some cases, may also provide health services; they focus on a very localized population. As a group, they generate a large amount of premium revenues but only one-tenth of the amount generated by the nonprofit and commercial health insurance companies.

Government health programs make up the largest source of third-party reimbursement in the country. The government's four largest third-party programs are Medicare, Medicaid, the Federal Employees Health Benefits Plan, and the Civilian Health and Medical Program of the Uniformed Services. Combined, they "account for more than 50 percent of the nation's hospital revenues and nearly a quarter of physician incomes" (Rapoport et al., 1982, p. 294). A third of the government's total third-party expenditures go for direct public medical services by the military, state hospitals, the Veterans Administration, public health activities, and other "socialized" health services. Their primary target is what Health and Human Services Secretary Margaret Heckler called "the most fragile Americans" ("Known Welfare Fraud," 1983, p. 42) — the elderly, the disabled, the poor, the very young, and the unemployed. A recent federal health insurance program — this one designated to be self-financing — protects the unemployed who have lost their benefits. Another, workers' compensation, is a state-administered program that protects workers from illness or injury associated with their jobs.

In addition to third-party reimbursement, the government offers some direct health services to selected populations. They include Native Americans, military personnel, veterans, merchant marines, and federal employees.

Claims payment agents administer the claims payment process of government third-party payments. That is, the government contracts with private agents to handle the claims payment process. More than 80 percent of the government's third-party payments are handled by these private contractors who are sometimes known as fiscal intermediaries (when processing Medicare hospital claims), carriers (when dealing with insurance under Medicare), or fiscal agents (as applied to Medicaid programs). As an example, Blue

Cross Plans, in addition to being private insurance companies, are also claims payment agents for Medicare.

Direct consumer reimbursement is a second major type of health care financing. This refers to individual out-of-pocket payments made for several different reasons. One is payments made by individuals who have no insurance coverage so that direct payment must be made for health and medical services. Another is for limited coverage and exclusions (services for which the consumer must bear the entire expense). For example, many individuals carry only major medical insurance and must pay directly for physician office visits, prescriptions, and dental care. In other instances, the insurance contract may include a deductible amount that must be paid by the insuree before reimbursement begins. The contract may be established on a co-payment basis that determines a percentage to be paid by the insurer and the rest by the individual. Or the individual may pay the remainder of a health service bill after the insurer has paid a previously agreed-upon fixed amount such as a fixed coverage for labor and delivery. Direct consumer payment accounts for approximately one-third of total personal health care expenditures in the United States (Gibson et al., 1984). See Figure 2-7.

Voluntary support, the third type, contributes both directly and indirectly to health care financing. Many voluntary agencies, as discussed earlier in this chapter, fund programs and provide benefits for individuals who would otherwise go without services. Volunteerism, the efforts of numerous individuals who donate their time and services, provides tremendous cost savings to health care institutions. It also enables many individuals to receive services, such as home-delivered meals or transportation to health care facilities, at no charge. Continued voluntary support is essential, particularly during an era when large amounts of federal monies for social programs have been withdrawn (Hanlon and Pickett, 1984).

ISSUES AND TRENDS

Federal Regulation

Between the 1950s and 1970s the federal government assumed a much stronger role in the financing and regulation of health services. First, federal subsidy of health care costs increased. There was greater federal control of state programs. Health services became regionalized and more comprehensive. Federal appropriations supported operational as well as capital and planning costs. There was greater federal support for health research. Federal support for health manpower training increased. Group medical practice multiplied as a cost-saving measure. Over 60 percent of the population was covered by some form of prepaid health insurance, largely because of the effects of Medicare and Medicaid. There was an increase in interagency health planning cooperation and improved health program evaluation. Neighbor-

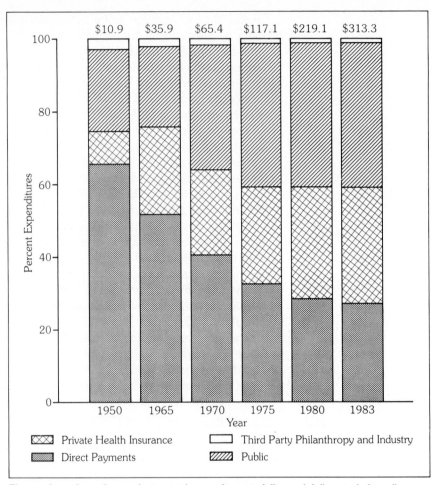

Figure 2-7
*Percent distribution of
personal health care
expenditures by direct and
third party payments
(U.S.A. selected years
1950–83).*

The numbers above the graph give total expenditures in billions of dollars, including all
expenditures other than expenses for prepayment and administration, for government public
health activities, and for expenditures of private voluntary agencies for other health services.

Source: R. M. Gibson, K. R. Levit, H. Lazenby, and D. R. Waldo. (1983). National health care
expenditures. *Health Care Financing Review* 1984 Winter; 6: Table 6, p. 14.

hood health centers, community mental health centers, and other programs
developed to improve health care access for everyone. It was a period of
economic prosperity that emphasized quality of care, and during it the federal government assumed a major role in the regulation of planning, use,
and reimbursement of health care services.

Cost Escalation

Accompanying these trends, however, was an insidious escalation in health
care costs. The early national effort to increase health resources, in the form
of facilities, programs, and manpower, concomitantly increased the public's

demand for health care. An even greater contribution to cost increases occurred through the system of third-party reimbursement. Third-party payment shielded consumers from the real costs of health care, encouraging consumer demand. More important, third-party reimbursement created a mood of unlimited spending because someone else was paying the bill. Hospitals and other providers could rely on payment regardless of what they spent, adding to the incentive to spend even more.

Government-financed programs, often unwieldy and expensive, fell prey to these escalating costs and to the pressures of inflation. Medicare, for example, which is financed through government trust funds, had so depleted its resources that its insolvency was predicted for the late 1980s ("Known welfare fraud," 1983). Later measures in the form of prospective payment legislation and Social Security recommendations were taken to extend the solvency of Medicare funds (Davis, 1983).

Currently, health care costs have been growing at a rate of 19 percent per year (Davis, 1983). In the period from 1950 to 1980, real per capita health care spending tripled, and total health care spending (government, insurance companies, and private individuals) was well over 10 percent of the gross national product in the early 1980s, rising to 11.4 percent in 1988 (Davis, 1983; Francis, 1988). (The gross national product [GNP] is the total value of all goods and services produced in the United States economy in one year [Health: U.S., 1985].) The Department of Health and Human Services has grown exponentially to the point that today it administers the third largest budget in the world, behind only the budgets of the United States and the Soviet Union (Davis, 1983), and it accounts for 34 percent of all federal spending ("Known welfare fraud," 1983).

Preferred Provider Organizations

Preferred Provider Organizations (PPOs) are a type of alternative delivery system that recently came into being (Ellwood, 1985). A PPO is an organization of health care providers that contracts on a fixed fee-for-service basis with a third-party payer to provide comprehensive health services to subscribers. Because of contractual fixed costs, employing organizations who subscribe can offer medical services to their employees at discounted rates (Roble, Knowlton, and Rosenberg, 1984).

Early use of PPOs appears to promote cost savings, but the long-range cost-effectiveness of this option is difficult to measure and has yet to be determined.

Health Maintenance Organizations

In recent years traditional fee-for-service practice has experienced serious competition in the form of comprehensive prepaid services. The concept of prepayment, or consumers paying in advance of health care, has existed for many years. As far back as 1933, prepaid medical groups were advocated to reduce costs and make services more accessible (Hyman, 1982). This pattern of prepayment for comprehensive services has continued ever since in a variety of forms. Examples of early plans were the Health Insurance Program of greater New York City and the Kaiser Plan. The success of these two plans, in particular, helped influence the growth of health maintenance organizations (HMOs), another alternative delivery system. (See Figure 2-8). HMOs, as discussed earlier, are prepaid systems that, for a monthly premium, provide comprehensive health services to plan participants.

From 1930 to 1965, the HMO movement, supported initially by the private sector, gradually gained federal backing. Group plans were a part of Medicare and Medicaid bills and the Partnership for Health Act. The HMO Act of 1973 demonstrated stronger federal support. Amendments to this act in 1976 lifted restrictions and further encouraged HMOs.

Today the chief characteristics of an HMO are the following (Rapoport et al., 1982, p. 257):

1. There is a contract between the HMO and the consumers (or their representative), who are the "enrolled population."
2. A regular (usually monthly) premium to cover specified (and typically broad) services is paid for or by each enrollee to the HMO; few addi-

Figure 2-8
A community health nurse works collaboratively with another health team member to promote client health in a health maintenance organization.

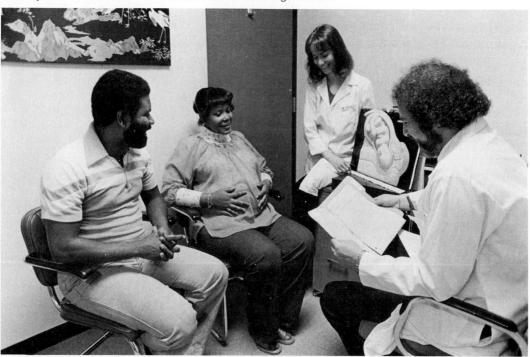

tional charges are levied because the payment mechanism is not basically fee-for-service.
3. The HMO contracts with professional providers to deliver the services due the enrollees; the basis for reimbursing those providers varies among HMOs.

Despite official encouragement and government subsidies, the growth of HMOs has been slower than expected. Yet they are strongly endorsed as an alternative delivery system because of their potential for conserving costs owing to their greater emphasis on prevention, health promotion, and ambulatory care, with a concomitant reduction in hospital and medical care utilization (Somers, 1986; Booth, 1985).

National Heath Insurance

Growing concern over the cost and accessibility of health services led in the 1960s and again in the mid-1970s to a renewed focus on national health insurance (NHI) as a solution. NHI, as an issue, had been debated since 1912, its proponents seeking comprehensive health care protection for the aged and needy, in particular. Numerous attempts to pass some form of NHI resulted in piecemeal legislation adding various benefits for Social Security recipients. The Kerr-Mills bill (1960) set a precedent of public financing for elderly persons who were "medically needy" but not on public assistance. Medicare (1965) was the first compulsory NHI program in the United States. However, it reached only 10 percent of the population (Somers and Somers, 1977).

In the 1970s the debate over NHI revived in full force. Many proposed NHI bills were considered by Congress. The seeming consensus over the need for government to assure access to needed health services for the total population was misleading. Divergent interests and conflicting philosophies led to heated debate, with four issues emerging as core areas of controversy. First was the public-private mix. What should be the amount and nature of private health insurance involvement in the public program? Second was the cost-sharing issue. To what extent, if any, should consumers share in the cost of the coverage? Third, what should be the amount and nature of cost and quality controls built into the program? And fourth, should the NHI program be used as a vehicle for reform of the health care provision system (Somers and Somers, 1977)? Resolution, to date, has not been reached, and experts are predicting that a viable NHI program is not likely in the near future (Somers and Somers, 1977). First, we must reconcile the major roles of our large private health insurance industry, hospitals, and the medical profession along with our nation's inherent aversion to direct government intervention.

Recommendations for National Health Insurance.   In the decade of the 1980s, study of NHI as an important concept continued. Somers and Somers (1977) recommended that NHI in its ideal form include the following:

1. Universal coverage regardless of income
2. Equitable financing using multiple sources but channeled through one mechanism
3. Comprehensive and balanced benefit structure
4. Incentives for efficient and effective use of resources and discouragement of health care price inflation
5. Controlled competition in the underwriting and administration of the program
6. Appropriate and feasible consumer options
7. Administrative simplicity
8. Flexibility
9. Acceptability to providers and consumers

Problems of Uninsured and Underinsured. With the numbers of people uninsured and underinsured rising dramatically, the need for national health insurance with some form of national health program is becoming paramount (Semmel, 1987). The poor, nearly poor, unemployed, and others who comprise the uninsured and underinsured make up between 15 and 20 percent of the United States population (Relman, 1987). More than half of uninsured adults (17 million in 1986) are workers whose employers offer no group-based health insurance (Swartz, 1987). The current system has failed to provide even minimum basic care for these groups (Figure 2-9). Further, the system has yet to adequately protect the elderly from financial disaster associated with the costs of long-term care and catastrophic illness. Advocates for the medically indigent, the disadvantaged, and the elderly are speaking out (Bergman, 1988). New groups have formed in recent years to study the issues and make policy recommendations (Relman, 1987). Among the issues being debated are controversial questions about organ transplants: who should receive them, and who will pay for them. NHI with a national health system will likely be a major consideration for the 1990s and beyond. Meanwhile, individual states are considering passage of statewide health insurance policies to address some of these difficult problems.

Competition and Regulation

Dramatic changes affecting health care occurred in the early 1980s. The federal government, failing to contain health care costs, shifted responsibility for the public's health and welfare back to state and local governments, emphasizing a decentralized system. Large amounts of federal support for health research, health manpower training, and public health programs were withdrawn. Continued escalation of health care costs prompted a concentrated effort among public and private providers alike to find cost-containment measures. Competition, encouraged by passage of the Budget Reconciliation Bill, was seen as a solution. Out of all this grew the competition versus regulation debate.

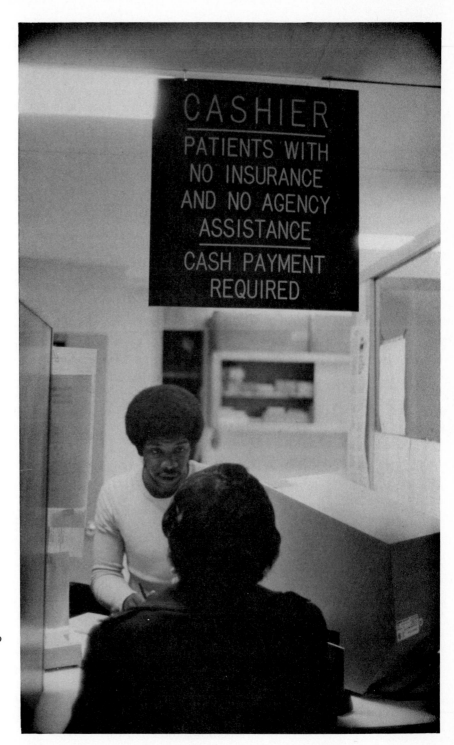

Figure 2-9
*People who have little or no
health insurance coverage
make up between 15 and
20 percent of the U.S.
population. National
health insurance is being
considered as a way to
alleviate the problem.*

Competition, its proponents say, offers wider consumer choice and positive incentives for cost containment. That is, consumers have freedom to select among various health plans on the basis of cost, quality, and range of services. Competing providers must develop efficient production and distribution methods to stay in business, and consumers, because of required cost sharing that is part of the competition model, are more likely to use only necessary services. Examples of competition are increasingly evident as a growing number of health plans, including HMOs and PPOs, vie with insurance companies for subscribers. Many hospitals, too, aggressively compete for patients. Advertisements depicting the new mother and father having a candlelight dinner with their new infant in the crib beside them in the hospital testify to hospital competition for obstetrical patients.

Ideally, competition offers the best service for the least cost. Regulation advocates, on the other hand, point out some of the problems associated with the competition model. Consumers often don't know how to make proper choices because they have limited knowledge of health services. Competition, they argue, leads to discriminate selection of consumers, especially low-risk, low-cost patients, thus excluding those who may need services the most. The competition model may not encourage teaching and research, because these tend to be expensive elements of our present system. And because of its concern with costs, competition could likely sacrifice quality (Weiss, 1982). Regulation, they say, is needed for standardization and controls, especially for quality and equal access. Leaders in the field have concluded that both are needed (Ehlinger, 1982; Somers, 1986). According to McNerney (1980, p. 1091), "It is rapidly becoming apparent that what we need is a proper balance between competition and regulation with more effective links . . . regulation [should be] used as a force to keep the market honest."

Prospective Payment

Prospective payment has evolved within the past ten years in response to the health care system's desperate need for cost containment. Under this concept, rate setting is done prospectively, or in advance of treatment, rather than retrospectively. Providers receive payment for services according to fixed rates set in advance (Shaffer, 1983). To correct unlimited reimbursement patterns and counteract disincentives to contain costs, the concept involves four steps (Dowling, 1979):

1. An external authority is empowered (by statute, market power, or voluntary compliance by providers) to set provider charges, third-party payment rates, or both.
2. Rates are set in advance of the prospective year during which they will apply and are considered fixed for the year (except for major, uncontrollable occurrences).

3. Patients, third-party payers, or both pay the prospective rates rather than the costs actually incurred by providers during the year (or charges adjusted to cover these costs).
4. Providers are at risk for losses or surpluses.

Prospective payment, then, imposes constraints on spending and gives incentives for cutting costs. For these reasons the federal government enacted into law its diagnosis related group (DRG) prospective payment plan in 1983 in an effort to curb Medicare spending in hospitals and to extend the program's solvency period. Prospective payment system (PPS) incentives have indeed reduced hospital stays and unnecessary admissions and created a boom in home health care (Fackelmann, 1987). A spinoff, however, is fierce competition among providers and mounting concern over quality.

Although PPS offers some solutions, it also raises some questions. Do DRGs promote premature discharge of hospitalized patients, and what effect may that have on their health and on the delivery of services outside the hospital? What is PPS's ongoing effect on quality of care in the hospital, in ambulatory settings, and in the home?

EFFECTS ON COMMUNITY HEALTH PRACTICE

Health care financing has significantly affected community health and community health practice by advancing (1) disincentives for efficient use of resources, (2) incentives for illness care, and (3) conflict with public health values.

Disincentives for Efficient Use of Resources

Disincentives for efficient use of resources include all the system structures that promote cost escalation and prevent cost containment. For example, retrospective financial reimbursement, with its lack of limit setting, encourages spending and drives costs up. Tax-deductible employer contributions for health care coverage and nontaxable employee health benefits encourage unnecessary use of services and raise costs. Lack of cost sharing by consumers and no financial risk for provider decision making create further disincentives to keep costs down.

Community health is affected in several ways. Abuse of resources in some parts of the system means a depletion in other areas. Community health programs have suffered greatly in recent years with diminished federal and state allocations and severe budget cuts affecting even basic community health services. Competition from the private sector in home care and other community services, such as health education programs, has forced traditional public health agencies to reexamine their programs and seek new avenues for service and new revenue sources. Costs indirectly affect even appropriate use of nursing personnel in community health. Failing to recognize the differences in skills of community health nurses and less prepared personnel, the proliferating agencies in community health often hire persons underqualified to give the high-caliber and comprehensive care needed in many instances. Finally, the advent of prospective payment and payment by DRGs is encouraging early hospital discharge and an increasing number of more acutely ill people needing home care. The immediate effect is to increase the demand for home care services of a highly skilled and more costly nature requiring changes in community health care provision patterns. The long-range effects of this phenomenon on family stress and caregiver health, on community health care reimbursement, and on the nature and structure of community health services provision has yet to be determined.

Incentives for Illness Care

Because of its financial incentives, the traditional American health care system tends to promote illness. Health care providers are primarily rewarded for treating problems, not for preventing them. The surgeon who advises a patient who is a potential candidate for hemorrhoidectomy to increase the fiber in his diet may be losing a surgical fee. Hospitals have more income when their beds stay full of sick or injured people. The bulk of most reimbursable health services centers around hospital, physician, nursing home, ambulatory care, and skilled nursing care in the home. These services are mostly illness oriented; the individual must play the role of patient in these settings. Health promotional activities such as comprehensive prenatal, maternal, and infant care; health education; childhood immunizations; and home services to enable the elderly to live independently are not covered by many insurers.

A system that financially supports illness care affects community health practice in several ways. The number and severity of health problems in a community increase when individuals postpone care because visits to the doctor or clinic mean greater expense — expense that they often cannot afford. Illness-oriented incentives create a basic societal valuing of illness care that, conversely, devalues wellness care. Health promotion and disease prevention efforts become second-ranked priorities in competition for scarce resources. In response to increased illness care, a greater proportion of community health practice is spent on treatment of disorders and rehabilitation, thus limiting the time and resources for prevention and health promotion. Prepayment methods and the growth of HMOs are positive moves in the direction of a more wellness-oriented financial incentive structure. An HMO has the incentive to offer preventive and health-promoting services such as early detection and treatment of symptoms, regular physical examinations, and health teaching.

Conflict with Public Health Values

Competition in health care is a reality with which community health practice must cope. Although competition offers a number of benefits, it poses some dilemmas for community health that are not easily resolved. Values underlying the competition model are in direct conflict with several basic public health values (Ehlinger, 1982). Competition, for example, encourages service providers to be adversarial — to win. Public health operates on the basis of collaboration and cooperation (Ray and Flynn, 1980). Competition serves a selected market determined, in part, by those able to purchase products or services. Public health is committed to serving all persons in need, regardless of ability to pay (Beauchamp, 1975). The competition model focuses on individuals and is present-oriented; public health is concerned with aggregates and is future-oriented, emphasizing prevention. Competition establishes relatively fixed limits for service, while public health must remain flexible if it is to be responsive to the total population's health needs.

The effect of those philosophical differences plus the constraints, such as civil service restrictions and political influences, under which most public health agencies must operate, make it very difficult for them to compete. They must still remain committed to providing the health promotion and disease prevention services that are their public trust. Yet competition seems necessary if they are to stay in business. Exclusion from health care competition, freedom from constraints, or some kind of special support may be needed to keep many of these programs alive. Competition may also serve as a stimulus for new and innovative community health services and the possible introduction of new roles and revenue sources for traditional public health agencies.

Summary

Many factors and events have influenced the current structure, function, and financing of community health services. Understanding these gives the community health nurse a stronger base for planning for the health of community populations.

Historically health care has progressed unevenly, marked by numerous influences. Primitive practices of early centuries were replaced with more advanced sanitary measures by the Greeks and Romans. The Middle Ages saw a serious health decline, with raging epidemics, leading to extensive nineteenth-century reform efforts in England and later in the United States.

Organized health care in the U.S. developed slowly. Public health problems, such as need for isolation of communicable disease and control of environmental pollution, prompted the gradual development of official interventions. For example, quarantines to control the spread of communicable disease were imposed in the late 1700s. Sanitary reform was pursued more vigorously during the 1800s. Local, then state, health departments were formed starting in the late 1700s. By the early 1900s the federal government had assumed a more active role in public health with a proliferation of health, education, and welfare services.

For many years efforts to address community health needs have been made by private individuals and public agencies. These two arms of service have not been coordinated in the past and only gradually during this century have begun to work together to form an emerging health care system.

The public arm of health services includes all government, tax-supported health agencies and occurs at four levels: local, state, national, and international. Each level deals with the health needs of the population that its boundaries encompass. Each level has a different structure and set of functions.

Private health services are the unofficial arm of the community health system. They include voluntary nonprofit agencies as well as privately owned (proprietary) and for-profit agencies. Their financial support comes from voluntary contributions, bequests, or fees. Private health organizations often supplement and complement the work of official agencies.

The delivery and financing of community health services has been significantly affected by various legislative acts. These acts have prompted such innovations as health insurance and assistance for the poor, monies to train health personnel and conduct health research, standards for health planning and delivery, and health protection for workers on the job.

Health care financing falls into three categories: third-party payers, direct consumer payment, and voluntary support. Several issues and trends have influenced community health care financing and delivery. They include early federal regulation, escalating health care costs, PPOs, the HMO movement, attempts to institute national health insurance, increased competition in health care, and prospective reimbursement.

The changing nature of health care financing has affected community health and its practice in three important ways. It has created disincentives for efficient use of resources; it has promoted incentives for illness care; and it has generated a conflict with basic public health values.

Study Questions

1. Debate the pros and cons of a strong federal role in health care provision as opposed to decentralized (state and local) control.
2. Describe three ways that escalating health care costs are influencing community health practice.
3. How does prospective reimbursement affect health care provision from the hospital's perspective? From a community health perspective?
4. Why does the competition model of health care provision pose problems for community health? Discuss the potential impact of competition on the poor and medically indigent.

References

American Public Health Association. (1975). The role of official local health agencies. *American Journal of Public Health* 65: 189–92.

Balinsky, W., and J. L. Starkman. (1987). The impact of DRGs on the health care industry. *Health Care Management Review* 12(3): 61–74.

Beauchamp, D. E. (1975). Public health: Alien ethic in a strange land? *American Journal of Public Health* 65: 1338–39.

Bergman, G. (1988). Standing alone: Why the U.S. has no national health system. *Grey Panther Network* 17(1): 13, 18.

Booth, R. (1985). Financing mechanisms for health care: Impact on nursing services. *Journal of Professional Nursing* 1(1): 34–40.

Davis, C. K. (1983). The federal role in changing health care financing. *Nursing Economics* 1(1): 10–17.

Dowling, W. L. (1979). Prospective rate setting: Concept and practice. *Topics in Health Care Financing* 3(2): 35–42.

Ehlinger, E. (1982). Implications of the competition model. *Nursing Outlook* 30: 518–21.

Ellwood, P. (1985). Alternative delivery systems: Health care on the move. *Journal of Ambulatory Care Management* 8(4): 1–2.

Fackelmann, K., and R. Sorian. (1987). Perspectives: Florida uproar shakes HMO movement. *McGraw-Hill's Medicine and Health,* May 4; 41(18), Suppl. 4.

Francis, S. (1988). U.S. industrial outlook 1988. *Medical Benefits: The Medical Economic Digest* 5(3): 1–2.

Gibson, R. M., K. R. Levit, H. Lazenby, and D. R. Waldo. (1984). National health care expenditures, 1983. *Health Care Financing Review* 6: 14.

Hanlon, J. J., and G. E. Pickett. (1984). *Public health: Administration and practice.* 8th ed. St. Louis: Times Mirror/Mosby.

Health: United States. (1985). DHEW Pub. No. (PHS) 86–1232. Washington, D.C.: Department of Health and Human Services, December 1985.

Hyman, H. (1982). *Health planning: A systematic approach.* 2nd ed. Rockville, Md.: Aspen Systems.

Joel, L. A. (1983). DRGs: The state of the art of reimbursement for nursing services. *Nursing and Health Care* 4: 560–63.

"Known welfare fraud is only the tip of the iceberg." (1983, November). *U.S. News & World Report:* 42–43.

Lewis, R. A. (1952). *Edwin Chadwick and the public health movement, 1832–1854.* New York: Longman's.

McNerney, W. J. (1980). Control of health care costs in the 1980s. *New England Journal of Medicine* 303: 1088–95.

Milio, N. (1984). Chains of impact from Reaganomics on primary care policies. *Public Health Nursing* 1(2): 65–73.

Rapoport, J., R. L. Robertson, and B. Stewart. (1982). *Understanding health economics.* Rockville, Md.: Aspen Systems.

Ray, D., and B. Flynn. (1980). Competition vs. cooperation in community health nursing. *Nursing Outlook* 28(10): 626–30.

Relman, A. S. (1987). The National Leadership Commission on Health Care. *The New England Journal of Medicine* 317(11): 706–7.

Roble, D. T., W. A. Knowlton, and G. A. Rosenberg. (1984). Hospital-sponsored Preferred Provider Organizations. *Law, Medicine Health Care* 12(5): 204–9.

Roemer, M. I. (1984). The value of medical care for health promotion. *American Journal of Public Health* 74: 243–48.

Semmel, H. (1987). Towards a national health program. *Health/PAC Bulletin* 17(5): 4–7.

Shaffer, F. (1983). DRGs: History and overview. *Nursing and Health Care* 4: 388–96.

Somers, A. R., and H. Somers. (1977). *Health and health care: Policies in perspective.* Germantown, Md.: Aspen Systems.

Somers, A. R. (1986). The changing demand for health services: A historical perspective and some thoughts for the future. *Inquiry* 23(4): 395–402.

Swartz, K. (1987). Workers needing insurance: Who are they? *Medical Benefits,* Sept. 30, 1987: 3–4.

A Washington Seminar Report. (1987). *For profit and nonprofit health care: Are the distinctions blurring?* Washington, D.C.: National Health Council, Inc.

Weiss, R. J. (1982). Competition in health care. *American Journal of Public Health* 72: 655.

World Health Organization. (1986). *Basic documents.* 36th ed. Geneva: WHO.

World Health Organization. (1988). *World Health Statistics Annual.* Geneva: WHO.

Selected Readings

Barger, S. G., D. G. Hinman, and H. R. Garland. (1985). *The PPO handbook.* Rockville, Md.: Aspen Systems.

Bergman, G. (1988). Standing alone: Why the U.S. has no national health system. *Grey Panther Network* 17(1): 13, 18.

Clark, E. J. (1981). The role of the states in the delivery of health services. *American Journal of Public Health* 71(Supp.): 59–69.

Davis, C. K. (1983). The federal role in changing health care financing. *Nursing Economics* 1(1): 10–17.

Ehlinger, E. (1982). Implications of the competition model. *Nursing Outlook* 30: 518–21.

Enthoven, A. C. (1978). Consumer-choice health plan: Inflation and inequity in health care today. Alternatives for cost control and an analysis of proposals for national health insurance. *New England Journal of Medicine* 298: 650–58.

Freeland, M., G. Calat, and C. Schendler. (1980). Projections of national health expenditures, 1980, 1985, and 1990. *Health Care Financing Review* 1(3): 17.

Fuchs, V. R. (1987). The counterrevolution in health care financing. *The New England Journal of Medicine* 316(18): 1154–56.

Ginzberg, E. (1987). A hard look at cost containment. *The New England Journal of Medicine* 316(18): 1151–54.

Hanlon, J. J., and G. E. Pickett. (1984). *Public health: Administration and practice.* 8th ed. St. Louis: Times Mirror/Mosby.

Hyman, H. (1982). *Health planning: A systematic approach.* 2nd ed. Rockville, Md.: Aspen Systems.

Jain, S. C. (1981). Introduction and summary: Role of state and local governments in relation to personal health services. *American Journal of Public Health* 71(Supp.): 5–8.

Joel, L. A. (1983). DRGs: The state of the art of reimbursement for nursing services. *Nursing and Health Care* 4: 560–63.

"Known welfare fraud is only the tip of the iceberg." (1983, November). *U.S. News & World Report:* 42–43.

Lewis, R. A. (1952). *Edwin Chadwick and the public health movement, 1832–1854.* New York: Longman's.

Luft, H. B. (1982). Health maintenance organizations and the rationing of medical care. *Milbank Memorial Fund Quarterly/Health and Society* 60: 268.

McNerney, W. J. (1980). Control of health care costs in the 1980s. *New England Journal of Medicine* 303: 1088–95.

Moran, D. W. (1982). HMOs, competition, and the politics of minimum benefits. *Milbank Memorial Fund Quarterly/Health and Society* 59: 190.

Morris, R. (1983). Will the growth of health and welfare services be resumed? *American Journal of Public Health* 73: 732–33.

Navarro, V. (1985). The public/private mix in funding and delivery of health services: An international survey. *American Journal of Public Health* 75(11): 1318–20.

Nutter, D. O. (1987). Medical indigency and the public health care crisis: The need for a definitive solution. *The New England Journal of Medicine* 316(18): 1156–58.

Powell, P. (1983). Fee-for-service. *Nursing Management* 14(3): 13–15.

Rapoport, J., R. L. Robertson, and B. Stewart. (1982). *Understanding health economics.* Rockville, Md.: Aspen Systems.

Ray, D., and B. Flynn. (1980). Competition vs. cooperation in community health nursing. *Nursing Outlook* 28(10): 626–30.

Relman, A. S. (1987). Practicing medicine in the new business climate. *The New England Journal of Medicine* 316(18): 1150–51.

Roemer, M. I. (1984). The value of medical care for health promotion. *American Journal of Public Health* 74: 243–48.

Shaffer, F. (1983). DRGs: History and overview. *Nursing and Health Care* 4: 388–96.

Somers, A. R. (1986). The changing demand for health services: A historical perspective and some thoughts for the future. *Inquiry* 23(4): 395–402.

Wasserman, P. (ed.). (1981). *Health organizations of the United States, Canada, and the world: A directory of voluntary associations, professional societies, and other groups concerned with health and related fields.* 5th ed. Detroit, Mich.: Gale Research.

Weiss, R. J. (1982). Competition in health care. *American Journal of Public Health* 72: 655.

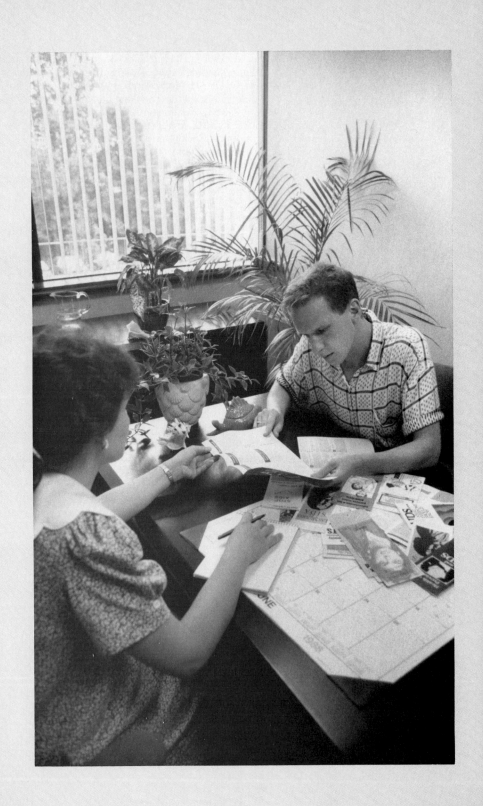

3 Community Health Nursing Foundations: Past and Present

Within the family of nursing specialties, community health nursing plays a unique and challenging role. Unlike other kinds of nursing, it focuses on promoting and protecting the health of populations, not just individuals. Operating within an environment of rapid change and increasingly complex challenges, this field of nursing holds the potential for positively shaping the quality of community health services and improving the general health of the public. In this chapter we examine the dynamic nature of community health nursing. After defining the field, we describe a conceptual framework for understanding community health nursing and explore the attributes of systems that form its theoretical base. Next, we trace the historical development of community health nursing and analyze several influential factors in its development. Finally, we discuss the major characteristics of contemporary community health nursing.

DEFINING COMMUNITY HEALTH NURSING

Any nursing specialty combines nursing theory with knowledge and skills germane to the specialty area (National League for Nursing, 1980). Community health nursing combines nursing with public health (American Nurses Association, 1980). It "synthesizes the body of knowledge from the public health sciences and professional nursing theories" (American Public Health Association, 1982). The purpose of this synthesis is to improve the health of the entire community. Thus, community health nursing can be defined as a field of practice that synthesizes knowledge and skills from nursing and public health and applies them toward the promotion of optimal health for the total community.

Contrary to one popular image, community health nursing does not serve only clients in the community (those outside the acute care setting). It is not a setting-based practice but a knowledge-based practice. As we shall see, nurses with other specialties have moved into the community, while some community health nurses work in hospitals. Community health nursing, or public health nursing (the terms are used synonymously in this text) makes its unique contribution to health care by the nature of its practice, which combines basic concepts from nursing and public health. Community health nursing is grounded in both public health science and nursing science, which makes its philosophical orientation unique. In the past it has been recognized as a subspecialty of both fields (Ruth and Partridge, 1978). That recognition continues today with an even clearer conception of the respective contributions made by the fields of public health and nursing to community health nursing practice (Hanchett and Clarke, 1988).

CONCEPTUAL FRAMEWORK FOR COMMUNITY HEALTH NURSING

Community health nursing combines theories, concepts, and principles to form the basis for its practice. A set of concepts can be integrated into a meaningful configuration called a conceptual framework, or model (Fawcett, 1984) that helps us interpret behaviors or situations. We shall summarize the concepts underlying community health nursing to evince a conceptual framework for understanding its nature and practice.

PRACTICE PRIORITIES

Three fundamental concepts underlie public health practice: prevention, protection, and promotion. *Prevention* includes activities aimed at avoiding the occurrence of illness or injury, such as enforcement of seat belt use, or at minimizing the effects of illness as much as possible, as with worker rehabilitation programs. *Protection* involves efforts to shield the public from harmful health effects of elements in the environment. These elements can range from obviously harmful physical agents, such as cigarette smoke or lead in furniture paint that may be ingested by teething toddlers, to less obvious agents, such as work stress and bereavement. *Promotion* refers to activities that maintain and enhance the community's level of wellness. These, too, cover a wide range, from such efforts as a community-wide parks improvement program to family planning. White describes these concepts as "practice priorities" (White, 1982, p. 528). They make up one aspect of community health nursing's distinctive emphasis, the long-range goal and priority of moving people ever nearer wellness on the wellness-illness continuum.

PRACTICE INTERVENTIONS

To accomplish the practice priorities, we can identify three categories of interventions: education, engineering, and enforcement (White, 1982). They provide varying degrees of "persuasion" for enhancing the accomplishment of public health goals. By *education* we mean the nursing actions of providing information to encourage people to voluntarily modify their behavior in health-promoting ways. Typical is encouraging proper diet and exercise. *Engineering* is a stronger form of persuasion. Nursing actions directly or indirectly manage the variables in the environment to reduce health risks. That is, specific actions are taken, such as immunization against disease, to prevent health problems. *Enforcement* uses more coercive measures, such as laws prohibiting child abuse or intake of harmful chemicals. Community health nursing employs all three interventions to protect the public, prevent illness or disability, and promote health. These varying levels of persuasion are discussed in Chapter 22 as three types of strategies for community health nursing management of change.

SCOPE OF PRACTICE

The extent of community health nursing's activity and influence still must be clarified. What does it encompass? We can understand the scope of community health nursing practice by answering the questions, "What is practiced?" and "For whom?" We have addressed the first question, "What?" as protection from health-endangering agents, prevention of illness and disability, and promotion of wellness. These practice priorities represent a trend, as we have seen in our historical review of community health nursing, away from a curative emphasis to a strong emphasis on the preventive and promotive end of the scale. The "For whom?" dimension covers a broad range from individuals to worldwide aggregates. Community health nursing, drawing on its public health foundations, maintains a conscious aggregate commitment. Wherever the nurse is engaged in practice along the individual-to-aggregate scale, the nurse still asks, "What populations are affected or at risk? What are their needs? How can those needs best be served?" For example, a community health nurse working with a day care center, when truly population focused, does not limit practice to the individuals in that center. Instead, the nurse considers the day care staff, its children, and their parents as three related population groups for assessment and intervention. Furthermore, the nurse with an aggregate orientation looks beyond the single day care center to clusters of day care centers in the community as potential populations for service. It is the goal of public health to reduce premature death, disease, disability, and discomfort and to protect, restore, and promote people's health for the good of the entire community (Institute of Medicine Committee, 1988).

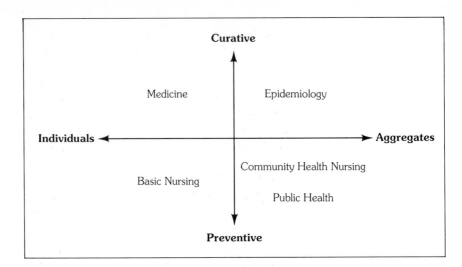

Figure 3-1
The scope of community
health nursing practice.

Figure 3-1 describes the scope of community health nursing practice on two axes. The horizontal axis shows the range from individuals to aggregates. The vertical axis exhibits the curative-preventive range. Placement of basic nursing, medicine, epidemiology, and public health — community health nursing in their respective quadrants evinces a clearer picture of the various disciplines' primary practice fields. Basic nursing and medicine both emphasize interventions at the individual end of the horizontal axis. Medicine is mostly curative; nursing emphasizes restorative and preventive services. Epidemiology, originally a branch of medicine, shifted its focus from acute disease to include chronic and disabling conditions and some preventive efforts. Its concern is always with aggregates. Public health and community health nursing emphasize aggregates and the promotion of high-level wellness.

HEALTH DETERMINANTS

We have discussed community health nursing's practice priorities, interventions, and scope. A further set of variables in our conceptual framework must be considered — the factors that influence health positively or negatively. Four contributing elements were identified by the Canadian government in 1974 and studied in the United States (Public Health Service, 1979). They form the basis for the health determinants in our conceptual framework (White, 1982). First are human biological factors, those physiological defenses and vulnerabilities that influence who is at risk. Second are environmental factors, any external agents or conditions (including economic ones) capable of enhancing or inhibiting health. Third are the adequacies and inadequacies of the health care system, the medical-technological-organizational determinants. Finally, there are psycho-socio-cultural factors, such as behaviors and life-styles, that influence health. Study of these variables suggests that the largest contributor to death in the United States (based on ten leading causes) is unhealthy behaviors or life-style (accounting for about 50 percent of deaths). The other determinants are environmental factors (20 percent), human biologic factors (20 percent), and inadequacies in the health care system (10 percent) (Public Health Service, 1979; Hanlon and Pickett, 1984).

COMMUNITY HEALTH NURSING DYNAMICS

Two dynamics, or driving forces, energize community health nursing practice. They are the nursing process and the valuing process (White, 1982).

The nursing process, which includes assessment, diagnosis, planning, implementation, and evaluation, provides the means for analyzing health needs and solving health problems. In Chapter 8 we explore the nursing process in greater depth as a tool for enhancing community health. Its application to community health problem solving and management of community health nursing practice can be seen throughout the book.

The valuing process, a second dynamic, guides community health nursing actions. To value something is to judge it worthy. What we value determines our priorities, commitments, and behavior. Public health holds to several significant values, some of which are discussed in Chapters 2 and 6. For example, public health subscribes to the greatest good for the greatest number, a concept that conflicts with our society's emphasis on individualism (Beauchamp, 1976). It bases its practice on collaboration and cooperation and believes in advocacy for the underserved and disadvantaged (Ehlinger, 1982). Values also influence consumers' attitudes and behaviors and dictate their responses to health care interventions. In Chapter 6 we examine values and health.

We now have the variables needed to describe the nature of community health nursing practice. Figure 3-2 exhibits them in a conceptual model that incorporates the practice priorities, interventions, scope, and health determinants with the nursing process and valuing dynamics.

SYSTEMS THEORY AND COMMUNITY HEALTH NURSING

Underlying the practice of community health nursing is a systems theory base. That is, systems theory, which is "the scientific exploration of wholes and wholeness" (von Bertanlanffy, 1968, p. 30), provides the foundation for understanding how communities function as living systems. A considerable body of literature treats systems theory in depth. Selected reference sources are listed at the close of this chapter.

A review of systems theory as it applies to community health nursing includes the following attributes. A *system* is "a whole which functions as a

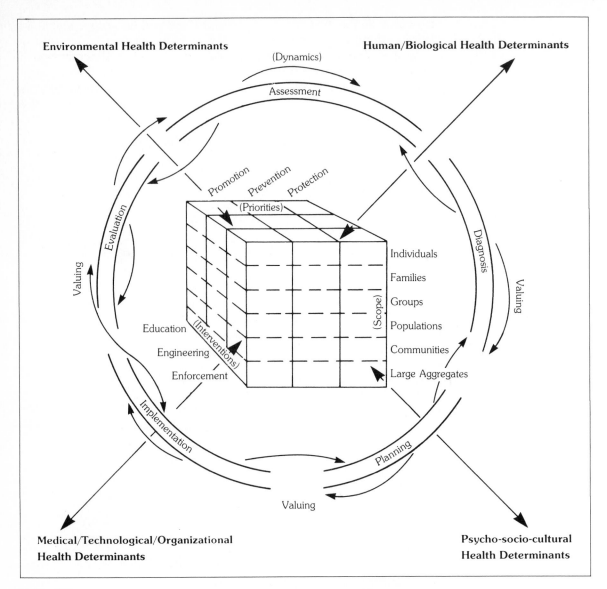

Figure 3-2
A conceptual model of
community health nursing
(adapted from White, 1982).

whole by virtue of the interdependence of its parts" (Buckley, 1968, p. xvii; Helvie, 1981, p. 6). In community health nursing the scope of practice addresses many sizes of systems, ranging from individuals and families to populations and larger aggregates. Each is a whole that functions as such by virtue of the relationships between its parts. Living systems, such as humans, animals, plants, or organizations, are known as *open systems* because they exchange matter, energy, and information with their environment. A *closed system,* such as a rock, does not have such an exchange and remains self-contained, isolated, and relatively unaffected by its environment. Community health nursing deals with systems that are open.

Open systems experience *hierarchical ordering* with other systems from simple to complex and from small to large. Such order is interlocking and interacting (Putt, 1978). For example, various human cells together make up larger systems such as the musculoskeletal or circulatory systems that, in turn, make up the body as a system. Similarly, people organize themselves into groups, such as the health system or the legal system, which are subunits of a larger community. Communities themselves are parts of larger systems in the same way that a school of fish is part of undersea life.

Living systems form *boundaries,* or lines of demarcation, that distinguish them from other systems and from their environment. Boundaries may be visible, such as human skin or a county line, or they may be understood, such as the composition of a group or community. A system's boundary serves as a means of identifying the system and acts as a filter for exchanging energies, in the form of materials or information, with its environment. Four sets of health determinants described in the community health nursing conceptual model form the environmental influences with which a community engages in this exchange. They are human biological factors, environmental factors, medical/technological/organizational factors, and psycho-socio-cultural factors. *Energy exchange* is a critical attribute of living systems, since the input-output phenomenon enables the system to function toward the purpose for which it exists. Energy exchange occurs at varying rates depending on the ability of the system to absorb energy from and release energy to its environment. Through energy absorption all living systems may potentially increase their order or complexity. The reverse is also true. A boundary may contract or expand depending on the system's goals and needs, thus establishing one of a system's functions, that of *boundary maintenance.* Systems need to monitor the input-output exchange with the environment to assure adequate functioning. A community, for example, may increase its health and social services as its population grows but may decrease these at a later date if emigration occurs. Community health nurses assess and seek to facilitate their client systems' ability to maintain their boundaries and engage in healthy exchanges with their environment.

All systems have *structure,* which may be described as the "arrangement of the component parts" (Putt, 1978, p. 2). The structure of a group, for instance, may consist of its leadership and a described set of followers. A community's structure is generally much more complex and consists of some kind of overall governance by an authority such as a president, governor, or mayor, coexisting with many subsystems, such as education or social services, that have their own internal structures. The parts of a system, sometimes called subparts or subsystems, are *interrelated* and interdependent and function together to maintain the whole. Thus, a change in one part can affect the operation of other parts or the total system. A change in one family member's life-style, such as unemployment, will likely affect the entire family system. Nurses, as change agents, seek to introduce many positive changes in community systems and need to understand the effects of these changes on system functioning. They also need to understand how to manage these changes most effectively. In Chapter 22, we will deal specifically with the community health nurse's role as an agent of change.

Systems may be stable or adaptive. As a system grows and learns, its ability to adapt increases. Too much flexibility, however, can lead to instability and disruption of functioning. Living systems need *quasi-equilibrium,* a relative steady state to which they return after adaptation. An example is the human body's return to normal temperature after a fever or a community's rebuilding after a devastating flood. To accomplish this adaptation, systems often employ a feedback loop for *self-correction.* That is, they retain some portion of the energy exchanged to enable them to adjust.

Although living systems may be very different from one another, they often share similar components. This attribute, known as *isomorphism* (Putt, 1978), enables nurses to use knowledge of one system as a basis for understanding another system. Community health nurses can generalize from their knowledge of the "universal traits" of individuals, families, and groups to increase their effectiveness in working with larger community systems.

NEUMAN'S HEALTH CARE SYSTEMS MODEL

Drawing on systems theory, Neuman has proposed a model for understanding and assisting clients (Neuman, 1980) that can enhance our use of the community health nursing conceptual framework just presented. (Our discussion of Neuman's model here is adapted to viewing clients as aggregates or population groups.) Neuman provides a holistic, or total system, view of clients receiving nursing care.

With the Neuman model, each client is seen as a whole system that is greater than the sum of its parts. Four sets of variables, or influences, make up each client's "whole." These are physiological, psychological, sociocultural, and developmental variables, similar to the health determinants presented in our conceptual framework. Given these variables, each client has a unique response to *stressors,* which are tension-producing stimuli that may potentially cause disequilibrium or illness.

A client's response to stressors is depicted as a series of concentric circles. In the center is a *core* of basic survival abilities, such as an individual's genetic responses and normal system functioning or a community's ability to make the best use of its natural resources. Surrounding the core are three boundaries. The first, or innermost, boundary is a set of flexible *lines of resistance.* These are the client's internal defense mechanisms against stress, such as an individual's immune response or a community's collective sense of responsibility. The second boundary is the *normal line of defense.* This describes the client's learned pattern for maintaining equilibrium over time, such as an individual's coping behaviors and adaptive life-style or a community's development of police and fire-fighting systems. The third boundary is a dynamic outer ring called the *flexible line of defense,* a protective buffer that prevents stressors from invading the normal line of defense. Examples of this boundary are adequate sleep and nutrition for an individual or regular maintenance of roads and support of schools within a community.

Neuman's model describes stressors as originating from a two-part environment. One part is the client's internal environment, where factors within the client become stressors. Examples of these *intrapersonal stressors* might be age level, maladaptive responses, or poor system maintenance. The second part of the environment, or external environment, produces two types of stressors. One is *interpersonal stressors* arising from interaction with other people or systems. For a population group, these might include such factors as stressful intergroup relationships, inadequate support systems, or maladaptive cultural patterns. The second type of stressor originating within the external environment is *extrapersonal stressors* which arise from the environment itself, such as economic problems, tornado damage, or a nuclear spill.

Neuman describes people as open systems who constantly interact with their environment, both influencing and being influenced by it. People respond to environmental stressors by either adapting themselves to the environment or changing the environment to meet their needs. People are healthy, according to Neuman (1982), when they have achieved a state of harmony between themselves and their environment—when they have successfully adapted to or changed their environment to meet their needs.

Nursing interventions in this model focus on assisting clients to remain stable within their environment (Neuman, 1983). Corresponding to our conceptual framework, nursing's goals include (1) *prevention:* helping clients to remove or minimize environmental stressors; (2) *health promotion:* strengthening clients' defenses; and (3) *protection:* promoting recovery (stability) when clients have responded to a stressor.

An adaptation of Neuman's model (Ross and Helmer, 1988) provides a useful means for applying the nursing process to population-focused practice. The community health nurse assesses and collects data on the population's perception of its situation. What are the perceived stressors impinging on their health and what are the population's reactions and lines of defense against the stressors? The nurse identifies her or his own perceptions of the stressors and then interprets and summarizes all the data in terms of their interpersonal, intrapersonal, and extrapersonal dimensions. Next, the nurse organizes the data into categories of influence: —physiological, psychological, sociocultural, and developmental. Using our conceptual framework, we would incorporate all four health determinants (biological, psycho-socio-cultural, medical/technological/organizational, and environmental) into this data categorization. The nursing diagnosis clarifies the differences in perception between the client population and the nurse and, based on the diagnosis, the nurse works collaboratively with other health professionals to design a care plan. Throughout the design, implementation, and evaluation of the plan, the nurse seeks to reduce the effect of stressors through primary, secondary, and tertiary prevention.

HISTORICAL DEVELOPMENT OF COMMUNITY HEALTH NURSING

Community health nursing as practiced today is the product of growth and adaptation. It has amended its structure to accommodate the needs of a changing society, yet it has always maintained its initial goal of improved community health. Its development, which has been influenced by changes in nursing, public health, and society, can be traced through several stages. In this section we examine these stages and their societal causes.

STAGES OF DEVELOPMENT

The history of public health nursing in the United States encompasses continuing change and adaptation (Frachel, 1988). The historical record reveals a professional nursing specialty that has been on the cutting edge of innovations in public health practice and has provided leadership to public health efforts. William Welch has been quoted as saying, "America's two greatest contributions to public health were the Panama Canal and the public health nurse" (cited in Hanlon and Pickett, 1984, p. 533).

We can identify three general stages in the development of community health nursing: (1) the district nursing stage, (2) the public health nursing stage, and (3) the community health nursing stage.

District Nursing (1860–1900)

Organized home nursing care started as a voluntary service for the poor. In 1859, William Rathbone, an English philanthropist, became convinced of the value of home nursing as a result of private care given to his wife (Kalisch and Kalisch, 1986). He was the first to promote the establishment of a visiting nurse service for the sick poor in Liverpool. In the United States, the first community health nurse, Frances Root, pioneered home visits to the poor in New York City. Immediately following this, the first visiting nurses were employed by the New York City Mission in 1877. In 1885, district nursing associations were founded in Buffalo and, in 1886, in Boston and Philadelphia. These district associations served the sick poor exclusively, because patients with enough money had private home nursing care. Before the establishment of district nursing, care of the sick poor had fallen to various religious and charitable groups that delivered sporadic and limited health care.

Although district nurses primarily cared for the sick, they also taught cleanliness and wholesome living to their patients, even in that early period. Florence Nightingale, who assisted William Rathbone by training home visiting nurses, referred to them as health nurses. Her ideas and methods helped influence home nursing practice in England and the United States. The work of district nurses focused almost exclusively on the care of individuals. District nurses recorded temperatures and pulse rates and gave simple treatments under the immediate direction of a physician. They also instructed family members in personal hygiene, healthful living habits, and the care of the sick (Figure 3-3). Nursing educational programs at that time did not truly prepare nurses for these functions.

The early district nursing services were formed by voluntary organizations. Funding came from contributions and, in some instances, from fees charged to patients on an ability-to-pay basis. The nursing services were administered by lay boards; even the actual nursing care was supervised by lay persons. In 1893, Lillian Wald initiated a district nursing service in New York City that, in contrast, provided nursing care under the supervision of nurses.

Figure 3-3
Examination of infants was part of early health department programs in which district nurses played a major role.

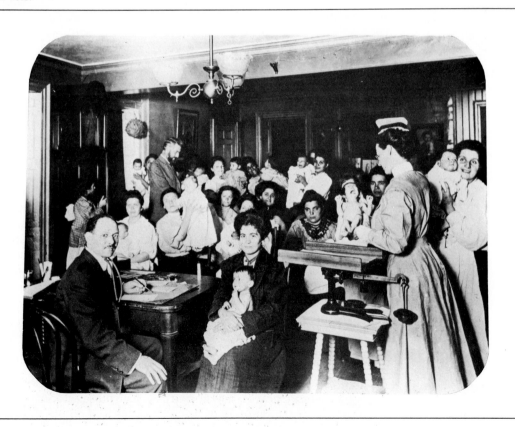

Her service was associated administratively with the health department, an official agency, although most district nursing services at that time remained voluntary.

Public Health Nursing (1900–1970)

By the turn of the century, district nursing began to broaden its focus to include the health and welfare of the general public, not just the poor. This new emphasis was part of a broader consciousness about public health. A growing sense of urgency about improving the health of all people led to an increase in the number of voluntary health agencies. These agencies supplemented the often ineffective work of government health departments. Specialized programs such as infant welfare, tuberculosis clinics, and venereal disease control were developed, causing a demand for nurses in establishments that included factories and schools. In 1902, the first school nurse in the United States was employed by the New York City Board of Education. By 1910, new federal laws made states and communities accountable for the health of their citizens.

The role of the district nurse expanded during this stage. Lillian Wald, a leading figure in this expansion, was the first to use the term *public health nursing* (Bullough and Bullough, 1979). District nursing had pioneered in health teaching (Brainard, 1922, p. 208), disease prevention, and promotion of good health practices. Now, with a growing recognition of familial and environmental influences on health, public health nurses broadened their practive even more. Nurses working outside the hospital setting increased their knowledge and skills in specialized areas such as tuberculosis, school health, and mental disorders.

Next, the family began to emerge as the unit of service. The multiple problems faced by many families started the trend toward nursing care generalized enough to meet a diversity of needs and provide continuity of care. By the 1920s public health nursing was acquiring more professional stature, in contrast to its earlier linkage with charity. It assumed greater leadership in improving and expanding health services and in increasing the standards of nursing education and practice. Public health nurses gradually gained more autonomy in such areas as bedside care and instruction of good health practices to families and community groups. Their collaborative relationships with other community health groups grew as the need to avoid gaps and duplication of services became apparent. Public health nurses also started to keep better records of their caregiving.

During this stage, the institutional base for public health nursing shifted to the government. Public health nursing services, which emphasized health guidance but also provided care for the ill, were offered through local health departments. As a result, rural public health nursing also expanded. Some of the district nursing services, now known as visiting nurse associations (VNAs), remained under the direction of voluntary agencies and offered their own nursing services of bedside care. In some places, city or county health departments joined administratively and financially with VNAs to provide a combination of services, such as bedside care and health guidance, to families.

The public health nursing stage was characterized by service to the public, although the family was recognized as a primary unit of care (Figure 3-4). Official health agencies, which placed greater emphasis on disease prevention and health promotion, provided the chief institutional base.

Community Health Nursing (1970–Present)

The emergence of the title *community health nursing* heralded a new era, as the strengths of traditional public health nursing combined with a new consciousness of service to communities or populations. By the mid-1960s a number of events had occurred to cause concern about the nature of public health nursing.

First, nursing education, recognizing the importance of public health content, began to require course work in public health for all baccalaureate graduates. This prerequisite meant that graduates were expected to incorporate public health principles such as health promotion and disease prevention into

Figure 3-4
The public health nurse, carrying her bag of equipment and supplies, made regular home visits to provide physical and psychological care as well as health teaching to families.

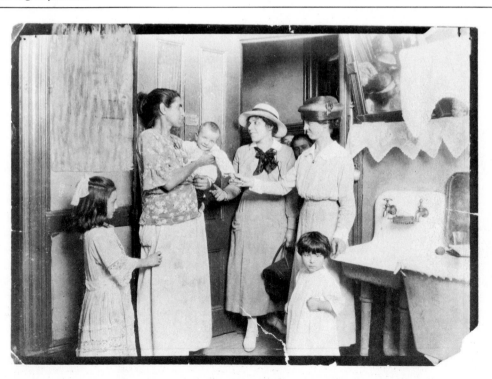

nursing practice, regardless of their sphere of service. Consequently, some people questioned whether public health nursing retained any unique content.

A second source of confusion over the definition of community health nursing arose from the fact that hospital nurses followed community cases and public health nurses followed hospital cases. Hospital walls seemed permeable, for community health nurses were not the only nurses practicing in the community.

Third, many new kinds of community health services appeared, and demands on community health nurses expanded their role. Furthermore, other community health professionals assumed responsibilities that had traditionally been the domain of public health nursing. Some school counselors in Oregon, for example, began coordinating home visits previously done by school nurses, and health educators, who are part of a discipline that has developed in the last decade, took over large segments of client education (Chavigny and Kroske, 1983). Social workers, too, provided services that appeared to overlap with community health nursing roles. Health educators, counselors, social workers, and others working in community health came prepared with different backgrounds and emphases in their practice. Their contributions were and still are important. Their presence, however, forced community health nurses to reexamine their own contribution to the public's health and incorporate stronger interdisciplinary and collaborative approaches into their practice. These developments raised several important questions. Should community health nursing, which had become generalized in practice, carve out a new specialization? Should it incorporate more specialized skills, such as physical assessment, into its generalized practice?

Fourth, accelerated changes in health care provision, technology, and social issues made increasing demands on community health nurses' ability to adapt to new patterns of practice. By the mid-1970s various community health nursing leaders had identified knowledge and skills needed for more effective community health nursing practice (Roberts and Freeman, 1973); this information had only begun to be incorporated in nursing school curricula.

Still, the direction in which community health nursing was moving had become clear—to care for, not simply in, the community (Freeman, 1973). Its primary responsibility was the health of aggregates (Williams, 1977); thus, its focus turned to more comprehensive community health care and diversity of programs. This shift made the term *community health nursing* more functional than the term *public health nursing;* in this text, however, we use the two interchangeably. Community health nursing meant population-oriented nursing of problems along the entire range of the wellness-illness continuum, although health promotion was increasingly emphasized. Community health nurses were carving out new roles for themselves, including independent practice. Collaboration and interdisciplinary teamwork were recognized as crucial to effective community nursing. Practitioners served in many kinds of agencies and institutions, such as senior citizen centers, ambulatory services,

Table 3-1
Development of Community Health Nursing

Stages	Focus	Nursing Orientation	Service Emphasis	Institutional Base (Agencies)
District nursing (1860–1900)	Sick poor	Individuals	Curative; beginning of preventive	Voluntary; some government
Public health nursing (1900–1970)	Needy public	Families	Curative: preventive	Government; some voluntary
Emergence of community health nursing (1970–present)	Total community	Populations	Health promotion; illness prevention	Many kinds: some independent practice

mental health clinics, and family planning programs, as well as in many other settings; they followed clients before, during, and after hospitalization. Documentation of nursing care, program evaluation, agency accreditation, peer review, and definitive community nursing research became high priorities. This field of nursing had begun to assume its responsibility as a full professional partner in community health.

Table 3-1 summarizes the most important changes that have occurred during community health nursing's three stages of development. It shows these changes in terms of focus, nursing orientation, service emphasis, and institutional base.

SOCIETAL INFLUENCES

Many factors influenced the growth of community health nursing. To understand better the nature of this field, we must recognize the forces that began and continue to shape its development. Six are particularly significant: advanced technology, progress in causal thinking, changes in education, the changing role of women, the consumer movement, and economic factors.

Advanced Technology

Advanced technology has contributed in many ways to shaping the practice of community health nursing. For example, technological innovation has greatly improved health care, nutrition, and life-style and caused a concomitant increase in life expectancy. Consequently, community health nurses direct much of their effort toward meeting the needs of older persons and working with chronic conditions. Advanced technology has also been a strong force behind industrialization, large-scale employment, and urbanization. We are now primarily an urban society; health planners project that 75 percent of the world's population will live in urban areas by the year 2000 (United Nations, 1987). Population density leads to many health-related problems, particularly the spread of disease and increased stress. Community health nurses are learning how to combat these urban health problems. In addition, changes in transportation and high job mobility have affected the health scene. As people travel and relocate, they are separated from families and traditional support systems; community health nurses frequently help people cope with the accompanying stress. New products, equipment, methods, and energy sources in industry have also increased environmental pollution and industrial hazards. Community health nurses have become involved in related research, occupational health, and preventive education. Technological innovation has helped promote medicine's complex diagnostic and treatment procedures, thus making illness-oriented care more dramatic and desirable, as well as more costly. Community health nurses face a challenge to demonstrate the physical and economic value of wellness-oriented care.

Finally, innovations in communications and computer technology have shifted America from an industrial society to an "information society" (Naisbitt, 1982). Our economy is now built on information — the production and marketing of knowledge. Community health nurses, now more than ever, are in the business of information distribution and use new computer technologies to enhance the efficiency and effectiveness of their services. Associated with high use of technology, societal needs for "high touch" (greater human contact), stress management, and treatments for other technology-induced health problems will continue to shape the role of community health nursing in the future (Powell, 1984).

Progress in Causal Thinking

Progress in causal thinking in the health sciences, particularly in epidemiology, has significantly affected the nature of community health nursing, (Turner and Chavigny, 1988). The germ theory of disease causation, established in the late 1800s, was the first real breakthrough in control of communicable disease. Nurses incorporated the teaching of cleanliness and personal hygiene into basic nursing care. A second advance in causal thinking was initiated by the tripartite view that called attention to the interactions between a causative agent, a susceptible host, and the environment. This information offered community health nursing new ways to control and prevent health disorders. For example, nurses could decrease the vulnerability of an individual (host) by teaching the person a healthier life-style. They could instigate measles vaccination programs as a means of preventing the organism (agent) from infecting children. They could promote proper disinfection of a school's swimming pool (environment) to prevent disease. Further progress in causal thinking led to the recognition that not just one single agent but many factors — a multiple causation approach — contribute to a disease or health disorder. A food poisoning outbreak that is associated with a restaurant might be caused not only by the salmonella organism but also by improper food handling and storage, lack of adherence to minimum food preparation standards, and lack of adequate health department supervision and enforcement.

Community health nurses can control health problems by examining all possible causes and then attacking strategic causal points. Current causal thinking has led to a broader awareness of unhealthy conditions; in addition to disease, problems such as accidents and environmental pollution are major targets of concern. As a result, work-related stress, environmental hazards, chemical food additives, and alcohol and nicotine consumption during pregnancy are all examples of concerns in community health nursing practice. Nursing's contribution to public health adds a further application of causal thinking. That is, nursing seeks to identify and implement the causes, or contributing factors, of wellness. Community health nurses do more than prevent illness; they seek to promote health. By conducting research and applying research findings, community health nurses promote health-enhancing behaviors, including healthier life-style practices such as eating low-fat diets, exercising, and maintaining social support systems.

Changes in Education

Changes in education, especially those in nursing education, have had an important influence on community health nursing practice. Education, once an opportunity for a privileged few, has become widely available; it is now considered a basic right and a necessity for a vital society. When people's understanding of their environment grows, an increased understanding of health is usually involved. For the community health nurse, health teaching has steadily assumed greater importance in practice. For the learner, education has led to much more responsibility. As a result, people feel that they have a right to know and question the reasons behind the care they receive. Community health nurses have had to shift from planning *for* clients to collaborating *with* clients.

Education has had other effects. The scientific approach, considered basic to progress, has created a dramatic increase in knowledge. The wealth of information relevant to community health nursing practice means that nursing students have more content to assimilate, and practicing community health nurses have to make greater efforts to keep abreast. In contrast to earlier times when nurses were trained to work as apprentices in hospitals or health agencies and perfunctorily follow orders, today's educational programs, including many in continuing education, prepare nurses to think for themselves in the application of theory to practice. Community health nursing has always required a fair measure of independent thinking and self-reliance; now community health nurses need skills in such areas as family and community assessment, policy making, political advocacy, research, management, and collaborative functioning. As the result of expanding education, community health nurses have had to reexamine their practice and clarify their roles.

Changing Role of Women

The changing role of women has profoundly affected community health nursing. In the past century, the women's rights movement has made considerable progress. Women have achieved the right to vote and have gained greater economic independence by entering the labor force. Women today have more education and consequently more influence than did women of the past. The percentage of women in professions such as medicine (17.6 percent), law (18.1 percent), and engineering (6 percent) has increased, although it is proportionately smaller than that of men (Bureau of Labor Statistics, 1987). Many women are managing the dual careers of job and family. These gains have decreased the number of women entering nursing, a profession whose responsibilities and recognition have improved but whose ability to compete with higher-paying and higher-status careers remains a problem.

Changes resulting from the women's rights movement continue to occur. Nurses still struggle for equality — equality of job selection, equal pay for equal work, and equal opportunity for advancement in the health field. If community health nurses are to influence the field of community health, they need status and authority equal to that of their colleagues. This step will require nurses to demonstrate their competence and learn to be assertive in assuming roles as full professional partners. In community health, as in society generally, women hold fewer administrative (39 percent) or policy-making positions than men do (Bureau of Labor Statistics, 1989). Although the majority of nurses are female, a higher proportion of male than female nurses serve in leadership capacities. This may be influenced by a larger proportion of women in nursing having less than full-time careers (Christman, 1988). The women's movement has contributed to community health nursing's gains in assuming leadership roles, but a need for much greater influence and involvement remains.

Consumer Movement

The consumer movement has also affected the nature of community health nursing. Consumers have become more militant, as evidenced in various boycotts and tax revolts. They are demanding their rights in many areas, including health care, regardless of sex, race, color, or socioeconomic level. Consumers now assert their right to be informed about and to participate in decisions that affect them. This movement has stimulated some basic changes in the philosophy of community health nursing. Health care consumers are viewed as active members of the health team, rather than as passive recipients of care. They may contract with the community health nurse for personal or family care, represent the community on the local health board, or act as ombudsmen: for example, to investigate complaints and report findings in order to protect the quality of care in a local nursing home.

This assumption of consumers' responsibility for their own health means that the community health nurse supplements, more often than supervises, clients' care.

The consumer movement also has contributed to increased concern for the quality of health services. Quality assurance programs, peer review, and tighter evaluation are now part of most health care accreditation requirements. Community health nursing has been led to improve its evaluation of services and programs. Many community health nursing agencies have begun to implement forms of peer review. In Chapter 23 we discuss these changes in greater detail.

The consumer movement has increased the demand for more humane, personalized health care. Dissatisfied with fragmented services offered by impersonal health workers, consumers now seek holistic care. A group of senior citizens living in a high-rise apartment building need more than a series of social workers, nutritionists, recreational therapists, nurses, and other callers ascertaining a variety of specific needs and starting a proliferation of programs. Community health nurses, as members of the health team, increasingly aim to provide coordinated, comprehensive, and personalized services—a case management approach.

Economic Forces

Various economic forces have affected community health nursing practice. Among these are changing health care financing patterns (including prospective payment and DRGs), decreased federal subsidy of public health programs, pressures for cost containment in health care, and increased competition among providers of health services. Each of these factors has significantly influenced the nature and delivery of community health nursing services and has been discussed in detail in Chapter 2.

Global economic forces also influence community health nursing practice. As the United States experiences increasing interdependence with foreign countries for trade, investments, and production of goods, we see growing population mobility and increased immigration, particularly among Hispanic and Asian populations. Under these conditions, the spread of AIDS poses a serious threat, as do problems associated with unemployment and poverty. The fastest growing sector of the job market is in technical areas that require new or retrained workers, and these jobs are frequently accompanied by high-tech and stress-related health problems.

Community health nursing has responded to economic forces in several ways. One is by assuming new roles, such as health educators in industry or case managers for Alternative Care or other government-sponsored programs for the elderly. Another is by directly competing with other community health service providers, particularly in such areas as ambulatory care or home care. Still another is by developing new programs and service emphases such as elder day care and respite care, in response to changing community needs created by economic forces. Yet another community health nursing response has been to develop new revenue-generating services, such as workplace wellness or health screening programs, to augment depleted budgets.

Economic factors continue to play a significant role in shaping community health nursing practice. Limited dollars for health promotion services and increased demands for home care have drawn some public health agencies into more illness-oriented than wellness-oriented services. Yet community health nurses continue to be resourceful in finding ways to foster the community's optimal health while adapting to changing economic conditions.

CHARACTERISTICS OF COMMUNITY HEALTH NURSING

Thus far in this chapter we have defined community health nursing and examined events and influences that have shaped its present practice. Now we will observe more closely the nature of community health nursing. Six characteristics of community health nursing are especially salient: (1) it is a field of nursing; (2) it combines public health with nursing; (3) it is population-oriented; (4) it emphasizes wellness; (5) it involves interdisciplinary collaboration; and (6) it promotes client responsibility and self-care.

FIELD OF NURSING

Community health nursing is a field of nursing; its basic knowledge and skills are those of professional nursing practice. It seeks to give humanistic, accessible, and holistic care. For instance, community health nurses are nursing when they express concern for a group of mothers and tired children sitting on hard chairs for three hours in a clinic hallway, or when they consequently change the appointment scheduling policy and establish a comfortable waiting area. They engage in nursing when they institute a discharge planning system with local hospitals to provide continuity of care. When they visit older clients in their homes to give personal care, instruction, and comfort, they are again nursing.

Community health nursing is a nursing specialty; nursing theory forms its foundation and the nursing process is one of its basic tools, but community health nursing synthesizes concepts, knowledge, and skills from public health to become a distinctive practice (Hanchett and Clarke, 1988).

ELEMENTS OF PUBLIC HEALTH

Knowledge of the following elements of public health is essential to community health nursing (Hanlon and Pickett, 1984; White, 1982; Williams, 1977, 1983):

1. The history and philosophy of public health, including the emphasis on the greatest good for the greatest number
2. The concept of aggregates — assessing needs, planning and providing services, and evaluating services' impact on population groups — including aggregate-level decision making
3. Priority of preventive and health-promoting strategies over curative strategies
4. The means for measurement and analysis of community health problems, including epidemiologic concepts and biostatistics
5. Influence of environmental factors on aggregate health
6. Principles underlying management and organization for community health, since the goal of public health is accomplished through organized community efforts
7. Public policy analysis and development

There are many ways in which community health nursing incorporates public health knowledge into its practice. For example, prior to immunization laws, some school nurses who were working with Cincinnati city health authorities were concerned with the failure of many children to receive adequate immunization. They used health statistics, specifically a review of school immunization records, to determine immunization needs of schoolchildren. Next, they set up an immunization program that successfully met the needs of the community (Anthony, Reed, Leff, Huffer, and Stephens, 1977). They effectively combined biostatistics with a community focus to carry out their goals.

Another group of community health nurses designed an experimental study to test the effectiveness of breast self-examination (BSE) instruction given to healthy women in their community (Shamian and Edgar, 1987). They tested the women's knowledge of the signs and symptoms of breast cancer and how to do BSE. They also examined how frequently these women did BSE. After they obtained this information the women received a BSE education session. Findings obtained after the educational program indicated that education provided by the nurses positively influenced the women's knowledge base and frequency of BSE practice. This epidemiologic study combined public health and nursing practice to show that nurses can be agents for change in community health.

As community health nurses carefully analyze their caseloads, assess group and community needs, establish priorities, and plan, implement, and evaluate services, they are utilizing public health management and organizational principles. For example, one community health nurse discovered a concern in the community whose needs she was assessing about the high incidence of dental decay among its schoolchildren. Because of the relationships she had already established within the community, she was able to help form a committee that studied the problem and initiated in one school a pilot dental health program that was to be evaluated a year later. She then continued to assist this committee in its efforts (Flynn, Gottschalk, Ray, and Selmanoff, 1978).

Each of the nurses mentioned here has demonstrated an important characteristic of community health nursing—the combination of fundamental public health concepts and nursing.

POPULATION EMPHASIS

The central mission of public health practice is to improve the health of population groups (Last, 1987). Community health nursing shares this essential feature: it is population-oriented, concerned with the personal and environmental health of population groups. A population may consist of a community health nurse's caseload or all the patients in a clinic. It may be a scattered group with common characteristics, such as people at high risk of developing coronary heart disease, or all the unwed mothers in a county. It may include all the people living in a district, census tract, city, or nation. In fact, the terms *population* and *community* (as defined in Chapter 1) can be used interchangeably.

Working with individuals and families as parts of aggregates is also common in community health nursing; however, such work must incorporate a population-oriented focus, a feature that distinguishes it from other nursing specialties. The difference is in orientation. Basic nursing focuses on individuals, and community health nursing focuses on aggregates (Williams, 1977; Hanchett and Clarke, 1988), but the many variations in client needs and nursing roles inevitably cause some overlap. Figure 3-5 shows these distinctions between basic and community health nursing.

Figure 3-5
Difference in client focus between basic nursing and community health nursing.

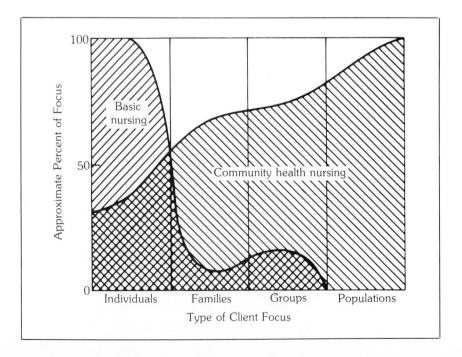

A population-oriented focus requires the observation of relationships. When working with individuals, families, or groups, the community health nurse does not consider them separately but rather in relationship to the rest of the community. When a case of hepatitis is diagnosed, for example, the community health nurse does more than simply treat it. The nurse tries to stop spread of the infection, locate the possible source, and prevent its recurrence in the community. As a result of their population-oriented focus, community health nurses seek to discover possible groups with a common health need, such as expectant mothers, or groups at high risk of developing a common health problem, such as potential diabetics or child abuse victims. Community health nurses continually look for ways to increase environmental quality. They work to prevent health problems by measures such as promoting safety in school playgrounds or offering more nourishing, easily prepared meals for nursing home residents. A population-oriented focus involves a whole new outlook and set of attitudes. The community is the client; service is provided to multiple and overlapping groups.

WELLNESS EMPHASIS

Another distinguishing characteristic of community health nursing is its emphasis on positive health, or wellness (Hanchett and Clarke, 1988). In Chapter 1 we discussed the wellness-illness continuum. Acute care nursing and medicine deal primarily with the illness end of that continuum because they treat health problems. In contrast, community health nursing has a primary charge to prevent health problems from occurring and to promote a higher level of health. For example, although a community health nurse may assist a woman at home with postpartum fatigue and depression, the nurse also works to *prevent* such problems among other mothers by engaging in health teaching, establishing prenatal classes, and encouraging proper rest, nutrition, adequate help, and stress reduction (see Figure 3-6). Individualized care is important, but prevention of aggregate problems in community health practice reflects more accurately its philosophy and benefits a larger number of people.

Community health nurses concentrate on the wellness end of the wellness-illness continuum in a variety of ways. They teach proper nutrition or family planning, demonstrate aseptic technique for home care of a wound, encourage regular physical and dental checkups, start exercise classes or physical fitness programs, and promote healthy interpersonal relationships. Their goal is to help the community reach its optimal level of wellness.

This emphasis on wellness changes the community health nursing role from a reactive to a proactive stance. It places a greater responsibility on community health nurses to find opportunities for intervention. In clinical nursing and medicine, the patients seek out professional assistance because they have health problems. As Williams (1977) puts it, "Patients select themselves into the care system, and the providers' role is to deal with what the patients bring to them." Community health nurses, in contrast, seek out poten-

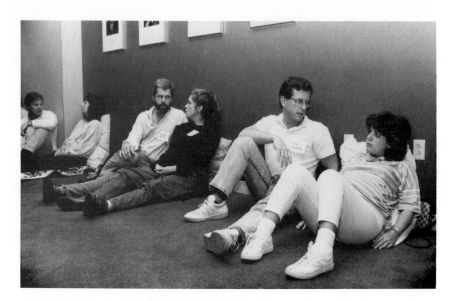

Figure 3-6
This prenatal class offers couples an opportunity to prepare physically and emotionally for delivery and their new roles as parents.

tial health problems. They identify high-risk groups and institute preventive programs. They watch for early signs of child neglect or abuse and intervene when any occur, often long before a request for help is made. They look for possible environmental hazards in the community, such as smoking in public places, and work with appropriate authorities to correct them. A wellness emphasis requires taking initiative and making sound judgments, which are characteristics of an *effective community health nurse.*

INTERDISCIPLINARY COLLABORATION

Community health nurses work as full members of a health care team. Such coordination and cooperation are required in a practice that deals with population groups. Individualized efforts and specialized programs, when planned in isolation, can lead to fragmentation and gaps in health services. For example, without collaboration, a well-child clinic may be started in a community that already has a strong early and periodic developmental screening and testing program; at the same time, community prenatal services may be nonexistent. Interdisciplinary collaboration is also important in individualized practice, since nurses need to plan with the physician, social worker, physical therapist, or other involved health professional and keep them informed of clients' health status; however, it is an even greater necessity in working with population groups.

Effective collaboration requires team members who are strong individuals. A variety of expertise and ideas, together with a commitment to team goals, leads to the best solutions. Community health nurses who think and act independently make a great contribution to the team effort. In appropriate situations, community health nurses function autonomously, making independent judgments. They also function interdependently, working with members of other disciplines on community advisory boards or health planning committees, for example.

Interdisciplinary collaboration requires clarification of each team member's role, a primary reason for community health nurses to understand the nature of their practice. When planning a city-wide immunization program with a community group, for example, community health nurses can explain the ways they might contribute to the program's objectives. They can offer to contact key lay individuals, with whom they have established relationships, in order to help influence community acceptance of the program. They can share their knowledge of the public's preference about times and locations to offer the program. They can help organize and give the immunizations, and they can influence planning for follow-up and continuity of care.

CLIENT RESPONSIBILITY

A characteristic of community health nursing that is sometimes overlooked is the encouragement of client responsibility in health care. Our examination of the consumer movement discussed consumers' rights to health care and to involvement in health care's decision making. However, consumers are frequently intimidated by health professionals and uninformed about health and health care. They do not know what information to ask for and are hesitant to act assertively. For example, a woman brought her two-year-old son, who had symptoms resembling those of scurvy, to a clinic. Recognizing a vitamin C deficiency, the physician told her to feed the boy large quantities of orange juice but gave no explanation. Several weeks later, she returned; the child was much worse. After questioning her, the nurse discovered that the mother had been feeding the child large amounts of an orange soft drink, not knowing the difference between that and orange juice. Obviously, the quality of care is affected when the consumer does not understand and cannot participate in the health care process.

PARTICIPATION

The goal of public health, "to protect, promote, and restore people's health" (Institute of Medicine Committee, 1988), requires a partnership effort. Just as learning cannot take place in schools without student participation, the goals of public health cannot be realized without consumer participation. Community health nursing's efforts toward health improvement can go only so far. Clients' health status and health behavior will not change unless they accept and apply community health nurses' proposals.

Community health nurses can encourage clients' participation by promoting clients' autonomy, rather than letting clients become too dependent on them. For example, an elderly couple had been receiving three visits a week from a community health nurse for assistance with the wife's surgical dressing changes and baths. During the visits the nurse taught the husband how to perform these procedures. She also showed him how to prepare simple, nutritious meals, and together they arranged with a Meals on Wheels service to bring the couple's dinners for a few weeks. She encouraged them to contact other community resources for assistance with shopping, housework, and transportation to the doctor's office. She reduced her visits to once a week, then to once a month, and, when the couple agreed that they were able to manage on their own, the relationship ended. Independence and feelings of self-worth are closely related. By treating people as independent adults, with trust and respect, community health nurses help promote self-reliance and the ability to function independently.

Self-Care

Community health nurses encourage clients to take responsibility for their own health. When consumers feel that their health and that of the community are their own responsibility, not that of health professionals, they will take a much more active interest in promoting it (Watkin, 1978). The process of taking responsibility for developing one's own health potential is called *self-care* (Levin, 1978; Norris, 1979; Goeppinger, 1982), a concept that has gained considerable prominence in recent years. As people maintain their own life, health, and well-being they are engaging in self-care (Figure 3-7). Some examples of self-care activities at the aggregate level are building safe playgrounds, developing teen employment opportunities, and providing senior exercise programs. When people's ability to continue self-care activities drops below their need, they experience a self-care deficit. At this point nursing may appropriately intervene. However, nursing's goal is to assist clients to return to or reach a level of functioning where they can attain optimal health and assume responsibility for maintaining it (Orem, 1985). To this end, community health nurses foster self-care by treating clients as adults capable of managing their own affairs, not, as Norris puts it, "as weak, needy, unintelligent, . . . bad, irresponsible children" (1979, p. 486). Nurses can encourage their clients to negotiate health care goals and practices, make their own appointments, contact their own resources (such as support groups or transportation services), identify and implement life-style changes that promote wellness, and learn ways to monitor their own health.

Consumer participation is promoted when clients serve as partners on the health care team. The goal of community health nurses is collaborating with clients rather than working for clients. As consumers are treated with respect and trust and, as a result, gain confidence and skill in self-care—promoting their own health and that of their community—their contribution to health care services will become increasingly valuable. The consumer perspective in

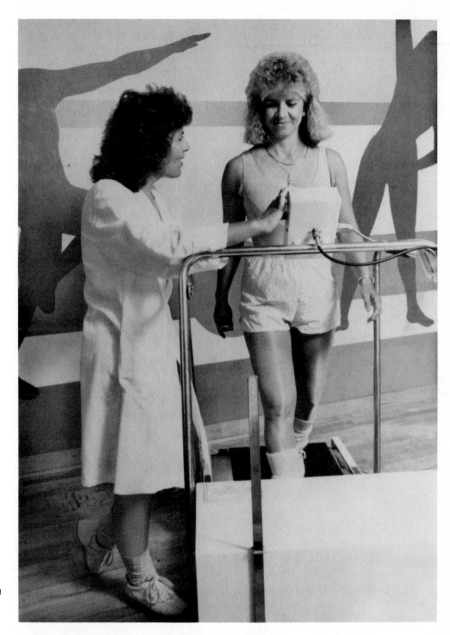

Figure 3-7
Health promotion and
illness prevention can
be enhanced through
participation in programs
that monitor health status.
Here, a woman exercises on
a treadmill while the nurse
checks her vital signs.

planning and delivering health services makes those services relevant to consumer needs. Community health nurses encourage the involvement of health care consumers by soliciting their ideas and opinions, by inviting them to participate on health boards and committees, and by using contracts for care that give them equal authority and responsibility in choosing services.

Summary

Community health nursing works to promote optimal health for aggregates. It achieves this goal by applying knowledge and skills from nursing and from public health.

A conceptual framework for community health nursing includes five sets of variables. Its practice priorities are prevention, protection, and promotion. Its interventions are education, engineering, and enforcement. Its scope of practice encompasses the range from individuals to aggregates, emphasizing the aggregate end of the individual-to-aggregate scale and the preventive end of the curative-preventive scale. Four health determinants are factors to be considered in designing practice interventions. They are human biological determinants, environmental determinants, medical-technological-organizational determinants, and social-behavioral determinants. Finally, two essential dynamics, the nursing process and the valuing process, guide community health nursing practice.

Systems theory, the study of wholes and wholeness, forms the theoretical base for community health nursing practice. Systems are interrelated and have interdependent parts. Systems may be open to exchange energy with their environments, or they may be closed. Systems experience hierarchical ordering; they form boundaries; they have structure; they need a relative state of equilibrium in order to function; and they have self-correcting, or adaptive, qualities.

Neuman's health care system model, which draws on systems theory, provides additional useful information for application of the community health nursing conceptual framework. The Neuman model focuses on stressors and people's reaction to them. Clients are seen as wholes composed of interacting variables. Each client has a core of basic survival abilities and three surrounding concentric boundaries called (1) lines of resistance, (2) normal line of defense, and (3) flexible line of defense. Stressors produce tension and can cause disequilibrium, or illness, in the client system. Stressors come from within the client (intrapersonal stressors) or from the client's environment (interpersonal and extrapersonal stressors). Nursing assessment and intervention draws on the client's and the nurse's perceptions of stressors and client responses. Nursing's goal is to help clients remain stable in their environment and to accomplish this goal, nurses use primary, secondary, and tertiary preventive measures.

Historically, the subspecialty of community health nursing developed through three stages. The district nursing stage began in 1860 with voluntary home nursing care for the poor. Sometimes called *health nurses,* these specialists treated the sick, and taught wholesome living to patients. The public health nursing stage began in 1900 and lasted until about 1970. It was characterized by a consciousness of the general public and its health care. The institutional base shifted to the government. The family became the primary unit of care. The community health nursing stage began around 1970 and has continued to the present. Nursing schools began to require course content in public health for all baccalaureate graduates. This stage made it clear that community nursing involved more than merely working in the community. Roles expanded in many different directions.

Six major societal influences have shaped the development of community health nursing. Advanced technology has solved some health care problems and created others; thus nurses' practice has focused greater attention on aging, chronic illness, and prevention. Progress in causal thinking has broadened nurses' perspective to multiple causes, including stress, environmental hazards, and the community structure. Changes in education have led community health nurses to emphasize collaborating with clients rather than planning for clients. The changing role of women has helped to open new avenues of leadership for nurses in community health. The consumer movement has increased the public's concern for quality health service. As consumers have assumed responsibility for their own health, community health nurses have become, in many instances, catalysts to assist clients toward autonomy in health. Finally, economic factors have affected community health nursing practice. These include limited funds for public health, cost containment pressures, and increased competition among health service providers. In response to these economic forces, community health nursing has developed innovative programs and new revenue sources to continue its commitment to promoting the public's health.

There are six important characteristics of community health nursing:

1. It is a field of nursing, a specialty within the larger discipline.
2. It combines the specialized knowledge of public health with nursing practice.
3. It has a population-oriented focus.
4. It emphasizes wellness rather than disease or illness.
5. It involves interdisciplinary collaboration (that is, teamwork) with other professionals.
6. It promotes client self-care by fostering a sense of responsibility among people for their own health.

Study Questions

1. What is one area of public health knowledge that makes community health nursing a nursing specialty? Describe how you might use it in actual practice.
2. Select one societal influence on the development of community health nursing and discuss its continuing impact. What other events are occurring today that shape community health nursing practice?
3. Describe a situation in community health nursing practice in which use of the practice intervention of education would be most appropriate. Do the same with engineering and enforcement. Discuss what made you match each situation with that intervention.

4. Assume you have received a referral to make a home visit to a 75-year-old man living alone whose wife recently died. Besides assessing his individual needs, what additional factors might you consider for assessment that would indicate an aggregate orientation?

References

American Nurses Association, Community Health Nursing Division. (1980). *A conceptual model of community health nursing* (Pub. No. CH-10 2M 5/80). Kansas City, Mo.: Author.

American Public Health Association. (1982). Definition and role of public health nursing in the delivery of health care (Policy Statement No. 8132). *American Journal of Public Health* 72: 210–12.

Anthony, N., M. Reed, A. Leff, J. Hoffer, and B. Stephens (1977). Immunization: Public health programming through law enforcement. *American Journal of Public Health* 67: 763–64.

Beauchamp, D. E. (1976). Public health as social justice. *Inquiry* 13: 3–14.

Brainard, A. M. (1922). *The evolution of public health nursing.* Philadelphia: W. B. Saunders.

Buckley, W. (ed.). (1968). *Modern systems research for the behavioral scientist.* Chicago: Aldine.

Bullough, V. and B. Bullough. (1979). *The care of the sick: The emergence of modern nursing.* New York: Neale, Watson.

Bureau of Labor Statistics. (1987). Labor force, employment, and earnings. *Employment and Earnings* 34(1): 376. U.S. Department of Labor.

Bureau of Labor Statistics. (1989). Employed civilians by occupation, sex, and age. *Employment and Earnings* 36(2): 31. U.S. Department of Labor.

Chavigny, K. H. and M. Kroske. (1983). Public health nursing in crisis. *Nursing Outlook* 31: 312–16.

Christman, L. (1988). Men in nursing. *Imprint* 35(3): 75.

Ehlinger, E. (1982). Implications of the competition model. *Nursing Outlook* 30: 518–21.

Fawcett, J. (1984). *Analysis and evaluation of conceptual models of nursing.* Philadelphia: F. A. Davis.

Flynn, B., J. Gottschalk, D. Ray, and E. Selmanoff. (1978). One masters curriculum in community health nursing. *Nursing Outlook* 26: 633–37.

Frachel, R. R. (1988). A new profession: The evolution of public health nursing. *Public Health Nursing* 5(2): 86–90.

Freeman, R. (1973). The dilemma of public health nursing today. In D. Roberts and R. Freeman (eds.), *Redesigning nursing education for public health: Report of the conference.* (Pub. No. [HRA] 75–75) (pp. 9–17) Bethesda, Md.: U.S. Department of Health, Education and Welfare.

Goeppinger, J. (1982). Changing health behaviors and outcomes through self-care. In J. Lancaster and W. Lancaster, (eds.), *Concepts for advanced nursing practice: The nurse as a change agent.* St. Louis: C. V. Mosby.

Hanchett, E. S., and P. N. Clarke. (1988). Nursing theory and public health science: Is synthesis possible? *Public Health Nursing* 5(1): 2–6.

Hanlon, J. J., and G. E. Pickett. (1984). *Public health: Administration and practice.* 8th ed. St. Louis: Times Mirror/Mosby.

Helvie, C. O. (1981). *Community health nursing: Theory and process.* Philadelphia: Harper & Row.

Kalisch, P., and B. Kalisch. (1986). *The advance of American nursing.* 2nd ed. Boston: Little, Brown.

Institute of Medicine Committee for the Study of the Future of Public Health. (1988). *The future of public health.* Washington D. C.: National Academy Press (August 1988, prepublication copy).

Last, J. M. (1987). *Public health and human ecology.* East Norwalk, Conn.: Appleton & Lange.

Levin, L. (1978). Self-care: An emerging component of the health care system. *Hospital & Health Services Administration* 23: 17.

Naisbitt, J. (1982). *Megatrends.* New York: Warner Books.

National League for Nursing. (1980). *Community health nursing: Education and practice* (Pub. No. 52-1834). New York: Author.

Neuman, B. (1980). The Betty Neuman health care systems model: A total person approach to patient problems. In J. Riehl and S. Roy (Eds.), *Conceptual models for nursing practice.* 2nd ed. New York: Appleton-Century-Crofts.

Neuman, B. (1982). *The Neuman systems model: Application to nursing education and practice.* Norwalk, Conn.: Appleton-Century-Crofts.

Neuman, B. (1983). Family intervention using the Betty Neuman health care systems model. In I. W. Clements and F. Roberts, *Family health: A theoretical approach to nursing care.* New York: Wiley.

Norris, C. M. (1979). Self-care. *American Journal of Nursing* 79: 486–89.

Orem, D. (1985). Nursing: Concepts of practice. 3rd ed. New York: McGraw-Hill.

Powell, D. J. (1984). Nurses—"High touch" entrepreneurs. *Nursing Economics* 2(1): 33–36.

Public Health Service. (1979). *Healthy people: The surgeon general's report on health promotion and disease prevention* (DHEW Publication No. PHS 79–55071). Washington, D.C.: U.S. Government Printing Office.

Putt, A. M. (1978). *General systems theory applied to nursing.* Boston: Little, Brown.

Roberts, D. and R. Freeman (eds.). (1973). *Redesigning nursing education for public health: Report of the conference* (Pub. No. [HRA] 75-75). Bethesda, Md.: U.S. Department of Health, Education and Welfare.

Ross, M. M., and H. Helmer. (1988). A comparative analysis of Neuman's model using the individual and family as the units of care. *Public Health Nursing* 5(1): 30–36.

Ruth, M. V., and K. Partridge. (1978). Differences in perception of education and practice. *Nursing Outlook* 26: 622–28.

Shamian, J., and L. Edgar. (1987). Nurses as agents for change in teaching breast self-examination. *Public Health Nursing* 4(1): 29–34.

Turner, J. G., and K. H. Chavigny. (1988). *Community health nursing: An epidemiologic perspective through the nursing process.* Philadelphia: J. B. Lippincott.

United Nations. (1987). *The prospects of world urbanization.* New York: United Nations Publication #ST/ESA/SER.A/101, Department of International Economic and Social Affairs.

von Bertalanffy, L. (1968). General systems theory: A critical review. In W. Buckley (ed.), *Modern systems research for the behavioral scientist.* Chicago: Aldine.

von Bertalanffy, L. (1972). The history and status of general systems theory. In Klir, G. J. (ed.), *Trends in general systems theory.* New York: Wiley.

Watkin, D. (1978). Personal responsibility: Key to effective and cost-effective health. *Family and Community Health* 1(1): 1–7.

White, M. S. (1982). Construct for public health nursing. *Nursing Outlook* 30: 527–30.

Williams, C. A. (1977). Community health nursing—What is it? *Nursing Outlook* 25: 250–54.

Williams, C. A. (1983). Making things happen: Community health nursing and the policy arena. *Nursing Outlook* 31: 225–28.

Selected Readings

American Nurses Association. (1981). *Standards: Community health nursing practice.* Kansas City, Mo. Author.

American Nurses Association, Community Health Nursing Division. (1980). *A conceptual model of community health nursing* (Pub. No. CH-10 2M 5/80). Kansas City, Mo. Author.

American Public Health Association. (1982). Definition and role of public health nursing in the delivery of health care (Policy Statement No. 8132). *American Journal of Public Health* 72: 210–12.

Anderson, E. (1983). Community focus in public health nursing: Whose responsibility? *Nursing Outlook* 31: 44–49.

Archer, S. (1982). Synthesis of public health science and nursing science. *Nursing Outlook* 30: 442–46.

Archer, S. E., and R. P. Fleshman. (1975). Community health nursing: A typology of practice. *Nursing Outlook* 23: 358.

Beauchamp. D. E. (1984). What is public about public health? *Health Affairs* 2(4): 76–87.

Brainard, A. M. (1922). *The evolution of public health nursing.* Philadelphia: W. B. Saunders.

Deloughery, G. L. (1977). *History and trends of professional nursing.* 8th ed. St. Louis: C. V. Mosby.

Dolan, J. A. (1978). *Nursing in society: A historical perspective.* Philadelphia: W. B. Saunders.

Frachel, R. R. (1988). A new profession: The evolution of public health nursing. *Public Health Nursing* 5(2): 86–90.

Freeman, R. (1973). The dilemma of public health nursing today. In D. Roberts and R. Freeman (eds.), *Redesigning nursing education for public health: Report of the conference* (Pub. No. [HRA] 75-75) (pp. 9–17) Bethesda, Md.: U.S. Department of Health, Education and Welfare.

Freeman, R., and J. Heinrich. (1981). *Community health nursing practice.* 2nd ed. Philadelphia: W. B. Saunders.

Fromer, M. J. (1983). *Community health care and the nursing process.* 2nd ed. St. Louis: C. V. Mosby.

Gardner, M. S. (1919). *Public health nursing.* 3rd ed. New York: Macmillan.

Goeppinger, J., P. G. Lassiter, and B. Wilcox. (1982). Community health is community competence. *Nursing Outlook* 30: 464–67.

Goodson, J. (1978). Demonstrating excellence in a community nursing service. In A. Warner (ed.), *Innovations in community health nursing* (pp. 16–22). St. Louis: C. V. Mosby.

Grissum, M. and C. Spangler. (1976). *Womanpower and health care.* Boston: Little, Brown.

Hanchett, E. S., and P. N. Clarke. (1988). Nursing theory and public health science: Is synthesis possible? *Public Health Nursing* 5(1): 2–6.

Hanlon, J. J., and G. E. Pickett. (1984). *Public health: Administration and practice.* 8th ed. St. Louis: Times Mirror/Mosby.

Hays, B. J., and N. R. Mockelstrom. (1977). Consumer survey: An approach to teaching consumer participation in community health. *Journal of Nursing Education* 16: 30.

Heide, W. S. (1973). Nursing and women's liberation: A parallel. *American Journal of Nursing* 73: 824–27.

Helvie, C. O. (1981). *Community health nursing: Theory and process.* Philadelphia: Harper & Row.

Kalisch, P., and B. Kalisch. (1986). *The advance of American nursing.* 2nd ed. Boston: Little, Brown.

Leahy, K., M. Cobb, and M. Jones. (1982). *Community health nursing.* 4th ed. New York: McGraw-Hill.

Naisbitt, J. (1982). *Megatrends.* New York: Warner Books.

National League for Nursing. (1980). *Community health nursing: Education and practice* (Pub. No. 52-1834). New York: Author.

Neuman, B. (1982). *The Neuman systems model: Application to nursing education and practice.* Norwalk, Conn.: Appleton-Century-Crofts.

Novello, D. J., et al. (1978). *Consumerism and health care.* New York: National League for Nursing.

Orem, D. (1985). *Nursing: Concepts of practice.* 3rd ed. New York: McGraw-Hill.

Public Health Service. (1979). *Healthy people: The surgeon general's report on health promotion and disease prevention* (DHEW Publication No. 79-55071). Washington, D.C. U.S. Government Printing Office.

Putt, A. M. (1978). *General systems theory applied to nursing.* Boston: Little, Brown.

Rathbone, W. (1890). *History and progress of district nursing.* New York: Macmillan.

Spradley, B. (1990). *Readings in community health nursing.* 4th ed. Glenview, IL: Scott, Foresman.

Turner, J. G., and K. H. Chavigny. (1988). *Community health nursing: An epidemiologic perspective through the nursing process.* Philadelphia: J. B. Lippincott.

Wald, L. (1934). *Windows on Henry Street.* Boston: Little, Brown.

Wales, M. (1941). *The public health nurse in action.* New York: Macmillan.

Watkin, D. (1978). Personal responsibility: Key to effective and cost-effective health. *Family and Community Health* 1(1): 1–7.

White, M. S. (1982). Construct for public health nursing. *Nursing Outlook.* 30: 527–30.

Williams, C. A. (1977). Community health nursing—What is it? *Nursing Outlook* 25: 250–54.

Williams, C. A. (1983). Making things happen: Community health nursing and the policy arena. *Nursing Outlook* 31: 225–28.

Winslow, C. E. A. (1946). Florence Nightingale and public health nursing. *Public Health Nursing* 38: 330–32.

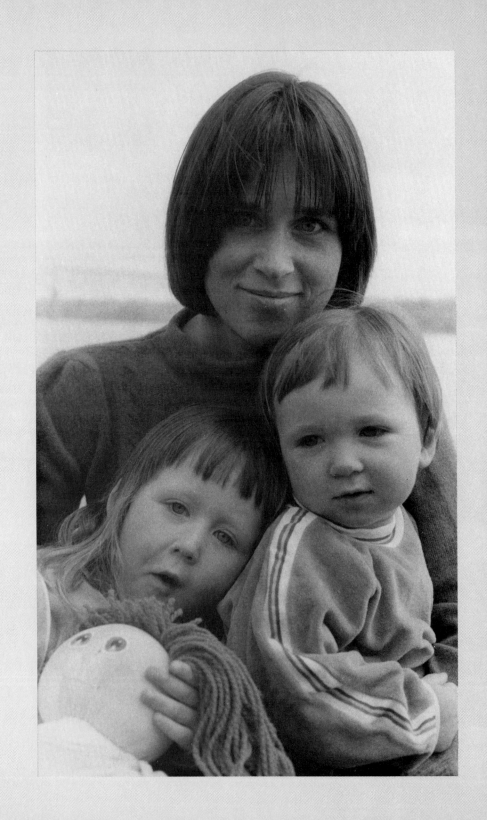

4 Family Theory

Imagine that you are employed as a community health nurse by an agency in Los Angeles. In a single day you might visit five families, each with different health problems. A young single mother seeks help in caring for her sick infant. Another family has an elderly parent recently discharged from the hospital after a stroke. The third family, Vietnamese refugees, needs instruction on the purchase and preparation of food. In the other two visits, you will check the progress of a serious burn on the arm of a ten-year-old, develop a contract for weight control with his mother, and assist a recently retired couple in adjusting to their new stage of life.

As you set out for a day of work, what kinds of things will you need to know? You will have to deal with specific health problems such as strokes, burns, and retirement. You need to know your goals — the promotion of health and self-care. You will have to rely on your knowledge of cultural differences when working with the Vietnamese family and perhaps other clients. You will need to know how to use certain tools such as problem solving and contracting. You will need to understand communication and know how to develop a helping relationship.

But do you need to know something about the nature of families? What should you know about the five families you will visit, apart from their individual members and problems? Do families, as basic units of a community, have characteristics that affect community health nursing service? The answer is an unqualified yes. As a community health nurse, your effectiveness depends on knowing how to work with family units. In this chapter we examine the nature of families and draw from various theories to strengthen your understanding of families as clients.

DEFINITION OF FAMILY

We might begin by asking, What is a family? Many different definitions exist, but most family theorists seem to agree that a family consists of a group of two or more individuals who share a residence, possess some common emotional

99

bond, and engage in interrelated social positions, roles, and tasks (Duvall and Miller, 1985; Baranowski and Nader, 1985; Leavitt, 1982). We can summarize these characteristics with the following definition: A family consists of two or more persons who live in the same household (usually), share a common emotional bond, and perform certain interrelated social tasks.

As this definition suggests, families may assume many different types of structures. A growing body of research on family structure and function shows that families have changed dramatically from the time when the nuclear family was the dominant form. Today's community health nurse needs to understand and work with many types of families. Later in the chapter we will examine variant family structures, but before doing so we will discuss the general characteristics of families and the features that make a family operate as a unit.

CHARACTERISTICS OF FAMILIES

We can make several observations about families in general. First, all families are unique. The five families mentioned earlier have their own distinct problems and strengths. None will be exactly like any other family. As you approach the door of a house or push the buzzer of an apartment, you cannot assume that you know what the family inside will be like. Consequently, you will have to gather information about each particular family in order to achieve your nursing objectives.

Second, every family is like every other family. The five families you visit share certain features with all families. These universal characteristics provide an important key to understanding each family's uniqueness. Five of the most important family universals for community nursing are listed below:

1. Every family is a small social system.
2. Every family has its own cultural values and rules.
3. Every family has structure.
4. Every family has certain basic functions.
5. Every family moves through stages in its life cycle.

No matter how many families you might visit in the course of a year, each one will have these universal features. It will be important to know how the social system, cultural values, structure, function, and stage of development affect health care provision. These five universals of family life provide the framework of this chapter and are based on systems theory, sociological theories, and theories of family development.

Third, some families are more alike than others. Between the extremes of complete uniqueness and universal features, certain similarities among some families permit a classification of structural subtypes. For example, although all families have structure, the five you visit may consist of four types — two nuclear families (husband, wife, children), one nuclear dyad (husband and wife), one multigenerational family, and one single-parent family. Knowing the range of variation within the family universals will help prepare you for the families you encounter. As we consider the universals of family life, we will also discuss those structural subtypes that characterize our own society; if we took a worldwide perspective, subtypes in family life would greatly proliferate, although the universals would still exist.

FAMILIES AS SOCIAL SYSTEMS

All of us fall into the trap of viewing families merely as collections of individuals. Caused partly by our cultural emphasis on strong individualism, this error also occurs because we encounter families through the individual members. We seldom think of the ways in which a family operates as a unit. When a community health nurse sits in a living room talking with a young mother about her new infant, it is difficult to realize that all the other family members are present by way of their influence. Systems theory offers some insights about how families operate as social systems. The attributes of living, or open, systems (discussed in Chapter 3) provide a helpful theoretical framework for strengthening our understanding of family structure and function. Let us begin by reviewing five attributes of open systems that shed light on the nature of families. Families (1) are interdependent, (2) maintain boundaries, (3) exchange energy with their environment, (4) are adaptive, and (5) are goal-oriented.

INTERDEPENDENCE AMONG MEMBERS

First, all the members of a family, because they are units within a system, are interdependent (Helvie, 1981). One member's actions affect the other members. For example, the community health nurse cannot expect that a father's change in life-style to reduce his risk of coronary heart disease will not affect the rest of the family. If he cuts back on working overtime, the family's income will be reduced. If he begins to eat different foods, food preparation and eating patterns in the family will be altered. A new exercise program may upset other family routines. Furthermore, as this one member adjusts to the demands of a change in life-style, his ability to carry out his usual roles as husband and father may be affected.

The interdependence of family members involves a set of internal relationships that influences the effectiveness of family functioning (Aldous, 1978). There is a complex network of communication patterns among family members. It is possible to diagram the network as a family map of all the dyads, triads, and combinations of interactions that occur within families (Satir, 1972). The way parents relate to each other, for instance, influences the quality of their parenting. When the bond between them is strong and nurturant, they

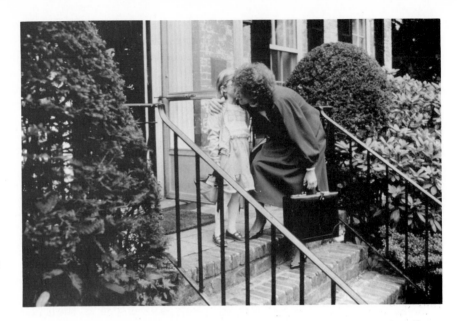

Figure 4-1
Strong affectional ties promote the quality of this working mother's relationship with her daughter.

have more to offer their children. Marital, parent-child, and sibling relationships all significantly influence family functioning (Figure 4-1). They determine how well the family as a system handles conflict, provides a support system for its members, copes with crises, solves daily problems, and capitalizes on its own resources.

FAMILY BOUNDARIES

Second, families, as systems, set and maintain boundaries (Aldous, 1978). Family closeness, which results from shared experiences and expectations, links family members together in a bond that excludes the rest of the world. A greater concentration of energy exists within the family than between the family and its external environment, thereby creating a family system boundary (Helvie, 1981). Witness an example of family unity as the Pedrocelli extended family gathers for a Sunday afternoon backyard picnic. Witness, too, the distinctiveness of this family from all the others in the neighborhood. Because of the things they have in common, the Pedrocellis set and maintain boundaries that unite them and also differentiate them from others.

Families, however, are not closed systems. Their boundaries are semipermeable, providing protection and preservation of family unity and autonomy while also allowing selective linkages with external associations. This leads us to consider the next attribute of systems that applies to families—energy exchange.

ENERGY EXCHANGE

Third, as systems, families exchange energy in the form of materials or information with their environment (Putt, 1978). A family must receive from and give to its environment in order to function adequately. All normally functioning living systems engage in such an input-output relationship. This occurs so that proper nutrients may be absorbed and wastes eliminated or information shared to promote a healthy ecological balance between the system and its environment. For a family system this means an exchange between the family and its immediate community.

A family's successful progress through its developmental stages depends on how well the family manages this energy exchange. For example, a child-bearing family, like the Pedrocellis, needs adequate food, shelter, and emotional support as well as information on how to accomplish its developmental tasks. In addition, the family needs community resources such as health care, education, employment, and other forms of environmental input. In return, the family contributes to the community through such activities as participation in work and consumption of goods and services. When a family does not have adequate income or emotional support (Clark, 1986) or does not utilize community resources, that family is not experiencing a proper energy exchange with its environment. An inadequate exchange can lead to dysfunctioning and poor health (Neuman, 1983).

ADAPTIVE BEHAVIOR

Fourth, families are equilibrium-seeking and adaptive systems. In accordance with their very nature, families never stay the same (Scanzoni, 1983). They shift and change in response to internal and external forces. Internally, the family composition changes as new members are added or members leave through death or divorce. Roles and relationships change as members advance in age and experience, and normative expectations change as members resolve their tensions and differing points of view. Externally, families are bombarded by influences from sources such as school, work, peers, neighbors, church, and government; consequently, they are forced to accommodate to new demands. Adapting to these influences may require a family to change its behavior, goals, and even its values. Like any system, the family needs a state of quasi equilibrium in order to function (Helvie, 1981). Thus, with each new set of pressures, the family shifts and accommodates as a means of regaining balance and a normal life-style. There are times when a family's capacity for adaptation is taxed beyond its limits. At this point the system may be in danger of disintegrating; that is, family members will leave or become dysfunctional because of unresolved stress. It is then that families may need some form of intervention, such as extended family mediation or external professional help, to provide a supplemental resource for restoring family equilibrium.

Community health nurses play an influential role in family equilibrium-seeking. Neuman describes the major goal of nursing as keeping the individual and family client systems stabilized within their environment (Neuman, 1983; Ross and Helmer, 1988). In Chapter 15 we will explore the community health nurse's stabilizing interventions with families.

GOAL-DIRECTED BEHAVIOR

Finally, families as social systems are goal directed. Families exist for a purpose—to establish and maintain a milieu that promotes the development of their members. In order to fulfill this purpose, a family must perform basic functions such as providing love, security, identity, a sense of belonging, preparation for adult roles in society, and maintenance of order and control. In addition to these functions, each family member engages in tasks to maintain the family as a viable unit. Duvall and Miller describe specific functions and tasks for each stage of the family's development (1985). We shall examine these functions and tasks in more detail shortly.

FAMILY CULTURE

The concept of family culture arises from a significant body of literature in the social and behavioral sciences. Research done by sociologists and anthropologists, in particular, sheds considerable light on the nature of families. Cross-cultural comparisons and in-depth analyses of families (Bott, 1971; Carter and McGoldrick, 1980; Farber, 1973; Gordon, 1978; Lancaster et al., 1987; Olson and McCubbin, 1983; Stephens, 1963; van den Berghe, 1979) demonstrate that each family has a "culture" that strongly influences its structure and function. Culture, "the acquired knowledge that people use to interpret experience and to generate behavior" (Spradley and McCurdy, 1980, p. 2) explains why a family behaves the way it does. It also gives the community health nurse a basis for assessing family health and designing appropriate interventions.

Three aspects of family culture deserve special emphasis. First, family members share certain values that affect family behavior. Second, certain roles are prescribed and defined for family members. Third, a family's culture determines its distribution and use of power. We shall examine these aspects of family culture now. Two additional aspects, family structure and function, follow for separate discussion.

SHARED VALUES AND THEIR EFFECT ON BEHAVIOR

Because every family has its own set of values and rules for operation (Getty and Humphreys, 1981), we can speak of family culture. Although families share many broad cultural values drawn from the larger society in which they live, they also develop unique variants. Some values will be explicitly stated: "Family matters must always stay within the family." Such values may give rise to specific operating rules: "Don't tell any of your friends how much money Daddy earns."

Like all cultural values, however, many family values will remain at a tacit level, outside the conscious awareness of family members. These values become powerful determinants of what the family believes, feels, thinks, and does. A family that values free expression for every member engages comfortably in loud, noisy debates, while another family that values quietness, order, and control will not tolerate its members raising their voices. One family uses birth control based on beliefs about human life and parental responsibility; another family chooses not to use birth control because it holds a different set of values. How a family views education, health care, life-style, child rearing, sex roles, or any of the myriad other issues requiring choices depends upon the cultural values of that family.

Family values include those beliefs transmitted by previous generations, religious influences, immediate social pressures, and the larger society. The combination of all these influences may lead a family to decide, perhaps unconsciously, that it is important to compete and succeed. Conversely, it may feel it is important to "hang loose" and never worry about tomorrow. Values become an integral part of a family's life and are very difficult to change.

PRESCRIBED ROLES

Roles, the assigned or assumed parts that members play during day-to-day family living, are bestowed and defined by the family (Goode, 1977; Miller and Janosik, 1980). That is, the family determines who will play which roles (prescribing roles) and generally what each role will comprise (defining roles). For instance, in one family the father role assigned to the male adult may be defined as an authoritative one that includes establishing rules, judging behavior, and administering punishment for violation of rules. In another family, the father role may be defined primarily as that of a loving benefactor. If there is an absence of an immediate male parent, a grandfather, uncle, friend, or mother may take over the father role. Selection of specific roles to be played in any given family will vary depending on the family's structure, needs, and patterns of functioning. In a single-parent family, for example, the parent may need to assume the roles of mother, father, and breadwinner, as well as other roles.

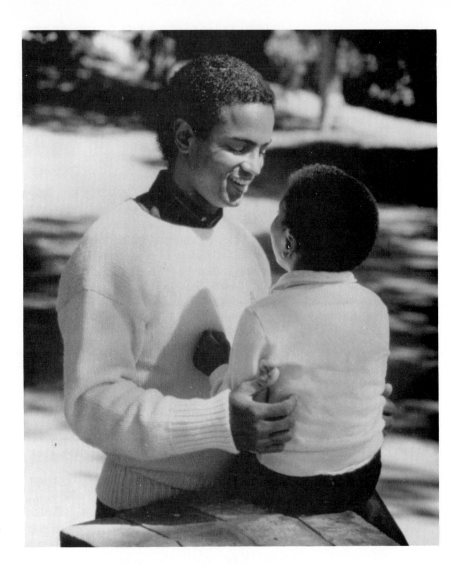

Figure 4-2
This single father enjoys the responsibility of child care during an outing with his son.

Families distribute among the roles all the responsibilities and tasks necessary to conduct family living (Figure 4-2). The responsibilities of breadwinner and homemaker, for example, with their accompanying tasks, may belong to husband and wife, respectively, or may be shared if both husband and wife hold jobs outside the home.

Family members often play several roles at the same time (Satir, 1972; Miller and Janosik, 1980). A woman, for instance, may play the role of wife to her husband, daughter to her mother living in the same home, and mother to each of her children. Even her mother role may involve wearing several different hats because it varies slightly with each child. A single-parent family often combines the roles of father and mother in one person but may distribute responsibilities and tasks more widely. A grandmother or children may assume responsibility for some chores and thus relieve the demands placed on the single parent. Among families, there is great variation in expectations for each role and the degree of flexibility in role prescriptions. Consequently, a family may place great demands on some members, although at the same time, members may interpret their roles differently. Confusion and conflict can develop unless roles are clarified.

POWER DISTRIBUTION

Power, the possession of control, authority, or influence over others, assumes different patterns in each family. In some families, power is concentrated primarily in one member, while in others it is distributed on a more egalitarian basis. The traditional patriarchal family, in which the father holds absolute authority over the other members, is rare in American society. However, the pattern of husband as head of the household and dominant member of the family is still frequently seen. Whether male or female, the dominant partner holds the majority of the decision-making power, particularly over the more important family affairs, such as employment, financial matters, and sexual activity. Other areas of decision making, including choices about vacations, housing, leisure activities, household purchases, and child rearing, may be shared or delegated. With changing societal influences, however, the present trend among American families is toward egalitarian power distribution. Rudolf Dreikurs long ago advocated that families form a "family council" for shared decision making and distribution of tasks (Dreikurs, 1964). Today many families practice joint decision making and equal participation by all members.

Roles often influence power distribution within the family. Along with the responsibilities attached to a role, a family may assign decision-making authority. The mother role frequently includes decision-making power regarding household management. A responsibility related to a son's role, such as lawn mowing, may empower him to decide when and how often he does the job.

Family power structure is also influenced by the amount of personal power residing in each member (Robischon and Smith, 1977). A mother or eldest son, for example, may exercise considerable influence over the family by virtue of personality and position rather than delegated authority. Even a child who throws temper tantrums may wield considerable power in a family.

We have viewed families as social systems and examined their cultural dimensions. We know that a family is tied biologically through kinship and probably socially through choice. We know that it exists for a purpose. Duvall's definition nicely summarizes these aspects of the family: "The family is a unity of interacting persons related by ties of marriage, birth, or adoption, whose central purpose is to create and maintain a common culture which promotes the physical, mental, emotional, and social development of each of its members" (Duvall and Miller, 1985, p. 6).

FAMILY STRUCTURES

For many people, the term *family* evokes a picture of a husband, wife, and children living under one roof with the male as breadwinner and the female as homemaker.

This nuclear family is often seen as the norm for everyone. Variations from this pattern often have been treated as deviant and abnormal, even in recent studies of the family (Olson, McCubbin, and Associates, 1983). The traditional nuclear family has been sacrosanct because it is such a fundamental part of our cultural heritage, an ideal reinforced by religion, education, and other influential social institutions. Recent changes in the nuclear family have led some to predict the demise of the family itself, yet reality insists that the nuclear model is not the only valid family form. The pressures of social conditions such as emerging new life-styles, increasing significance of work for women, and changing sexual roles have effected changes in the American family. We now see a growing number of households of cohabiting adults, single parents, and single persons. Although the classic nuclear family continues to exist, there are now many variations of the nuclear model as well as emerging new patterns of family structure. Each requires recognition and acceptance by professionals who wish to help families achieve optimal health.

Families come in many shapes and sizes. We can place these varying family structures into two general categories, traditional and nontraditional.

TRADITIONAL FAMILIES

Traditional family forms are the forms most familiar to us. There is generally no question that these are families; society sanctions their legitimacy. The most obvious are husband, wife, and children living together (nuclear family), or husband and wife living as a couple, either childless or with children launched (nuclear dyad). Community health nurses also work with many families that have one parent as a result of divorce, separation, or death. The nurse may visit an elderly man living alone in a high-rise apartment (single-adult family) or a home where a grandmother and a divorced older granddaughter with her baby are living with the daughter's nuclear family (multigenerational family). Sometimes, particularly among ethnic groups, we find a group of relatives that consists of several nuclear families who live close to each other and share goods and services. Perhaps they own and run a family business together, sharing income and expenses, eat many meals together, and all have some responsibility for raising the children (kin network). Table 4-1 lists a number of traditional family structures.

Career patterns, particularly for women, further characterize traditional family structures. Scanzoni (1983, p. 85) distinguishes between three types of nuclear families in which women and men are either "workers," "achievers,"

Table 4-1
Traditional and Nontraditional American Family Structures

Structure	Participants	Living Arrangements
Traditional		
Nuclear family	Husband Wife Children	Common household
Commuter family	Husband Wife Children sometimes	Divided household between two cities
Nuclear dyad	Husband Wife	Common household
Single-parent family	One adult (separated, divorced, widowed) Children	Common household
Single adult	One adult	Living alone
Multigenerational family	Any combination of the first four traditional family structures	Common household
Kin network	Two or more reciprocal households (related by birth or marriage)	Close geographic proximity
Nontraditional		
Commune family	Two or more monogamous couples Shared children	Common household
Group marriage commune family	Several adults "married" to each other Shared children	Common household
Group network	Reciprocal nuclear households or single members	Close geographic proximity
Unmarried single- parent family	One parent (never married) Children	Common household
Unmarried couple	Two adults (heterosexual, homosexual, or "just friends")	Common household
Unmarried couple and child family	Two adults (as above) Children	Common household

Source: Adapted from M. B. Sussman (1971).

or "partners." In the first type, husband and wife are both earners; each holds a full- or part-time job. The second type describes couples in which both partners have careers and are usually employed full-time. Equal partners, the third type, refers to a shared, interdependent relationship in which "all work and domestic arrangements are open to negotiation and continual renegotiation." Nuclear dyads may be any of these three types. Some single-parent families include a working adult; others may have a single parent, such as a woman deserted by her husband and without any employable skills, who has no career. These variant structures remind us that even traditional families can assume many forms.

One variant of traditional families that is seen with greater frequency today is the "commuter marriage." In this type of family, the partners hold jobs in two different cities. The pattern is usually for one partner (married or unmarried) to live and work and perhaps raise children in the "home" city while the other works in a distant city. The second partner generally lives in the other city and commutes home for weekends or less frequent visits, depending on the distance. Sometimes this arrangement is temporary, as when one partner is going to school or gets transferred through work and the couple chooses not to move the rest of the family until the end of the school year. In other instances the "commuting" may continue for years. Clearly this arrangement influences family roles and functions, challenging a family's ability to maintain healthy relationships. A traditional family in which one partner must take numerous business trips will experience similar effects on family roles and functioning.

NONTRADITIONAL FAMILIES

Nontraditional family structures include a variety of family forms; some of these forms are accepted by society and others are strongly questioned on the basis of illegitimate union. Table 4-1 lists some of the prominent nontraditional structures. One of the more well-known nontraditional family forms is composed of several unrelated, monogamous (married or committed to one person) couples living together and collectively rearing their children (commune family). A variation of the commune family is the common household in which several adults are all "married" to each other; they share everything, including sex and child rearing (group marriage). Occasionally a group of nuclear families, not related by birth or marriage but bound by a common set of values such as a religious system, live close to each other and share goods, services, and child-rearing responsibilities (group network). Some commune and group network families select one of their members, usually a male, to be their leader, or head.

Some nontraditional families clearly form outside marriage. One example, seen more and more in community health, is the single, unmarried parent (most often a young, unwed mother) and child (Figure 4-3). Many adult couples form a family alliance outside marriage or through a private ceremony not legally recognized as marriage (unmarried couple). They may range from young adults living together to an elderly couple sharing their lives outside of marriage to avoid tax penalties. Such cohabiting couples may be heterosexual, homosexual, or the same sex without a sexual relationship. In some instances, these couples have their own biological or adopted children (unmarried couple and child family).

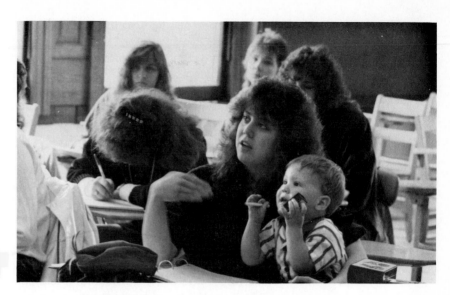

Figure 4-3
The teen mother with her child represents a family form seen frequently by community health nurses. Each type of family structure has its own unique set of resources and needs.

Families that do not fit the traditional nuclear model make up an increasing proportion of the American population. For instance, in 1960, legally married couples made up 75 percent of American households. That figure had declined to 65 percent by 1975, and by 1988 had dropped to nearly 55 percent (U. S. Bureau of Census, 1989). Less than 20 percent of American families now have a working father, a full-time homemaker mother, and one or more children (*A Growing Crisis*, 1983). The number of couples who share a household without marrying more than doubled between 1970 and 1979 (Cherlin, 1981) and had reached 2.6 million (3 percent) in 1988 (U. S. Bureau of Census, 1989). As of 1986, approximately 12 percent (over 10 million) of all families in the United States had a woman as head of the household; more than half (or over 6 million) of these female-headed households included children under 18 (U. S. Bureau of Census, 1988). The number of households headed by men with no spouse present increased from 1.7 million (2.1 percent) in 1980 to 2.4 million (2.7 percent) in 1986. Of these male-headed households with no spouse present, nearly half (almost one million homes) included children under 18 (U. S. Bureau of Census, 1988). The proportion of children under 18 years of age who lived with one parent increased from 12 percent in 1970 to 24 percent in 1988 (U. S. Bureau of Census, 1989). Divorce is also changing family structures; nearly half of all marriages now end in divorce (higher for teenage marriages) and the median duration of marriages is approximately seven years (U. S. Bureau of Census, 1988).

Varying family structures raise three important issues for consideration. First, community health nurses can no longer hold to the myth that idealizes the traditional nuclear family (Getty and Humphreys, 1981). Societal changes force them (and all who work with families) to accept many variations in family forms as valid and functional. Unless community nurses adopt this posture and avoid judging by standards appropriate to the idealized nuclear family, they are in danger of creating even more problems for the families they attempt to serve. To hold to an ideal that parents must meet all their children's needs, for example, can lead to a conclusion that parenting is defective when children have personality deficits. This expectation may be unrealistic and unattainable for dual-career and, perhaps even more so, for single-parent families, who require supplemental resources to meet children's needs.

Second, the structure of an individual's family may change several times over a lifetime. A girl may be born into a kin network, shift to a nuclear family when her parents move and become part of a single-parent family when her parents are divorced. As she matures, she may choose to become a single adult living alone, later to become a part of a cohabiting couple, and still later to marry and form a nuclear family. For the individual, each variant family form involves changes in roles, interaction patterns, socialization processes, and linkages with external resources (President's Commission, 1981).

Finally, each type of family structure creates different issues and problems that, in turn, influence a family's ability to perform its basic functions. (Scanzoni, 1983). Each particular structure determines the kind of support needed from nursing or other human service systems (Olson and McCubbin, 1983). A single adult living alone, for instance, may lack companionship or a sense of being needed by other family members. A kin network family provides broad, extended family support and security but may have problems in power distribution and decision making. An unmarried couple raising a child may be parenting well but not receiving needed external support from the community in the form of recognition, approval, or assistance. Variations in structure, then, create differing family strengths and needs, an important consideration for community health nurses.

FAMILY FUNCTIONS

Families in every culture throughout history have engaged in the same basic functions. In different societies these tasks have been performed in different ways. Nonetheless, families always have produced children, physically maintained their members, and provided social placement, socialization, emotional support, and social control (Goode, 1977; Miller and Janosik, 1980). Some societies have experimented with separation of these functions, allocating activities such as child care, socialization, or social control to a larger group. The Israeli kibbutz and Chinese commune are examples. Yet, for most peoples, the individual family unit (in its variant forms) persists, accompanied by most of the same basic functions. In American society, certain social institutions perform some aspects of traditional family functions. Schools, for example, help socialize children; professionals supervise health care; and churches influence values. Thus we see some modifications and overlap in patterns of functioning. Six functions are typical of American families today. Families provide (1) affection, (2) security, (3) identity, (4) affiliation, (5) socialization, and (6) controls (Duvall and Miller, 1985; Sussman, 1971).

AFFECTION

The family functions to give members affection and emotional support (Figure 4-4). Love brings couples together initially in our society and later produces children. In some cultures affection comes after marriage. Continued affection creates an atmosphere of nurturance and care for all family members that is necessary for health, development, and survival (Aldous, 1978). It is common knowledge that infants cannot survive without love. Indeed, human beings of any age require love as sustenance for growth and find it

Figure 4-4
An important family function is to demonstrate affection in order to promote members' growth. A child, recognizing his father's love, responds with confidence.

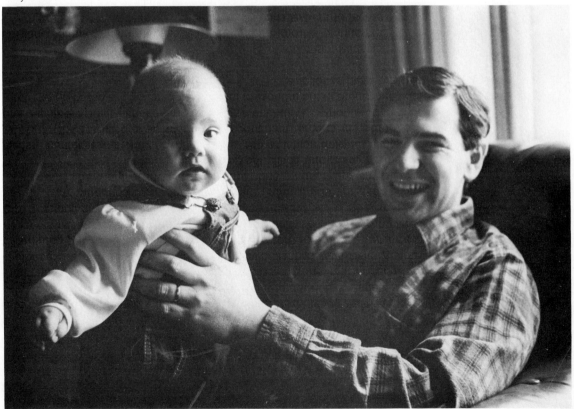

primarily in the family. Families, unlike many other social groups, are bound by affectional ties whose strength determines family happiness and closeness. Consider how the sharing of gifts on a holiday or the loving concern of a family for a sick member draws the family together. Positive sexual identity and sexual fulfillment are also influenced by a loving atmosphere. Early students of the family emphasized sexual access and procreation as basic family functions. Now we recognize that families exist not only to regulate the sex drive and perpetuate the species but also to sustain life and foster human potential through a strong affectional climate (Lancaster et al., 1987).

SECURITY AND ACCEPTANCE

Families meet their members' physical needs by providing food, shelter, clothing, health care, and other necessities; in so doing, they create a secure environment. Members need to know that these basics will be available and that the family is committed to providing them.

The stability of the family unit also gives members a sense of security. The family offers a safe retreat from the competition of the outside world, a place where its members are accepted for themselves. They can learn, make mistakes, and grow in a secure environment. Where else does the toddler, after repeated falls, receive the encouragement to keep trying to walk; or the child, teased by a bully, regain his courage; or a parent, feeling burned out on a job, find comfort and renewal? The dependability of the family unit promotes confidence and self-assurance among its members, contributing to their mental and emotional health and equipping them with the skills necessary to cope with the outside world.

IDENTITY AND SATISFACTION

The family functions to give members a sense of social and personal identity. From infancy on, the individual gains a sense of identity and worth from the family. Like a mirror, the family reflects back to its members a picture of who they are and how valuable they are to others. Positive reflections provide the individual with a sense of satisfaction and worth, such as that experienced by a girl when her family applauds her efforts in a swimming meet. Need fulfillment in the home determines satisfaction in the outside world; it particularly affects other interpersonal relationships and career choices. Roles learned within the family also give members a sense of identity. A boy growing up and learning his family's expectations for the male role soon develops a sense of the kind of person he must strive to be; often, he is expected to be strong, competitive, successful, and unemotional.

Families influence their members' social placement. That is, as a result of genetics, social class, race, economic position, and many other factors, families determine where their members will be placed in the social order.

Social placement is a way of telling members who they are. For example, the members of a wealthy, influential family will be expected to follow in that family's tradition of attending Ivy League schools, mixing in upper-class social circles, and selecting high-status careers. A poor family, with its contrasting value system and social heritage, may influence its members to receive very little formal education and move into a trade at an early age. In fact, families influence their members' physical characteristics, intellectual abilities, educational experiences, social positions, economic levels, and religious and political affiliations. All these factors help to shape member identity.

AFFILIATION AND COMPANIONSHIP

The family functions to give members a sense of belonging throughout life. Because families provide associational bonds and group membership, they help satisfy their members' needs for belonging. We all know that we are integral—that we belong—to our families. However, the quality of a family's communication influences its closeness. If communication patterns are effective, then affiliation ties are strong and needs for belonging are met. One family handles conflict over financial expenditures, for instance, by discussing differences and making compromises. A second family never resolves its financial conflicts. Instead, one member makes a selfish purchase and another member retaliates with an equally expensive personal expenditure. The healthier interactional pattern of the first family contributes to its strong sense of affiliation.

The family, unlike other social institutions, involves permanent relationships. Long after friends from school, the old neighborhood, work, or church have come and gone, we still have the family. The family provides its members with affiliation and fellowship that are unbroken by distance or time. Even when scattered across the country, family members will gather to support each other and to share in a holiday, wedding, graduation, or funeral. After separation, there is no need to reestablish ties; it is taken for granted that we belong and that we can take up where we left off. It is to the family that we turn in times of happiness or need. We know we can freely share our distress and joy, call at any time, and borrow a shoulder to cry on or money to get us out of a financial bind. The durability of this affiliation remains a resource for life.

SOCIALIZATION

The family functions to socialize the young. Families transmit their culture—their values, attitudes, goals, and behavior patterns—to their members. Members, socialized into a way of life that reflects and preserves that cultural heritage, pass that heritage on, in turn, to the next generation (Figure 4-5). From infancy on, we learn to control our bowels, eat with utensils, dress our-

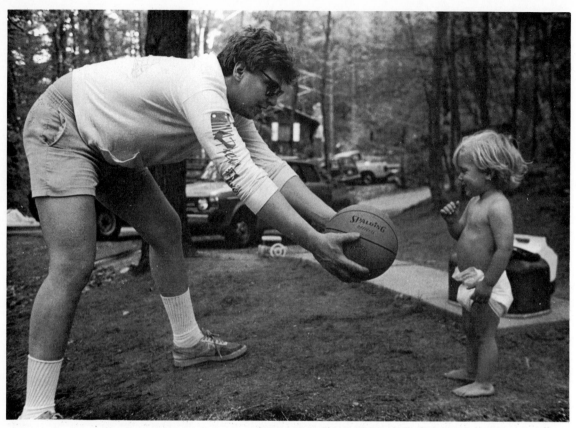

Figure 4-5
This little boy learns early that sports are an important part of the male role.

selves, manage our emotions, and behave according to sociocultural prescriptions for our age and sex. Through this process, we learn our roles in the family. Our life-styles, the foods we prefer, our relationships with other people, our ideas about child rearing, and our attitudes about religion, abortion, equal rights, or euthanasia are all strongly influenced by our families. Although experiences outside of the family also have a strong influence on roles, they are filtered through the perceptions we acquired during early socialization.

The socialization process also influences the degree of independence experienced by growing children. Some families release their maturing members by degrees, preparing them early for adult roles. Other families promote dependent roles and find release painful and difficult.

CONTROLS

The family functions to maintain social control. Families maintain order through establishment of social controls both within the family and between family members and outsiders. Members' conduct is controlled by the family's definition of acceptable and nonacceptable behaviors. From minor points such as keeping one's elbows off the table to larger issues, such as standards of home cleanliness, appropriate dress, children's proper address of adults, or a teenager's curfew, the family imposes limits. Then it maintains those limits by a system of rewards for conformity and punishments for violations. Children growing up in a family quickly learn what is "right" and what is "wrong" by family standards. Gradually family control shifts to self-control as members learn to discipline their own lives; later on, they will adopt or modify many of the same standards to use with their own children.

Division of labor is another aspect of the family's control function. Families allocate various roles, responsibilities, and tasks to their members in order to assure provision of income, household management, child care, and other essentials (Figure 4-6).

Families also regulate the way internal and external resources are used. The family identifies internal resources, such as member abilities, financial income, or material assets, and decides how they will be utilized. For instance, a man with artistic skills may be the member to landscape the yard, and a woman with mechanical aptitude the member to repair appliances. This same family may choose to drive an old car in order to spend a fair portion of its income on entertainment, such as eating in restaurants or going to movies. Families also determine the external resources used by their members. Some families take advantage of the many religious, health, and social services available to them in the community. They seek regular medical care, encourage their children to participate in scouting programs, become in-

Figure 4-6
Family members all have assigned responsibilities. Older children often help with the care and training of their younger siblings. Here a young girl reads a bedtime story to her little sister.

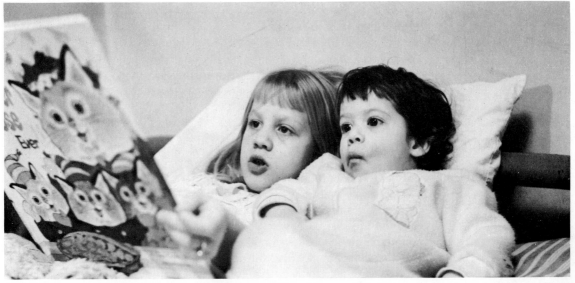

Table 4-2
Family Functions and Tasks

Family Functions	Associated Developmental Tasks
Affection	Establishment of climate of affection Promotion of sexuality and sexual fulfillment Addition of new members
Security and acceptance	Maintenance of physical requirements Acceptance of individual members
Identity and satisfaction	Maintenance of motivation Self-image and role development Social placement and satisfying activities
Affiliation and companionship	Development of communication patterns Establishment of durable bonds
Socialization	Internalization of culture (values and behavior) Guidance for internal and external relationships Release of members
Controls	Maintenance of social control Division of labor Allocation and utilization of resources

volved in church activities, or join a bowling league. Other families, not recognizing or valuing external resources, limit their members' use of them.

Each of the six functions just described is an ongoing family responsibility, essential for the maintenance and promotion of family health (Duvall and Miller, 1985). Incorporated into these functions are specific tasks that a family must do to promote its growth and development. These activities are a family's developmental tasks, summarized in Table 4-2.

FAMILY LIFE CYCLE

Our examination of the nature of families has shown that they are social systems with cultural values, structures, roles, and functions. Another way to understand families is to view them developmentally.

DEVELOPMENTAL THEORY

Knowledge of the family life cycle comes from developmental theory. From the early work of Erikson (1963), Piaget (1973), Havighurst (1972), and others, we know that individuals, as they grow and mature, progress through certain stages of development. Erikson, for instance, described eight developmental levels, each with its accompanying basic task and its negative counterpart if the task was not achieved (1963). Infants, at level one, must learn basic trust or else they will acquire basic mistrust. Toddlers, at level two, need to learn autonomy or they will acquire shame and guilt. Preschoolers focus on initiative, and school-agers on industry, or else they feel guilt and inferiority respectively. Adolescents are concerned with identity as opposed to role confusion, and young adults with intimacy as opposed to isolation. Middle-aged people are involved with generativity and older adults with ego-integrity, or else they will experience stagnation and despair, respectively. Progress through each stage, Erikson said, varied for each person and was influenced by many factors, both genetic and environmental. Failure to achieve the basic task of each level would lead to its negative counterpart and result in mental illness.

Havighurst (1972) listed many developmental tasks accompanying six basic life phases — from infancy through later maturity. He believed development was based on cognitive learning stemming from the individual's physical, social, and psychic readiness.

Piaget (1973) described four levels of cognitive development from birth to 15 years of age. During the sensori-motor stage (0–2 years), thought is based on physical manipulation of objects and events. In the preoperational stage (2–7 years), the individual acquires knowledge through the symbolism of language. Concrete operations (7–11 years) describes the stage when individuals attempt solution of concrete problems with logical reasoning. Finally, formal operations (11–15 years) is the stage when individuals begin to practice true logical thought and to deal with abstract concepts. They begin to think deductively, synthesize material and solve problems scientifically. Piaget proposed that each stage incorporated and built on learning from the previous stage, with modifications continuing throughout life.

Just as individuals progress through defined developmental stages, so do families. Many of the characteristics of individual growth also apply to families. For example, we know that families, while maintaining themselves as entities, change continuously. These changes occur in a sequential pattern of stages known as the family life cycle (Duvall and Miller, 1985), sometimes called the "family career" (Aldous, 1978). Families inevitably grow and develop as the individuals within them mature and adapt to the demands of successive life changes. A family's composition, set of roles, and network of interpersonal relationships change with the passage of time (Friedman, 1986). Family structures, too, vary with each stage of the family life cycle.

Consider the following example. The Jordans, a young married couple, concentrated on learning their respective roles of husband and wife and building a mutually satisfying marriage relationship. With the birth of their first child, Scott, the family composition and relationships changed, and role transitions occurred. The Jordans were not only husband and wife but father, mother, and son; the family had added three new roles. Within the next four years, two daughters, Lisa and Tammy, were born. The introduction of each new member not only increased family size but significantly reorganized family living. As Duvall and Miller (1985) point out, no two children are ever born into precisely the same family. One by one the children entered school; Mrs. Jordan went to work for a florist; and soon Scott was leaving for college. The Jordans, like every family, were moving through the family life cycle and, in so doing, were experiencing a series of developmental changes.

FAMILY DEVELOPMENTAL STAGES

Family development through the life cycle occurs in a predictable pattern of recognizable stages. Gross examination of family development shows two broad stages: *expansion* of the family as new members are added and roles and relationships are increased, and *contraction* of the family as members leave to start lives of their own. Within this framework of the expanding-contracting family are more specific stages that mark changing patterns in family growth and development. Family theorists describe similar stages in the family life cycle, which begins when two people become committed to each other, thereby forming their own family, and continues through the years of having, rearing, and launching children, to the empty nest stage, retirement years, and finally the death of both partners.

Family developmental stages, as outlined by various researchers, reflect three different criteria, first suggested by Duvall and Hill (1948) and described by Aldous (1978). One way to determine family life cycle stages is to look at changes in the number of family members. Stages based on this criterion are listed as follows:

1. Establishment
2. Expanding—from the time the first child enters the family, until the arrival of the last child
3. Stable—child rearing until the first child leaves
4. Contracting—period until the last child leaves
5. Couple alone

A second criterion bases family life cycle stages on the age and school placement of the oldest child.

1. Family with infant (0–2 years)
2. Family with preschooler (3–5 years)
3. Family with school-aged child (6–12 years)
4. Family with adolescent (13–20 years)
5. Family with young adult (21 years to oldest child leaving)

A third criterion focuses on family changes connected with the husband/father's occupational retirement. After family establishment and children leaving home there were middle and aging phases, with aging lasting from the father's retirement until the death of one spouse (Aldous, 1978).

Duvall eventually combined all three criteria into eight stages, which are depicted graphically in Figure 4-7 (Duvall and Miller, 1985).

In this model the age of the oldest child serves as a criterion for demarcation between stages. A family enters the preschool stage, for instance, when the oldest child is 2½ years of age and moves into the school stage when the oldest child is 6 years of age, even though the family may have other younger children. The size of each wedge in the circle reflects that stage's relative

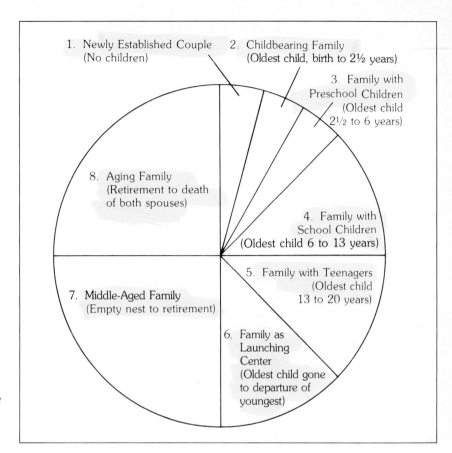

Figure 4-7
Duvall's eight stages of the nuclear family life cycle. Size of wedge reflects relative percent of total life cycle spent in each stage.

length. As a result of societal changes (particularly increased life span and changing roles and career patterns for women), families are having fewer children, the child-rearing period is shorter, and the median length of marriage has increased to 43.6 years (Aldous, 1978). In addition, an increasing number of couples are waiting to start their families (Wilkie, 1981). Many women desire to complete a higher degree or other training, gain more work experience, become more firmly established in a career ladder, or have a stronger financial base before having children. Because of these and other patterns mentioned earlier, couples are spending a longer portion of their lives together alone, thus expanding stages 1, 7, and 8.

FAMILY DEVELOPMENTAL TASKS

To progress through the stages of the life cycle, a family must carry out its basic functions and the developmental tasks associated with those functions (see Table 4-2). Unlike individual developmental tasks, which are specific to each age level, family developmental tasks are ongoing throughout the life cycle. All families, for instance, must provide for the physical needs of their members at every stage. The manner and degree to which each function is carried out will vary, however, depending on how well members are meeting their individual developmental tasks and on the demands of each particular stage. Physical maintenance, for example, will be affected by parents' ability to accept responsibility and seek out the necessary resources to provide food, clothing, and shelter for their children. At early stages, children will usually be dependent on their parents for meeting these needs; at the school, teenage, and launching stages, however, children may increasingly contribute to home management and family income. The responsibility for these tasks shifts from parents to other family members as well.

Some functions require greater emphasis at certain stages. Socialization, for example, consumes much of a family's time during the early years of member development. These same functions and their associated developmental tasks can be further broken down into actions specific to certain stages. A family, for example, while carrying out its function of maintaining controls, sets clearly defined limits for children at the preschool stage: "Do not cross the street," "You may have dessert only after you finish your vegetables," "Bedtime is at 8:00 P.M." During the school stage, control activities may center around allocating responsibilities and division of labor within the family: "Feed the dog," "Clean your room," "Take out the trash." When a family reaches the teenage stage, its control function increasingly focuses on the relationships between family members and outsiders. It may regulate some activities through means such as setting a "home by midnight" limit. In other areas, such as moral conduct, controls may use family values and thus be more subtle. A family at this stage must recognize the need for young people to assume increasing responsibility for their own behavior as well as realize its own diminishing control over members. Duvall and Miller (1985) describe these activities as "stage-critical" family developmental tasks (see Table 4-3).

EMERGING FAMILY PATTERNS

Up to this point, our discussion of the family life cycle has focused primarily on the nuclear family. Since we encounter many nuclear families in community health, the family life cycle provides a useful means for analyzing their growth and development. However, other family structures, such as single adults living alone, single-parent families, newly merged families after death or divorce, or couples who never have children, follow different life cycle patterns. They do not fit the framework just presented and require different criteria for analysis. Researchers in family theory have yet to describe nonnuclear family stages in any systematic fashion. Stein (1981) suggests the notion of a "life-spiral" rather than a life cycle pattern to more realistically describe the fluctuations of contemporary nontraditional families. Aldous (1978) has suggested the following stages for families of divorced mothers who have custody of their children and do not remarry.

Stage 1 Establishment of the single-parent family

Stage 2 Mother institutes or reinstitutes her work-life career

Stage 3 Mother with adolescents

Stage 4 Mother with young adults

Stage 5 Mother in the middle years

Stage 6 The retirement of mother from work-life career or parental responsibilities

Carter and McGoldrick (1980) suggest phases for divorce and remarriage and propose that each phase is accompanied by emotional transitions and certain developmental concerns. Tables 4-4 and 4-5 show these phases.

Table 4-3
Selected Stage-Critical Family Developmental Tasks

Stage of Family Life Cycle	Family Position	Stage-Critical Family Developmental Tasks
Married couple	Wife Husband	Establishing a mutually satisfying marriage Adjusting to pregnancy and the promise of parenthood Fitting into the kin network
Childbearing	Wife-mother Husband-father Infant daughter, or son, or both	Having and adjusting to infants, and encouraging their development Establishing a satisfying home for both parents and infant(s)
Preschool-age	Wife-mother Husband-father Daughter-sister Son-brother	Adapting to the critical needs and interests of preschool children in stimulating, growth-promoting ways Coping with energy depletion and lack of privacy as parents
School-age	Wife-mother Husband-father Daughter-sister Son-brother	Fitting into the community of school-age families in constructive ways Encouraging children's educational achievement
Teenage	Wife-mother Husband-father Daughter-sister Son-brother	Balancing freedom with responsibility as teenagers mature and emancipate themselves Establishing outside interests and careers as growing parents
Launching center	Wife-mother-grandmother Husband-father-grandfather Daughter-sister-aunt Son-brother-uncle	Releasing young adults into work, military service, college, marriage, etc., with appropriate rituals and assistance Maintaining a supportive home base
Middle-aged parents	Wife-mother-grandmother Husband-father-grandfather	Rebuilding the marriage relationship Maintaining kin ties with older and younger generations
Aging family members	Widow or widower Wife-mother-grandmother Husband-father-grandfather	Coping with bereavement and living alone Closing the family home or adapting it to aging Adjusting to retirement

Source: Adapted from Duvall and Miller (1985).

Table 4-4
Life Cycle Phases in Divorce

Phase	Emotional Transitions	Developmental Issues
Divorce		
1. Decision to divorce	Accepting of inability to resolve marital tensions	Acceptance of one's own part in the failure of the marriage
2. Planning breakup of the system	Supporting viable arrangements for all parts of the system	a. Working cooperatively on problems of custody, visitation, finances b. Dealing with extended family about the divorce
3. Separation	a. Willingness to continue cooperative coparental relationship b. Work on resolution of attachment to spouse	a. Mourning loss of intact family b. Restructuring marital and parent-child relationships; adaptation to living apart c. Realignment of relationships with extended family; staying connected with spouse's extended family
4. Divorce	More work on emotional divorce: Overcoming hurt, anger, guilt	a. Mourning loss of intact family: giving up fantasies of reunion b. Retrieval of hopes, dreams, expectations from the marriage c. Staying connected with extended families
Post-Divorce Family		
1. Single-parent family	Willingness to maintain parental contact with ex-spouse and support contact of children with ex-spouse and his or her family	a. Making flexible visitation arrangements with ex-spouse and his or her family b. Rebuilding own social network
2. Single-parent (Noncustodial)	Willingness to maintain parental contact with ex-spouse and support custodial parent's relationship with children	Finding ways to continue effective parenting relationships with children

Source: Carter and McGoldrick (1980).

Because of recent societal changes, today's community health nurses increasingly need to understand and help families that fall into three main types. One type includes growing numbers of adolescent unwed mothers whose own developmental needs as well as limited parenting skills present a challenge to the community health nurse. A second type comprises a great number of couples who, after widowhood or divorce, have remarried and merged two families. Merged families require considerable adjustment and relearning of roles, tasks, communication patterns, and relationships (Papernow, 1984). The community health nurse needs to understand the complex dynamics of such situations and offer support and encouragement as family members work through these problems. The third family type is made up of elderly couples, or more frequently, elderly individuals (most often women) living alone. As the population ages, an increasing number of elderly people live alone. Even when an elderly person moves to a retirement home or a home with assisted living, he or she often feels isolated, cut off from meaningful contacts with friends and family. Many of these aging families do not understand or practice the appropriate stage-specific functions and develop-

Table 4-5
Life Cycle Phases in Remarriage

Steps	Emotional Transitions	Developmental Issues
1. Entering new relationship	Recovery from loss of first marriage (adequate "emotional divorce")	Recommitment to marriage and to forming a family; readiness to deal with complexity and ambiguity
2. Conceptualizing and planning new marriage and family	Accepting one's own fears and those of new spouse and children about remarriage and forming a stepfamily Accepting need for time and patience for adjustment to complexity and ambiguity of a. multiple new roles b. boundaries: space, time, membership, and authority c. affective issues: guilt, loyalty conflicts, desire for mutuality, unresolvable past hurts	a. Working on openness in the new relationships to avoid pseudomutuality b. Planning for maintenance of cooperative coparental relationships with ex-spouses c. Planning to help children deal with fears, loyalty conflicts, and membership in two systems d. Realignment of relationships with extended family to include new spouse and children e. Planning maintenance of connections for children with extended family of ex-spouse(s)
3. Remarriage and reconstitution of family	Final resolution of attachment to previous spouse and ideal of "intact" family Acceptance of a different model of family with permeable boundaries	a. Restructuring family boundaries to allow for inclusion of new spouse-stepparent b. Realignment of relationships throughout subsystems to permit interweaving of several systems c. Making room for relationships of all children with biological (noncustodial) parents, grandparents, and other extended family d. Sharing memories and histories to enhance stepfamily integration

Source: Carter and McGoldrick (1980).

mental tasks that would help them adjust and experience positive aging. Again, the community health nurse can offer assistance by understanding family developmental theory and tailoring family interventions accordingly.

Summary

Community health nurses' effectiveness in working with families depends on their understanding of family theory and characteristics.

Every family is unique; its needs and strengths are different from those of every other family. At the same time, each family is alike because all share certain universal characteristics. Five of these universals have particular significance for community health nursing.

First, every family is a small social system. All the members within a family are interdependent; what one does affects the others and, ultimately, influences total family health. Families, as social systems set and maintain boundaries that unite them and preserve their autonomy while also differentiating them from others. Because these boundaries are semipermeable, families engage in an input-output energy exchange with external resources. Families are equilibrium-seeking and adaptive systems that strive to adjust to internal and external life changes. Also, like other systems, families are goal directed. They exist for the purpose of promoting their members' development.

Second, every family has its own culture, its own set of values and rules for operation. Family values influence member beliefs and behaviors. These same values prescribe the types of roles that each member assumes. A family's culture also determines its power distribution and decision-making patterns.

Third, every family has structure that can be categorized as either traditional or nontraditional. The most common traditional family structure is the nuclear family, consisting of husband, wife, and children living together. Other traditional structures include husband and wife living as a couple alone, single-parent families, single-adult families, multigenerational families, and kin networks. Nontraditional family structures incorporate many family forms, some recognized as legitimate by society and others not easily accepted. These variations include commune families, group marriages, group networks, unmarried single-parent families, and unmarried couples living together with or without children. Variant family structures remind us that the nuclear family is no longer the only viable family form, that people experience many family structures during their lifetimes, and that a family's ability to perform its basic functions is influenced by its structure.

Fourth, every family has certain basic functions. A family gives its members affection and emotional support. It promotes security through provision of an accepting, stable environment in which physical needs are maintained. A family gives its members a sense of social and personal identity, and it influences their placement in the social order. It provides members with affiliation, a sense of belonging. It socializes its members by teaching basic values and attitudes that determine their behavior. Finally, the family maintains order through establishment of social controls.

Fifth, every family moves through stages in its life cycle. Families develop in two broad stages: a period of expansion when they add new members and roles and a period of contraction when members leave. More specific developmental stages within this expanding-contracting framework can also be identified. For the nuclear family we see eight stages ranging from the newly established couple through childbearing, child rearing, and child launching to middle and old age.

While advancing through each developmental stage in the life cycle, a family must continue to perform all of its basic functions. It must also accomplish certain tasks specific to each stage. Life cycle stages and developmental tasks vary for families with differing structures.

Study Questions

1. Select a family (other than your own) that you know well and analyze it, answering the following questions:
    a. If the major breadwinner in this family became permanently disabled and unable to work, how would the family most likely respond—immediately and in the long run?

    b. What are some of this family's rules for operating and the values underlying those rules?

    c. Structurally, what kind of family is it?

    d. What are the strongest and weakest functions performed by this family and why do you think so?

    e. In what developmental stage is this family and how does that affect its functioning?

2. Describe the major differences that you see between a nuclear family and a single-parent family. How do these differences affect the families' roles and functions?

3. Discuss the pros and cons of a married couple both working at full-time careers. Should they have children? In what ways could a community health nurse assist this couple? Whose values should be considered in making decisions about their family life?

References

Aldous, J. (1978). *Family careers: Developmental change in families.* New York: Wiley.

Baranowski, T., and P. Nader. (1985). Family health behavior. In D. Turk and R. Kerns (eds.), *Health, illness, and families.* New York: Wiley.

Bott, E. (1971). *Family and social network: Roles, norms, and external relationships in ordinary urban families.* 2nd ed. New York: Macmillan.

Carter, E. A., and M. McGoldrick (eds.). (1980). *The family life cycle.* New York: Gardner.

Cherlin, A. J. (1981). *Marriage, divorce, remarriage.* Cambridge: Harvard University Press.

Clark, J. (1986). Supporting the family . . . heading off a breakdown. *Nursing Times* 82(32): 33–34.

Dreikurs, R. (1964). *Children: The challenge.* New York: Meredith.

Duvall, E. M., and R. Hill, cochairs. (1948). Report of the Committee on the Dynamics of Family Interaction, prepared at the request of the National Conference on Family Life. Washington, D.C. (mimeographed).

Duvall, E. M., and B. Miller. (1985). *Marriage and family development.* 6th ed. New York: Harper & Row.

Erikson, E. (1963). *Childhood and society.* 2nd ed. New York: Norton.

Farber, B. (1973). *Family and kinship in modern society.* Glenview, Ill.: Scott, Foresman.

Friedman, M. M. (1986). *Family nursing: Theory and assessment.* 2nd ed. New York: Appleton-Century-Crofts.

Getty, C., and S. Humphreys. (eds.). (1981). *Understanding the family: Stress and change in American family life.* New York: Appleton-Century-Crofts.

Goode, W. J. (1977). The family as a social institution. In W. J. Goode (ed.), *Principles of sociology.* New York: McGraw-Hill.

Gordon, M. (ed.) (1978). *The American family in social-historical perspective.* New York: St. Martin's.

A growing crisis: Disadvantaged women and their children. (1983). Washington, D.C.: U.S. Commission on Civil Rights.

Havighurst, R. J. (1972). *Developmental tasks and education.* 3rd ed. New York: McKay.

Helvie, C. O. (1981). *Community health nursing: Theory and process.* New York: Harper & Row.

Lancaster, J. B., J. Altmann, A. S. Rossi, and L. R. Sherrod. (1987). *Parenting across the life span.* New York: Aldine de Gruyter.

Leavitt, M. (1982). *Families at risk: Primary prevention in nursing practice.* Boston: Little, Brown.

Miller, J. R., and E. H. Janosik. (1980). *Family-focused care.* New York: McGraw-Hill.

Neuman, B. (1983). Family intervention using the Betty Neuman health care model. In I. W. Clements and F. B. Roberts, *Family health: A theoretical approach to nursing care.* New York: Wiley.

Olson, D., H. I. McCubbin, and Associates. (1983). *Families: What makes them work.* Beverly Hills, Calif.: Sage.

Papernow, P. (1984). The stepfamily cycle: An experiential model of stepfamily development. *Family Relations* 33: 355.

Pearce, D. M., and H. McAdoo. (1981). *Report of the National Advisory Commission on Economic Opportunity.* Washington, D.C.: U.S. Government Printing Office.

Piaget, J. (1973). *The psychology of intelligence.* Totowa, N. J.: Littlefield, Adams.

President's Commission for a National Agenda for the Eighties. (1981). Helping families — To help themselves. *International Journal of Family Therapy* 3: 208–233.

Putt, A. M. (1978). *General systems theory applied to nursing.* Boston: Little, Brown.

Robischon, P., and J. A. Smith. (1977). Family assessment. In A. Reinhardt and M. Quinn (eds.), *Current practice in family-centered community nursing.* St. Louis: C. V. Mosby.

Ross, M. M., and H. Helmer. (1988). A comparative analysis of Neuman's model using the individual and family as the units of care. *Public Health Nursing* 5(1): 30–36.

Satir, V. (1972). *Peoplemaking.* Palo Alto, Calif.: Science and Behavior Books.

Scanzoni, J. (1983). *Shaping tomorrow's family: Theory and policy for the 21st century.* Beverly Hills, Calif.: Sage.

Spradley, J. P., and D. W. McCurdy. (1980). *Anthropology: The cultural perspective.* 2nd ed. New York: Wiley.

Stein, P. J. (ed.). (1981). *Single life: Unmarried adults in social context.* New York: St. Martin's.

Stephens, W. W. (1963). *The family in cross-cultural perspective.* New York: Holt, Rinehart & Winston.

Sussman, M. B. (1971). Family systems in the 1970s: Analysis, policies, and programs. *Annals of the American Academy* 396: 216–35.

U.S. Bureau of Census. (1988). *Statistical abstract of the U.S.* 108th ed. Washington, D.C.: U.S. Department of Commerce.

U.S. Bureau of Census. (1989). *Current population reports: Marital status and living arrangements.* Washington, D.C.: U.S. Department of Commerce, Series P-20, No. 433.

van den Berghe, P. L. (1979). *Human family systems: An evolutionary view.* New York: Elsevier North Holland.

Wilkie, J. (1981). The trend toward delayed parenthood. *Journal of Marriage and the Family* 43(3): 583.

Selected Readings

Aldous, J. (1978). *Family careers: Developmental change in families.* New York: Wiley.

Baranowski, T., and P. Nader. (1985). Family health behavior. In D. Turk and R. Kerns (eds.), *Health, illness, and families.* New York: Wiley.

Cherlin, A. J. (1981). *Marriage, divorce, remarriage.* Cambridge: Harvard University Press.

Colon, F. (1980). The family life cycle of the multi-problem poor family. In E. Carter and M. McGoldrick (eds.), *The family life cycle: A framework for family therapy.* New York: Gardner.

Combrinck-Graham, L. (1985). A developmental model for family systems. *Family Process* 24(2): 139–50.

Duvall, E. M., and B. Miller. (1985). *Marriage and family development.* 6th ed. New York: Harper & Row.

Friedman, M. M. (1986). Family nursing: Theory and assessment. 2nd ed. New York: Appleton-Century-Crofts.

Getty, C., and S. Humphreys. (1981). *Understanding the family: Stress and change in American family life.* New York: Appleton-Century-Crofts.

Goode, W. J. (1977). The family as a social institution. In W. J. Goode (ed.), *Principles of Sociology.* New York: McGraw-Hill.

Howard, J. (1978). *Families.* New York: Simon & Schuster.

Hymovich, D., and M. Barnard (eds.). (1973). *Family health care.* New York: McGraw-Hill.

Knafl, K. A., and H. K. Grace. (1978). *Families across the life cycle.* Boston: Little, Brown.

Lancaster, J. B., J. Altmann, A. S. Rossi, and L. R. Sherrod. (1987). *Parenting across the life span.* New York: Aldine de Gruyter.

Leavitt, M. (1982). *Families at risk: Primary prevention in nursing practice.* Boston: Little, Brown.

Martin, E. P., and J. M. Martin. (1978). *The black extended family.* Chicago: University of Chicago Press.

Masnick, G., and M. J. Bane. (1980). *The nation's families: 1960–1990.* Boston: Auburn.

McCubbin, H. I. (1979). Integrating coping behavior in family stress theory. *Journal of Marriage and the Family* 41: 237–44.

Mendes, H. A. (1979). Single-parent families: A typology of lifestyles. *Social Work* 24: 193.

Miller, J. R., and E. H. Janosik. (1980). *Family-focused care.* New York: McGraw-Hill.

Mills, D. (1984). A model for stepfamily development. *Family Relations* 33: 365.

Nelson, M., and G. Nelson. (1982). Problems of equity in the reconstituted family: A social exchange analysis. *Family Relations* 31: 223.

Neuman, B. (1983). Family intervention using the Betty Neuman health care model. In I. W. Clements and F. B. Roberts, *Family health: A theoretical approach to nursing care.* New York: Wiley.

Norton, A. (1980). The influence of divorce on traditional life cycle measures. *Journal of Marriage and the Family* 42: 63.

Olson, D., H. I. McCubbin, and Associates. (1983). *Families: What makes them work.* Beverly Hills, Calif. Sage.

Papernow, P. (1984). The stepfamily cycle: An experiential model of stepfamily development. *Family Relations* 33: 355.

Pratt, L. (1976). *Family structure and effective health behavior: The energized family.* Boston: Houghton Mifflin.

Putt, A. M. (1978). *General systems theory applied to nursing.* Boston: Little, Brown.

Scanzoni, J. (1983). *Shaping tomorrow's family: Theory and policy for the 21st century.* Beverly Hills, Calif.: Sage.

Schulman, G. (1981). Divorce, single parenthood, and stepfamilies: Structural implications of these transitions. *International Journal of Family Therapy* 3:87–112.

Stein, P. J. (ed.). (1981). *Single life: Unmarried adults in social context.* New York: St. Martin's.

Turk, D., and R. Kearns (eds.). (1985). *Health, illness, and families.* New York: Wiley.

Wilkie, J. (1981). The trend toward delayed parenthood. *Journal of Marriage and the Family* 43(3): 583.

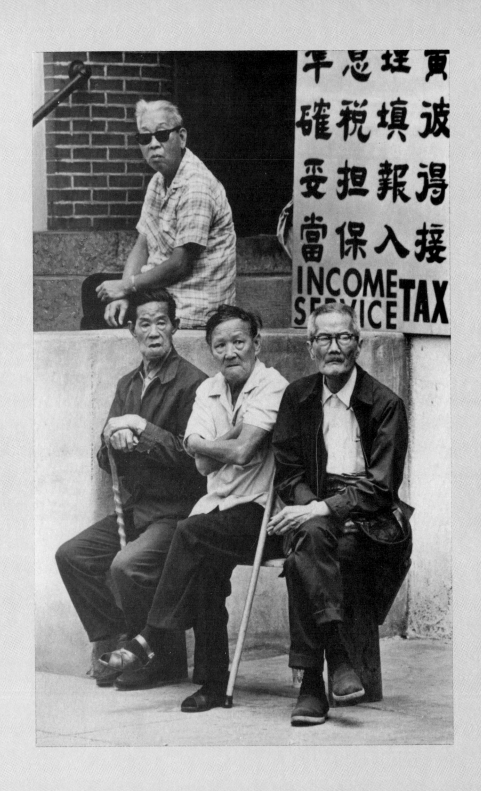

5 Culture and Community

Most health professionals value individuality. We are delighted to see children grow and develop in unique ways. We applaud someone's creative achievement. We each have preferences about the kind of food we eat, the way we dress, and how we decorate our living quarters. The right to be ourselves and different from others is highly valued. But although individuality is part of our culture, we recognize limits to the range of acceptable differences. People whose behavior falls outside that range become deviants or misfits. Our culture approves moderate social drinking but not alcoholism. Why are some behaviors acceptable and others not? Why do so many health professionals have difficulty trying to convince their clients to accept new ways of thinking and acting? Explanations can be found by examining the concept of culture and its application to community health nursing practice.

THE MEANING OF CULTURE

Culture refers to the ideas, values, and behavior that are shared by members of some social group. It is a design for living, a way of life.

As we defined it in Chapter 4, culture is "the acquired knowledge that people use to interpret experience and to generate behavior" (Spradley and McCurdy, 1980, p. 2). More than simply custom or ritual, culture is a way of organizing and thinking about life. It gives people a sense of security about their behavior; without having to consciously think about it, they know how to act. Culture also provides the underlying values and beliefs upon which people's behavior is based. For example, culture determines the value we place on achievement, independence, work, and leisure. It forms the basis for our definitions of male and female roles and determines our responses to authority figures. As anthropologist Edward Hall says, "Culture controls our lives" (1959, p. 38).

INFLUENCE ON BEHAVIOR

Every community, every social or ethnic group, has its own culture. Furthermore, all the individual members behave in the context of that specific culture. Each of us belongs to a group or set of overlapping groups that influences our thoughts and actions. Even very small elements of everyday living are influenced by our culture. For instance, culture determines the distance we stand from another person while talking (Meisenhelder, 1982). A comfortable talking distance for Americans is at least two and a half feet (Figure 5-1), while Latin Americans prefer a shorter distance, often only 18 inches, for dialogue. Consider how culture influences our perception of time. When we make an appointment to see someone, we expect the other person to be on time or not more than a few minutes late. To keep a person waiting (or to be kept waiting) for 45 minutes or an hour is insulting and intolerable. Yet there are other cultures and subcultures, including Native American and Asian groups, whose response to time is much more flexible; their members think nothing of waiting or keeping someone else waiting for an hour or two. Clearly, culture, as Benjamin Paul puts it, "is a blueprint for social living" (cited in Landy, 1977, p. 233).

RELATIONSHIP TO HEALTH CARE

Culture, because it so profoundly influences thinking and behavior, is an essential dimension of health care. Just as physical and psychological factors determine clients' needs and attitudes toward health and illness, so too does

Figure 5-1
Culture influences everyday behavior by giving people a prescribed set of norms for their conduct. It has taught these people how far apart to stand during a casual conversation.

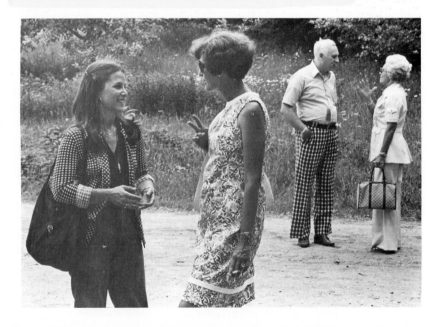

culture. Kark emphasizes that "culture is perhaps the most relevant social determinant of community health" (1974, p. 149). Culture influences diet and eating practices. In fact, Hanlon and Pickett comment that because of culturally derived preferences, "one of the most difficult problems is changing eating habits" (1984, p. 283). Culture determines how people rear their children, react to pain, cope with stress, deal with death, respond to health practitioners, and value the past, present, and future, yet the concept of culture is not always clearly understood or incorporated into health care. Many nursing care plans omit consideration of clients' cultural and social needs. Others may include them only after some painful experience at the client's expense, as is shown in the following illustration.

Maria Juárez, a 53-year-old Mexican-American widow, was referred to a community health nursing agency by a clinic. Her married daughter reported that Mrs. Juárez was having severe and prolonged vaginal bleeding and needed medical attention. The daughter had made several appointments for her mother at the clinic, but Mrs. Juárez had refused at the last minute to keep any of them.

After two broken home visit appointments, the community health nurse made a drop-in call and found Mrs. Juárez at home. The nurse was greeted courteously and invited to have a seat. After introductions, the nurse explained that she and the others were only trying to help. Mrs. Juárez had caused a lot of unnecessary concern to everyone by not cooperating, she scolded in a friendly tone. Mrs. Juárez quickly apologized and explained that she had felt fine on the days of her broken appointments and saw no need "to bother" anyone. Questioned about her vaginal bleeding, Mrs. Juárez was evasive. "It's nothing," she said, "it comes and goes like always, only maybe a little more." She listened politely, nodding in agreement as the nurse explained the need for her to see a physician. Her promise to come to the clinic the next day, however, was not kept. The staff labeled Mrs. Juárez unreliable and uncooperative.

Mrs. Juárez had been brought up in a traditional Mexican-American culture (Reinert, 1986) that taught her to be submissive and interested primarily in the welfare of her husband and children. She had learned long ago to ignore her own needs and, in fact, found it difficult to identify any personal wants. Her major concern was to avoid causing trouble for others. To have a medical problem, then, was a difficult adjustment. The pain and bleeding had caused her great apprehension. Many Mexican-Americans have a particular dread of sickness and especially hospitalization (Herrera and Wagner, 1977). Furthermore, Mrs. Juárez's culture had taught her the value of modesty. "Female problems" were not discussed openly. This cultural orientation meant that the sickness threatened her modesty and created intense embarrassment. Conforming to Mexican-American cultural values, she had first turned to her family for support. Often it is only under dire circumstances that members of this cultural group seek help from others; to do so means sacrificing pride and dignity (Erkel, 1985). Mrs. Juárez agreed to go to the clinic because refusal would have been disrespectful, but her fear of physicians as well as her extreme reluctance to discuss such a sensitive problem kept her from going. Mrs. Juárez was being asked to take action that violated a number of deeply felt cultural values. Her behavior was far from unreliable and uncooperative. With no opportunity to discuss and resolve the conflicts, she had no other choice.

CULTURAL DIFFERENCES

A major barrier to meeting Mrs. Juárez's needs was a failure by the nurse to recognize cultural differences. In fact, many of the health care system's failures result from this shortsightedness (Patrick et al., 1985). It is most obvious that every group has its own culture when we contrast our way of life with a vastly different one, for example, that of a New Guinea tribe. We easily recognize culture when we see people sleep on the floor together in large extended family groups, eat monkey meat with their fingers from a common bowl, or seldom discipline young children.

Cultural differences, however, are equally strong in the United States (Bullough and Bullough, 1982). Although broad cultural values are shared by many of us, a rich diversity of subcultures also exists. Immigration patterns in recent years have changed the United States' population composition. During the 1970s, roughly half a million immigrants legally entered the United States.

In the first half of the 1980s (1980–1985) over a million had already entered the United States. As shown in Figure 5-2, Asian and Spanish-speaking immigrants were by far the largest groups to enter the United States in the 1980s. The *Harvard Encyclopedia of American Ethnic Groups* (Thernstrom et al., eds., 1980) lists one hundred different ethnic groups living in the United States, 50 of which are significant in size. According to the United States Census Bureau (1989), two of the largest minorities include Spanish-speaking Americans, numbering eighteen million officially (with many more entering illegally), representing approximately 7 percent of the population, and Asian-Americans, numbering roughly 5 million, or approximately 2 percent of the population. (According to informal predictions, half of all Americans will be Spanish-speaking by the year 2000.) The largest minority group in the United States continues to be blacks, numbering close to 30 million, or about 12 percent of the population (U.S. Census Bureau, 1989).

The increase in and great variety of cultural groups reinforces the need to understand and appreciate cultural differences. It also presents a significant challenge to community health nurses, requiring, among other things, that we develop new communication skills to cross language barriers and that we be ready to explore traditional ethnic health and curing practices to determine their effectiveness and safety.

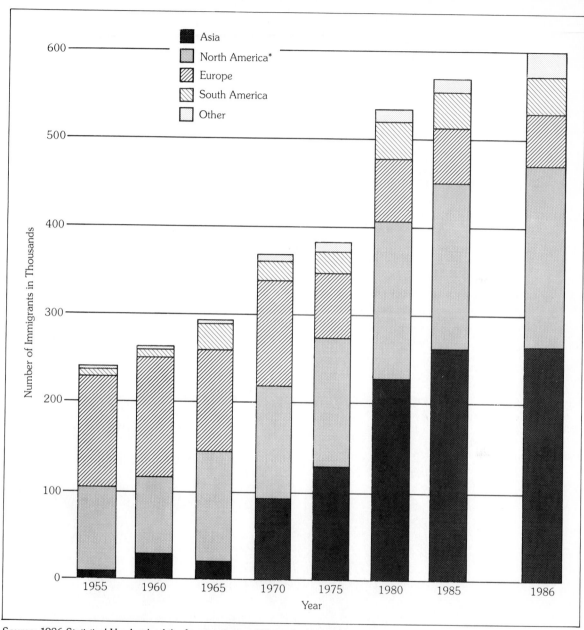

Source: 1986 Statistical Yearbook of the Immigration and Naturalization Service: United States Immigration and Naturalization Service, Washington, D.C.

*North America includes Canada, Mexico, the Caribbean, and Central America.

Figure 5-2
Immigrants admitted by region of birth: selected fiscal years 1955–86.

The members of each subculture retain some of the characteristics of the society from which they came or in which their ancestors lived (Mead, 1960). Some of their beliefs and practices, such as the food they eat, the language they speak at home, the way they celebrate holidays, or their ideas about sickness and healing, remain an important part of their everyday life (Figure 5-3). Native American groups have retained some aspects of their traditional cultures. Mexican-Americans, Irish-Americans, Swedish-Americans, Italian-Americans, Afro-Americans, Puerto Ricans, Chinese-Americans, Japanese-Americans, Vietnamese-Americans, and many other ethnic groups have their own subcultures. Furthermore, certain customs, values, and ideas are unique to the poor, the rich, the middle class, women, men, youth, and the elderly. Many deviant groups, such as narcotic addicts, criminals, and skid row alcoholics, have developed their own subcultures. Regional subcultures, such as that of the Kentucky mountain people, also have distinctive ways of defining the world and coping with problems. Other subcultures, such as those of rural migrant farm workers and urban homeless street people, acquire their own sets of values and patterns for dealing with their environments. Even occupational and professional groups develop their own special languages and outlooks. Nurses, for example, have a special culture with unique vocabulary, values, clothes, and customs. Recognizing such cultural differences is a first step toward cultural understanding.

Figure 5-3
A religious Jewish family lights candles on the sabbath in keeping with their traditional beliefs.

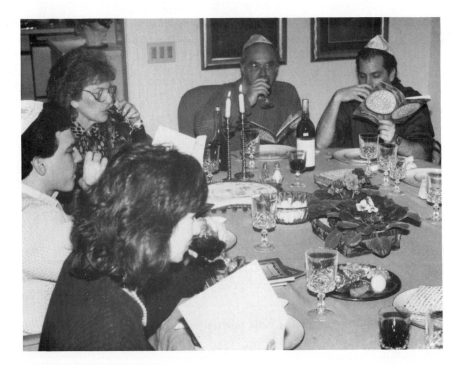

ETHNOCENTRISM

Another barrier to effective care for Mrs. Juárez was judging her behavior by middle-class standards. Good patients, many people believe, appreciate help from health professionals and comply with their requests. This kind of thinking is based on the assumption that "my way is right." It is easy to view one's own way of life as the best and to reject those whose ideas differ as inferior, ignorant, or irrational. Such a belief is called *ethnocentrism* (Leininger, 1970). According to one definition, "ethnocentrism is a mixture of belief and feeling that your own way of life is desirable and actually superior to [that of] others" (Spradley and McCurdy, 1980, p. 27). Ethnocentrism creates biases and misconceptions about human behavior that can cause irreparable damage to interpersonal relationships. Ethnocentrism, as Gagnon (1983, p. 127) points out, "interferes with [nurses'] perception of the knowledge received from others." Mrs. Juárez was labeled unreliable and uncooperative because she failed to conform to prescribed patterns of correct behavior, yet these same patterns contradicted Mrs. Juárez's value system. From her perspective, American health culture must have seemed equally strange and irrational. It is one thing to believe that your way is good for you, and it is another to insist that everyone else conform to it. Here lies the distinction between healthy cultural identification and ethnocentrism. Here also is another clue to the mystery of bridging cultural gaps; rather than apply moral judgments, one should understand and appreciate cultural differences.

Overcoming ethnocentrism requires a concerted effort on the nurse's part to see the world through the eyes of clients. It means learning to set aside, as much as possible, the nurse's own biases and preconceptions. It means attempting to understand the meaning of other people's culture for them, and it means appreciating their culture as important and useful.

CHARACTERISTICS OF CULTURE

In their study of culture, anthropologists and sociologists have made significant contributions to the field of community health. Five characteristics of culture are especially pertinent to our efforts to improve community health: culture is (1) learned, (2) integrated, (3) shared, (4) tacit, and (5) dynamic.

CULTURE IS LEARNED

Patterns of cultural behavior are acquired, not inherited. As Spradley and McCurdy explain, rather than being genetically determined, "human social relations in every society are governed by acquired cultural knowledge" (1980, p. 15). Each of us learns a cultural heritage through the process of socialization, sometimes called *enculturation*. As a little girl grows up in a given society, she acquires certain attitudes, beliefs, and values. She learns how to behave in ways appropriate to that society's definition of the female role. She is learning that culture (Figure 5-4). Ruth Benedict, a noted anthropologist, summarizes this learning process (1934, p. 2):

> The life-history of the individual is first and foremost an accommodation to the patterns and standards traditionally handed down in his community. From the moment of his birth the customs into which he is born shape his experience and behavior. By the time he can talk, he is the little creature of his culture, and by the time he is grown and able to take part in its activities, its habits are his habits, its beliefs his beliefs, its impossibilities his impossibilities.

Figure 5-4
This child at her father's knee learns early to enjoy and value music.

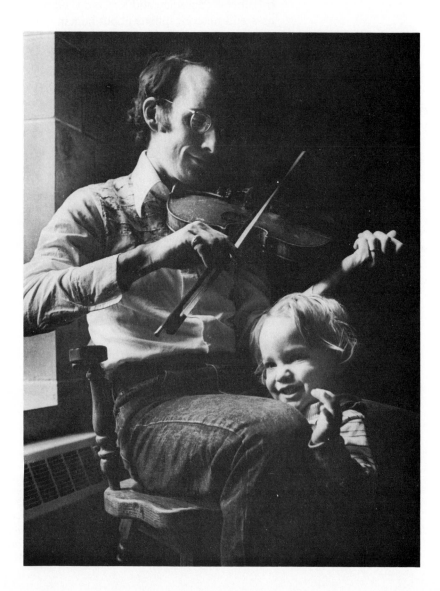

Although culture is learned, the process and results of that learning are different for each person. Each individual has a unique personality and experiences life in a singular way; both these factors influence acquisition of culture. Families, social classes, and other groups within a society differ from one another, and this social variation has important implications for planned change. Since culture is learned, it is possible for parts of it to be relearned. People might change some cultural elements or adopt some new behaviors or values. In addition, George Foster (another well-known anthropologist) points out, "There will be differences in the ease and ability with which [people] continue to learn and in their flexibility in casting off old forms of behavior that conflict with new forms" (1962, p. 18). Some individuals and groups will be more willing than others to try new ways and thus potentially influence change.

CULTURE IS INTEGRATED

Rather than an assortment of various customs and traits, a culture is a functional, integrated whole. As in any system, all the parts of a culture are interrelated and independent. Ruth Benedict, who first examined the systemic nature of culture, says, "A culture, like an individual, is a more or less consistent pattern of thought and action" (1934, p. 46). The various components of a culture, such as its social mores or religious beliefs, perform separate functions that depend upon and articulate in relative harmony with each other to form an operating whole. Benedict emphasizes that this cultural whole is greater than the sum of its individual parts (1934). In other words, to understand culture, one cannot simply describe single traits. Each part must be viewed in terms of its relationships to other parts and to the whole.

Our own culture is an integrated web of ideas and practices. For example, we promote the consumption of three balanced meals a day, a practice tied to our belief that nutrition leads to good health and that prevention is better than cure. These cultural traits, in turn, are related to our values about health. Health, we say, is essential for, among other conditions, maximum energy output and productivity at work. Productivity is important because it enables us to compete effectively. These values are linked to religious beliefs about hard work and taboos against laziness. Nutrition, health, economics, religion, and family are the fibers of a web whose design and usefulness depends upon their integration.

Another person's culturally determined behavior can be understood, therefore, by considering it in the context of that person's larger culture. For example, when parents who are Jehovah's Witnesses refuse blood transfusions for their child, their action is neither irrational nor ignorant. Rather, it represents behavior consistent with the couple's cultural values and beliefs and, in regard to their child's health, results from deeply held religious convictions. The single behavior of refusing blood transfusions, when viewed in context, is part of a larger religious belief system and a basic component of their culture.

The recognition that culture is integrated, that introducing a change in one part of a cultural system will affect other parts, influences community health nursing practice. Mrs. Juárez's cultural beliefs about modesty and self-effacement were related to her culture's definition of the woman's role that, in turn, influenced her interpersonal relationships. To change one practice was to affect many others. Likewise, the request from a nurse to submit to a pelvic examination by a male physician was equal to saying, "Stop behaving like a woman!" Asking certain Native American groups to accommodate to rigid appointment scheduling means requiring them to reframe their concept of time. It also violates their values of patience and pride. Before nurses attempt a change in a person's or group's behavior, they need to ask how that change will affect the clients through its influence on other parts of their culture. Extra time and patience or different strategies may be needed if change is still indicated. Nurses may often find that their own practice system can be modified to preserve the client's cultural values.

CULTURE IS SHARED

Culture is the product of aggregate behavior, not individual habit. Certainly, individuals practice a culture, but customs are phenomena shared by all members of the group (Figure 5-5). Because it is collectively shared, culture has been called *superindividual*. As Murdock explains (1972, p. 258),

> Culture does not depend on individuals. An ordinary habit dies with its possessor, but a group habit lives on in the survivors, and is transmitted from generation to generation. Moreover, the individual is not a free agent with respect to culture. He is born and reared in a certain cultural environment, which impinges upon him at every moment of his life. From earliest childhood his behavior is conditioned by the habits of those around him. He has no choice but to conform to the folkways current in his group.

Knowing that culture is shared helps us to understand human behavior. For example, a community health nurse tried unsuccessfully to persuade an American mother to stop heavily oiling her infant's skin (Taylor, 1973). She discovered that the mother was acting in a tradition of her subculture that held that oil promoted good health. The fact that all the other mothers in that religious group also used oil on their babies proved a powerful deterrent to the change requested by the nurse. Individual health behavior is always influenced by other people of the same culture. Thus, it becomes very difficult for one person to ignore some cultural practice when it will continue to be reinforced by other group members. In fact, group acceptance and a sense of membership almost always depend on conforming to shared cultural practices (Harwood, 1981).

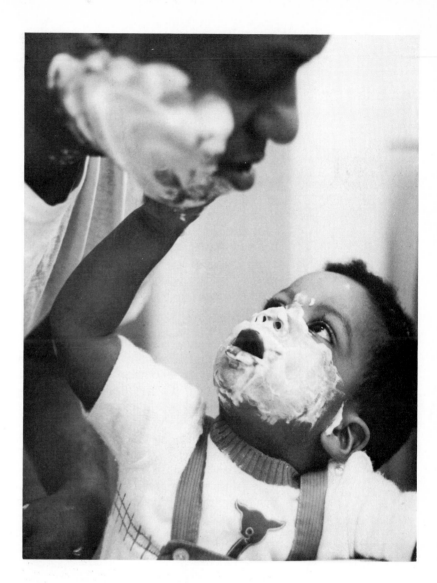

Figure 5-5
Children learn much of
their culture and future
roles through observation
and imitation of adult
behavior. As this little boy
imitates his father shaving,
he is learning to identify
with the male sex role.

Effect on Community Health Nursing

Community health nursing practice with groups and communities takes on added significance when it recognizes that culture is shared. Attempting to provide health care to one individual at a time limits community health nurses' effectiveness. Once a nurse leaves, the client must face all the informal cultural pressures that come from friends and family. On the other hand, focus on an entire group can change that group's health behavior positively and thus affect individual practices. The pattern of oiling young infants, for instance, ceased when the nurse worked with the entire church group. She began with a well-recognized cultural strategy: to work through formal or informal leaders. She contacted the minister and discussed the cultural practice. He admitted that anointing with oil, a Biblical teaching, was one of their beliefs. When she explained her concerns, he agreed that a drop of oil on the head was all that was needed. He clarified this teaching in his next sermon, and as a result, additional health problems also cleared up when other members of the group stopped rubbing oil into wounds and infections (Taylor, 1973).

In another example, a community health nursing instructor with several groups of nursing students successfully developed a series of health classes for a group of Indian women who lived on the northwest coast of Washington state (Aichlmayr, 1969). As the group accepted teaching on subjects such as child care, treatment of burns, and prevention of colds, individual behavior was affected. A group focus also gives the nurse a broader picture of the culture being served and a better understanding of its health needs. Respect and trust of the entire group can be won, thus increasing the chance to improve health practices.

Shared Values

One of the most important elements shared by a culture is its values. Each culture classifies phenomena "into good and bad, desirable and undesirable, right and wrong" (Foster, 1962, p. 18). When people respond in favor of or against some practice, they are reflecting their culture's values about that practice. One man may eagerly anticipate eating a steak for dinner. Another, who believes that eating meat is sacrilegious, will experience revulsion at the idea. Some American subcultures think that loud, vocal expressions are a necessary way to deal with pain. Others value silence and stoicism. Either way, values serve a purpose. Shared values give a culture stability and security; they provide a standard for behavior. Members know what to think and how to act. Values are more deeply rooted than behaviors and consequently change more slowly.

CULTURE IS TACIT

Culture provides a guide for human interaction that is mostly unexpressed, or tacit. Members of a cultural group, without the need for discussion, know how to act and what to expect from one another. Culture provides an implicit set of cues for behavior, not a written set of rules. As Spradley and McCurdy explain, "Much of our culture is outside of awareness. We have learned elaborate cultural rules for acting, feeling, and even thinking, but the rules remain hidden from view" (1980, p. 16). It is like a memory bank where we store knowledge for recall when the situation requires it, but this recall process is generally outside of our consciousness. Culture teaches us the proper tone of voice to use for each occasion. It tells us how close to stand when talking with someone (see Figure 5-1). We learn to make responses that are appropriate to our sex, role, and status. We know what is right and wrong. All of these attitudes and behaviors are so ingrained, so tacit, that we seldom, if ever, need to discuss them. We know. The same is true for each culture.

The difficulty comes when we cross cultural boundaries. No longer does our culture provide a guide for behavior. The cues given by a person in another culture may mean something entirely different. Silence in a group meeting with Native American women was uncomfortable for some nurses but enjoyed by the Indian women, who valued patience and listening (Primeaux and Henderson, 1981). Offering food to a guest, in many cultures, is not merely a social gesture but an important symbol of hospitality and acceptance. To refuse, for any reason, is an insult and a rejection. Thus our behavior, albeit completely well intentioned and appropriate for our own culture, can cause misunderstanding and damage to our relationships with people of another culture.

Because culture is tacit, it is difficult to realize which of our own behaviors may be offensive to people from other groups. It is also difficult to know the meaning and significance of their practices. Consequently, community health nurses have a twofold task in developing cultural awareness; not only must they understand clients' culture, but they must also maintain awareness of the aspects of their own culture they take for granted. Cross-cultural conflict can be resolved through conscious efforts at developing awareness, patience, and acceptance of cultural differences.

CULTURE IS DYNAMIC

Every culture experiences constant change; none is entirely static. Within every cultural group are individuals who generate innovations. More important, there are members who see advantages in other people's ways and are willing to adopt new practices. Each culture, including our own, is an amalgamation of ideas, values, and practices from a variety of sources. This process depends of course, on the extent of exposure to other groups. Nonetheless, every culture is in a dynamic state of adding or deleting components. Functional aspects are retained; less functional ones are eliminated. When this does not occur the cultural group may face serious difficulty. For example, many Southeast Asian refugees in the United States have continued to prepare and eat food in their traditional fashion. As a result, a recent study showed that "between 1975 and 1984, the incidence of trichinosis in the United States was 25 times greater for the Southeast Asian refugee population than for the general United States population" (Stehr-Green and Schantz, 1986, p. 1238).

The dynamic nature of culture is useful to community health nursing for several reasons. Cultures and subcultures do indeed change over time. Patience and persistence are probably key attributes to cultivate when working toward improvement of health behaviors. Another point to remember is that cultures change as their members see greater advantages in the "new ways." Convincing them of these advantages will have to be done in a language they understand and in the context of their own cultural value system. This is an important reason for nurses to develop an understanding of their clients' culture (Leininger, 1977, Orque et al., 1983). Furthermore, change within a culture is usually brought about by certain key individuals who are receptive to new ideas and able to influence their peers. Tapping this resource becomes imperative for successful change. Finally, the health culture can change, too. Consider its changes in the past. Nurses can learn a great deal from their clients and their cultures. And as practitioners discover more effective ways of working with clients, they can and may choose to modify their own practices.

CULTURE AND NURSING PRACTICE

Our examination of the meaning and nature of culture has shown the need to recognize cultural differences and understand clients in the context of their cultural backgrounds. Practically speaking, however, how can the concept of culture be applied to everyday community health nursing practice? The following case studies give some insights.

CULTURE OF THE POOR

This first case study represents a community of people whose way of life is not often considered as a separate subculture (Figure 5-6).

The Jacksons came to the city health center through a welfare referral. Albert, 42 years of age, had left each of his last three jobs after only a few days of employment. The caseworker made a home visit and found Vera Jackson, a shy, thin, 38-year-old woman, with three of her children. The other three were in school. The small, two-bedroom apartment, part of a multiracial, low-income housing project, was "shabby, dirty, and cluttered," according to the referral. Albert seldom came home. Vera held the family together, supplementing the welfare checks through occasional day housework and a night cleaning job in an office building. She didn't know where Albert was, maybe somewhere drunk again. They had been in the city for eight months. Before that, Albert had done itinerant farm labor. Neither had finished high school. "We ain't stayed long anywheres, I guess," Vera told the caseworker. Two of the children had bad colds, one of which was complicated by a deep, chesty cough. The boy felt feverish, and the caseworker, concerned, arranged for Vera to take him to the health center.

The center's waiting room was crowded and noisy; staff hustled impatiently through the hallways. Vera's neighbor at the housing project had warned her, "That place don't like us poor folks." She and the children

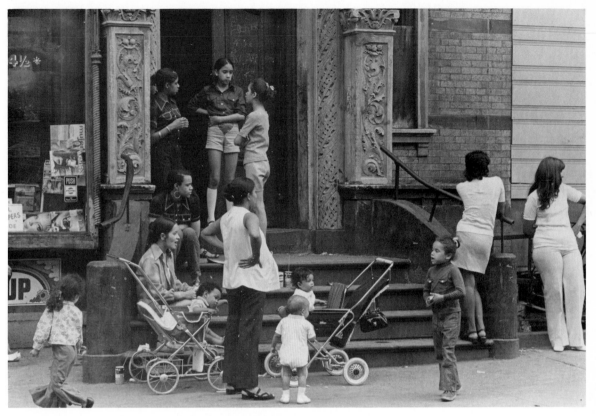

Figure 5-6
The economically disadvantaged population has beliefs and practices that
form a separate subculture and provide its members with a guide for
interaction and daily living.

waited anxiously and then started when the loudspeaker blared out "Jackson." The nurse was friendly but brisk. "Mrs. Jackson," she inquired, "how are you?" There was no time for Vera to reply as the nurse launched into an explanation of the care and prevention of colds while checking the boy and taking his temperature. The physician, too, had many instructions. "These children should be on supplemental vitamins," he commented. "Are they eating well-balanced meals?" Vera was confused. "Do you have any questions?" the nurse asked, handing her the antibiotics and some pamphlets on child growth and development. Vera shook her head. She felt too stupid to say anything, too embarrassed to admit she did not understand. A well-balanced meal, she thought, must mean not overfeeding the kids. That was no problem, considering the little they had to eat. She saw no point in vitamins. Why should they take something when they were well? She could not afford them anyway. She guessed that giving her son the medication at supper, their one "meal" a day, was what the doctor meant when he directed that the boy take it with each meal. Several days later the Jackson boy was hospitalized with pneumonia. Although he recovered, the Jacksons never returned to the health center.

Poverty and Health

The culture of the low-income population can easily be misunderstood by health professionals. Rather than sharing the same values and practices as middle-class professionals, the poor exist in a separate subculture that is diverse and unique. People who are economically disadvantaged come from many backgrounds and bring the values, beliefs, and customs of their backgrounds with them. Because of this diversity, some have challenged the notion of a culture of poverty, warning of the dangers of stereotyping (Pesznecker, 1984; Martin and Henry, 1989). As in any culture, individual variations exist because people belong to overlapping groups even within a specified culture. The nurse needs to be careful to avoid stereotyping the poor, as this may lead to inaccurate assessments and interventions. What, then, is the culture of the poor? We all understand the concept of poverty as a state of being economically disadvantaged or, because of extremely limited resources, being unable to obtain the diet, living conditions, activities, or amenities that fit the general "norms" of society. But the culture of the poor is more than economic. Culture, as we have already discussed, is the ideas, values, and behaviors that a group shares and that provide a design for living. Once a person or group of persons is poor, regardless of the circumstances leading to that poverty, those individuals learn a set of behaviors and adopt a set of values in order to cope with life. It is these values and practices that make up the culture of the poor.

Two attributes, in particular, characterize the culture of the poor. One is that the poor "live strictly and whole-heartedly in the present" (Strauss, 1967, p. 10). Much of the health practitioner's emphasis tends to be preventive and thus future-oriented. Taking vitamins, eating right, and preventing colds all involve a future-orientation, a value conflicting with values in Mrs. Jackson's realm of experience. Economically disadvantaged persons may have an orientation to the present because frequently they must meet immediate needs at the expense of long-term gains.

A second cultural attribute is that the lives of the poor "are uncertain, dominated by recurring crises" (Strauss, 1967, p. 10). Our larger society espouses a value of ordered, controlled, and well-planned lives. We advocate crisis prevention. For the poor, including migrant farm workers and urban homeless people, the demands of daily living with limited resources require adaptation on a day-to-day and even moment-by-moment basis. In many instances, positive health may be valued by this group but unattainable; thus they learn to live with illness and crisis (Pesznecker, 1984).

Many of the poor have learned to accept their life conditions and to make the most of them. Despite limited resources and often limited education, many have positive health practices (Pratt, 1971). Differences in life-style, dress, and behavior can easily lead the nurse to make assumptions about this group that are not necessarily correct. For instance, the poor have been characterized as having low self-esteem (Robertson, 1969). While this may be true in some instances, it is not fair or accurate to make such a generalization. Mrs. Jackson's behavior was less likely caused by low self-esteem than by a number of interacting variables including the confusing, depersonalized atmosphere of the health center.

Mrs. Jackson's cultural differences deserved recognition and acceptance. Her point of view should have been explored, her questions and concerns discussed. She required a relationship of trust with a caring person who understood and appreciated her culture and who offered health assistance within the context of that culture.

The Homeless

Street people, or the homeless, are a subgroup of the poor. This group includes some people who choose this way of life (Spradley, 1988) and many more who are thrust into it through unfortunate circumstances. Unemployment and recent restrictions in health and social welfare programs have given rise to an increasing number of homeless people of all ages, including families with small children. These individuals eke out an existence in the streets; they sleep in subways, cars, missions, or wherever they can find shelter; and they eat scraps or wait in free food lines. Because they lack adequate resources, the homeless population has adopted the culture of the poor.

A large segment of the homeless population comprises dysfunctional individuals and families. Fewer rehabilitative services for the discharged mentally ill and the stresses of modern society contribute to this problem. A study comparing "normal" and homeless persons showed that the latter had "higher amounts of psychiatric disorder, poor health care utilization patterns, and high social dysfunction" (Fischer et al., 1986, p. 519). Another study, conducted in Boston, compared 49 homeless female-headed families to 81 housed female-headed families. The homeless mothers more often had a history of abusive relationships, use of drugs and alcohol. They also had many more serious psychological problems. More supportive relationships, better housing, and income were among the needed solutions offered for addressing their situation (Bassuk and Rosenberg, 1988).

The health status of the homeless is often fair to poor. A study of urban homeless reported that 53 percent had no regular source of health care and 81 percent had no health insurance. Lack of money and health insurance were cited as major barriers to care (Robertson and Cousineau, 1986).

The plight of the homeless has caught public attention in recent years, and new programs are being developed to address their problems. Jonas admonished, "The American Way should not tolerate homelessness" (1986, p. 1084), but much work remains to be done. Community health nurses will have increasing opportunities in the future to provide assistance to the homeless population. At the same time, nurses need to recognize this population's culture and respect their differences before substantive changes can occur.

CULTURE OF IMMIGRANT AND REFUGEE POPULATIONS

The next case study involves clients transplanted from one culture to an entirely different culture; it presents an interesting challenge to the community health nurse (Figure 5-7).

Armed with enthusiasm and pamphlets on pregnancy and prenatal diet, the community health nurse began home visits to the Kim family. Her initial plan was to discuss pregnancy and fetal development, teach diet, and prepare the mother for delivery. Mr. Kim, a graduate student, was present to interpret since Mrs. Kim spoke very little English. Their two boys, three years and one and one half years of age, played happily on the kitchen floor. The family offered tea to the nurse and listened politely as she explained her reasons for coming and added, "How can I be most helpful to you? What would you like from my visits?"

The Kims were grateful for this approach. Hesitant at first, they hinted at Mrs. Kim's fears of American doctors and hospitals; her first two children

Figure 5-7
Clients transplanted from completely different cultures will continue to adhere to their own beliefs and practices. This Vietnamese family enjoys eating a traditional meal with chopsticks—one of many customs it will maintain until selected aspects of the new culture are gradually absorbed.

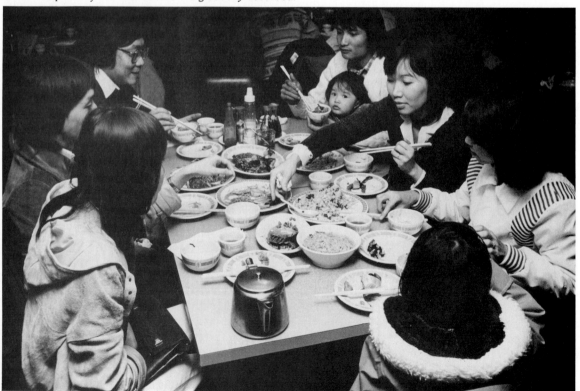

had been born in Korea. None of the family had any experience with Western medicine. They shared some concerns about adjustment to living in the United States. It was difficult to shop in American food stores with their overwhelming variety of foods, many of which the Kims found unfamiliar. Mrs. Kim, who had come from a family whose servants prepared the food, was an inexperienced cook. Servants had also cared for the children, and her role had been that of an aristocrat in hand-tailored silk gowns.

Listening carefully, the nurse began to realize the striking differences between her own and her clients' culture. Her care plans changed. In subsequent visits she determined to learn about Korean culture and base her nursing intervention on that knowledge. She learned about their traditional ways of raising children, male and female roles, and practices related to pregnancy and lactation. She respected their value of "saving face" and attempted never to offend their pride or dignity. As time went on, her interest and respect for their way of life won their trust. She inquired about their cultural practices before attempting any intervention. As a result, the Kims were receptive to her suggestions. Appropriate changes were made in Mrs. Kim's diet, for example, that were still compatible with her food preferences and cultural eating patterns. Because she was not accustomed to drinking milk, she increased her calcium intake by learning to prepare custards (which disguised the milk flavor) and by eating more green, leafy vegetables. After five months, a strong, positive relationship had been established between this family and the nurse. Mrs. Kim delivered a healthy baby girl and looked forward to continued supportive visits from the community health nurse.

Although she had not initially considered the possibility of cultural barriers, the nurse soon recognized that subtle but important differences existed and thus changed her objectives. She proceeded to gain understanding and respect of this family's culture as a means toward improving their health. Whenever possible, she adapted her teaching and suggestions to comply with the Kims' culture. Implicitly, her message was, "Your culture is valuable and necessary for you. The parts of that culture that can continue to be useful, I will help preserve. The parts that are not functional for you in this new society, I will help you change, over time."

An increasing number of immigrants and refugees, like the Kims, from many different countries have been assimilated into American culture in recent years. While they quickly adapt in many respects, learning the language and seeking housing and employment, they continue to operate within the framework of their own cultural beliefs and behaviors. The initial conflict between their culture and American culture often causes *culture shock,* "a form of anxiety that occurs when one is required to interact with others in a cross-cultural situation" (Spradley and McCurdy, 1980, p. 25). Immigrants and refugees find themselves in a strange community with people who act in unfamiliar ways. The same is true for nurses working overseas in unfamiliar countries. No longer are the small but important cues available that orient them to appropriate behavior. Instead they may feel isolated and anxious and even become dysfunctional or ill. Time and learning the new culture are the major remedies. As adjustment occurs, old beliefs and practices that are still functional in the new culture can be retained while others that are not functional must be replaced.

CULTURE OF A NATIVE AMERICAN GROUP

A third case study portrays another distinct culture. Its members were born and live in the United States, assume many American values and practices, yet preserve large aspects of their own culture (Figure 5-8).

As she drove up the dirt road and parked her car next to the community hall, Sandra felt apprehensive. She had been warned by the previous community health nurse that these Indian people were hard to work with: "They're all lazy and unappreciative. You can't get anywhere with them." It was only through the urging of an Indian community aide, Mrs. Brown, that a group of the women had reluctantly agreed to meet with the new nurse. They would see what she had to say.

Sandra's steps echoed hollowly as she walked across the wooden floor of the large room to the far corner where a group of women sat silently in a circle. Only their eyes turned; their faces remained impassive. Mrs. Brown rose slowly, greeted the nurse, and introduced her to the group. Swallowing

Figure 5-8
Many Americans, such as these Native Americans, come from culturally diverse backgrounds and retain many aspects of their original culture.

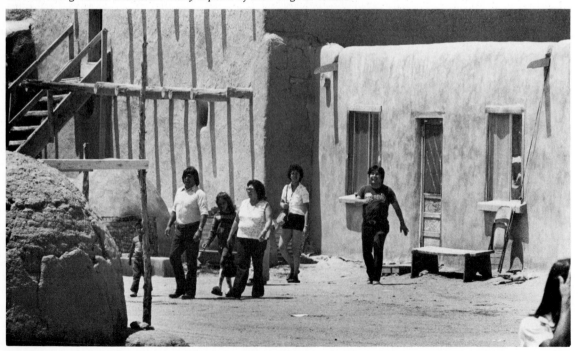

her fear, Sandra smiled. She told them of her background and explained that she had not worked with Indian people before. There was a long silence. No one spoke. Sandra continued, "I'd like to help you if I can, maybe with problems about care of your children when they are sick or questions about how to keep them healthy, but I don't know what you need or want." Silence fell again. She would like to learn from them, she repeated. Would they help her? Again an uncomfortable silence ensued.

Then one woman began to speak. Quietly, but with deep feeling, she described several bad experiences with the previous nurse and the county social worker. Then others spoke up: "They *tell* us what we should do. They don't listen. They say our way is not good." Seeing Sandra's interest and concern, the women continued. One of their main concerns was their children's health. Another was the high incidence of accidents and injuries on the reservation. They wanted to learn how to give first aid. Other concerns were expressed. The group agreed that Sandra could help them by teaching a first-aid class.

In the weeks that followed, Sandra taught several classes on first aid and emergency care. She then began a series of sessions on child health. Each time she would ask the women to choose a topic or problem for discussion and elicit from them their accustomed ways of dealing with each problem, for example, how they handled toilet training or taught their children to eat solid foods. Her goal was to learn as much as she could about their culture and incorporate that information into her teaching, which preserved as many of their practices as possible. Sandra also visited informally with the women in their homes and at community gatherings. She learned about their way of life, their history and their values. For example, patience was highly valued. It was important to be able to wait patiently, even if a scheduled meeting was delayed as much as two hours. It was also important for others to speak, which explained the Indian women's comfort with silences during a conversation. Other values influenced their way of life. Courage, pride, generosity, and honesty were all important determinants of behavior. These were also values by which they judged Sandra and other professionals. Sandra's honesty in keeping her promises enabled the women to trust her. Her generosity in giving her time, helping them occasionally with some household task, and arranging for child care during classes won their respect.

The women came to accept her, and Sandra was invited to eat with them and share in tribal get-togethers. The women criticized and advised her on acceptable ways to speak and act. Her openness and patience to learn and her respect for them as a people had paved the way to improving their health. At first, Sandra felt that her progress was very slow, but this slowness was actually an advantage. She had built a solid foundation of cross-cultural trust, and in the months that followed, she saw many changes in their health practices.

Native Americans, or American Indians, are a diverse group made up of many different tribes scattered throughout the United States. Each tribe or nation has its own distinct language, beliefs, customs, and rituals. Thus the community health nurse cannot assume that knowledge of one group can be generalized to others. Knowledge of certain similarities among the various groups, such as dignity, patience, the importance of the family, and integration of religion into everyday life, can assist the nurse in working with the members of a specific tribe (Primeaux and Henderson, 1981).

PRINCIPLES FOR PRACTICE

In the context of these cases and our earlier discussion of culture, several principles for nursing practice can be identified: (1) recognize and appreciate cultural differences, (2) understand cultural reasons for client behavior, (3) listen and learn before advising, (4) empathize with culturally different clients, (5) show respect for clients and their culture, (6) be patient, and (7) analyze your behavior.

RECOGNIZE AND APPRECIATE CULTURAL DIFFERENCES

Our beliefs and ways of doing things frequently contrast with those of our clients. A first step toward bridging cultural barriers is recognition of those differences. Mrs. Jackson's values and health practices sharply contrasted with those of the center's staff. Failure to recognize these differences led to a breakdown in communication and ineffective care. Another group, black Americans, while diverse and heterogenous, in some respects form a subculture of their own (Jackson, 1981). Many black Americans are caught in a cycle of discrimination and poverty that may account for higher mortality and morbidity rates for this group (Bullough and Bullough, 1982). Their subcultural differences, such as the importance of women's roles and religion in the black family, need to be recognized. Once differences in culture are recognized, it is important to accept and appreciate them. A nurse's ways are valid for the nurse; clients' ways work for them. The nurse visiting the Kims avoided the dangerous ethnocentric trap of assuming that her way was best, and she consequently developed a fruitful relationship with her clients.

UNDERSTAND CULTURAL REASONS FOR CLIENT BEHAVIOR

Each of the client's actions, like our own, is based on underlying culturally learned beliefs and ideas. Mrs. Kim did not like milk because her culture had taught her that it was distasteful. The Indian women's response to waiting or keeping someone else waiting was influenced by their value of patience. Instead of making assumptions or judging client behavior, first learn about the culture that guides that behavior (Calhoun, 1986). Some culturally based reason is causing clients to engage in (or avoid) certain actions. The nurse can collect data about clients' cultures through questioning, observation, and reading. Several cultural assessment guides are available to assist in this activity (Bloch, 1983; Brownlee, 1978; Leininger, 1977; Orque, 1983; Tripp-Reimer, 1985). Tripp-Reimer et al. (1984) suggest that a thorough cultural assessment may be too time-consuming and costly. Instead, they propose the two-phase assessment process outlined in Table 5-1.

Categories to explore in the assessment include values, beliefs, customs, and social structure components.

Conducting a "community cultural assessment" (Gagnon, 1983, p. 128) is another way to enhance understanding of a cultural group. This involves gathering cultural data such as the following in the context of a community assessment (Gagnon, 1983, p. 130).

1. Community value systems
   a. customs (dress, nutritional habits, matriarchy versus patriarchy, emotional reactions)
   b. beliefs (religious and otherwise)
   c. taboos
2. Goals and expectations of the community
3. Community's definition of health
4. Values and attitudes toward health
5. Existing preventive health behavior
6. Perception of health problems
7. Acceptability of health program(s)
8. Perception of the purpose of health program(s)

Table 5-1
Two-phased Cultural Assessment Process

Phase I – Data Collection

Stage 1 Assess values, beliefs, and customs (e.g., ethnic affiliations, religion, decision-making patterns).

Stage 2 Collect problem-specific cultural data (e.g., cultural beliefs and practices related to diet and nutrition).
Make nursing diagnosis.

Stage 3 Determine cultural factors influencing nursing intervention (e.g., child-rearing beliefs and practices that might affect nurse teaching toilet training or child discipline).

Phase II – Data Organization

Step 1 Compare cultural data with
– standards of clients' own culture (e.g., clients' diet compared to cultural norms);
– standards of the nurse's culture
– standards of the health facility providing service.

Step 2 Determine incongruities in above standards.

Step 3 Seek to modify one or more systems (clients', nurse's or the facility's) to achieve maximum congruity.

We describe community assessment in more detail in Chapter 13. Two other methods that have proven effective for study in greater depth of cultural groups are ethnographic interviewing and participant observation (Spradley, 1979, 1980).

LISTEN AND LEARN BEFORE ADVISING

We do not change people's behavior by just giving suggestions or instructions. For Mrs. Jackson as well as the Native American women, this approach had, in fact, the opposite effect. Health teaching must be geared to the client's level of understanding and frame of reference. We accomplish this by finding out about the client first. Asking questions, listening, and observing help us to understand clients and their culture (Orque, 1983). Consequently, nursing intervention can be tailored to their needs.

One study showed that client behavior was interpreted differently by professionals of a different culture than by professionals of the clients' culture (Tripp-Reimer, 1982). Learning clients' culture first is critical to effective nursing care. Interviewing members of a subcultural group, as in Robertson and Cousineau's study of the homeless, provides valuable data for planning interventions (1986).

EMPATHIZE WITH CULTURALLY DIFFERENT CLIENTS

In addition to learning their culture or subculture, we need to understand clients' points of view. We need to stand in their shoes, to identify with them. As the nurse listens, observes, and gradually learns clients' culture, she or he must add a further step of choosing to avoid ethnocentrism. Otherwise the nurse's view of that culture will remain distorted. The ability to show interest, concern and compassion enabled Sandra to win the affection and respect of the Native American women. It told the Kims that their nurse cared about them. These nurses participated in the feelings and ideas of their clients. Empathizing, or identifying intellectually, with clients gives them needed reassurance and often provides the motivation to adopt new health behaviors (Robertson, 1969).

SHOW RESPECT FOR CLIENTS AND THEIR CULTURE

Respect is shown in many ways. When Sandra involved the Native American women in decisions and gave them choices, she was showing respect. When the nurse gave positive recognition to the importance of the Kims' culture, she was showing respect. Within the United States, people of different cultures and subcultures particularly need respect. Their ways are in contrast to the dominant culture. It is difficult for them to retain pride in their life-styles, or in themselves, when constantly reminded that their ways are inferior. The message may be only implied or even unintentional. Such was the case for Mrs. Jackson. The health center's routine and the manner of the staff were certainly not meant intentionally to show disrespect. They did, nevertheless, and Mrs. Jackson was intimidated and unable to receive the help she needed. Everyone needs respect to enhance pride, dignity, and self-esteem; it is an important contributor to good mental health. Showing respect is also an important means for breaking down barriers in cross-cultural communication.

BE PATIENT

It takes time to build trust and effect cultural change. It can be difficult to establish the nurse-client relationship when it involves two different cultures. Trust must be won, and winning it may take weeks, months, or even years. Patience is essential. Time must be allowed for both the nurse and the client to learn how to communicate with one another, to test each other's trustworthiness, and to learn about each other. Change in behavior (learned aspects of the culture) occurs gradually. Some aspects of both the nurse's and the client's cultures can, and probably will, change. The Kims' nurse, for example, modified some of her usual practices and adapted them to the Kims' culture and needs. They, in turn, began to assume some American practices and values. However, the process took several months. Time and patience help to break down cultural barriers.

ANALYZE YOUR BEHAVIOR

Self-awareness is crucial for the nurse working with people from other cultures (Leininger, 1970). Remember that your culture is different from theirs. Are you aware of your own values, habits, and typical responses? How would you appear to clients? The nurse who assisted Mrs. Jackson probably thought she was being friendly, efficient, and helpful. In terms of her own culture, this nurse's behavior was intended to reassure clients and meet their needs. Unaware of the negative consequences of her behavior, she caused damage rather than met needs.

To gain skill in analyzing their own behavior, nurses should keep in mind two points. First, knowledge of the clients' culture helps nurses to know how clients will interpret various behaviors. It tells nurses what responses are most appropriate to make. Second, establishing a relationship of trust with clients of different cultures opens doors of communication. As in Sandra's experience, trust creates a willingness to share reactions and constructively criticize behavior.

Summary

In community health, each client, whether a family, group, or community, has its own culture. A culture is a design for living, and every culture is different. The unique culture of each group is essential for the functioning of that group. It serves as a guide for behavior, a map telling the people of that group how to live. Culture provides a set of norms and values, which are the threads holding together the fabric of a society. It offers stability and security.

Several characteristics of culture are significant for community health nursing practice. It is *learned*, not acquired. Thus some elements can be re-learned, and some practices changed. It is *integrated*. All of the many traits making up a culture work together as a functioning whole. Specific cultural practices must be considered in the context of the client's larger culture. Changing one set of traits will affect other aspects of the culture. It is *shared*. Culture is a group phenomenon; it controls all the members' values and behavior. Attempts to change individual behavior may be ineffective; a group approach might be more productive. It is *tacit*. Culture tells people how to behave without the need for conscious thought. A collision between two different cultures can create considerable conflict and misunderstanding. Conscious effort is required to understand and accept cultural differences. It is *dynamic*. Every culture preserves its integrity by deleting nonfunctional practices and acquiring new components that will better serve the group. Consequently, it is possible to introduce improved health practices that are presented in a manner consistent with the clients' cultural values.

Some principles, drawn from an understanding of the concept of culture, can guide community health nursing practice:

1. Recognize and appreciate the differences between your clients' culture and your own.
2. Understand the cultural basis for your clients' behavior.
3. Listen and learn before giving advice.
4. Empathize with clients of different cultural backgrounds.
5. Show respect for clients and their culture.
6. Be patient. It takes time to build trust and effect cultural change.
7. Analyze your behavior in the context of the clients' culture.

Study Questions

1. Based on your own cultural background, how would you feel and what behaviors would you exhibit if you were:
   a. A client sitting in a clinic waiting room in a foreign country whose language you didn't know?
   b. Part of a nutrition class being told to eat foods you had never heard of before?

c. Visited in your home by a nurse who told you to discipline your child in a way that contradicted everything you had been reared to believe about parenting?

2. Describe three tacit cultural rules that govern your own behavior. How might these affect your interaction with clients from another culture?

3. What does the term *ethnocentrism* mean to you? Have you ever experienced someone else being ethnocentric in their attitude toward you? If so, describe that experience.

References

Aichlmayr, R. H. (1969). Cultural understanding: A key to acceptance. *Nursing Outlook* 17: 20–23.

Bassuk, E. L., and L. Rosenberg. (1988). Why does family homelessness occur? A case control study. *American Journal of Public Health* 78(7): 783–88.

Benedict, R. (1934). *Patterns of culture.* Boston: Houghton Mifflin.

Bloch, B. (1983). Bloch's assessment guide for ethnic/culture variations. In M. Orque and B. Bloch (eds.), *Ethnic nursing care.* St. Louis: C. V. Mosby.

Brownlee, A. T. (1978). *Community, culture, and care.* St. Louis: C. V. Mosby.

Bullough, V. L., and B. Bullough. (1982). *Health care for the other Americans.* New York: Appleton-Century-Crofts.

Calhoun, M. A. (1986). Providing health care to Vietnamese in America: What practitioners need to know. *Home Healthcare Nurse* 4(5): 14–22.

Erkel, E. A. (1985). Conceptions of community health nurses regarding low-income black, Mexican-American, and white families, Parts I and II. *Journal of Community Health Nursing* 2(2): 99–107, 109–18.

Fischer, P. J., S. Shapiro, W. R. Breakey, J. C. Nathony, and M. Kramer. (1986). Mental health and social characteristics of the homeless: A survey of mission users. *American Journal of Public Health* 76(5): 519–24.

Foster, G. M. (1962). *Traditional cultures and the impact of technological change.* New York: Harper & Row.

Gagnon, A. T. (1983). Transcultural nursing: Including it in the curriculum. *Nursing and Health Care* 4(3): 127–31.

Hall, E. T. (1959). *The silent language.* Garden City, N.Y.: Doubleday.

Hanlon, J. J., and G. E. Pickett. (1984). *Public Health: Administration and Practice.* St. Louis: Times Mirror/Mosby.

Harwood, A. (ed.). (1981). *Ethnicity and medical care.* Cambridge, Mass.: Harvard University Press.

Herrera, T., and N. Wagner. (1977). Behavioral approaches to delivering health services in a Chicano community. In A. Reinhardt and M. Quinn (eds.), *Current practice in family-centered community nursing.* St. Louis: C. V. Mosby.

Jackson, J. J. (1981). Urban black Americans. In A. Harwood (ed.), *Ethnicity and medical care.* Cambridge, Mass.: Harvard University Press.

Jonas, S. (1986). On homelessness and the American Way. *American Journal of Public Health* 76(9): 1084–86.

Kark, S. L. (1974). *Epidemiology and community medicine.* New York: Appleton-Century-Crofts.

Landy, D. (1977). *Culture, disease and healing: Studies in medical anthropology.* New York: Macmillan.

Leininger, M. (1970). *Anthropology and nursing: Two worlds to blend.* New York: Wiley.

Leininger, M. (1977). Transcultural nursing: A promising subfield of study for nurses. In A. Reinhardt and M. Quinn (eds.), *Current practice in family-centered community nursing* (pp. 36–50). St. Louis: C. V. Mosby.

Martin, M.E., and M. Henry. (1989). Cultural relativity and poverty. *Public Health Nursing* 6(1): 28–34.

Mead, M. (1960). Cultural contexts of nursing problems. In F. C. MacGregor (ed.), *Social science in nursing.* New York: Wiley.

Meisenhelder, J. B. (1982). Boundaries of personal space. *Image* 14(1): 16–19.

Murdock, G. (1972). The science of culture. In M. Freilich (ed.), *The meaning of culture: A reader in cultural anthropology* (pp. 252–66). Lexington, Mass.: Xerox College Publishing.

Orque, M. S. (1983). Orque's ethnic/cultural system: A framework for ethnic nursing care. In M. S. Orque, B. Bloch, and L. S. Montroy (eds.), *Ethnic nursing care.* St. Louis: C. V. Mosby.

Patrick, D. L., Y. Sittampalam, S. Somerville, W. Carter, and M. Bergner. (1985). A cross-cultural comparison of health status values. *American Journal of Public Health* 75(12): 1402–7.

Pesznecker, B. L. (1984). The poor: A population at risk . . . multidimensional model of poverty . . . practice implications. *Public Health Nursing* 1(4): 237–49.

Pratt, L. (1971). The relationship of socioeconomic status to health. *American Journal of Public Health* 61: 281–91.

Primeaux, M., and G. Henderson. (1981). American Indian patient care. In G. Henderson and M. Primeaux (eds.), *Transcultural health care.* Philadelphia: F. A. Davis.

Reinert, B. R. (1986). The health care beliefs and values of Mexican-Americans. *Home Healthcare Nurse* 4(5): 23–31.

Robertson, H. R. (1969). Removing barriers to health care. *Nursing Outlook* 17: 43–46.

Robertson, M. J., and M. R. Cousineau. (1986). Health status and access to health services among the urban homeless. *American Journal of Public Health* 76(5): 561–63.

Spradley, J. P. (1979). *The ethnographic interview.* New York: Holt, Rinehart and Winston.

Spradley, J. P. (1980). *Participant observation.* New York: Holt, Rinehart and Winston.

Spradley, J. P. (1988). *Your owe yourself a drunk: An ethnography of urban nomads.* Lanham, Md.: University Press of America.

Spradley, J. P., and D. W. McCurdy. (1980). *Anthropology: The cultural perspective.* 2nd ed. New York: Wiley.

Stehr-Green, J. K., and P. M. Schantz. (1986). Trichinosis in Southeast Asian refugees in the United States. *American Journal of Public Health* 76(10): 1238–39.

Strauss, A. L. (1967). Medical ghettos. *Trans-Action* 4(62): 7–15.

Taylor, C. (1973). The nurse and cultural barriers. In D. Hymovich and M. Barnard (eds.), *Family health care* (pp. 119–27). New York: McGraw-Hill.

Thernstrom, S., et al. (eds.). (1980). *Harvard encylopedia of American ethnic groups.* Cambridge, Mass.: Harvard University Press.

Tripp-Reimer, T. (1982). Barriers to health care: Variations in interpretation of Appalachian client behavior by Appalachian and non-Appalachian health professionals. *Western Journal of Nursing Research* 4(2): 179–91.

Tripp-Reimer, T. (1985). Cultural assessment. In J. Bellack and P. Bamford (eds.), *Nursing assessment.* North Scituate, Mass.: Duxbury.

Tripp-Reimer, T., P. J. Brink, and J. M. Saunders. (1984). Cultural assessment: Content and process. *Nursing Outlook* 32(2): 78–82.

United States Bureau of Census. (1989). *Current population reports.* Washington, D.C.: U.S. Department of Commerce.

Selected Readings

Aichlmayr, R. H. (1969). Cultural understanding: A key to acceptance. *Nursing Outlook* 17: 20–23.

Alvarez, W. F., J. Doris, and O. Larson, III. (1988). Children of migrant farm work families are at high risk for maltreatment: New York State study. *American Journal of Public Health* 78(8): 934–36.

Bassuk, E. L., and L. Rosenberg. (1988). Why does family homelessness occur? A case control study. *American Journal of Public Health* 78(7): 738–88.

Bauwens, E. (ed.). (1978). *The anthropology of health.* St. Louis: C. V. Mosby.

Benedict, R. (1934). *Patterns of culture.* Boston: Houghton Mifflin.

Bernal, H., and R. Froman. (1987). The confidence of community health nurses in caring for ethnically diverse populations. *Image* 19(4): 201–3.

Bloch, B. (1983). Bloch's assessment guide for ethnic/cultural variations. In M. S. Orque, B. Bloch, and L. S. Montroy (eds.), *Ethnic nursing care.* St. Louis: C. V. Mosby.

Brownlee, A. T. (1978). *Community, culture, and care.* St. Louis: C. V. Mosby.

Bullough, V. L., and B. Bullough. (1982). *Health care for the other Americans.* New York: Appleton-Century-Crofts.

Butler, F. R. (1987). Minority wellness promotion: A behavioral self-management approach. *Journal of Gerontological Nursing* 13(8): 23–28.

Calhoun, M. S. (1986). Providing health care to Vietnamese in America: What practitioners need to know. *Home Healthcare Nurse* 4(5): 14–22.

Davitz, L. J., Y. Sameshima, and J. Davitz. (1976). Suffering as viewed in six different cultures. *American Journal of Nursing* 76: 1296–97.

DeGracia, R. (1979). Cultural influences on Filipino patients. *American Journal of Nursing* 79: 1412–14.

Erkel, E. A. (1985). Conceptions of community health nurses regarding low-income black, Mexican-American, and white families, Parts I and II. *Journal of Community Health Nursing* 2(2): 99–107, 109–18.

Fischer, P. J., S. Shapiro, W. R. Breakey, J. C. Nathony, and M. Kramer. (1986). Mental health and social characteristics of the homeless: A survey of mission users. *American Journal of Public Health* 76(5): 519–24.

Gagnon, A. J. (1983). Transcultural nursing: Including it in the curriculum. *Nursing and Health Care* 4(3): 127–31.

Gordon, V., I. M. Matousek, and T. A. Lang. (1980). Southeast Asian refugees. *American Journal of Nursing* 80: 2031–36.

Hall, E. T. (1959). *The silent language.* Garden City, N.Y.: Doubleday.

Harwood, A. (ed.). (1981). *Ethnicity and medical care.* Cambridge, Mass.: Harvard University Press.

Iskander, R. (1987). Developing a black consciousness . . . health needs of black communities. *Nursing Times* 83(42): 66, 69.

Jackson, J. J. (1981). Urban black Americans. In A. Harwood (ed.), *Ethnicity and medical care.* Cambridge, Mass.: Harvard University Press.

Jacobson, M. L., M. A. Mercer, L. K. Miller, and T. W. Simpson. (1987). Tuberculosis risk among migrant farm workers on the Delmarva Peninsula. *American Journal of Public Health* 77(1): 29–32.

Jonas, S. (1986). On homelessness and the American Way. *American Journal of Public Health* 76(9): 1084–86.

Kemp, C. (1985). Cambodian refugee health care beliefs and practices. Public Health Nursing 2(1): 41–52.

Kleinman, A. (1980). *Patients and healers in the context of culture*. Berkeley: University of California Press.

Kneip-Hardy, M., and M. Burkhardt. (1977). Nursing the Navajo. *American Journal of Nursing* 77: 95–96.

Koshi, P. T. (1977). Symposium on cultural and biological diversity and health care. *Nursing Clinics of North America* 12: 1.

Kramer, M., and C. Schmalenber. (1977). *Path to biculturalism*. Wakefield, Mass.: Contemporary Publishing.

Kubricht, D. W., and J. A. Clark. (1982). Foreign patients: A system for providing care. *Nursing Outlook* 30(1): 55–57.

Kunitz, I. J., and J. E. Levy. (1981). Navajos. In A. Harwood (ed.), *Ethnicity and medical care*. Cambridge, Mass.: Harvard University Press.

Kunstadter, P. (1985). Health of Hmong in Thailand: Risk factors, morbidity, and mortality in comparison with other groups. *Culture, Medicine and Psychiatry* 9(4): 329–51.

Leininger, M. (1970). *Anthropology and nursing: Two worlds to blend*. New York: Wiley.

Leininger, M. (1978). *Transcultural nursing*. Somerset, N.J.: Wiley.

Martinez, R. A. (ed.). (1978). *Hispanic culture and health care*. St. Louis: C. V. Mosby.

Mead, M. (1960). Cultural contexts of nursing problems. In F. C. MacGregor (ed.), *Social science in nursing* (pp. 74–78). New York: Wiley.

Mei-Li, L. (1976). Folk beliefs of the Chinese and implications for psychiatric nursing. *Journal of Psychiatric Nursing* 14: 38–41.

Meisenhelder, J. B. (1982). Boundaries of personal space. *Image* 14(1): 16–19.

Meleis, A. I. (1981). The Arab-American in the health care system. *American Journal of Nursing* 81: 1180–83.

Milio, N. (1973). Values, social class and community health services. In A. Reinhardt and M. Quinn (eds.), *Family-centered community nursing: A sociocultural framework* (pp. 187–97). St. Louis: C. V. Mosby.

Mitchell, A. C. (1978). Barriers to therapeutic communication with black clients. *Nursing Outlook* 26: 109–112.

Moccia, P., and D. J. Mason. (1986). Poverty trends: Implications for nursing. *Nursing Outlook* 34(1): 20–24.

Montero, D. (1978). The Vietnamese refugees in America: Patterns of socioeconomic adaptation and assimilation. College Park, Md.: Institute of Urban Studies, University of Maryland.

O'Brien, M. E. (1983). Reaching the migrant worker. *American Journal of Nursing* 83: 895–97.

Orque, M. S. (1983). Orque's ethnic/cultural system: A framework for ethnic nursing care. In M. S. Orque, B. Bloch, and L. S. Montroy (eds.), *Ethnic nursing care*. St. Louis: C. V. Mosby.

Patrick, D. L., Y. Sittampalam, S. Somerville, W. Carter, and M. Bergner. (1985). A cross-cultural comparison of health status values. *American Journal of Public Health* 75(12): 1402–7.

Paul, B. D. (1955). *Health, culture and community*. New York: Russell Sage Foundation.

Pesznecker, B. L. (1984). The poor: A population at risk . . . multidimensional model of poverty . . . practice implications. *Public Health Nursing* 1(4): 237–49.

Primeaux, M. H. (1977). American Indian health care practices. *Nursing Clinics of North America* 12: 55–65.

Primeaux, M. H., and G. Henderson. (1981). American Indian patient care. In G. Henderson and M. Primeaux (eds.), *Transcultural health care.* Philadelphia: F. A. Davis.

Reinert, B. R. (1986). The health care beliefs and values of Mexican-Americans. *Home Healthcare Nurse* 4(5): 23–31.

Robertson, M. J., and M. R. Cousineau (1986). Health status and access to health services among the urban homeless. *American Journal of Public Health* 76(5): 561–63.

Smith, K. G. (1986). The hazards of migrant farm work: An overview for rural public health nurses. *Public Health Nursing* 3(1): 48–56.

Sobralski, M. (1985). Perceptions of health. *Topics in Clinical Nursing* 7(3): 32–39.

Spector, M. (1979). Poverty: The barrier to health care. In R. E. Spector (ed.), *Cultural diversity in health and illness.* New York: Appleton-Century-Crofts.

Spradley, J. P. (1979). *The ethnographic interview.* New York: Holt, Rinehart and Winston.

Spradley, J. P. (1980). *Participant observation.* New York: Holt, Rinehart and Winston.

Spradley, J. P., and D. W. McCurdy. (1980). *Anthropology: The cultural perspective.* 2nd ed. New York: Wiley.

Stern, P. N. (1981). Solving problems of cross-cultural health teaching: The Filipino child-bearing family. *Image* 13: 47–50.

Strasser, J. A. (1978). Urban transient women. *American Journal of Nursing* 78: 2076–79.

Stumpf, P. S. (1983). The culture of poverty: An overused conceptual model. In P. L. Chinn (ed.), *Advances in nursing theory development.* Rockville, Md.: Aspen Systems.

Taylor, C. (1973). The nurse and cultural barriers. In D. Hymovich and M. Barnard (eds.), *Family health care.* New York: McGraw-Hill, 119–27.

Tripp-Reimer, T., P. J. Brink, and J. Saunders. (1984). Cultural assessment: Content and process. *Nursing Outlook* 32(2): 78–82.

Wagner, N., and M. Haug. (eds.). (1971). *Chicanos: Social and psychological perspectives.* St. Louis: C. V. Mosby.

Waren, R., and M. Hoefer. (1987). 1986 Statistical Yearbook of the Immigration and Naturalization Service. Washington, D.C.: United States Immigration and Naturalization Service.

Weeks, H. A. (1977). Income and disease—The pathology of poverty. In L. Corey, M. Epstein, and S. E. Saltman (eds.), *Medicine in a changing society.* (2nd ed.). St. Louis: C. V. Mosby.

Westermeyer, J., T. F. Vang, and J. Neider. (1983). Migration and mental health among Hmong refugees. *Journal of Nervous and Mental Disorders* 171(2): 92–96.

Wissow, L. S., A. M. Gittelsohn, M. Szklo, B. Starfield, and M. Mussman. (1988). Poverty, race, and hospitalization for childhood asthma. *American Journal of Public Health* 78(7): 777–82.

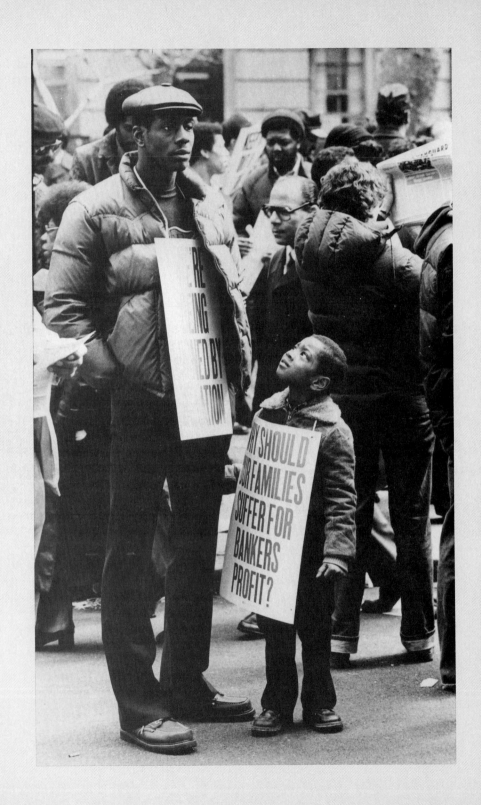

6 Values and Ethical Decision Making in Community Health

Sara T. Fry

Barbara W. Spradley

Today's community health nurses, together with other health care professionals, face an expanding number of ethical, or moral, dilemmas. Scientific and technological advances have created many of these dilemmas. Computerized record-keeping systems, for instance, make patient information readily accessible and raise issues of confidentiality and patients' rights. Intubation and resuscitation in terminal disease, and when (as well as how) to prolong life raise additional ethical questions. Numerous other issues, such as informed consent, organ transplants, experimental therapy, decision making for incompetent patients, or the right to refuse care to an AIDS patient, force us to deal with an endless barrage of ethical decisions. Underlying every issue and influencing every ethical decision are values. In fact, ethics and values are inextricably intertwined.

Community health nurses encounter value differences every day, and value differences, in turn, create ethical dilemmas. Consider, for example, the dilemma one nurse in Seattle faced on her first home visit to an elderly man whom we shall call Mr. Bates. Referred by concerned neighbors, this 78-year-old gentleman was homebound and living alone with severe arthritis under steadily deteriorating conditions. Overgrown shrubs and vines covered the yard and house, making access impossible except through the back door. A wood-burning stove in the kitchen was the sole source of heat and that room plus a corner of the dining room were Mr. Bates' living quarters. The remainder of the once lovely three-bedroom house, including the bathroom, was layered with dust, unused. His bed was a cot in the dining room, his toilet a two-pound coffee can placed under the cot. Unbathed, unshaven, and existing on food and firewood brought in by neighbors, Mr. Bates seemed to be living in deplorable and unsafe conditions. Yet he valued his independence so highly that he adamantly refused to leave.

The conflict in values between Mr. Bates' choice to live independently and the nurse's value of having him in a safer living situation raises several ethical questions. When do health practitioners or family members have the right to override an individual's preferences? When do neighbors' rights (Mr. Bates' home was an eyesore and his care was a source of anxiety for his neighbors) supersede one homeowner's rights? Should the nurse be responsible when family members can help but won't take action? Mr. Bates had one son living in a neighboring state.

Values and the valuing process strongly shape the nature of community health nursing practice. Values determine nurses' as well as clients' decisions and responses. The concept of value is a familiar topic to nurses. The function and meaning of values and value systems have been a part of their educational preparation in the humanities and the sciences. Values are widely discussed in history, philosophy, and literature. Theoretical consideration and empirical studies about values and value systems are also well documented in the literature of sociology, psychology, and the applied sciences such as nursing.

Values serve as the criteria or standards by which evaluations are made. In order to understand the relationship between values and health and the influence of values on ethical decision making, it is necessary to describe the nature or function of values and value systems in human behavior. Once it is clear how values and value systems affect behavior, then we can understand the role of values in choices related to health. In this chapter, we will explore (1) the nature and function of values and value systems, (2) the role of values and value systems in ethical decision making, (3) the central values related to health care choices and their potential conflicts, and (4) the implications of values and ethics for community health nursing practice.

VALUES AND VALUE SYSTEMS

Social psychologist Milton Rokeach (1973) has explained values and value systems in a particularly useful manner. A *value* is a lasting belief that a certain way of acting or being is personally or socially preferable to an opposing or different way of acting or being. Building on this definition, we can describe a *value system* as a lasting, organized set of beliefs about a preferred way of acting or being. This set of beliefs ranges along a continuum from minimum to maximum importance. With these definitions in mind, we can explore the nature and function of values and value systems and their relationship to health.

THE NATURE OF VALUES

The nature of values can be described according to five qualities: endurance, relativity, belief, reference, and preference.

Endurance

Values endure in the sense that they are sufficiently stable to provide continuity to personal and social existence. Religious beliefs, for example, offer stability to many people. For Mr. Bates, independence was a long-term value. This is not to say that values are completely stable over time, because we know that values do change throughout one's life. Yet social existence requires standards within the individual as well as an agreement on standards among groups of individuals. As Kluckhohn (1951, p. 400) points out, without values, "the functioning of the social system could not continue to achieve group goals; individuals . . . could not feel within themselves a requisite measure of order and unified purpose." Thus, by adding an element of collective purpose in social life, values guarantee endurance and stability in social existence.

Relativity

Isolated values are usually organized into a hierarchical system. As an individual confronts social situations throughout life, isolated values learned in early childhood come into competition with other values, requiring a weighing of one value against another (Figure 6-1). Concern for others' welfare, for instance, competes with self-interest. Through experience and maturation, the individual integrates values learned in different contexts into systems in which each value is ordered relative to other values.

Figure 6-1
Values are learned and endure as they are reinforced by the significant people around us. This boy imitates his father's smoking behavior.

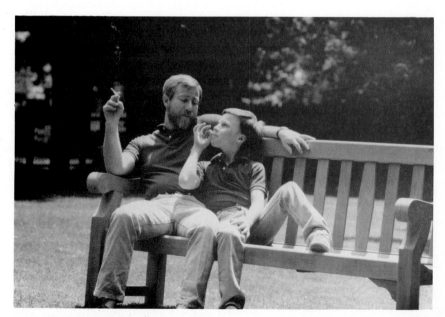

Belief

Rokeach (1973) describes values as a subcategory of beliefs. He argues that some beliefs are descriptive, or capable of being true or false; other beliefs are evaluative, involving judgments of good and bad; and still other beliefs are prescriptive-proscriptive, determining whether an action is desirable or undesirable. Values, he says, are prescriptive-proscriptive beliefs. They are concerned with what ought to be. Parents' values about child behavior, for example, determine their choices for disciplinary measures. Sharing the characteristics of all beliefs, values have cognitive, affective, and behavioral components. Rokeach (1973, p. 7) writes: "(1) A value is a cognition about the desirable.... To say that a person has a value is to say that cognitively he knows the correct way to behave or the correct end-state to strive for. (2)... he can feel emotional about it, be affectively for or against it.... (3) A value has a behavioral component in the sense that it is an intervening variable that leads to actions."

Reference

Values also have a reference quality. That is, they may refer to end-states of existence called *terminal values* (e.g., religious salvation, peace of mind, world peace), or they may refer to modes of conduct called *instrumental values* (e.g., confidentiality, promise-keeping, and honesty). The latter can have a moral focus or a nonmoral focus, and these values may conflict. For example, a nurse may experience a conflict between two moral values such as whether to act honestly or to act respectfully. Similarly, she or he can experience conflict between two competence (nonmoral) values such as whether to plan logically or to plan creatively. The nurse can also experience conflict between a competence value and a moral value such as whether to act efficiently or to act fairly.

Preference

A value is something preferred over other alternatives. It is a preference for one mode of behavior over another, such as exercise over inactivity, or for one end-state over another, such as trimness over obesity. We simply prefer one over the other, like Mr. Bates' preference for independence over personal comfort. The preferred end-state or mode of behavior is located higher in our personal value hierarchy.

The qualities of values — endurance, relativity, belief, reference, and preference — indicate that values have the potential for an extensive range of application in human existence. Unfortunately, very little is known about the conditions under which people employ values. Theorists can suggest only that values enjoy a central place of importance within people's value-attitude-belief systems. Thus, an exploration of value systems and the priority of values within those systems is the next step in understanding how values are ultimately related to individual and aggregate-level choices concerning health.

THE NATURE OF VALUE SYSTEMS

Contrasting value systems may be seen in many community health nursing practice settings. One nurse experienced such a contrast on her first home visit to a family. Referred by a social worker for recurring problems with head lice and staphylococcal infections, the family was living in the worst conditions the nurse had ever seen. Papers, moldy food, soiled clothing, and empty beer cans covered the floors. The nurse recoiled in horror. The children, home from school, were clustered around the television. Their mother, a divorced, single parent, unkempt and obese, sat smoking a cigarette with a can of beer in her hand. She had been unable to earn enough money waitressing to support herself and the children, so the family was now on welfare. Her main pleasure in life was television soap operas. The nurse was interpreting the situation through the framework of her own value system (as we all do), yet the family clearly had its own value system as well.

Value systems are generally considered organizations of beliefs that are of relative importance in guiding individual behavior (Rokeach, 1973). Instead of being guided by single or isolated values, however, behavior at any point in time (or over a period of time) is influenced by multiple or changing clusters of values. Thus, it is important to understand how values are integrated into a person's attitude-value-belief system, how values assume a place in a hierarchy of values, and how this hierarchical system changes over time.

As mentioned previously, Rokeach (1973) indicates that learned values are integrated into an organized system of values and that each value has an ordered priority with respect to other values. For the welfare family, television entertainment apparently held a higher value than order and cleanliness. This system of ordered priority is stable enough to reflect the continuity of one's personality and behavior within culture and society, yet it is sufficiently flexible to allow a reordering of value priorities in response to changes in the environment, social setting, or personal experiences. Behavioral change would, of course, be regarded as the visible response to a reordering of values within an individual's hierarchical value system.

Adults generally possess only a few, perhaps a dozen and a half, *terminal values,* such as peace of mind or achievement. These are influenced by complex physiological and social factors. Human needs, such as physiological needs, security, love, self-esteem, and self-actualization, proposed by Maslow (1969), are believed to be the greatest influences on terminal values. While a person may have only a few terminal values, the same person may possess as many as five or six dozen *instrumental values.* The latter, singly or in combination with other instrumental values, also help determine terminal values. For example, instrumental values of acceptance, taking it easy, living one day at a time, or not being concerned about the future, can help to shape the terminal value of peace of mind. Or instrumental values of hard work, driving oneself to compete, or not letting anyone get in one's way, can influence the terminal values of achievement. Figure 6-2 illustrates the influence of instrumental values as well as human needs on the development of terminal values.

FUNCTIONS OF VALUES AND VALUE SYSTEMS

Values and value systems have different functions. Values function primarily as standards for behavior, and value systems function as plans for conflict resolution and decision making.

Standards for Behavior

In general, values function as standards that guide actions and behavior in daily situations. Once internalized by an individual, a value such as honesty becomes a criterion for that individual's personal conduct. Values may func-

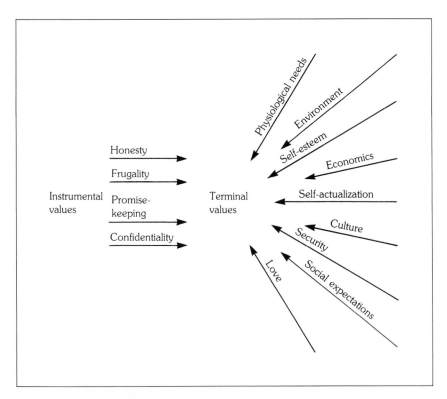

Figure 6-2
Factors influencing personal values.

tion as criteria for developing and maintaining attitudes toward objects and situations or for justifying one's own actions and attitudes. Values also may serve as the standards by which we pass moral judgment on ourselves and others (Rokeach, 1968).

Values have a long-term function in giving expression to human needs. According to Rokeach (1973), the strong motivational component of a value helps a person adjust to society, defend ego against threat, and test reality. In addition, values are employed as standards to guide presentation of the self to others, to ascertain whether we are as moral and as competent as others, and to persuade and influence others by indicating which beliefs, attitudes, and actions of others are worth trying to reinforce or change.

Plans for Conflict Resolution and Decision Making

When an individual encounters a social situation, several values within his or her value system are activated rather than just a single value. For example, the nurse entering Mr. Bates' home applied her values of health protection, safety, cleanliness, and respect for the individual and his right to autonomy. Clearly, all the activated values will not be compatible with one another. Thus, conflict between values is inevitable in social existence, depending on the situation and the specific values activated.

Obviously, some values will triumph over others when conflicting values are activated. It is not known why some values consistently triumph over others and are stronger directives for individual behavior. Even though a value system is a hierarchy of values that slowly changes and adjusts to social existence over time, some values, such as the value placed on high achievement in the United States, seem to consistently remain in higher positions than other values. Other values do, of course, lose their positions of importance in a value hierarchy. It is this changing arrangement of values in a hierarchical system that determines, in part, how conflicts will be resolved and decisions will be made. Thus, an individual's value system functions as a learned organization of principles and rules that helps him or her choose between alternative courses of action and reach decisions (Figure 6-3).

VALUES CLARIFICATION AND ETHICAL DECISION MAKING

One way to understand the influence and priority of values in our own as well as clients' behavior is to employ various values clarification techniques in decision making. According to Steele and Harmon (1983, p. 13), values clarification is a process of discovery that "attempts to bring to conscious awareness the values and underlying motivations that guide one's actions." Since individuals are largely unaware of the motives underlying their behavior and choices, values clarification is potentially important to the kind of decisions individuals make. Only by understanding our own values and their

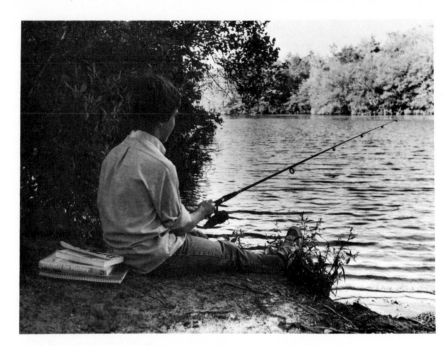

Figure 6-3
Our hierarchical value
system helps us choose
between alternative courses
of action. This boy's love
of fishing is clearly more
important to him than
getting his schoolwork done.

priority or importance can we be certain that our choices are more the result of rationality and less the result of other influences, such as cultural, social, or other kinds of previous conditioning. Values clarification by itself does not yield a set of rules for future decision making and does not indicate the right or wrong of alternative actions. Values clarification does, however, help guarantee that any course of action chosen by an individual is consistent and in accordance with that individual's beliefs and values.

VALUES CLARIFICATION

Although there are several approaches to values clarification, all approaches seem to agree on (1) the process of valuing, and (2) strategies used in values clarification (Simon and Clark, 1975; Simon and Kirschenbaum, 1972; Steele and Harmon, 1983; Uustal, 1977a, 1977b, 1978).

Process of Valuing

Before values clarification can take place, an understanding of the process of valuing is necessary. Uustal (1977b) lists seven steps. During the process of valuing, the person

1. Chooses the value freely and individually.
2. Chooses the value from among alternatives.

3. Carefully considers the consequences of the choice.
4. Cherishes or prizes the value.
5. Publicly affirms the value.
6. Incorporates the value into behavior so that it becomes a standard.
7. Consciously employs the value in decision making.

These steps provide specific actions for the discovery and identification of individual values. They also assist the decision-making process by explicating the process of valuing itself.

Strategies in Values Clarification

Uustal (1978) offers several strategies of values clarification that are ultimately useful to the decision-making process in community health nursing practice. Strategy 1 is a means by which nurses can come to know themselves and their values better (see Figure 6-4). Strategy 2 assists in discovering value clusters and the priority of values within personal value systems (see Figure 6-5). Strategy 3 can be used to examine one's responses to selected issues in nursing practice. Each response helps establish priorities of values by asking the nurse to choose among the alternatives presented or to indicate degree of agreement or disagreement (see Figure 6-6).

Other values clarification strategies are included in the study questions at the end of this chapter to assist nurses in understanding their ordering of values and to help them consider directions for change.

All of these strategies can be used to analyze and understand how values are meaningful to people and ultimately influence their choices and behavior. Clarification of one's values is the first step in the decision-making process and affects the ability of individuals to make ethical decisions. Values clarification also promotes understanding and respect for values held by others, such as patients and other health care providers. As pointed out by

Figure 6-4
Values clarification
strategy 1.

Name Tag

Take a piece of paper and write your name in the middle of it. In each of the four corners, write your responses to these four questions:

1. What two things would you like your colleagues to say about you?
2. What single most important thing do you do (or would you do) to make your nurse-client relationships positive ones?
3. What do you do on a daily basis that indicates you value your health?
4. What are the three values you believe in most strongly?

In the space around your name, write at least six adjectives that you feel best describe who you are.

Take a closer look at your responses to the questions and to the ways in which you described yourself. What values are reflected in your answers?

Patterns

Which of the following words describe you? Draw a circle around the seven words that best describe you as an individual. Underline the seven words that most accurately describe you as a professional person. (You may circle and underline the same word.)

ambitious   reserved   assertive   opinionated

    concerned   generous   independent

easily hurt   outgoing   reliable   indifferent

    capable   self-controlled   fun-loving

suspicious   solitary   likable   dependent

    intellectual   argumentative   dynamic   unpredictable

compromising   thoughtful   affectionate   obedient

    logical   imaginative   self-disciplined

moody   easily led   helpful   slow to relate

Reflect on the following questions:

1. What values are reflected in the patterns you have chosen?
2. What is the relationship between these patterns and your personal values?
3. What patterns indicate inconsistencies in attitudes or behavior?
4. What patterns do you think a nurse should cultivate?

Figure 6-5
Values clarification
strategy 2.

Figure 6-6
Values clarification
strategy 3.

Forced Choice Ranking

How do you order the following alternatives by priority? (There is no correct set of priorities.) What values emerge in response to each question?

1. With whom on a nursing team would you become most angry? The nurse who
   _____ never completes assignments.
   _____ rarely helps other team members.
   _____ projects his or her own feelings on clients.

2. If you had a serious health problem, you would rather
   _____ not be told.
   _____ be told directly.
   _____ find out by accident.

3. You are made happiest in your work when you use
   _____ your technical skills in caring for clients with complex needs.
   _____ your ability to compile data and arrive at a nursing diagnosis.
   _____ your ability to communicate easily and skillfully with clients.

4. It would be most difficult for you to
   _____ listen to and counsel a dying person.
   _____ advise a pregnant adolescent.
   _____ handle a situation of obvious child abuse.

Uustal (1977b, p. 10), "Nurses cannot hope to give optimal, sensitive care to any patient without first understanding their own opinions, attitudes, and values." With this process in mind, we can now explore the role of values in ethical decision making.

ETHICAL DECISION MAKING

Values are central to any consideration of ethics or ethical decision making. Yet it is not at first obvious what counts as an ethical problem in health care or in the practice of nursing. Most nurses easily recognize the moral crisis in decisions, for example, to let an abnormal newborn infant die, to terminate a pregnancy resulting from rape, or to help a terminally ill and suffering client to end his life. These decisions clearly seem to involve ethical components, yet it is not immediately evident why we call these decisions ethical while others that are faced in the routine practice of community health nursing are not considered ethical in nature.

What is "ethics" and what is "ethical"? Webster defines ethics as "the study of standards of conduct and moral judgment... the system or code of morals of a particular... religion, group, profession, etc." (1983, p. 627). Ethics, Bandman and Bandman explain, "is concerned with doing good and avoiding harm" (1985, p. 4). For a decision to be ethical, then, means that one makes a choice to do the greatest good and avoid the most harm in any given situation. Of necessity the decision maker must exercise moral judgment. Let us examine how a nurse makes these moral judgments, or evaluations.

Moral and Nonmoral Evaluations

A key requirement of ethical decision making is distinguishing between evaluative statements and statements presenting nonevaluative facts. Ethics necessarily involves making evaluative judgments. Moving from the judgment that we *can* do something to the judgment that we *ought* to do something involves incorporating a set of norms — of judgments of value, right, duties, and responsibilities. Thus, in order to be ethically responsible in the practice of nursing, it is important to develop the ability to recognize evaluative judgments as they are made in nursing practice.

One approach is to reflect upon one's recent experiences. Select an experience that, at first, seems to involve no particular value judgments. Begin describing what occurred and watch for evaluative words. Among the words to watch for are verbs such as *want, desire, prefer, should,* or *ought.* The evaluations may also be expressed in nouns such as *benefit, harm, duty, responsibility, right,* or *obligation.*

Sometimes the evaluations are expressed in terms that are not direct expressions of evaluations but are clearly functioning as value judgments. For example, the American Nurses Association (ANA) *Code for Nurses* (1985, p. 5) states that "the nurse provides services...unrestricted by considerations of social or economic status, personal attributes, or the nature of health problems." In this statement the ANA could be describing the facts about the way all nurses behave. It is not the case, however, that all nurses behave in this manner. Rather, this statement prescribes that nurses *ought* to provide services without discrimination and that the ethical nurse does provide services in this manner.

Another approach to ethical decision making is to distinguish between moral and nonmoral evaluations (Veatch, 1977). Moral evaluations are prescriptive-proscriptive beliefs having certain characteristics that separate them from other evaluations such as aesthetic judgments, personal preferences, or matters of taste. The differences between the evaluations lies in the grounds on or the reasons for which the evaluations are being made (Frankena, 1973).

Moral evaluations are evaluations of human actions, institutions, or character traits rather than inanimate objects such as paintings or architectural structures. Moral evaluations also have distinctive characteristics. First, the evaluations are ultimate. They have a preemptive quality, meaning that other values or human ends cannot, as a rule, override them (Beauchamp and Childress, 1983; Fried, 1978). Second, they possess universality or reflect a standpoint that applies to everyone. They are evaluations that everyone in principle ought to be able to make and understand, even if some individuals, in fact, do not (Baier, 1958; Rawls, 1971). Third, moral evaluations avoid giving a special place to one's own welfare. They have a focus that keeps others in view, or at least considers one's own welfare on a par with that of others (Beauchamp and Childress, 1983; Rawls, 1971).

Judgments possessing the above characteristics are moral judgments. Because these judgments involve moral values, however, conflicts among them are inevitable. Hence, it is easy to see that any clinical decision in nursing practice that involves a conflict over values potentially involves a moral conflict. The nurse may be faced with the choice between preserving the client's welfare or the welfare of someone else. With Mr. Bates, for example, the nurse chose to honor his desire for independence at the risk of his own physical safety. Not until he fell and broke a hip did he reluctantly agree to be moved out of his home. The nurse may have to choose whether to keep a promise of confidentiality or to provide needed assistance for a client even though a confidence would have to be broken. The nurse may have to decide to protect the interests of colleagues or the interests of the employing institution, whether to serve future clients by striking for better conditions or to serve present clients by refusing to strike. Each decision involves a potential conflict between moral values and creates a decision-making problem in quite ordinary nursing situations.

Decision-Making Frameworks

In attempts to resolve the conflict between moral values in community health nursing practice and to provide morally accountable nursing service, several frameworks for ethical decision making have been proposed. In each framework, the role of values is a key element in the decision-making process. For example, the list of questions below from Stanley (1980) demonstrates the use of values clarification techniques as a preliminary step to decision making:

1. What is going on in this case situation?
    a. Separate scientific facts from questions of values and morals.
    b. Identify the nurse's value system.
2. By what criteria should decisions be made?
    a. Professional codes
    b. Religious perspectives
    c. Philosophical reasoning or works
3. Who should decide?
4. For whose benefit is the decision made?
5. How should professionals decide and act?
    a. Alternative actions
    b. Response to ethical principles

The separation of questions of fact from questions of value and the identification of the nurse's value system are considered fundamental to choosing alternative courses of action.

The identification of clients' values and those of other persons involved in conflict situations is also an important part of ethical decision making. For example, what are Mr. Bates' values, what are the values of neighbors who are concerned but feel they can no longer care for him, and what are the nurse's values? An ethical decision-making framework that includes the identification and clarification of all values impinging on the making of ethical decisions is outlined below (Thompson and Thompson, 1981):

1. Review the situation.
    a. What health problems exist?
    b. What decisions need to be made?
    c. Separate ethical components of the decisions from those decisions that can be made solely on a scientific knowledge base.
    d. Identify all individuals/groups affected by the decision.
2. Decide what further information is needed before a decision can be made.
3. Identify ethical issues. Discuss historical, philosophical, and religious bases for these issues.

4. Identify your own values and beliefs. Identify professional responsibilities dictated by the ANA *Code for Nurses.*
5. Identify values and beliefs of other people involved in the situation.
6. Identify value conflicts, if any.
7. Decide who should make the decision. Determine nurse's role in making the decision.
8. Identify range of decisions or actions that are possible. Determine implications for all people involved. Identify how suggested actions conform to the *Code for Nurses.*
9. Decide on a course of action and follow through.
10. Evaluate the results of the actions or decisions. Generalize for future situations.

In a different consideration of values, the framework in Figure 6-7 advocates keeping multiple values in tension before resolution of conflict and action on the part of the nurse. This framework apparently does not view value conflict as capable of resolution until all possible alternative actions have been explored. Final resolution of the ethical conflict would then occur through conscious choice of action even though some or even many values would be overridden by stronger, presumably moral values. The triumphant values would apparently be those values located higher in the decision maker's hierarchy of values.

Figure 6-7
Ethical decision-making
framework 3.

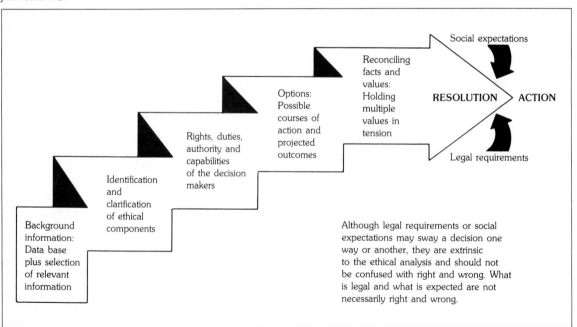

VALUES AND HEALTH CARE

The relationship between values and health has been studied extensively by the President's Commission for the Study of Ethical Problems in Medicine and Biomedical and Behavioral Research. Created by the U.S. Congress in November 1978, the President's Commission had the responsibility to study and report on the ethical and legal implications of a number of issues in medicine and research. Between 1981 and 1983, the Commission published most of its findings and conclusions in a series of nine reports on the following topics: definition of death, informed consent, genetic screening and counseling, access to health care, life-sustaining treatment, privacy and confidentiality, genetic engineering, compensation for injured research subjects, and whistle-blowing.

In all of its reports, the Commission discussed the importance of three basic human values—self-determination, well-being, and equity (President's Commission, 1983b). These values are considered the key values that ought to guide decision making in the provider-client relationship and are the criteria by which the success of a particular interaction is judged.

SELF-DETERMINATION

The value of self-determination or individual autonomy is defined by the Commission (1983a, p. 44) as "an individual's exercise of the capacity to form, revise, and pursue personal plans for life." Self-determination is instrumentally valued because self-judgment about one's goals and choices is conducive to an individual's sense of well-being. Thus, respecting self-determination is based on the belief that better outcomes will result when self-determination is respected and encouraged. Those outcomes that apparently will be maximized by respecting self-determination seem to include enhanced self-concept, enhanced health-promoting behaviors, and enhanced quality of care.

Yet self-determination is also intrinsically valued. It is valued (1) for the freedom from outside control it provides, and (2) because it indicates that the individual chooses his own actions or the actions that affect him. To not respect this value of self-determination is to demonstrate disrespect to persons or to fail to provide them with adequate protection against arbitrary domination by others. Those desiring to be self-determining express the desire to be instruments of their own acts of will, not the will of other persons.

The Commission noted that in health care contexts this desire was of such high ethical importance that self-determination actually overrides practitioner determinations in most situations. This position was supported by the results of a survey undertaken by the Commission (1982): 72 percent of those surveyed said they would prefer to make decisions jointly with their physicians after treatment alternatives had been explained. Physician responses in the same survey, however, indicated that the majority of physicians (88 percent) believe that patients want doctors to make decisions for them. The wide difference between patient expectations regarding self-determination and physician beliefs indicates that self-determination on the part of patients is at high risk in most health care contexts. Physicians and possibly other health practitioners simply fail to recognize the high value attributed to self-determination by patients.

The Commission (1982) also noted that respect for self-determination promotes personal integration within a chosen life-style and is important for creative self-agency. Thus, the value of self-determination is a value that should be nourished in the provision of health care. Noting that "personal responsibility for decision-making is one of the wellsprings of a democracy," the Commission (1983a, p. 46) said the concept of health care decision making includes informing patients of alternative courses of treatment and of the reasoning behind all recommendations.

Yet it is important to note that self-determination cannot be respected at all times and in all situations. There are times when self-determination is impermissible or even impossible. For example, there are times when society must impose restrictions on the range of acceptable client choices, as in cases of child abuse; and there are times when clients are not competent to exercise self-determination, as is true for certain levels of mental illness or dementia. Thus, the Commission recognized two instances in which restrictions might be put on self-determination: (1) when some objectives of individuals are contrary to the public interest or the interests of others in society, and (2) when a person's decision making is so defective or mistaken that the decision fails to promote the person's own values or goals. As an example of the first instance, restriction might occur when clients request professional help in carrying out criminal activities or when a client's request entails depleting of health care resources for other individuals. As an example of the second instance, restriction might occur when clients refuse life-saving treatment for trivial reasons. In these situations, self-determination is justifiably overridden on the basis of the promotion of well-being, another important value in health care decision making.

WELL-BEING

The Commission's reports defined the value of individual well-being in terms of health or the client's subjective preferences concerning health. It is noted that therapeutic interventions offered by health professionals are intended to improve a client's health. Health care is, therefore, considered a means of promoting clients' well-being.

Unfortunately, interventions believed to promote health, health care decisions, and an individual's sense of well-being are not necessarily causally related. Sometimes there are no objective medical criteria (or nursing criteria) for determining if some proposed intervention will promote health. In the case of alternative methods of providing health care, the proffered method may simply reflect the health professional's values or subjective choice. Thus the value of client well-being may be more a matter of professional choice than client choice in many situations.

Determining what constitutes health and how the client's well-being can be promoted often requires a knowledge of the client's subjective preferences. It is generally recognized that clients may be inclined to pursue different directions in treatment procedures based on individual goals and interests. Community health nurses, on the other hand, are committed to helping clients and avoiding harm to them. Thus they are obliged to understand each client's needs and develop reasonable alternatives for treatment or care from which clients may choose. In addition, when individuals are not capable of making a choice, the nurse is obliged to make health care decisions that promote the value of well-being. This may mean that the alternatives that the nurse presents for choice are only ones that will, in face, promote well-being. According to the Commission (1983a, p. 44), "Shared decision-making requires that a practitioner seek not only to understand each patient's needs and develop reasonable alternatives to meet those needs but also to present the alternatives in a way that enables patients to choose one they prefer." Well-being and self-determination are therefore two values that are intricately related in the provision of community health nursing service.

EQUITY

The third value important to decision making in health care contexts is the value of equity. It is a value of central importance to the provision of health care, but it poses many practical and philosophical difficulties.

Like the values of self-determination and well-being, equity has several facets. It is sometimes defined as the value that directs that like cases be treated alike. In other contexts, it is defined as the value that directs that all individuals be treated fairly. Both definitions include the notions that it is unjust (or inequitable) to treat people identically when they are in significant respects unalike. The need for health care and other goods differs among individuals. Equity means that all individuals should have access to health care according to benefit or needs. It also means that an adequate level of health care should be provided for all citizens.

Focus on an adequate level of health care for everyone makes equity a value that avoids unacceptable restrictions on individual liberty while not overcommitting resources to every citizen. The major problem with this definition of equity, of course, is that it assumes that an adequate level of health care can be economically available to all citizens. In times of limited technical resources and decreased financial resources, however, it may be impossible to respect the value of equity. In these situations, the value obligations of professional practice may well create conflicts of values that seem impossible to resolve.

In attempting to deal with the difficult problems posed by the distribution of available health goods in times of economic crisis, the Commission wisely refrained from definitive interpretations of the values of equity, well-being, and self-determination. It did, however, set terms of reference by which those who are responsible for formulating policy on health care could compare the ethical implications of alternative proposals. Considering the availability of health care services for all citizens, the justifications for claiming that health care services should, as a matter of national policy, be available to all, and the importance of the values involved, the Commission (1983b, pp. 29–30) reached several conclusions:

1. Society has an ethical obligation to ensure equitable access to health care for all. This obligation rests on the special importance of health care and is derived from its role in relieving suffering, preventing premature death, restoring functioning, increasing opportunity, providing information about an individual's condition, and giving evidence of mutual empathy and compassion.
2. The societal obligation is balanced by individual obligations. Individuals ought to pay a fair share of the cost of their own health care and take reasonable steps to provide for such care when they can do so without excessive burdens.
3. Equitable access to health care requires that all citizens be able to secure an adequate level of care without excessive burdens. Equitable access also means that the burdens borne by individuals in obtaining adequate care ought not to be excessive or to fall disproportionately on particular individuals.
4. When equity occurs through the operation of private forces, there is no need for government involvement. But the ultimate responsibility for ensuring that society's obligation is met, through a combination of public and private sector arrangements, rests with the Federal government.
5. The cost of achieving equitable access to health care ought to be shared fairly. The cost of securing health care for those unable to pay ought to be spread equitably at the national level and not allowed to fall more heavily on the shoulders of particular practitioners, institutions, or residents of different localities.
6. Efforts to contain rising health care costs are important but should not focus on limiting the attainment of equitable access for the least well-served portion of the public. Measures designed to contain health care costs that exacerbate existing inequities or impede the achievement of equity are unacceptable from a moral standpoint.

Considering the relationships among the values of self-determination, well-being, and equity, what are the implications of the Commission's conclusions for community health nursing? Specifically, how do these human values affect the practice of nursing and the provision of nursing services to the community?

IMPLICATIONS FOR COMMUNITY HEALTH NURSING PRACTICE

Values and their relationship to health have many implications for community health nursing. In Chapter 3, we discussed the valuing process as an essential dynamic in the conceptual model for community health nursing practice. Values underlie the nurse's evaluation of any given situation and influence her or his responses and decisions. Consider how the values described in the previous section influence nursing practice. The value of self-determination has implications for how community health nurses (1) respect the choices of clients, (2) protect privacy, (3) provide for informed consent, and (4) protect diminished capacity for self-determination. The value of well-being has implications for how community health nurses (1) reduce harm and provide benefits to client populations, (2) measure the effectiveness of nursing services, and (3) balance costs of services against real benefits. The value of equity has implications for community health nursing in terms of its priorities for (1) distributing health goods (macroallocation issues) and (2) deciding which populations will obtain available health goods and nursing services (microallocation issues).

Decisions based on one value will mean, of course, that this value will come in conflict with other values. For example, deciding on the basis of well-being may conflict with deciding on the basis of self-determination or equity. How community health nurses balance these values may even conflict with their own personal values or the values of the nursing profession. In these situations, values clarification techniques and the use of values clarification in decision making may assist the community health nurse in making decisions that are not only ethical but also promote the greatest well-being for clients without substantially reducing their self-determination or ignoring equity. As the number and complexity of ethical decisions in community health increase, so too does the need for ethical standards and mechanisms to help nurses make the best choices possible. The American Nurses Association's *Code for Nurses with Interpretive Statements* (1985) provides a helpful guide. Some health care organizations and community agencies, using the ANA Code or some other similar document, have developed their own specific standards and guidelines. More and more health care organizations are using ethics committees or ethics rounds to review cases and establish moral evaluations.

Summary

Values and the valuing process strongly influence community health nursing practice and ethical decision making. It is important that community health nurses understand the meaning of values and their relationship to health and health decisions.

A value is a lasting belief that a certain means or end-state is preferable over other choices. A value system organizes these beliefs into a continuum of relative importance that guides human behavior.

One can understand the nature of values by examining their qualities: endurance, relativity, belief, reference, and preference. Multiple values form changing clusters of values, or value systems, that shape people's behavior. People generally possess multiple *instrumental* values that help to determine their *terminal* personal values, such as what they believe about love or self-determination. Values function as standards for behavior, as criteria for attitudes, as standards for moral judgments, and give expression to human needs. Value systems order values by priority, provide a plan for conflict resolution, and organize principles.

Since values and value systems guide ethical decision making, nurses need to be aware of and understand their own underlying beliefs. The process of valuing goes through several steps from selection and prizing of a value to integration and conscious use of the value in decision makng. Various strategies can be employed to accomplish values clarification.

Understanding personal values assists the nurse in making ethical evaluations in practice. Responsible ethical decision making requires an effort on the nurse's part to make moral evaluations based on moral values. That is, the moral values used should reflect high-level priority, universality, and a focus on others rather than self. Ethical conflicts in nursing practice involve a conflict between moral values. Several frameworks for ethical decision making are available to guide the nurse.

Three key human values influence client health and the nurse-client relationship: self-determination, well-being, and equity. The community health nurse must, as often as possible, respect clients' self-determination to enhance their acting responsibly on their own behalf. The nurse seeks to promote clients' sense of well-being through interventions that respect clients' subjective preferences but reduce potential harm and offer benefits. The nurse also promotes equity — the value that everyone should have access to health care as needed. The nurse must keep these values in balance, using values clarification techniques when conflicts between values arise.

Study Questions

1. Where do you stand on the following issues? For each statement, decide whether you strongly agree, agree, disagree, strongly disagree, or are undecided.

a. Clients have the right to participate in all decisions related to their health care.
b. Nurses need a system designed to credit self-study.
c. Continuing education should be mandatory.
d. Clients should always be told the truth.
e. Standards of nursing practice should be enforced by state examining boards.
f. Nurses should be required to take relicensure examinations every five years.
g. Clients should be allowed to read their health record when they request to do so.
h. Abortion should be an option available to every woman.
i. Badly deformed newborns should be allowed to die.
j. There should be laws guaranteeing desired health care for each person in this country.

2. In a grid similar to the one below, write a statement of belief in the space provided and examine it in relation to the seven steps of the process of valuing. Some areas of confusion and conflict in nursing practice that you might want to examine are peer review, accountability, confidentiality, euthanasia, licensure, patients' rights, abortion, informed consent, and terminating treatment.

   To the right of your statements, check the appropriate boxes indicating when your beliefs reflect one or more of the seven steps in the valuing process. Is your belief a value according to the valuing process?

Statement	Freely chosen	Alternatives	Consequences	Cherished	Affirmed	Incorporated	Employed
	1	2	3	4	5	6	7

3. Rank in order the following 12 potential nursing actions by using 1 to indicate the choice that you feel is most important in a nurse-client relationship and 12 to indicate the choice you believe is least important.

Touching the client.

Empathetically listening to clients.

Disclosing yourself to clients.

Becoming emotionally involved with clients.

Teaching clients.

Being honest in answering clients' questions.

Seeing that clients adhere to medical therapy.

Helping to decrease the client's anxiety.

Making sure that medications and treatments are done on time.

Following doctors' orders.

Remaining "professional" with clients.

Choice. (Add an alternative of your own.)

Examine the way in which you have ordered these options. What values can you identify based on your responses in this exercise? How do these values emerge in your behavior?

References

American Nurses Association. (1985). *Code for nurses with interpretive statements.* Kansas City, Mo.: Author.

Baier, K. (1958). *The moral point of view.* Ithaca, N.Y.: Cornell University Press.

Bandman, E. L., and B. Bandman. (1985). *Nursing ethics in the life span.* Norwalk, Conn.: Appleton-Century-Crofts.

Beauchamp, T. L., and J. F. Childress. (1983). *Principles of biomedical ethics.* 2nd ed. New York: Oxford University Press.

Frankena, W. K. (1973). *Ethics.* Englewood Cliffs. N.J.: Prentice-Hall.

Fried, C. (1978). *Right and wrong.* Cambridge, Mass.: Harvard University Press.

Kluckhohn, C. (1951). Values and value-orientations in the theory of action: An exploration in definition and classification. In T. Parsons and E. A. Shils (eds.), *Toward a general theory of action* (pp. 388–433). Cambridge, Mass.: Harvard University Press.

Maslow, A. (1969). *Toward a psychology of being.* 2nd ed. New York: Van Nostrand.

President's Commission for the Study of Ethical Problems in Medicine and Biomedical and Behavioral Research of (1978), Pub. L. No. 95-622, 1978 U.S. Code Cong. & Ad. News (92 Stat.) 3438 (codified primarily at 42 U.S.C.A. §§ 300v.–300v.–3. [1982]).

President's Commission for the Study of Ethical Problems in Medicine and Biomedical and Behavioral Research. (1982). *Making health care decisions: Volume one report.* Washington, D.C.: U.S. Government Printing Office.

President's Commission for the Study of Ethical Problems in Medicine and Biomedical and Behavioral Research. (1983a). *Securing access to health care: Volume one report.* Washington, D.C.: U.S. Government Printing Office.

President's Commission for the Study of Ethical Problems in Medicine and Biomedical and Behavioral Research. (1983b). *Summing up.* Washington, D.C.: U.S. Government Printing Office.

Rawls, J. (1971). *A theory of justice.* Cambridge, Mass.: Harvard University Press.

Rokeach, M. (1968). *Beliefs, attitudes and values: A theory of organization and change.* San Francisco: Jossey-Bass.

Rokeach, M. (1973). *The nature of human values.* New York: Free Press.

Simon, S. B., and J. Clark. (1975). *More values clarifications: Strategies for the classroom.* San Diego, Calif.: Pennant Press.

Simon, S. B., and H. Kirschenbaum. (1972). *Values clarification: A handbook of practical strategies for teachers and students.* New York: Hart Publishing.

Stanley, T. (1980). Ethics as a component of the curriculum. *Nursing and Health Care* 1: 63–72.

Steele, S. M., and M. V. Harmon. (1983). *Values clarification in nursing.* 2nd ed. Norwalk, Conn.: Appleton-Century-Crofts.

Thompson, J. B., and H. O. Thompson. (1981). *Ethics in nursing.* New York: Macmillan.

Uustal, D. B. (1977a). Searching for values. *Image* 9 (February): 15–17.

Uustal, D. B. (1977b). The use of values clarification in nursing practice. *Journal of Continuing Education in Nursing* 8 (May–June): 8–13.

Uustal, D. B. (1978). Values clarification in nursing. *American Journal of Nursing* 78: 2058–63.

Veatch, R. M. (1977). *Case studies in medical ethics.* Cambridge, Mass.: Harvard University Press.

Williams, R. (1968). Values. In D. L. Sills (ed.), *International Encyclopedia of the Social Sciences* (p. 283). New York: Crowell, Collier and Macmillan.

Webster, N. (1983). *Webster's new universal unabridged dictionary.* 2nd ed. Cleveland, Ohio: New World Dictionaries/Simon & Schuster.

Selected Readings

American Nurses Association. (1985). *Code for nurses with interpretive statements.* Kansas City, Mo.: Author.

American Nurses Association. (1982). *Ethics references for nurses.* Kansas City, Mo.: Author.

Anderson, R. C., et al. (1987). Ethical issues in health promotion and health education. *American Association of Occupational Health Nurses Journal* 35(5): 220–23, 246–48.

Aroskar, M. A. (1979). Ethical issues in community health nursing. *Nursing Clinics of North America,* 14(1): 35–44.

Bandman, E. L., and B. Bandman. (1985). *Nursing ethics in the life span.* Norwalk, Conn.: Appleton-Century-Crofts.

Bayer, R. (1984). Ethical challenges of the movement for home care. *Caring* 3(10): 57–62.

Beauchamp, T. L., and J. F. Childress. (1983). *Principles of biomedical ethics.* 2nd ed. New York: Oxford University Press.

Benjamin, M., and J. Curtis. (1986). *Ethics in nursing.* 2nd ed. New York: Oxford University Press.

Cassidy, J. C. (1988). Access to health care: A clinician's opinion about an ethical issue. *American Journal of Occupational Therapy* 42(5): 295–99.

Childress, J. F. (1981). *Priorities in Biomedical ethics.* Philadelphia: The Westminister Press.

Churchill, L. R., and J. J. Simon. (1982). Abortion and the rhetoric of individual rights. *The Hastings Center Report* 9: 10–12.

Cruttenden, L. (1987). The right to reject care: How community nurses can help the elderly chronically sick. *Nursing Times* 83(5): 33–35.

Curtin, L. (1978). A proposed model for critical ethical analysis. *Nursing Forum* 17: 12–17.

Curtin, L. (1982). No rush to judgment. In L. Curtin and J. Flaherty (eds.), *Nursing ethics: Theories and pragmatics* (pp. 57–63). Bowie, Md.: Robert J. Brady.

Davis, A., and M. Aroskar. (1983). *Ethical dilemmas and nursing practice.* 2nd ed. Norwalk, Conn.: Appleton-Century-Crofts.

Dubos, R. (1968). *So human an animal.* New York: Scribner's.

Ethical issues in health promotion. *Hospital Ethics,* May/June: 5–6.

Ewing, W. A. (1987). Domestic violence and community health care ethics: Reflection on systemic intervention . . . AMEND, Abusive Men Exploring New Directions. *Family and Community Health* 10(1): 73–82.

Francoeur, R. T. (1983). *Biomedical ethics: A guide to decision making.* New York: Wiley.

Fried, C. (1978). *Right and wrong.* Cambridge, Mass.: Harvard University Press.

Illich, I. (1975). *Medical nemesis: The expropriation of health.* New York: Pantheon.

Jameton, A. (1984). *Nursing practice: The ethical issues.* Englewood Cliffs, N.J.: Prentice-Hall.

Kilner, J. F. (1988). Selecting patients when resources are limited: A study of U.S. medical directors of kidney dialysis and transplantation facilities. *American Journal of Public Health* 78(2): 144–47.

Lancaster, J. (1987). From the editor . . . cost constraints in health care precipitate numerous ethical questions. *Family and Community Health* 10(1): v.

Last, J. M. (1987). Ethical issues in public health. In *Public health and human ecology.* East Norwalk, Conn.: Appleton & Lange.

Last, J. M. (1987). Ethics, mores and values — and AIDS. *Canadian Journal of Public Health* 78(2): 75–76.

McLeroy, K. R., et al. (1987). The business of health promotion: Ethical issues and professional responsibilities. *Health Education Quarterly* 14(1): 91–109.

Matejski, M. P. (1981). Ethical issues, nursing and the health care system. *Nursing Leadership* 27: 33.

Muyskens, J. L. (1982). *Moral problems in nursing: A philosophical investigation.* Totowa, N.J.: Rowman & Littlefield.

Ostwald, S. K., et al. (1987). Community health nursing in workplace health programs: Rationale and ethics. *Journal of Community Health Nursing* 4(3): 121–29.

Pence, T. (1983). *Ethics in nursing: An annotated bibliography.* New York: National League for Nursing.

President's Commission for the Study of Ethical Problems in Medicine and Biomedical and Behavioral Research. (1982). *Making health care decisions: Volume one report.* Washington, D.C.: U.S. Government Printing Office.

President's Commission for the Study of Ethical Problems in Medicine and Biomedical and Behavioral Research. (1983a). *Securing access to health care: Volume one report.* Washington, D.C.: U.S. Government Printing Office.

President's Commission for the Study of Ethical Problems in Medicine and Biomedical and Behavioral Research. (1983b). *Summing up.* Washington, D.C.: U.S. Government Printing Office.

Sease, S. S. (1985). Ethical dimensions of community health: Increasing awareness. *Journal of Community Health Nursing* 2(3): 129–33.

Simon, S. B., and J. Clark. (1975). *More values clarification: Strategies for the classroom.* San Diego, Calif.: Pennant Press.

Simon, S. B., and H. Kirschenbaum. (1972). *Values clarification: A handbook of practical strategies for teachers and students.* New York: Hart Publishing.

Spaar, B. (1987). Final demands (a case study). *Nursing Times* 83(5): 58.

Stanley, T. (1980). Ethics as a component of the curriculum. *Nursing and Health Care* 1: 63–72.

Steele, S. M., and M. V. Harmon. (1983). *Values clarification in nursing.* 2nd ed. Norwalk, Conn.: Appleton-Century-Crofts.

Thompson, J. B., and H. O. Thompson. (1981). *Ethics in nursing.* New York: Macmillan.

Uustal, D. B. (1978). Values clarification in nursing. *American Journal of Nursing* 78: 2058–63.

Veatch, R. M., and S. T. Fry. (1987). *Case studies in nursing ethics.* Philadelphia: J. B. Lippincott.

TWO Tools for Practice

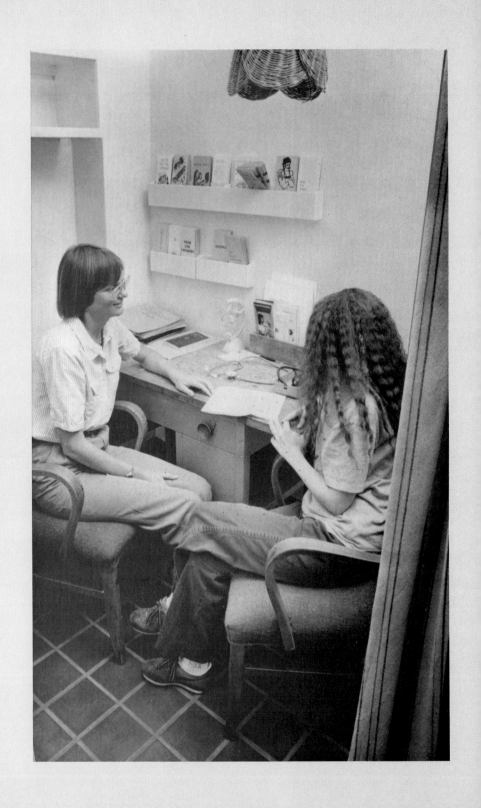

Roles and Settings for Community Health Nursing Practice

There was a day when uniformed public health nurses and home visits summed up the roles and settings of community health nursing, but that day is gone. Today we find professional community health nurses practicing in a wide variety of settings, such as family planning clinics, industrial plants, and elementary schools, and these nurses are no longer restricted to giving treatment. Instead, their roles range from educators and organizers to agents of change. In Chapter 3 we discussed the nature of community health nursing—how it developed and the characteristics that form a conceptual foundation for its practice. Now we shall consider the specific application of these concepts in the form of various roles assumed by community health nurses, as well as the kinds of settings in which these roles are practiced.

ROLES OF COMMUNITY HEALTH NURSES

Community health nursing incorporates a variety of roles; one could say that community health nurses wear many hats while conducting day-to-day practice. At times, one role is primary. For example, a community health nurse may assume a set of responsibilities in a specialized role such as that of full-time manager. More often, however, a number of roles are assumed simultaneously. Several factors influence the roles played by community health nurses. The organization with which the nurse is affiliated usually has policies that govern nursing activity. Consumers use community health nursing services differently, depending on their perceptions of nursing. Sociocultural norms, which vary from one group to another, will affect the roles of some community health nurses. For example, some groups' values about acceptable female behavior will influence role choices. Political and legal restrictions also set limitations and determine directions for community health nursing practice. Perhaps the most important factor in determining roles will be the community health nurse's own values and ability to adapt to changing health needs. To clarify and expand our understanding of the way community health nursing is practiced, we shall examine seven major roles: (1) care provider, (2) educator, (3) advocate, (4) manager, (5) collaborator, (6) leader, and (7) researcher.

CARE PROVIDER

The most familiar role is that of a clinician or provider of care; however, giving nursing care takes on new meaning in the context of community health. The target of service expands beyond the individual to include families, groups, and communities. Nursing care is still designed for the special needs of the client; however, when that client is a group of people, care takes different forms. It requires different skills to assess collective needs and tailor service accordingly. For instance, a community health nurse might receive a referral to visit a family with multiple problems. The call is triggered by the 11-year-old son's frequent absence from and misbehavior at school. Together, the nurse and family, in consultation with other public health professionals, design a plan of care that includes intervention for the whole family. It is a response to consideration of the family's resources and problems and the family members' perceptions of the situation.

Holistic Care

We recognize that clinical nursing is holistic, but in community health this approach means viewing the client as a larger system. The client, most often a family or group, is a composite of people whose relationships and interactions with each other must be considered in totality. Holistic care must emerge from this systems perspective (Anderson and McFarlane, 1988). For example, a community health nurse may be working with a group of pregnant teenagers living in a juvenile detention center. The nurse would consider the girls' relationships with each other, their parents, the fathers of their unborn children, and the detention center staff. The nurse would evaluate their age levels, developmental needs, and peer influences, as well as their knowledge of pregnancy, delivery, and issues related to the choice of keeping or giving up their babies. The girls' reentry into the community and their future plans for school or employment would also be considered. Holistic care would go far beyond the physical condition of pregnancy and childbirth.

Focus on Wellness

The role of care provider in community health is also characterized by its focus on wellness (Birmingham, 1987). As we discussed in Chapter 1, the community health nurse provides care along the entire range of the wellness-illness continuum but especially emphasizes promotion of health and prevention of illness. Nursing care includes seeking out clients in order to offer preventive services, rather than waiting for them to come for help after problems arise (Mullen, 1986). Community health nurses identify people who are interested in achieving a higher level of health and work with them to accomplish that goal. They may help a family or group learn how to live healthier life-styles, or they may work with a group that wants to quit smoking. They may hold seminars at a men's club on handling stress. They may assist a family with a terminally ill member at home in developing positive acceptance of dying and death.

Necessary Skills

The community health nurse uses many different skills in the care provider role. In nursing's early years, the skills most often used were those associated with physical care. (Such skills are still very important as earlier hospital discharges and a growing number of elderly persons in the population create more complex physical care demands.) As time went on, skills in observation, listening, communication, and counseling became integral to the care provider role. The role included an increased emphasis on psychological and sociocultural factors. Most recently, environmental considerations, such as awareness of problems caused by pollution or of emotional stress related to urban congestion, have created a need for new skills such as assessment and intervention at the community level. We address these skills in greater detail in later chapters.

EDUCATOR ROLE

It is widely recognized that health teaching is part of good nursing care and one of the major functions of the community health nurse (Brown, 1988). Health education is especially significant for two major reasons. First, the clients in the community are usually not in an acute state of illness and are better able to absorb and act on health information. For example, a class of expectant parents, unhampered by significant health problems, can grasp the relationship of diet to fetal development. They will understand the value of specific exercises to the childbirth process and then perform those exercises. Second, the health educator role is significant because people in the community have acquired a higher level of health consciousness. Through plans ranging from the president's physical fitness program to local antismoking campaigns, people are recognizing the value of health and are increasingly motivated to achieve higher levels of wellness. When a middle-aged businessman, for example, is discharged from the hospital following a heart attack, he is likely to be more interested than he was before in learning how to prevent occurrence of an attack. He can learn how to reduce stress, develop an appropriate and gradual exercise program, and alter his eating habits. Families with young children are often interested in learning about children's growth and development; many young parents want to raise happier, healthier children. In an increasing number of businesses and industries nurses are promoting the health of employees through active wellness programs (Kirkpatrick, 1985; Chen, 1988). The companies recognize that improved health of their workers means less absenteeism and higher production levels in addition to other benefits (White, 1986). Some companies even provide exercise areas and equipment for employee use.

All nurses teach patients about personal care, diet, and medications. Community health nurses, however, go beyond these topics to educate people in a great many areas. People in the community need and want to know about a wide variety of topics. How do you toilet train a two-year-old? What foods should you avoid when you have coronary atherosclerosis? How do you manage an alcoholic spouse? What do you do with adolescent rebellion? What is the best way to lose weight and keep it off? How can you organize the community to work for clean air? What are health consumers' rights? The range of topics taught by community health nurses extends from personal health care and management of leisure to environmental health and community organization.

As educators, community health nurses seek to facilitate client learning. They share information with clients informally, often in the clients' homes (Figure 7-1). They act as consultants to individuals or groups. They may hold formal classes to increase people's understanding of health and health care. Community health nurses utilize established community groups in their teaching. For example, they may teach parents at a PTA meeting about signs

Figure 7-1
Teaching this mother how to help her child is one of the many ways that community health nurses serve as health educators.

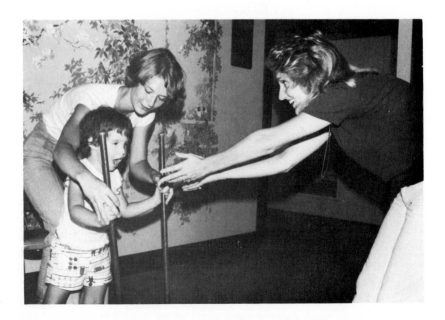

of drug abuse, discuss safety practices with a group of industrial workers, or give a presentation on the importance of early detection of child abuse to a health planning committee considering the funding of a new program. At times, the community health nurse facilitates client learning through referral to more knowledgeable sources or through use of experts on special topics. The community health nurse also facilitates clients' self-education; in keeping with the concept of self-care, clients are encouraged and helped to use appropriate health resources and to seek out health information for themselves. The emphasis throughout the health teaching process continues to be placed on illness prevention and health promotion. Health teaching as a tool for community health nursing practice is discussed in Chapter 11.

ADVOCATE ROLE

The issue of patients' rights is important in health care today. Every patient or client has the right to receive just, equal, and humane treatment. In our present society, the health care system is often characterized by fragmented and depersonalized services. Clients, especially poor and disadvantaged ones, are frequently unable to achieve their rights. They become frustrated, confused, and degraded, unable to cope with the system on their own.

Advocacy Goals

Kosik (1972) has described two underlying goals in client advocacy. One is to help clients gain greater independence. The community health nurse shows clients what services are available, which services they are entitled to, and how to obtain services, until they can discover this information for themselves. A second goal is to make the system more responsive and relevant to the needs of clients. By calling attention to inadequate or unjust care, the community health nurse can influence change.

Consider the experience of a family that we shall call the Martins. Gloria Martin and her three small children had gone to the Westside Clinic on Wednesday. On Tuesday morning, the baby, Tony, had suddenly started to cry. Nothing would comfort him. Gloria called the clinic and was told to come in the next day. The clinic did not take appointments and was too busy to see any more patients that day. The rest of that day and night Tony cried almost incessantly. On Wednesday there was a 45-minute bus ride and a wait of three and a half hours in the crowded reception room, a wait punctuated by intake workers' interrogations. The children were restless, and the baby was crying. Finally they saw the physician. Tony had an inguinal hernia that could be gangrenous. The doctor admonished the mother that the baby should have been brought in sooner. Now immediate surgery was necessary. Someone at the clinic told Gloria that Medicaid would pay for it. Someone else told her that she was ineligible because she was not a registered clinic patient. By now all the children were crying. Gloria had been up most of the night. She was frantic, confused, and felt that no one cared. This family needed an advocate.

Advocacy Actions and Characteristics

As an advocate, the community health nurse pleads the cause of another by speaking and acting on that person's or group's behalf. There are times when health care clients need someone to explain what services to expect and which services they ought to receive. They need someone to guide them through the complexities of the system and someone to assure the satisfaction of their needs.

The advocate role requires at least four important characteristics. First, advocates must be *assertive*. In the Martins' dilemma, a community health nurse took the initiative to identify their needs and find appropriate solutions. She contacted the right people and helped them establish eligibility for coverage of surgery and hospitalization costs. She helped Gloria make arrangements for the baby's hospitalization and the other children's care. A second characteristic of the advocate role is *willingness to take risks,* to go out on a limb if need be, for the client. The community health nurse was outraged at the kind of treatment that the Martins had received—the delays in service, the impersonal care, and the surgery that could have been prevented. She wrote a letter describing the details of the Martins' experience to the clinic director, the chairman of the clinic board, and the nursing director. It resulted in better care for the Martins and a series of meetings aimed at changing clinic procedures and providing better initial screening. A third characteristic of advocates is their ability to *communicate well,* to bargain thoroughly and convincingly. The community health nurse helping the Martins was able to state the problem clearly and argue for its solution. Finally, the advocate role requires the ability to *identify sources of power* and tap into them for the client's benefit. By contacting the most influential people in the clinic and appealing to their desire for quality service, the nurse concerned with the Martins was able to facilitate change.

MANAGER ROLE

Community health nurses, like all nurses, are managers of client care. Nurses are serving as managers when they supervise family care, run clinics, conduct community health planning projects, or manage caseloads. Case management, in particular, has become increasingly important in community health nursing. As patients leave hospitals earlier, as families struggle with multiple and complex health problems, as increasing numbers of elderly persons need alternatives to nursing home care, and as competition and scarce resources contribute to fragmentation of services, there is a growing need for someone to keep all the pieces together. Community health nurses, through case management, address this need (Hanlon and Pickett, 1984). As managers, community health nurses perform three main functions: planning, organizing, and coordinating.

Planning

Planning, the first and most basic function performed by the nurse as a manager, enables the nurse to decide on an objective (client care goals) and to achieve it (nursing process). The nurse begins by studying the situation and drawing up a detailed plan. Community health nurses, as managers, need time for planning, which involves determining client concerns and needs, establishing objectives, and deciding on an appropriate course of action. When starting a therapy group for recovering drug addicts, for example, the nurse sits down with the entire group to discuss the members' present situations and ambitions. What would they like to accomplish in group therapy? What topics would they like to cover? How would they like to approach them — through discussion or role playing? When and where would they like to meet? In the process of making these decisions, nurses are planning, that is, mapping out a course of action based on predetermined goals and objectives.

Organizing

The second function of the community health nurse's managerial role is organizing. Organizing means structuring activities and placing people into a functioning whole aimed at attaining stated objectives (Longest, 1976). A manager must arrange matters so that the job can be done. People, activities, and relationships have to be assembled in order to put the plan into effect (Rowland and Rowland, 1985). In the process of organizing, the nurse provides a framework for the various aspects of service so that each will run smoothly and accomplish its purpose. The framework is a part of service preparation. When a community health nurse manages a well-baby clinic, for instance, the organizing function involves making certain that all equipment and supplies are present, required staff are hired and on duty, and staff responsibilities are clearly designated.

Coordinating

Coordinating, the third function of the community health nurse's managerial role, means bringing people and activities together so that they function in harmony while pursuing desired objectives. Like the matching of a movie film's sound track with its pictures, coordination involves assembly and synchronization. It occurs during planning and implementation of service. On a nurse-patient or nurse-family level, some coordination is almost always necessary (Figure 7-2). The nurse may arrange an early demonstration of walking on

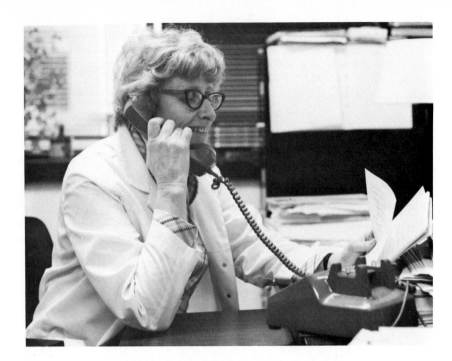

Figure 7-2
As a manager, the nurse coordinates client care so that needed resources are available at the right time.

crutches by the physical therapist, time a home health aide's visit to coincide with an older woman's preferred bath schedule, or bring an eight-year-old boy and his parents together with his teacher and the learning disabilities specialist to discuss ways to approach his learning problems.

Coordinating becomes a more complex activity at the community level. Consider a community health nurse working with a group of citizens and health professionals who are interested in starting a mobile health center for a two-county area. Their objective is to make health service more accessible to residents. The nurse will need to contact many individuals, arrange meetings, explore funding sources, talk with community leaders, and help maintain the group's focus on its objective. Once the project is in operation, the nurse, as manager, will have a continuing responsibility to coordinate it.

The manager role, at times, involves other functions, such as leading, staffing, supervising, motivating, and controlling service activities (Rowland and Rowland, 1985). While performing all these functions, community health nurses most often are participative managers; that is, they participate with clients, staff, or both, in planning and carrying out services.

COLLABORATOR ROLE

Community health nurses seldom practice in isolation. Their work involves many other people, including other nurses, physicians, social workers, physical therapists, nutritionists, attorneys, and secretaries. As a member of the health team (Williams, 1986), the community health nurse assumes the role of collaborator. To collaborate means to work jointly with others in a common endeavor, to cooperate as partners. Successful community health practice depends on this multidisciplinary collegiality (Turner and Chavigny, 1988). Everyone on the team, including the community health nurse, has an important and unique contribution to make to the health care effort. As on a championship football team, the better each member plays his position and cooperates with other members, the more likely the health team is to win.

Interdisciplinary collaboration has been discussed in Chapter 3 as a vital characteristic of community health nursing. The collaborator role is simply an application of that concept. For example, one family needed to find a good nursing home for their 83-year-old grandfather. The community health nurse and family, including the grandfather, made a list of desired features that included a shower. He did not like baths. The daughter, son-in-law, and community health nurse, working with a social worker, located and visited several homes. The grandfather's physician was contacted for medical consultation, and the grandfather made the final selection. In another situation, the community health nurse collaborated with the city council, police department, neighborhood residents, and manager of a senior citizens' high-rise apartment building to help a group of elderly people organize and lobby for safer streets. In a third example, a school nurse noticed a boy with a high absentee record and low grades. Counseling was started after joint planning with his parents, teacher, school psychologist, and family physician.

The community health nurse's collaborator role requires skills in communicating, in interpreting the nurse's unique contribution to the team, and in acting assertively as an equal partner. The collaborator role may also involve functioning as a consultant (Figure 7-3).

Figure 7-3
The nurse often has unique knowledge about clients that as a collaborator she shares with other health team members.

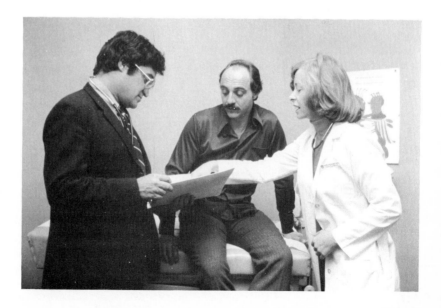

LEADER ROLE

Community health nurses are increasingly becoming active leaders. When they guide decision making, stimulate interest in health promotion, initiate therapy, direct a preventive program, and influence health policy, they are assuming leadership roles. As leaders, nurses usually influence and persuade, rather than direct, others.

The role of leader, as distinguished from the role of manager, serves a unique purpose. Its main function is to effect change; thus, the community health nurse becomes an agent of change. (Chapter 22 elaborates on this role.) As leaders, nurses influence people to think and behave differently about their health and the factors contributing to it. For example, a community health nurse who made home visits to a young mother suggested that the mother invite her neighbors over for coffee and discussion about health topics of interest. The group met once a month and grew as the community health nurse increased their desire for more information.

The role of leader assumes a different form in another situation. A community health nurse was eager to start a mental health program, which she and her nursing colleagues felt was needed, through the agency for which she worked. But certain individuals on the health board were opposed to adding any new programs because of cost. Her approach was to gather considerable supportive data to demonstrate the program's need and cost-effectiveness. She lunched individually with key board members in order to convince them of the need. She prepared written summaries, graphs, and charts and, at a strategic time, presented her case at a board meeting. The mental health program was approved and implemented.

As leaders, community health nurses also exert influence through health planning (McLemore, 1980). The need for coordinated, accessible, cost-effective health care services creates a challenge and an opportunity for community health nurses to become more involved in health planning at all levels—organizational, local, state, national, and even international. Nurses need to exercise their leadership responsibility and assert their right to share in health decisions (Edwards, 1983).

RESEARCHER ROLE

The researcher role is an integral part of community health nursing practice. But, it may be asked, how can research be combined with practice? It is true that research in the strictest sense involves a complex set of activities conducted by persons with highly developed and specialized skills. But there is another way to view research, that is, as an investigative process. From this perspective, all community health nurses are researchers, or investigators.

Research literally means to search—to investigate, discover, and interpret facts. All research in community health, from the simplest inquiry to the most complex epidemiologic study, uses the same fundamental process. Most simply put, the research process involves the following steps: (1) identify an area of interest, (2) specify the research question or statement, (3) review the literature, (4) identify a conceptual framework, (5) select a research design, (6) collect and analyze data, (7) interpret the results, and (8) communicate the findings (see Chapter 24).

Investigation builds on the nursing process, that essential dynamic of community health nursing practice, using it as a problem-solving process (Polit and Hungler, 1983). That is, the nurse identifies a problem or question, collects and analyzes data by making an investigation, suggests and evaluates possible solutions, and selects a solution or rejects them all and starts the investigative process over again. In one sense the nurse is a health planner, investigating health problems in order to design wellness-promoting and disease-preventing interventions for community populations.

Attributes of the Researcher Role

A questioning attitude is a basic prerequisite to good nursing practice. There have probably been many times when a nurse revisited a patient and noticed some change in his condition such as restlessness or pallor. Consequently, the nurse wondered what was causing this change and what could be done about it. In everyday practice, community health nurses encounter numerous situations that challenge them to ask questions. Consider the following examples:

> "Mr. Hansen is still very weak on his right side since his CVA [cerebrovascular accident]. I wonder if he really understands how to do his exercises?"
> "Little Marc seems unusually quiet, and I see another bruise on his left arm. Could this possibly be the beginning of child abuse?"
> "This prenatal class is dragging; am I going too fast, is there some conflict in the group, or do the members need more opportunity for expressing themselves?"
> "While driving through this part of the city, I haven't seen a single playground for miles. I wonder where the kids play?"

Each of these questions places the community health nurse in the role of investigator. They express the fundamental attitude of every researcher: *a spirit of inquiry.*

A second attribute, careful *observation,* is also evident in the examples just given. The community health nurse develops a sharpened ability to notice things as they are, including deviations from the norm and even subtle changes that suggest the need for some nursing action.

Coupled with observation is *open-mindedness,* another attribute of the researcher role. After observing Mr. Hansen's weakness, the community health nurse postulates that Mr. Hansen may not understand how to do his exercises, but she keeps an open mind to other possibilities. He can demonstrate his exercises, and if that is not the problem, perhaps he needs some different activities to strengthen the weak muscles. In the case of little Marc, the community health nurse's observations suggest child abuse as the possible cause. But open-mindedness requires consideration of other alternatives, and as a good investigator, the nurse explores these as well.

The community health nurse also uses *analytic* skills in this role. In the prenatal class example, the nurse has already started to analyze the situation by trying to determine its cause-and-effect relationships. Successful analysis depends on how well the data have been collected. Insufficient information can lead to false interpretations, so the community health nurse is careful to seek out the needed data. Analysis, like a jigsaw puzzle, involves studying the pieces and fitting them together until the meaning of the whole picture can be described.

Finally, the researcher role involves *tenacity*. The community health nurse persists in an investigation until facts are uncovered and a satisfactory answer is found. Noticing an absence of playgrounds and wondering where the children play is only a beginning. The nurse, concerned about the children's safety and need for recreational outlets in the district, gathers data about location and accessibility of play areas as well as felt needs of community residents. A fully documented research report may result. If the data support a need for additional play space, the report can be brought before the proper authorities.

Levels in the Researcher Role

Community health nurses practice the researcher role at many levels. Up to this point we have focused primarily on simple kinds of investigations to emphasize that research is an essential and integral part of community health nursing practice; however, the attributes that have been described are basic to research practice at any level. In addition to everyday inquiries, community health nurses often participate in agency or organizational studies to determine such matters as the effectiveness of a screening program or the need for a new family planning clinic. Some community health nurses also initiate more complex research of their own or in collaboration with other health professionals, perhaps a full-scale epidemiologic study. The researcher role, at all levels, helps to determine needs, evaluate effectiveness of care, and develop theoretical bases for community health nursing practice. In Chapters 9 and 24 we explain community health research in greater detail.

SETTINGS FOR PRACTICE

We have just examined community health nursing from the perspective of its major roles. Now we can place the roles in context by viewing the settings in which they are practiced. The numbers and kinds of places for community health nursing practice are too varied for us to examine all of them here. For purposes of discussion, however, they can be grouped into six categories: (1) homes, (2) ambulatory care settings, (3) schools, (4) occupational health settings, (5) residential institutions, and (6) the community at large.

HOMES

One of the most frequently used settings for community health nursing practice is the home (Figure 7-4). In the home setting all of the community health nursing roles, to varying degrees, are performed. Clients discharged from acute care institutions, such as hospitals or mental health facilities, are regularly referred to community health nursing for continued care and follow-up. Here the nurse can see the client in a family and environmental context, and

Figure 7-4
A follow-up home visit by the community health nurse assures this couple that their new baby is doing well. Such visits provide opportunities for family health promotion.

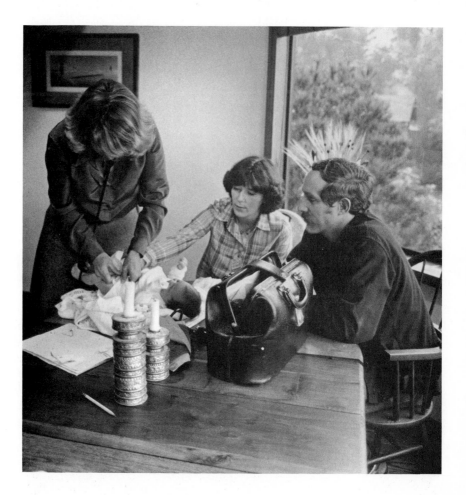

service can be individualized to the client's particular needs. For example, Mr. White, 67 years of age, was discharged from the hospital after undergoing a colostomy. Doreen, the community health nurse from the county public health nursing agency, immediately started home visits. She met with Mr. White and his wife to discuss their needs as a family and to plan for Mr. White's care and adjustment to living with a colostomy. Practicing the care provider and educator roles, she reinforced and expanded on the teaching started in the hospital for colostomy care, that is, bowel training, diet, exercise, and proper use of equipment. As part of a total family care plan, Doreen provided some forms of physical care for Mr. White as well as counseling, teaching, and emotional support for both the Whites. In addition to consulting with the physician and social services, she arranged and supervised home health aide visits that gave personal care and homemaker services. She thus utilized the manager, leader, and collaborator roles.

The home is a setting for health promotion as well. Many community health nursing visits focus on assisting families in understanding and practicing healthier living. They may, for example, include instruction in parenting, infant care, child discipline, eating right, getting proper exercise, coping with stress, or managing grief and loss.

The character of the home setting is as varied as the clients whom the community health nurse serves. In one day a community health nurse may visit an elderly, well-to-do widow in her luxurious home, a middle-income family in their modest bungalow, and a transient in his one-room fifth-story walk-up apartment. In each home situation, community health nurses can view their clients in perspective and, therefore, better understand their limitations, capitalize on their resources, and tailor health services to their needs. In the home, unlike most other health care settings, clients are on their own turf. They feel comfortable and secure in familiar surroundings and are often better able to understand and apply health information. Client self-respect can be promoted, since the client is host while the nurse is a guest.

AMBULATORY CARE SETTINGS

Ambulatory care settings include a variety of places in which community health nurses practice. Each is a place where clients *come* for day service; in other words, they seek out or are referred to these health services for care that does not include overnight stays. Clinics are an example of an ambulatory setting. Sometimes multiple clinics, offering medical, surgical, orthopedic, dermatologic, and many other services, are located in outpatient departments of hospitals or medical centers. They may also be based in comprehensive neighborhood health centers. A single clinic, such as a family planning or well-child clinic, may be found in a location more convenient for clients, such as a church basement or empty storefront. Some kinds of day care centers, such as those for physically handicapped or emotionally disturbed adults, utilize community health nursing services. Additional ambulatory care settings include health departments and community health nursing agencies where clients may come for assessment and referral or counseling.

Offices are another type of ambulatory care setting. Some community health nurses provide service in conjunction with medical practice; for example, a community health nurse associated with a HMO sees clients in the office and undertakes screening, referrals, counseling, health education, and group work. Others establish independent practices by seeing clients in nursing centers as well as making home visits (Goodson, 1978; Gloss and Fielo, 1987; Thibodeau, 1987).

Another type of ambulatory care setting includes places where services are offered to selected groups. For example, community health nurses practice in migrant camps, Native American reservations, prisons, children's day care centers, churches (Miller, 1987), and remote mountain and coal-mining communities. Again, in each ambulatory care setting all the community health nursing roles are utilized to varying degrees.

SCHOOLS

Schools of all levels make up a major group of settings for community health nursing practice. Nurses from community health nursing agencies frequently serve private schools of elementary and intermediate levels. Public schools are served by the same agencies or by community health nurses hired through the public school system. Community health nurses may work with groups of children in preschool settings, such as Montessori schools, as well as in vocational or technical schools, junior colleges, and college and university settings. Specialized schools, such as those for the handicapped, are another setting for community health nursing practice.

Community health nurses' roles in school settings are expanding. School nurses, whose primary role was initially that of care providers, are widening their practice to include more health education, collaboration, and client advocacy. For example, one school had been accustomed to utilizing the nurse as a first-aid giver and record keeper. Her duties were handling minor problems, such as headaches and cuts, and keeping track of such events as immunizations. This nurse determined to expand her practice and, after planning and preparation, implemented a series of classes on personal hygiene, diet, and sexuality; started a drop-in health counseling center in the school; and established a network of professional contacts for consultation and referral. Community health nurses in school settings are also beginning to assume managerial and leadership roles and to recognize that the researcher role should be an integral part of their practice. The nurse's role with preschool and school-age populations is discussed in greater detail in Chapter 17.

OCCUPATIONAL HEALTH SETTINGS

Business and industry provide another group of settings for community health nursing practice. Employee health has long been recognized as making a vital contribution to individual lives, productivity of business, and the well-being of the entire nation. Organizations now are expected to provide a safe and healthy work environment in addition to offering health insurance for health care. An increasing number of companies, recognizing the value of healthy employees, go beyond offering traditional health benefits to supporting health promotional efforts. Some businesses, for example, offer healthy snacks such as fruit at breaks and promote jogging during the noon hour. A few larger corporations have built exercise facilities for their employees, provided health education programs, and offered financial incentives for losing weight or staying well.

Community health nurses in occupational health settings practice a variety of roles. Early industrial nursing, which started in 1895 when the first nurse was hired by an industry, mostly involved visiting sick workers in their homes (Freeman and Heinrich, 1981). The care provider role was primary for many years as nurses continued to care for sick or injured employees at work. However, recognition of the need to protect employees' safety and later to prevent their illness led to inclusion of health education. Now industrial nurses also act as employee advocates, assuring appropriate job assignments for workers and adequate treatment for job-related illness or injury. They collaborate with other health care providers and company management to offer better services to their clients and act as leaders and managers in developing new health services in the work setting, endorsing programs such as hypertension screening or weight control. Occupational health settings range from industries and factories, such as an automobile assembly plant, to business corporations and even large department stores. The field of occupational health offers a challenging opportunity, particularly in smaller businesses where nursing coverage usually is not provided. In Chapter 18 we more fully describe the role of the nurse serving the working population.

RESIDENTIAL INSTITUTIONS

Facilities where clients reside form a fifth group of settings in which community health nursing is practiced. Clients may be housed temporarily in these institutions, as in a halfway house for recovering alcoholics, or on a relatively permanent basis, as in an inpatient hospice program for the terminally ill. Some of these institutions, such as hospitals, exist solely to provide health care. Community health nurses based in a community agency maintain continuity of care for their clients by collaborating with hospital personnel, visiting clients in the hospital, and helping plan care during and following hospitalization. As part of their caseloads, some community health nurses serve one or more hospitals on a regular basis by providing a liaison with the community, consultation for discharge planning, and periodic in-service programs to keep hospital staff updated on community services for their clients. Other community health nurses with similar functions are based in the hospital and serve the hospital community. A nursing home staffed with skilled nurses is another example of a residential facility providing health care that may utilize community health nursing services. In this kind of setting, where residents are usually elderly with many chronic health problems, community health nurses function particularly as advocates and collaborators to improve care. They will coordinate available resources to meet the needs of residents and their families and help safeguard the maintenance of proper nursing home operating standards. Sheltered workshops and group homes for mentally retarded adults are other examples of residential institutions that serve clients who share specific needs.

Community health nurses also practice in settings where residents are gathered for purposes other than receiving care. Health care is offered as an adjunct to the primary goals of the institution. For example, many nurses work with camping programs for children and adults offered by churches and other community agencies, such as the Boy Scouts, Girl Scouts, or the YMCA. As camp nurses, community health nurses practice all available roles, often under interesting and challenging conditions.

Residential institutions provide unique settings for community health nurses to practice health promotion. Their clients are a "captive" audience whose needs can be readily assessed and whose interests can be stimulated. These settings offer community health nurses the opportunity to generate an environment of caring and optimal-quality services.

COMMUNITY AT LARGE

Unlike the five settings already discussed, the sixth setting for community health nursing practice is not confined to a specific location or building. When nurses work with groups, populations, or the total community, they may practice in many different places. For example, a community health nurse, as care provider and health educator, may work with a parenting group in a church or town hall. Another nurse, as client advocate, leader, and researcher, may study the health needs of a neighborhood's elderly population by collecting data throughout the area and meeting with resource people in many places. Again, the community at large becomes the setting for practice of a nurse who serves on health care planning committees, lobbies for health legislation at the state capitol, or runs for a school board position.

Although the term *setting* implies place, it is important to remember that community health nursing practice is not limited to a specific arena. Community health nursing is a specialty of nursing defined by the nature of its practice (Anderson and Meyer, 1985), and it can be practiced anywhere.

Summary

Community health nursing incorporates many roles and is practiced in many settings. Seven major roles, when combined, describe community health nursing practice: care provider, educator, advocate, manager, collaborator, leader, and researcher. The types and number of roles that are practiced vary depending on the nurse, clients, and demands of the situation.

The settings of community health nursing practice are also many and varied, but they can generally be grouped into six categories: homes, ambulatory care settings, schools, occupational health settings, residential institutions, and the community at large.

Study Questions

1. What are some ways that a community health nurse can make care holistic and focused on wellness with a group of chemically dependent adolescents?
2. Select one community health nursing role and describe its application in meeting your next-door neighbor's needs.
3. Describe a hypothetical or real situation in which you, as a community health nurse, would combine the roles of leader, collaborator, and researcher (investigator). Discuss how each of these roles might be played.
4. If your community health nursing practice setting is the community at large, will your practice roles be any different from those of the nurse whose practice setting is the home? Why? What determines the roles played by the community health nurse?

References

Anderson, E., and J. McFarlane. (1988). *Community as client.* Philadelphia: J.B. Lippincott.

Anderson, E., and A. T. Meyer. (1985). Report of the Conference. *Consensus conference on the essentials of public health nursing practice and education.* Rockville, Md.: U.S. Department of Health and Human Services.

Birmingham, J. J. (1987). The wellness frontier: The community. *Nursing Administration Quarterly* 11(3): 14–18.

Brown, M. A. (1988). Health promotion, education, counseling and coordination in primary health care nursing. *Public Health Nursing* 5(1): 16–23.

Chen, M. S., Jr. (1988). Wellness in the workplace: Beyond the point of no return. *Health Values* 12(1): 16–22.

Edwards, L. (1983). Health planning: Opportunities for nurses. *Nursing Outlook* 31(6): 322–25.

Freeman, R., and J. Heinrich. (1981). *Community health nursing practice.* Philadelphia: W. B. Saunders.

Gloss, E. F., and S. B. Fielo. (1987). The nursing center: An alternative for health care delivery. *Family and Community Health* 10(2): 49–58.

Goodson, J. (1978). Demonstrating excellence in a community nursing service. In A. Warner (ed.), *Innovations in community health nursing* (pp. 16–22). St. Louis: C. V. Mosby.

Kirkpatrick, S. L. (1985). Nurses: Leaders in wellness health promotion at the worksite. *Occupational Health Nursing* 33(9): 450–52.

Kosik, S. H. (1972). Patient advocacy or fighting the system. *American Journal of Nursing* 72: 694–96.

Longest, B. (1976). *Management practices for the health professional.* Reston, Va.: Reston Publishing.

McLemore, M. (1980). Nurses as health planners. *Journal of Nursing Administration* 1: 13–17.

Miller, J. T. (1987). Wellness programs through the church: Available alternative for health education. *Health Values* 11(5): 3–6.

Mullen, K. D. (1986). Wellness: The missing concept in health promoting programming for adults. *Health Values* 10(3): 34–37.

Polit, D., and B. Hungler. (1983). Nursing research: Principles and methods. 2nd ed. Philadelphia: J. B. Lippincott.

Rowland, H. S., and B. L. Rowland. (1985). Nursing administration handbook. 2nd ed. Rockville, Md.: Aspen Systems.

Thibodeau, J. A., et al. (1987). Evolution of a nursing center. *Journal of Ambulatory Care Management* 10(3): 30–39.

Turner, J., and K. Chavigny. (1988). *Community health nursing: An epidemiologic perspective through the nursing process.* Philadelphia: J. B. Lippincott.

White, D. M. (1986). Health promotion pays: 3 to 1 return seen in stress management programs. *Occupational Health and Safety* 55(8): 18–19, 55.

Williams, E. (1986). Teamwork: Reinventing the wheel. *Community Outlook* (September): 36, 38.

Selected Readings

American Nurses Association. (1986). *Standards: Community health nursing practice.* Kansas City, Mo.: Author.

Anderson, E., and J. McFarlane. (1988). *Community as client.* Philadelphia: J. B. Lippincott.

Archer, S., and R. Fleshman. (1975). Community health nursing: A typology of practice. *Nursing Outlook* 23: 358–64.

Basch, C. E., et al. (1985). Promoting high-level wellness in a rural state: The Wellness Education Workshop. *Health Values* 9(4): 18–23.

Bernal, B. (1978). Levels of practice in a community health agency. *Nursing Outlook* 26: 364–69.

Birmingham, J. J. (1987). The wellness frontier: The community. *Nursing Administration Quarterly* 11(3):14–18.

Boomer, H. J. (1987). Health for all by the year 2000: The role of the health visitor. *Health Visitor* 60(1): 10–12.

Bremer, A. (1987). Revitalizing the district model for the delivery of prevention-focused community health nursing services. *Family and Community Health* 10(2): 1–10.

Brown, M. A. (1988). Health promotion, education, counseling and coordination in primary health care nursing. *Public Health Nursing* 5(1): 16–23.

Brown, M. L. (1981). *Occupational health nursing.* New York: Springer.

Buchanan, B. F. (1987). Human-environment interaction: A modification of Neuman Systems Model for aggregates, families, and the community. *Public Health Nursing* 4(1): 52–64.

Erickson, G. P. (1987). Public health nursing initiatives: Guideposts for future practice. *Public Health Nursing* 4(4): 202–211.

Fromer, M. J. (1983). Functions of the community health nurse. In M. J. Fromer (ed.), *Community health care and the nursing process.* 2nd ed. (pp. 155–172). St. Louis: C. V. Mosby.

Goodson, J. (1978). Demonstrating excellence in a community nursing service. In A. Warner (ed.), *Innovations in community health nursing* (pp. 16–22). St. Louis: C. V. Mosby.

Hanlon, J. J., and G. E. Pickett. (1984). *Public health: Administration and practice.* 8th ed. St. Louis: Times Mirror/Mosby.

Igoe, J. B. (1975). The school nurse practitioner. *Nursing Outlook* 23: 381–84.

Keller, M. J. (1979). Health needs and nursing care of the labor force. In M. J. Fromer (ed.), *Community health care and the nursing process.* St. Louis: C. V. Mosby.

Laffrey, S. C. (1985). Health promotion: Relevance for nursing. *Topics in Clinical Nursing* 7(2): 29–38.

Levin, L. S. (1978). Patient education and self-care: How do they differ? *Nursing Outlook* 26: 170–75.

Lunin, L. F. (1987). Where does the public get its health information? *Bulletin of New York Academy of Medicine* 63(10): 923–38.

Lurie, N., et al. (1987). Preventive care: Do we practice what we preach? *American Journal of Public Health.* 77(7): 801–4.

Maglacas, A. M. (1988). Health for all: Nursing's role. *Nursing Outlook* 36(2): 66–71.

Novak, J. C. (1988). The social mandate and historical basis for nursing's role in health promotion. *Journal of Professional Nursing* 4(2): 80–87.

Oda, D. (1979). Community nursing in schools: Developing a specialized role. In S. Archer and R. Fleshman (eds.), *Community health nursing: Patterns and practice.* 2nd ed. North Scituate, Mass.: Duxbury Press.

Pesznecker, B., M. A. Draye, and J. McNeil. (1982). Collaborative practice models in community health. *Nursing Outlook* 30: 298–302.

Porter-O'Grady, T. (1985). Health versus illness: Nurses can chart course for the future. *Nursing and Health Care* 6(6): 318–21.

Vance, C. (1979). Women leaders: Modern-day heroines or societal deviants? *Image* 11: 33–36.

Warner, A. (ed.). (1978). *Innovations in community health nursing.* St. Louis: C. V. Mosby.

Williams, C. A. (1977). Community health nursing—What is it? *Nursing Outlook* 25: 250–54.

Williams, C. A. (1983). Making things happen: Community health nursing and the policy arena. *Nursing Outlook* 31: 225–28.

Wyatt, G. K., et al. (1985). Interventions useful to the public health nurse: Improving health behaviors. *Journal of Nursing Education* 24(4): 168–70.

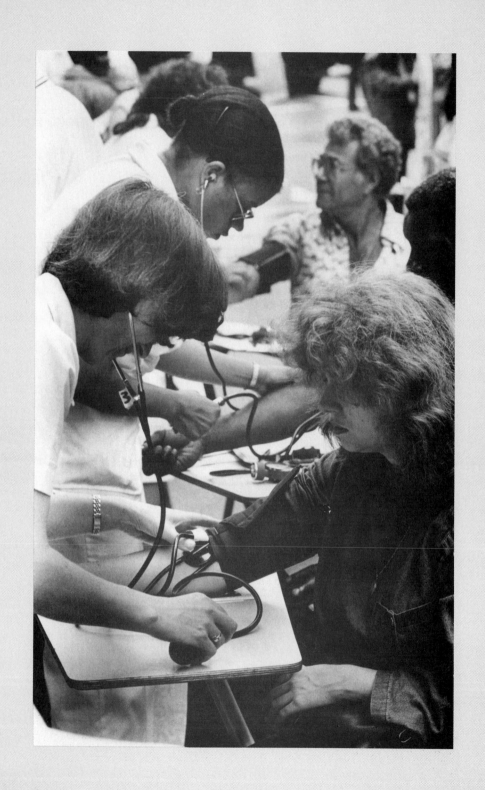

8 The Nursing Process in Community Health

Underlying all community health nursing practice flows one of its essential dynamics — the nursing process (White, 1982). Defined as a systematic, purposeful set of interpersonal actions (Mauksch and David, 1972), the nursing process provides the active, driving force for change that is the first and most important tool employed by the community health nurse.

Three characteristics emphasize the importance of this tool for community health nursing. First, the nursing process is a problem-solving process that addresses community health problems at all aggregate levels and aims to prevent illness and to promote the public's health. Second, it is a management process that requires analysis of a situation, decision making, planning, organizing, directing and controlling service efforts, and evaluating outcomes. As a management tool the nursing process addresses all aggregate levels. Third, it is a change process that works to improve various levels of health-related systems and the way people behave within those systems.

In this chapter we shall examine the nursing process: its components and dynamics for solving problems, managing nursing actions, and improving community health nursing practice.

COMPONENTS OF THE NURSING PROCESS

Process, the moving element of this tool, means forward progression in an orderly fashion toward some desired result. In community health, the nursing process involves a series of components, or steps, that enable the nurse to work with clients to achieve their optimal health. Nursing theorists attach different labels to these components, but all agree on the basic sequence of actions. The five major components are assessment, diagnosis, planning, implementation, and evaluation. All of these depend on a sixth component — interaction. Nursing literature and practice give increasing emphasis to this element of the process (Brill, 1973; Daubermire and King, 1973; Langford, 1978; Capers and Kelly, 1987). Nurse-client interaction is often an implied or assumed element in the process; for community health nursing, particularly, it is an essential first step.

INTERACTION

Community health nursing practice involves helping clients to help themselves. Listening to an elderly couple, teaching a class of expectant mothers, lobbying in the legislature for the poor, or working with parents to set up a dental screening program for children—all involve relationships. The nurse may establish an initial relationship, maintain an existing one, or redefine a previous one. Whatever its stage of development, a relationship involves reciprocal influence and exchange—in a word, interaction. This mutual give and take between nurse and clients, whether a family, a group of mothers on an Indian reservation, or school children, is the first step in the nursing process.

Need for Communication

Interaction requires communication. When a community health nurse initially contacts a family, for example, any information she may have in advance can give only partial clues to that family's needs and wants. Unless they begin by talking and listening, the later steps in the nursing process will go awry. By open, honest sharing, the nurse will begin to develop trust and establish lines of effective communication. For instance, she will explain who she is and why she is there. She will encourage the family members to talk about themselves. Nurse and family together will discuss their relationship and clarify the desired nature of that alliance. Does the family want help to identify and work on its health needs? Would its members like this nurse to continue regular contacts? What will their respective roles be? Effective communication, as a part of interaction, is essential to develop understanding and facilitate a free exchange of information between nurse and clients.

Interaction is reciprocal. Nurses must avoid the temptation either to do all the talking or merely to listen while a father or mother monopolizes the conversation. There is a dynamic exchange between two systems, with the community health nurse representing one system and the client the other. Whether the client is a handicapped family, a parent group, or an entire community, this exchange involves a two-way sharing of information, ideas, feelings, concerns, and ultimately self. The key elements of interaction are mutuality and cooperation.

Consider the following example: A dozen junior high school boys, most of whom were on the football team, met for several weeks with the school nurse to discuss physical fitness, nutrition, and other health topics. After their agreed-upon goals had been accomplished, the nurse wondered whether further meetings were needed. She raised the question and offered several topics, such as taking drugs and preventing injuries, for possible future sessions. The boys were not interested in these suggestions but, after more discussion, said they did want help with talking to girls. Renewed interaction was necessary as a first step in reapplying the nursing process.

Interaction paves the way for a helping relationship. As nurse and client interact, each is learning about the other. There is a period of testing before trust can be fully established. For the school nurse, establishing interaction had been more difficult at the time of her initial contact with the boys. They had been reluctant to talk, felt embarrassed to discuss personal subjects with a woman, and yet had strong interests in bodybuilding and personal appearance, strong enough to attract them to these optional sessions. Interaction began with a friendly exchange on nonthreatening topics and gradually deepened as the boys seemed ready to discuss personal subjects. Now it was relatively simple to talk about a new "problem" (to start the nursing process over again) because a helping relationship had already been developed. The nurse had a track record. The boys trusted, respected, and liked her, so they were happy to interact around a new need.

Group Level

Because community health practice focuses largely on the health of population groups, interaction goes beyond the one-to-one approach of clinical nursing (Williams, 1977). The challenge that faces the community health nurse is a one-to-group approach. A family, a group of concerned neighbors, and a group of handicapped persons are all collections of people with different concerns and opinions. Each person in a group is influenced by the thinking and behavior of the other group members. Nursing interaction with a group as the client demands an understanding of group behavior and group-level decision making, and it requires interpersonal communication at the group level. Thus, the task of interacting becomes more complex with a group than with an individual, but it also can be challenging and rewarding. Once community health nurses address themselves to understanding aggregate behavior, they can capitalize on the potential of group influence in order to make a far-reaching impact on the health of the total community. During this phase of the nursing process, however, the challenge lies with learning to interact effectively at the aggregate level. In later chapters we will look more closely at communicating and working with groups.

Interaction is more than a first step; it is an integral, ongoing part of the nursing process (see Figure 8-1). It is central to the process because nurse-client interaction forms the core of the relationship and information exchange. The effectiveness of each successive step—assessment, diagnosis, planning, implementation, and evaluation—depends on nurse-client interaction.

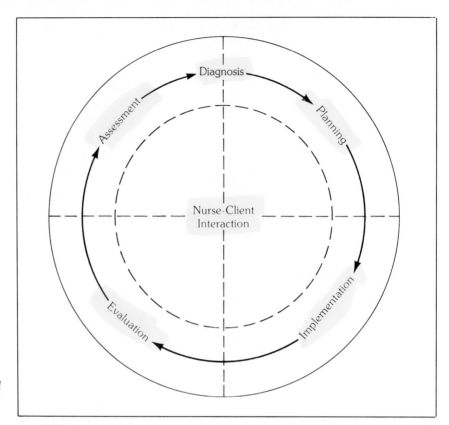

*Figure 8-1
Nursing process
components. Nurse-client
interaction, a permeable
structure, forms the core of
the process. As nurse and
client maintain a reciprocal
exchange of information
and trust through
interaction, they can
effectively assess client
needs; diagnose needs; and
plan, implement, and
evaluate care.*

ASSESSMENT

After establishing ongoing interaction, the community health nurse is ready to determine client needs; therefore, assessment is the next phase of the nursing process. According to Webster, *assessment* means judgment of the importance, size, or value of something; it is an act of appraisal. Nurses judge client health status to discover existing or potential needs as a basis for planning future action (Aggleton and Chalmers, 1986).

Assessment involves two major activities: (1) collection of pertinent data and (2) interpretation of data. These actions overlap and are repeated constantly throughout the assessment. Thus, while assessing a family's need for counseling, the nurse may simultaneously collect data on a persistent cough in a child and interpret previously collected data about nutritional deficiencies.

Collection of Data

The nurse can collect a wide range of data in the process of assessing community clients. What information and how much to collect depend, in the first place, on the initial reason for nurse-client contact. A specific health problem, such as Down's syndrome in the family, obesity among a group of teenagers, or widespread pediculosis in a grade school, focuses the data collection on information related to the present problem and its resolution. If the initial reason for nurse-client contact is health promotion, as for a normal postpartum family, data collection can be broadened to include information such as family history, constellation, present health status, coping abilities, support systems, and parenting skills.

A second consideration in data collection involves actual versus potential needs. Assessment of clients with multiple problems may force the community health nurse to focus only on existing (actual) needs because of limited time and resources. When possible, however, the community health nurse collects data aimed at uncovering potential needs in order to prevent problems from occurring (Figure 8-2). Early and periodic screening of children or health screening for hypertension, glaucoma, and diabetes are examples of preventive assessment.

Community health nurses utilize many sources in data collection. They begin by talking with clients because clients are closest to their own situation and can frequently offer the most accurate insights and comprehensive information. This is primary data because it is obtained directly from the client. A secondary source of data is people who know the client group well. In working with a family, the extended family members, friends, neighbors, and work associates may all be potential sources of information, pending client permission. Additional secondary sources include health team members, client records, community agencies, reference books, research reports, and

Figure 8-2
The nurse assesses individual, family, and community health through data collection. Here a free health screening program for hypertension gives the nurse important information on which to base future plans.

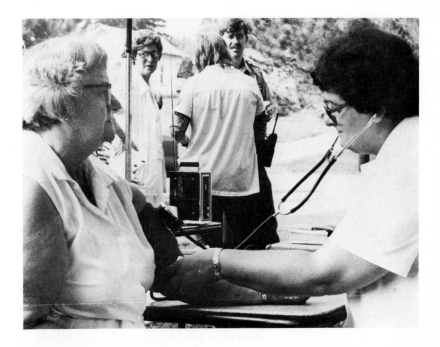

community health nurses themselves. Secondary data may not accurately describe the client or reflect client self-perceptions. Thus, secondary data may need further validation.

Data collection in community health requires the exercise of sound professional judgment, effective communication techniques, and special investigative skills. Observation is a basic method for gathering primary data. Seeing the family and its home environment tells the nurse something about its socioeconomic level and ability to cope using present resources. Hearing interpersonal conflict among the members of a weight control group can give the nurse clues about possible client concerns and stress levels. Noticing the absence of a caring atmosphere in a nursing home may suggest a need for intervention. Observation, as a data-gathering method, depends largely on nonverbal communication. The tone of a conversation may be friendly, hostile, or passive. A family may fail to keep appointments. A group's body language or a neighborhood's appearance conveys a message. All offer information about clients.

Another method for data collection is the interview. The interview involves a series of questions designed to elicit needed information. The community health nurse may conduct a formal interview during an early encounter to gather a health history and to encourage client expression. Informal directed questioning can sometimes provide even more data about client health status and needs. Communicating with clients serves as an important follow-up observation. If you observe children with bruises that suggest possible abuse, a carefully planned informal interview may be useful. You may discover a mother who is isolated and under emotional stress. Then you can undertake cooperative nurse-client planning for dealing with the problem.

Listening is an important data collection method. It is a skill that must be acquired through discipline and concentration. Too often we listen inattentively while we formulate our next question or allow our minds to wander. Good listening involves eye contact. It assures clients of sincere interest and encourages greater expression of ideas and feelings. The community health nurse who is a good listener can gain a wealth of information about clients.

Direct examination is still another method for collecting data. When working with individuals we think of percussion, auscultation, palpation, inspection, and measurement as means of direct examination. Applied to community groups and aggregates, direct examination assumes different forms such as surveys, screening instruments, epidemiologic research, or environmental testing for pathological determinants. Surveys, like interviews, provide specific information in response to selected questions. They can be especially useful for gathering data such as patterns of behavior among teenage alcoholics or battered women. Community health nurses also use surveys to assess neighborhood and community needs. Many kinds of standard screening instruments, including blood pressure apparatus, audiometers, scales, neurologic appraisal guides, and developmental tests, are useful for collecting data about clients. Epidemiologic research and environmental measurements add further data for community health analysis.

Interpretation of Data

This stage of assessment is analytic. Interpretation of data means analyzing the information gathered, drawing inferences or possible conclusions about the data's meaning, and validating those inferences to determine their accuracy. First, the nurse separates the data into categories such as physical, mental, social, and environmental. In many instances, data base sheets used in community agencies provide a structure for gathering and analyzing data. Second, the nurse examines each category to determine its significant meaning. At this point the nurse may need to search for additional information to clarify the meaning of the present data. Next, inferences are made. The nurse has analyzed the data base and come to a tentative conclusion about its meaning. But before making a diagnosis, the nurse must validate those assumptions. Are they accurate? Are they sound? The client should participate actively in data interpretation by clarifying feelings, explaining the circumstances surrounding the situation, and acting as a sounding board for testing assumptions. The nurse also uses other resources, such as other health team members, to check out and confirm inferences. An example of data interpretation follows.

A community health nurse had been collecting data about a group of mothers who regularly attended a well-child clinic. Their responses to child health information and parenting classes had been considerably less than enthusiastic, yet when questioned, they expressed no dissatisfaction with the teaching program. After examining all the data, the nurse concluded that their social and supportive needs were far greater than their need for child care information. Merely gathering weekly at the clinic served an important function for them. She sat down with the mothers and discussed her findings. All agreed that they needed to get out of the house and be with people who had similar kinds of problems and interests.

In the situation just cited, data analysis led to drawing an inference, which was then validated. These are the important activities in interpretation of data. There is an ever-present danger in data interpretation, however, of making inaccurate assumptions and diagnoses. Many nursing care plans and activities have been based on false ideas of clients' needs, resulting in wasted and sometimes detrimental efforts. Thus, the importance of validation cannot be overemphasized. Data collection and data interpretation are sequential activities, with validation serving as a bridge between them (see Figure 8-3). When performed thoroughly, these steps lead to an accurate diagnosis.

DIAGNOSIS

Diagnosis, the next step in the nursing process, is the conclusion the nurse draws from interpretation of collected data. It is a statement of client need, sometimes called the *problem statement*. In community health, however, nurses do not limit their focus to problems; they consider the client as a total

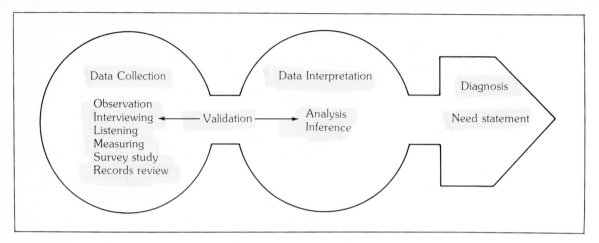

Figure 8-3
Assessment and diagnosis phases of the nursing process. Interpretation of data leads to diagnosis of client needs.

system and look for evidence of all kinds of needs that may influence the client's level of wellness. Needs cover the whole length of the health-illness continuum from a specific health problem, such as chemical dependency, all the way to opportunities for maximizing client health by filling needs such as improvement of parenting skills or development of better nutrition. Thus the statement of client need, the diagnosis, can focus on a wide range of topics.

Diagnoses differ in their scope. A *broad diagnosis,* such as the well-child clinic mothers' need for emotional support, must be further broken down to become manageable for planning care. The community health nurse in the above example did further data collection and interpretation to develop a list of specific needs or diagnoses. Together, she and the mothers identified their feelings of inferiority as housewives, feelings of limited sexual satisfaction, and feelings of powerlessness about family decision making and spending of family money. A broad diagnosis is useful as a starting point. It can serve as a summary, as in the diagnosis of culture shock, nonsupportive parenting, or an unsafe school playground. Using the broad diagnosis as a base, the nurse can ask further questions, gather more data, and with the client develop a set of *specific diagnoses* on which to act (Miaskowski, 1985; Wright, 1985). Diagnoses that are already specific are ready for the planning step.

The nursing diagnosis changes over time because it reflects changes in client health status; therefore, diagnoses need to be periodically reevaluated and redefined. The changing diagnosis can be a useful means of encouraging clients toward improved health because it gives them a clear standard against which to measure their progress.

PLANNING

The purpose of the planning phase is to determine how to meet client needs. Assessment discloses needs but does not prescribe the specific actions necessary to meet them. Knowing that the group of mothers at the well-child clinic needed emotional support did not tell the nurse what to do about it. A diagnosis of culture shock for a family newly arrived from Cuba does not reveal what action to take. The nurse must plan.

Planning is a logical, decision-making process. It means designing an orderly, detailed program of action around specific goals. There is a systematic approach to planning that guides the community health nurse during this phase of the nursing process: (1) list needs in order of priority, (2) establish goals and objectives, and (3) write the care plan. As they do in the rest of the nursing process, community health nurses collaborate with clients in each of these planning activities.

Setting Priorities

Setting priorities means assigning rank to client needs (diagnoses). One way to order needs is to group them into three categories—immediate, intermediate, and long-range—and then assign a priority to those in each group. Immediate needs are more urgent but not necessarily more important. For example, a meeting place was the most immediate need identified by a community health nurse and a group of senior citizens who wanted a class on exercise for the aging. Obviously their goal, to learn about appropriate exercises, was more important than finding a place to meet; however, the immediate need was requisite to accomplishing the long-range goal. Some needs are ranked as immediate because they are potentially hazardous or life-threatening, such as lack of eye protection in a school welding class. Other needs are ranked first because they are of the greatest concern to the client. One family could not see how they would manage to lift and move their grandfather, a man who had recently had a cerebrovascular accident (CVA). They selected his transportation as their highest priority. Other needs were identified but could not be addressed until this first concern had been addressed.

Establishing Goals and Objectives

Goals and objectives are as crucial to planning as a target is to a missile-firing team. The nurse without planned objectives who visits a needy family cannot expect to accomplish anything. Needs must be translated into goals to give direction and meaning to the nursing care plan. Goals can first be stated broadly to give an overview of the proposed end product and then divided into subgoals or objectives that describe specific desired outcomes and target dates. Objectives, as used here, are like stepping stones to help us reach the larger goal. For the family concerned about transporting their grandfather, their need, goal, and objectives were defined in the following manner:

Need
   Family members do not know how to help the grandfather, who recently had a CVA, move around the house after his discharge from the nursing home.

Goal
   Within a week after the grandfather comes home, the family will be able to help him move about the house.

Objectives
   1. On the grandfather's first day home, the community health nurse will determine with the family their capabilities (including the grandfather's) for helping him move about the house.
   2. A physical therapist, making a joint home visit on the first day with the community health nurse, will recommend needed equipment and procedures to be used for helping the grandfather move.
   3. Recommended equipment will be installed by the end of the second day.
   4. Each day, family members will practice lifting and moving procedures under the nurse's supervision.
   5. By the end of the first week, all family members will be able to help grandfather move safely in and out of bed and to the bathroom, kitchen, and living room.

Development of objectives depends on a careful analysis of all the ways one could accomplish the larger goal. One needs to first select the courses of action best suited to meeting the goals, and then build objectives. For the grandfather and family, other alternatives, such as keeping him in the nursing home longer, hiring an orderly to assist him at home, or confining him to bed with a strong exercise program, were considered and rejected. The grandfather's and family's choice was to rehabilitate him as soon as possible in his normal environment.

Some rules of thumb are helpful when writing objectives. Each objective should state a single idea. When more than one idea is expressed, as in an objective to obtain equipment and learn procedures, completion of the objective is much more difficult to measure. State each objective as an outcome. In other words, write the objective so that it describes one end result. For instance, objective 5 describes what the family will be able to do to help their grandfather move. This is a behavioral objective because it describes observable behaviors that can be measured. One can more readily evaluate objectives that include specifics such as what will be done, who will do it, and when it will be accomplished. Then everyone knows exactly what has to be done and within what time frame. Writing measurable objectives makes a tremendous difference in the success of planning.

Planning means thinking ahead. The nurse looks ahead toward the desired end product and then decides on all the intermediate actions necessary to meet that goal. Sometimes an objective itself describes the intermediate actions. At other times the nurse may wish to break down an objective further into several activities. For example, with objective 4, the nurse first explained the procedures, then demonstrated how they were done, and then helped each family member try them. Their ability to practice was dependent on this sequence of activities. Good planning requires this kind of detail.

Decision making is an important part of planning. Decisions must be made while establishing priorities. Selecting goals and, from a variety of possible solutions, choosing the best courses of action to meet the goals requires decisions. Further decision making is involved in selecting objectives and, when indicated, the specific actions to accomplish the objectives.

To facilitate planning and decision making, the community health nurse involves other people. Clients, of course, must be included at every step. They, after all, are the ones for whom the planning is being done and without whose insights and cooperation the plan may not succeed. At times the involvement of other nurses is important. Team meetings, nurse-supervisor conferences, or nurse-expert consultant sessions are all useful resources for planning. In addition, the community health nurse will frequently wish to confer with members of other health disciplines. Interdisciplinary team conferences are valuable for gaining a broader perspective and enlisting wider support for the evolving plan.

Recording the Plan

Recording the plan comes next. Until now, the planning phase has been a series of intellectual exercises done jointly with the client and perhaps with other health team members. The nurse has probably written notes on the decisions made about priorities, goals, objectives, and actions. Now the nurse can spell these out clearly in a format that meets the needs of the particular practice setting (see Figure 8-4 for an example). Regardless of the type of care plan form(s) used, certain items should be addressed:

1. *Data base* is all the subjective and objective information — physical, psychological, social, and environmental — collected about clients. It includes background health information (past and present); individual, family, group, and community assessment; and health history or systems review. The data base is usually kept on separate forms that allow space for ongoing entries and analysis.
2. *Needs* are the specific areas related to the client's health that have been identified for intervention. Preferably, they are areas that both client and nurse agree require action. In some settings, they are called *problems, problem list,* or *nursing diagnoses.* Goals are statements that describe the resolution of the need. For clarity in planning, both a written need statement and goal statement are helpful.
3. *Expected outcomes* are the objectives. They are specific statements that describe what the nurse and the clients hope to accomplish. It is often necessary to construct two or three expected outcomes (objectives) for each need or goal to achieve comprehensive results. These objectives provide the nurse planner with specific targets at which to aim and around which to design actions.
4. *Planned actions* are the activities or methods of accomplishing the expected outcomes. They are specific, planned interventions to meet the objectives. Plans should include appropriate actions by nurse and client.

NURSING CARE PLAN

Client _____ Jones Family _____

Date	No.	Need/Goal	Expected Outcomes	Planned Actions	Progress/Evaluation	Date
2/20	1.	Parents and 14-year-old daughter rarely have time to talk to each other. Goal: To increase amount and quality of communication between parents and daughter.	a. Family will eat together at least once a day on weekdays for 3 months.	a. Determine which meal will be eaten together and select appetizing menus.	a. Have eaten all but 2 dinners together since 2/26. Had breakfasts together instead on 4/6 and 4/13. Family feels objective has been accomplished. Plan to continue frequent meals together.	5/28
			b. Family conversation during meals will include discussion of everyone's activities.	b. Parents will show interest in daughter by asking questions and decreasing amount of discussion between themselves. Daughter will ask parents questions about their days.	b. Family states meal conversation is much more satisfying. All say they are learning much about each other. Conversation is free-flowing. Family interaction in front of nurse is relaxed, open. Objective accomplished.	5/28
			c. Family will have one activity together each month for next 3 months.	c. Family will go to a movie in March, eat dinner out in April, have a picnic in May.	c. Watched TV movie instead. Made popcorn. Had a good time.	3/24
					Ate at nice restaurant. Enjoyed being together.	4/21
					Daughter invited friend to picnic on 5/19. All played games together. Family is satisfied that communication goal is met and plans to continue monthly family activities.	5/28
				d. Family will meet with nurse monthly to evaluate progress.		

Figure 8-4
Partial sample of nursing care plan.

5. *Progress and evaluation* describe the actual outcomes or results and what they mean. What happened? How and when was each objective met, and if not met, why not? It is essential to include evaluation in the written care plan. Too often, progress notes become a substitute for evaluation. Progress notes are useful, periodic summaries; evaluation requires analysis and conclusions. Progress notes and evaluation may be combined if space is allowed on the care plan. Generally, it is best to enter progress notes on a separate page.

One way to record the plan is to list items 2–5 in columns with space for the nurse to record specifics (see Figure 8-4). An increasing number of nurses find it helpful to give a copy of the plan to clients. In many instances, having a copy promotes clients' sense of being equal partners in the responsibility of meeting goals.

IMPLEMENTATION

Implementation is putting the plan into action. It means that the activities delineated in the plan are carried out, some by the nurse and some by the client. In community health nursing, this is a point of particular emphasis. It is not just nursing action or nursing intervention but *collaborative* implementation. Certainly, the nurse's professional expertise and judgment provide a necessary resource to the client. The nurse is also a catalyst and facilitator in planning and activating the nurse-client action plan. But a primary goal in community health is to help people learn to help themselves toward their optimal level of health. To realize this goal, the nurse must constantly involve clients in the deliberative process and encourage their sense of responsibility and autonomy. Other health team members, too, may participate in carrying out the plan. Therefore, all are partners in implementation.

Preparation

The actual course of implementation, outlined in the plan, should be fairly easy to follow if goals, expected outcomes, and planned actions have been designed carefully. Nurse and clients should have a clear idea of the who, what, why, when, where, and how. Who will be involved in carrying out the plan? What is each person's responsibilities? Do all understand why and how to do their parts? Do they know when and where activities will occur? As implementation begins, nurses should review these questions for themselves as well as clients. This is the time to clarify any doubtful areas and thus facilitate a smooth implementation phase.

Even the best planning, though, may require adjustments. For example, the Jones family ran into a snag when they discovered that the three of them could not agree on what constituted an appetizing menu. To solve this unexpected conflict, they elected to take turns planning the menu so that each had a regular opportunity to eat favorite foods. This solution, they decided, would contribute to feelings of goodwill and enhance mealtime conversation. Thus, implementation requires flexibility and adaptation to unanticipated events.

Activities

Sometimes implementation is referred to as the action phase of the nursing process. In one sense, this is true because action is finally taken to solve the problem or meet the need. Up to this point, the nursing process has been largely background work. The early steps of the nursing process are much like preparing to build a bridge. Bridge construction requires initial negotiation (interaction); research on bridge construction, environmental considerations, and traffic use (assessment); and bridge design (planning). Implementation is actually building the bridge and seeing its completion.

The process of implementation requires a series of nursing actions. First, the nurse applies appropriate theories to the actions being performed. For the Jones family, the community health nurse used theories of communication and of adolescent behavior, among other theories, to guide the implementation process. Second, the nurse provides an environment that is conducive for carrying out the plan, such as a quiet room in which to hold a teaching session. Third, the nurse prepares the client for the care to be received. This step means building on the interaction established earlier so that open communication and trust are maintained. Client knowledge, understanding, and attitudes are assessed. The plan is carefully interpreted. Nurse and client form a contractual agreement about the content of the plan and how it is to be carried out. Fourth, the plan is carried out or modified and carried out by the nurse and client. Modification requires constant observation and interchange during implementation since these actions determine the success of the plan and the nature of needed changes. Finally, the nurse documents the implementation process through progress notes.

EVALUATION

Evaluation, the final component of the nursing process, is the last in a sequence of actions leading to the resolution of client health needs. The nursing process, as a professional tool for goal attainment, is not complete without measuring and judging the effectiveness of that goal attainment. Too often emphasis is placed primarily on assessing client needs and planning and implementing care. But how effective was the care? Were client needs truly met? Professional practitioners owe it to their clients, themselves, and to other health service providers to evaluate.

Evaluation is an act of appraisal. When one evaluates something, one judges its value in relation to a standard and a set of criteria. For example, when eating dinner in a restaurant, diners evaluate the dinner in terms of the standard of a satisfying meal. The criteria for their standard may include qualities such as a wide variety of choices on the menu, reasonable price, tasty food, nice atmosphere, and good service. They also evaluate the meal for a purpose. Were money and time well spent, and will they want to eat there again? Evaluation requires a purpose, standards and criteria, and judgment skills.

Purpose

The ultimate purpose of evaluating care in community health nursing is to determine whether planned actions met client needs; how well they were met; and if not, why not. In the pressure of daily practice, nurses are frequently limited to writing a quick progress note and a short final summary. This substitute for evaluation describes what occurred but does not judge its value. Evaluation is a critical component in the nursing process; without it, there is no basis for knowing whether previous actions were worthwhile and no evidence on which to base future plans. Therefore, nurses need evaluation to complete the series of activities that help them reach their goal of client health.

Standards and Criteria

Evaluation utilizes standards and criteria. In community health nursing, the standards are the intended results of the nursing care plan — the goals. The criteria for these standards are the specific, expected client behaviors that will demonstrate accomplishment of goals — the objectives. The Jones family had a standard that was their goal to increase the amount and quality of communication between parents and daughter (Figure 8-4). How did they and the nurse know when the goal was met? The expected outcomes (objectives) were written as specific behaviors; these became criteria for evaluation. When all of the conditions or criteria were met, they knew the goal had been accomplished.

Consider another example. Several diabetic women attending a clinic had a problem with obesity. A community health nurse working in the clinic helped them form a weight-loss group. Each woman set a goal of a specific number of pounds to lose in a year and then developed objectives (expected outcomes) to help her reach that goal. One of them, Mrs. Sanders, planned the following:

Goal (Standard)
    Lose 50 pounds by the end of the year (target date).

Objectives (Criteria)
1. Lose two pounds a week for the first 10 weeks.
2. Lose one pound a week for the next 30 weeks.
3. Maintain weight loss for 12 weeks.

The women planned ways to meet each of their objectives, such as a specific daily calorie limit and regular exercise program. Some added hobbies or a series of personal rewards (a new dress after losing 15 pounds) to serve as motivators and pleasure substitutes. Mrs. Sanders evaluated the completion of her goal by using the standard (50 pounds in a year) and the criteria spelled out in her objectives. To maximize group support and encourage healthy behavior patterns during weight loss, the nurse suggested having a group goal. This became their standard for measuring group success:

Group Standard
The group will stay healthy while accomplishing 90 percent of the weight loss goals.

Group Criteria
1. By the end of the year the group will lose at least 90 percent of the sum of the expected individual weight losses.
2. The group will have no diabetes-related infections during the year.
3. All of the group members will be exercising at least once a week by the end of the year.
4. No more than 10 percent of the group will have had an illness that kept them in bed more than one day during the year.

The prepared standard and set of criteria helped the group evaluate its success.

The above examples emphasize the relationship of good planning to evaluation. When nurse and client prepare clear, specific goals and objectives, then there is no question about how or what to evaluate. It will be obvious that the goal is either met or not met (Figure 8-5).

Judgment Skills

Evaluation requires judgment skills. The nurse compares real outcomes with expected outcomes and looks for discrepancies (Hegyvary, et al., 1987). When actual client behavior matches the desired behavior, then the goal, if well planned, is met. If it is not met, why not? The nurse will need to examine several possible explanations for the failure. Data collection may have been inadequate, the diagnosis incorrect, the plan unrealistic, or implementation ineffective. Circumstances, client motivation, or both may have changed. There may not have been enough client participation in one or more parts of the process. After determining the cause of the failure, the nurse can reassess, plan, and initiate corrective action.

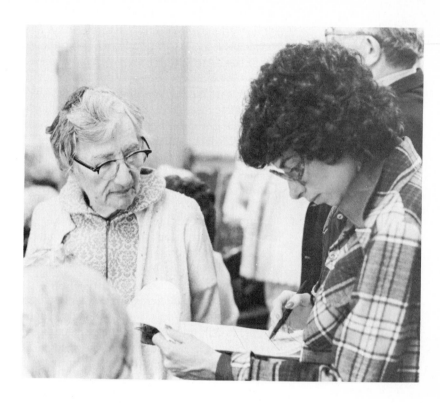

*Figure 8-5
Elderly clients in a
community health
education program are
being interviewed to
evaluate the outcomes of
the program.*

Quality Assurance

In community health nursing, evaluation is also done to measure the quality of client care, nurse performance, and programs and services (Decker, et al., 1979; Ingram, 1987; Schmele, 1985). These measurements reflect nursing's increasing concern with quality assurance. An ideal quality assurance system included the following (*Assessing Quality,* 1976), and this list remains valid today:

1. An organizational entity created for assessing quality
2. Establishment of standards or criteria against which quality is assessed
3. A routine system of gathering information
4. Assurance that such information is based on the total population or representative sample of patients or potential patients
5. A process that provides the results of review to patients, the public, providers, and sponsoring organizations, as well as methods to institute corrective actions

With the burgeoning emphasis on accountability in health care, community health nursing is being challenged to devise better ways of documenting service effectiveness and cost efficiency. A variety of methodologies and tools exists and is constantly being broadened to facilitate these evaluative processes. One method is the nursing audit, which evaluates quality of nursing care by analyzing client records. Another is peer review (American Nurses Association, 1988). All of these methods, however, operate on the same basic principle discussed earlier, that is, that evaluation requires a clear purpose as well as a standard and specific criteria against which outcomes are measured. We discuss quality assurance in depth in Chapter 23.

CHARACTERISTICS OF THE NURSING PROCESS

The nursing process provides a framework or structure upon which community health nursing actions are based. Application of the process varies with each situation, but the nature of the process remains the same. Certain elements of that nature are important for community health nurses to emphasize in their practice (see Figure 8-6).

The process is *deliberative* (Weidenbach, 1964). That is, it is purposefully, rationally, and carefully thought out. It requires the use of judgment. Community health nurses frequently practice in situations that demand independent thinking and difficult decision making. The nursing process is a tool to facilitate making these determinations.

Figure 8-6
*Nursing process
characteristics emphasized
in community health
nursing practice.*

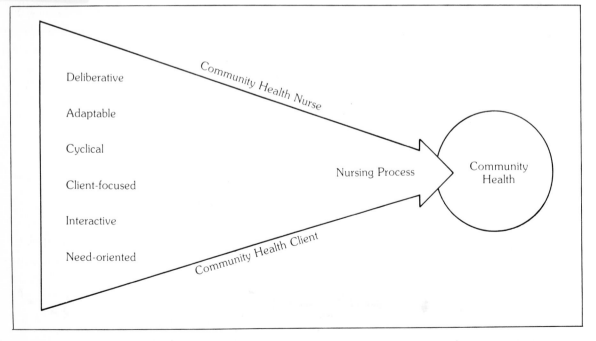

The process is *adaptable* (Lewis, 1988). Its dynamic nature enables the community health nurse to adjust appropriately to each situation, to be flexible in applying the process to client needs. The nurse adapts and individualizes service for each community client.

The process is *cyclical*. Although a sequence of actions constitutes the framework of the nursing process, these actions are in constant progression (Henley, 1986). The nurse in any given situation engages in continual interaction, data collection, analysis, intervention, and evaluation. Steps are repeated over and over in the nurse-client relationship, and as interactions between nurse and client continue, various steps in the process are used simultaneously.

The process, because it is used for and with clients, is *client focused*. Clients are nursing's reason for being. Nurses use the nursing process for the express purpose of helping clients, directly or indirectly, to achieve and maintain health (Cooper, 1986). The client as a total system, whether a family, group, or community, is the target of the nursing process.

The process is *interactive*. Nurse and client are engaged in a process of ongoing interpersonal communication, "a communicative interaction process" (Daubenmire and King, 1973, p. 512). Giving and receiving accurate information are necessary to promote understanding between nurse and client and foster effective use of the nursing process. Furthermore, as the consumer movement, patient's rights, and the self-care concept have gained emphasis, client and nurse have increasingly jointly assumed responsibility for promoting client health. The client-nurse relationship can and should be a partnership (Yura and Walsh, 1973). Called "peer practice" by some (Bayer and Brandner, 1977, p. 86), the nursing process is shared by nurse and client.

Finally, the nursing process, as applied in community health, is *need oriented* (Clark, 1985). Long association with problem solving has tended to limit the nursing process's focus to the correction of problems. Although problem solving is certainly an appropriate use of the nursing process, application of the nursing process in community health to anticipation of needs and prevention of problems assumes additional significance. This focus is needed if we are to realize the goals of community health, "to protect, promote, and restore the people's health" (Sheps, 1976, p. 3).

Summary

The effectiveness of community health nursing practice depends on how well the nursing process is used as a tool for enhancing aggregate health. The nursing process means appropriately applying a systematic series of actions toward helping clients achieve their optimal level of health. These actions or components of the process include interaction, assessment, diagnosis, planning, implementation, and evaluation.

Interaction is the first component, because nurse and clients must establish a relationship of reciprocal influence and exchange. It requires effective communication to assess needs and establish trust between nurse and clients as partners in the nursing process.

Assessment is a process of appraising client health status to determine existing or possible future needs. Community health nursing is not limited to identifying problems. Rather, there is a strong emphasis on exploring ways to help clients achieve optimal health. Assessment provides the basis for future nursing action. It involves collecting and interpreting data.

Diagnosis involves analyzing the collected data and determining what needs to be corrected or changed. It is a judgment of client needs.

Planning means designing a specific course of action to meet identified client needs. To plan, one must rank client needs, establish goals and objectives, design activities to meet the objectives, and write the care plan. The plan should include a data base, statements describing client needs and goals to be achieved, specific objectives, progress notes, and finally, an evaluation of each objective.

Implementation is activating the plan and seeing it through to completion. During implementation, the nurse applies appropriate theory; provides a facilitative environment; prepares the client for care; with the client, carries out or modifies and carries out a plan; and documents the implementation.

Evaluation measures and judges the effectiveness of the plan. Were client needs met? If not, why not? To evaluate, nurses need to understand clearly why they are evaluating. What is the purpose? They also need a standard (goal) and a specific set of criteria (objectives) for each goal to use in measuring the outcomes. There is an important relationship between good planning and evaluation, because well-prepared goals and objectives are essential for adequate evaluation. If goals are not met, the failure may result from inadequate assessment or planning. Determining the cause of the failure can lead to corrective action. Evaluation does not end the nursing process; rather, it documents what has been accomplished and what yet needs to be done in order that the process, a continuing cycle, can start again.

Certain characteristics of the nursing process should be emphasized by community health nurses in their practice. The process is *deliberative*, requiring and aiding the exercise of judgment in decision making. It is *adaptable*, encouraging flexibility in practice. It is *cyclical*, fostering a constant, ongoing use of the process. It is *client focused,* helping the nurse to keep the proper target of client health in view. It is *interactive*, promoting nurse-client communication and client participation. Finally, it is *need oriented,* encouraging identification of ways to help clients achieve optimal health.

Study Questions

You have been practicing the nursing process with individuals to effect change in their health status. Now consider how you can expand that application to aggregates. Select a population group in your community, such as preschoolers, unwed mothers, Southeast Asian refugees, or elderly home-bound persons.

1. As potential clients, how might you start the interaction phase with them?
2. What specific areas would you want to assess? Make a list of hypothetical symptoms that indicate a need.
3. Invent a diagnosis for this group that would be supported by the data you collected in your assessment.
4. What alternative courses of action should you consider for addressing this need? Select the most appropriate one.
5. Start a plan for implementation including an overall goal and at least one objective.
6. List the activities needed to meet your objective(s), and describe how you might carry them out.
7. How would you evaluate your nursing interventions with this population group?

References

Aggleton, P., and H. Chalmers. (1986). Nursing research, nursing theory, and the nursing process. *Journal of Advanced Nursing* 11(2): 197–202.

American Nurses Association. (1988). *Peer review guidelines.* Kansas City, Mo.: Author.

Assessing quality in health care: An evaluation (Final Report). (1976). Washington, D.C.: Institute of Medicine, National Academy of Sciences.

Bayer, M., and P. Brandner. (1977). Nurse/patient peer practice. *American Journal of Nursing* 77: 86–90.

Brill, N. I. (1973). *Working with people: The helping process.* Philadelphia: J. B. Lippincott.

Capers, C. F., and R. Kelly. (1987). Neuman nursing process: A model of holistic care. *Holistic Nursing Practice* 1(3): 19–26.

Clark, J. (1985). Delivering the goods... the nursing process in health visiting. *Community Outlook* (Jan.): 23–24, 26–28.

Cooper, I. (1986). The nursing process at work... occupational health nurses. *Nursing Times* 82(1): 32–35.

Daubenmire, M. J., and I. M. King. (1973). Nursing process models: A systems approach. *Nursing Outlook* 21: 512–17.

Decker, F., L. Stevens, M. Vancini, and L. Wedeking. (1979). Using patient outcomes to evaluate community health nursing. *Nursing Outlook* 27(4): 278–82.

Hegyvary, S., et al. (1987). *Outcome measures in home health care: Research.* National League for Nursing Publication #21-2194: 29–37.

Henley, M. (1986). The health visiting process... based on the nursing process. *Senior Nurse* 4(5): 23–24.

Ingram, H. H. (1987). Quality assurance in a public health agency. *Quarterly Review Bulletin* 12(11): 372–76.

Langford, T. (1978). Establishing a nursing contract. *Nursing Outlook* 26 (5): 386–88.

Lewis, T. (1988). Leaping the chasm between nursing theory and practice. *Journal of Advanced Nursing* 13(3): 345–51.

Marriner, A. (1979). *The nursing process.* 2nd ed. St. Louis: C. V. Mosby.

Mauksch, I. G., and M. L. David. (1972). Prescription for survival. *American Journal of Nursing* 72: 2189–93.

Miaskowski, C. A. (1985). Nursing diagnosis within the context of nursing process. *Occupational Health Nursing* 33(8): 401–4, 419–22.

Schmele, J. A. (1985). A method for evaluating nursing practice in a community setting. *Quality Review Bulletin* 11(4): 115–22.

Sheps, C. G. (1976). *Higher education for public health: Report of the Milbank Memorial Fund Commission.* New York: Neale, Watson.

Weidenbach, E. (1964). *Clinical nursing: A helping art.* New York: Springer.

White, M. S. (1982). Construct for public health nursing. *Nursing Outlook* 30: 527–30.

Williams, C. A. (1977). Community health nursing — What is it? *Nursing Outlook* 25: 250–53.

Wright, C. (1985). Computer-aided nursing diagnosis for community health nurses. *Nursing Clinics of North America* 20(3): 487–95.

Yura, H., and M. B. Walsh. (1973). *The nursing process: Assessing, planning, implementing, evaluating.* New York: Appleton-Century-Crofts.

Selected Readings

Aggleton, P., and H. Chalmers. (1985). Models and theories: Orem's self-care model. *Nursing Times* 81(1): 36–39.

Bloch, D. (1975). Evaluation of nursing care in terms of process and outcome: Issues in research and quality assurance. *Nursing Research* 24: 256–59.

Blum, H. (1981). *Planning for health: Generics for the eighties.* 2nd ed. New York: Human Sciences Press.

Bohm, S. M. (1978). Toward 2002: A community perspective. *New Zealand Nursing Journal* 71: 24–28.

Capers, C. F., and R. Kelly. (1987). Neuman nursing process: A model of holistic care. *Holistic Nursing Practice* 1(3): 19–26.

Clark, J. (1985). Delivering the goods. . . the nursing process in health visiting. *Community Outlook* (Jan.): 23–24, 26–28.

Cooper, I. (1986). The nursing process at work. . . occupational health nurses. *Nursing Times* 82(1): 32–35.

Cordes, S. M. (1978). Assessing health care needs: Elements and processes. *Family and Community Health* 1(2): 1–16.

Davidson, S. V. (1978). Community nursing care evaluation. *Family and Community Health* 1(1): 37–55.

Decker, F., L. Stevens, M. Vancini, and L. Wedeking. (1979). Using patient outcomes to evaluate community health nursing. *Nursing Outlook* 27: 278–82.

Donabedian, A. (1978). *The quality of medical care: Methods for assessing and monitoring the quality of care for research and for quality assurance programs in health.* Washington, D.C.: U.S. Government Printing Office.

Evaluation of quality of public health nursing. (1976). Washington, D.C.: American Public Health Association, Public Health Nursing Section.

Flynn, B., and D. Ray. (1979). Quality assurance in community health nursing. *Nursing Outlook* 27: 650–53.

Gilman, S., and P. Nader. (1979). Measuring the effectiveness of a school health program — Methods and preliminary analysis. *Journal of School Health* 49: 10–13.

Gordon, M. (1976). Nursing diagnosis and the diagnostic process. *American Journal of Nursing* 76: 1232–34.

Hadley, R. D. (1978). Nurses develop quality assurance program in community health setting. *American Nurse* 10: 3–6.

Henley, M. (1986). The health visiting process. . . based on the nursing process. *Senior Nurse* 4(5): 23–24.

Kermode, S. (1986). A conceptual framework for nursing practice. *Australian Journal of Advanced Nursing* 3(3): 27–34.

Langford, T. (1978). Establishing a nursing contract. *Nursing Outlook* 26: 386–88.

Marriner, A. (1979). *The nursing process*. 2nd ed. St. Louis: C. V. Mosby.

Mayers, M. G. (1972). *A systematic approach to the nursing care plan*. New York: Appleton-Century-Crofts.

National League for Nursing. (1975). *Accreditation of home health agencies and community nursing services* (No. 21-1306). New York: Author.

Parzick, J., and M. Nolan, Sr. (1978). POMR at work in a home health agency. *Family and Community Health* 1(1): 101–113.

Phaneuf, M., and M. Wandelt. (1974). Quality assurance in nursing. *Nursing Forum* 4: 328–45.

Scutchfield, F. D. (1975). Alternate methods for health priority assessment. *Journal of Community Health* 1(3): 29–38.

Shaffer, M. K., and I. L. Pfeiffer. (1978). Home visit: A gray zone in evaluation. *American Journal of Nursing 78*: 239–41.

Simmons, D. A. (1980). *A classification scheme for client problems in community health nursing* (DHEW 80-16, HRP 0501501). Springfield, Va.: National Technical Information Services, Nurse Planning Information Series No. 14.

Wandelt, M., and J. Ager. (1974). *Quality patient care scale*. New York: Appleton-Century-Crofts.

Wray, J. G. (1977). Problem-oriented recording in community nursing—A new experience in education. *Journal of Nursing Education* 16(9): 12–15.

Yura, H., and M. B. Walsh. (1973). *The nursing process: Assessing, planning, implementing, evaluating*. New York: Appleton-Century-Crofts.

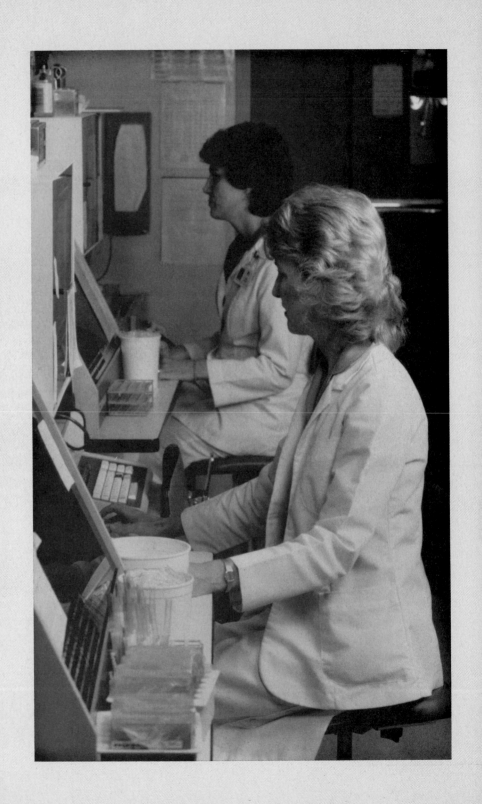

9 Epidemiology

The practice of nursing has traditionally rested on two important corner-stones of scientific knowledge — biophysical and psychosocial study. The biophysical basis involves the study of human anatomy and physiology, eti-ology and treatment of disease, and processes of physical development. The psychosocial basis includes the study of psychological and social develop-ment, psychiatric illness, and social aspects of nursing care.

Public health adds a third cornerstone of scientific knowledge: information on the health and illness characteristics of population groups. For example, suppose a community health nurse wants to develop a plan to prevent an outbreak of rubella, a communicable disease that affects the human fetus with congenital rubella syndrome. In order to develop such a prevention plan, information about population groups is required. Which members of a community have been immunized against rubella? What is the expected number of rubella cases (the morbidity rate)? What members of the commu-nity have the highest risk of rubella? Any program of screening, immunization, or health promotion regarding rubella must be based on this kind of informa-tion about population groups in order to be effective. This information comes from *epidemiology,* a specialized form of scientific research.*

DEFINITION OF EPIDEMIOLOGY

Epidemiology may be defined as the study of the distribution and determi-nants of health, disease, and injuries in human populations. Epidemiologists ask such questions as, What is the occurrence of health and disease in a population? Is there an increase or decrease in a health state over the years?

*The author is indebted to Shirley J. Thompson and Sara L. Turner, who contributed the epidemiology chapter for the second edition of this text and whose ideas have influenced the development of this chapter.

Does one geographical area have a higher frequency of disease than another? What characteristics of persons with a particular condition distinguish them from those without the condition? Is one treatment or program more effective than another in changing the health of individuals? Why do some people recover from a disease when others do not? The ultimate goal of epidemiology is to search for causes of health problems and identify solutions to prevent disease and improve the health of the entire population. In its search for causes, epidemiology provides health workers, including community health nurses, with a body of knowledge on which to base their practice, and methods for studying new and existing problems. This chapter describes these methods of study and their relevance to community health nursing. At the end of this chapter we include a glossary of terms most often used in epidemiology.

EPIDEMIOLOGY AND COMMUNITY HEALTH NURSING

As long as the nurse focuses on the individual as the client, epidemiology may have minimal usefulness. However, community health nursing and epidemiology have an important theme in common: the health of groups. Epidemiology offers community health nurses a specific methodology for assessing the health of families, groups, and entire communities (Figure 9-1). Furthermore, it provides a frame of reference for investigating and improving clinical practice in any setting. Whether the community health nurse's goals are to im-

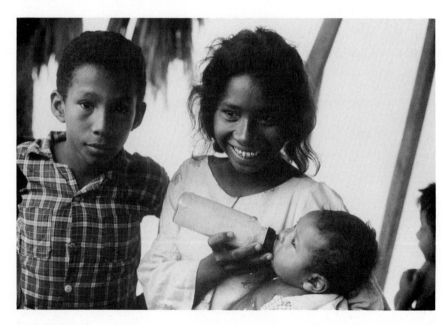

Figure 9-1
Epidemiologic research focuses on the health of population groups. This Colombian mother and her children represent a population with numerous health needs for study.

prove a family's nutrition, to control the spread of AIDS, to deal with health problems created by a tornado, or to assist mothers who choose to deliver their babies at home, epidemiologic data can be useful.

Consider one example. In Cali, Colombia, many potential clients were not using available child health services. In order to discover why some and not others used the services and to develop remedial actions, epidemiologic data was needed. How many children were in the target population? What characterized the mothers and children who did and did not use the services? What illness problems existed? How many children had been immunized for what illnesses? Dr. Beatrice J. Selwyn, a nurse and epidemiologist, selected a single *barrio* (a residential area) with a population of more than 50,000 people for epidemiologic study. Trained assistants interviewed a sample of 529 mothers with children under 5 years of age; among other findings, Selwyn discovered the characteristics of those who did not use the available child health services. This information laid a groundwork for identifying the target population and designing services to reach that population. For example, nonusers did not read newspapers but did listen to the radio, which suggested an effective line of communication about new services. Selwyn summarized the value of this kind of investigation: "Answers obtained in the interview suggest ways to structure delivery systems to the subculture of the population to be served, e.g., taking immunization services to the homes of mothers rather than waiting for them to come to the service" (Selwyn, 1978).

To conduct studies such as this, community health nurses need a basic understanding of epidemiologic principles. For more insight, we will review how these principles have been utilized in the past to significantly improve the health of numerous population groups.

HISTORICAL BACKGROUND OF EPIDEMIOLOGY

The roots of epidemiology can be traced to Hippocrates (460–477 B.C.). Sometimes referred to as the first epidemiologist, Hippocrates believed that disease not only affected individuals but was a mass phenomenon. He was one of the first people to associate the occurrence of disease with lifestyle and environmental factors. However, it was not until the late nineteenth century that modern epidemiology actually came into existence. The term is derived from the Greek words epi (upon) demos (the people) and logos (knowledge), thus meaning the knowledge or study of what happens to people.

Some of the most dramatic things that have happened to communities of people have been epidemic diseases. In past centuries cholera, bubonic plague, and smallpox swept through community after community, killing thousands of people, changing the community structure, and altering the life-style of masses of people. Epidemiology became a distinct branch of medical science through its concern with epidemics of infectious diseases. In 1348, the Black Death swept through Europe and England, killing millions of people. In

England alone, approximately one-fourth of the population died from the plague, which takes one of two forms. If the plague bacilli infect the lymph glands of armpit or groin, a lump or bubo develops (thus the name *bubonic plague*). If the bacilli lodge in the lungs, pneumonia, or *pneumonic plague,* results. The plague continued in Europe, but with less force, for three centuries and then waned, only to reappear in an epidemic in Hong Kong in 1896.

Kitasato, a Japanese bacteriologist, discovered the plague bacillus during this Hong Kong epidemic; within ten years, epidemiologists had traced its life cycle from rats to fleas to humans. Now intervention was possible, and public health officials declared war on rats, seeking to make ships and wharf buildings rat-proof. The first major campaign against rats took place in California after an outbreak of plague in 1900. Although successful, the bacillus appears to have spread to ground squirrels (Burnet, 1962), and cases still occur occasionally in the United States.

FLORENCE NIGHTINGALE'S INFLUENCE

The roots of epidemiology in nursing can be traced back to Florence Nightingale (1820–1910) (Cohen, 1984). Miss Nightingale often obtained advice on issues related to hospital statistics and disease classification from her close friend William Farr, who was chief statistician of England's General Register Office for health and vital statistics. Her detailed record keeping and careful description of the health conditions among the military in the Crimea represents one of the first systematic descriptive studies of the distribution and patterns of disease in a population. Changes made according to her suggestions brought dramatic proof of the authenticity of her observations and knowledge. Forty out of every 100 British troops were dying in the Crimea before Miss Nightingale instituted environmental and nutritional changes in the hospital and field. When her work in the Crimea was finished, the mortality rate was only 2 percent. Florence Nightingale's use of statistical data along with her commitment to environmental reform strongly influenced nursing's evolution into a profession whose service addressed public health problems as well as hospital care. As nursing has evolved, the community health nurse has continued to intervene at both the individual and aggregate level, working to improve the environment and focusing on high-risk groups and populations.

HOST, AGENT, ENVIRONMENTAL MODEL

Through their intensive study of infectious diseases, epidemiologists began to consider disease states in terms of causal agent, susceptible host, and environment. For example, the agent responsible for plague is the plague bacillus; humans are susceptible hosts, along with rats and a few other animals. But fleas that bite both rats and humans must be present in order to transfer the

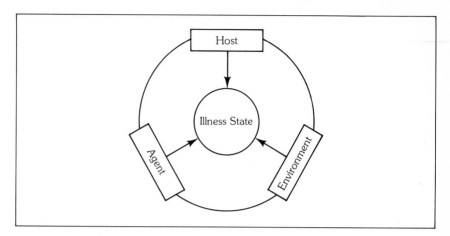

Figure 9-2
Epidemiologic model.
Epidemiologists study the
causal agent, the susceptible
host, and environmental
factors that contribute to an
illness state (or a wellness
state). Intervention may act
on any of these three to
prevent the spread of illness
or to improve health in a
population.

bacillus from rats to human hosts. Numerous environmental factors influence relationships between agents and hosts. The black rat, once native to India and a carrier of the plague, came to Europe with the Crusaders and spread the Black Death in 1348. Historic records even then indicated that certain people were more susceptible to the plague than others. Far more men died from this disease than women and children, who often were unaffected, or only mildly ill. The host, agent, and environment model, shown in Figure 9-2, offered the epidemiologist a plan for intervention. As soon as the agent was identified, measures could be taken to keep the bacillus from contacting human hosts; eradicating rats known to carry the disease was a major preventive measure.

As the threat of the great epidemic diseases declined, epidemiologists began to focus on other infectious diseases such as diphtheria, infant diarrhea, typhoid, tuberculosis, and syphilis. They also gathered data pertaining to host characteristics, agent, and environmental factors in diseases such as scurvy among sailors and the occupational disease of scrotal cancer among chimney sweeps. In recent years, epidemiologists have turned to the study of major causes of death and disability, such as cancer, cardiovascular disorders, mental illness, accidents, arthritis, and congenital defects. Equally important, they have moved from concentrating only on illness to focusing on how agent, host, and environment are involved in wellness at various levels. In response to an escalating demand for health promotion, health care and screening services have come under the scrutiny of epidemiology.

CAUSAL RELATIONSHIPS

The purpose of epidemiologic study has been to discover causal relationships in order to offer effective prevention and protection. Over the years, as scientific knowledge of health and disease has expanded, epidemiology has changed.

EARLY THEORIES

Early causal thinking was dominated by Sydenham's miasma theory. This theory held that disease was caused by noxious vapors associated with decaying organic matter. Prevention based on this theory attempted to eliminate the sources of the miasma (vapors). Despite its faulty reasoning, this type pf prevention has had positive consequences in our awareness that decaying organic matter can be a source of infectious diseases.

A contagion theory of disease had developed by the mid-eighteenth century. This theory inspired various concepts of immunity and even some initial attempts at vaccination against smallpox. Late in the nineteenth century, the germ theory of disease was established. Epidemiologic efforts then began to focus on identifying the microorganisms that caused disease as a first step in prevention. Once an agent had been identified, measures could be taken to contain its spread. Fumigating ships to kill rats, protecting wharf buildings and human habitations against rats, and removing rat food supplies from easy access were all measures to protect the public by further preventing spread of the plague bacilli.

Up to this point, epidemiologists viewed disease in terms of a simple cause-and-effect relationship. Finding a single cause (plague bacilli) and attacking it (eliminating rats) seemed the solution for preventing many diseases. In the case of bubonic plague, this approach appeared quite effective. However, scientific research revealed that disease causation was much more complex than was first suspected. For example, although most members of a group might be exposed to the plague, many did not contract the disease. With bubonic plague, as with many other infectious diseases, the characteristics of the host can determine the spread of the disease. Not everyone in a population is at risk; we now know that "untreated bubonic plague has a case fatality rate commonly reported to be about 50 percent; rarely it is no more than a localized infection of short duration (pestis minor). Plague organisms have been recovered from throat cultures of asymptomatic contacts of pneumonic plague patients" (Benenson, 1985, p. 285). Clearly, such evidence makes it difficult to speak of a single cause for plague and many other disease states.

Furthermore, even the agent and course of transmission can be quite complex. Although it is a flea that carries the bacilli from rat to human in bubonic plague, pneumonic plague can spread directly from one human being to another. The environment must also be considered as part of the cause in nearly every disease and health state. Considering the plague again, evidence suggests that it originated in the high steppes of Asia and spread to other parts of the world. After a rather successful attempt to control the spread of plague in California during the early part of this century, epidemiologists discovered that the ground squirrel also carried the bacillus. But the question arose as to whether the bacillus spread from the rat to the ground squirrel or whether it had always been part of the squirrel's ecology. Although this question has not been answered, we do know that the western United States offers an environment conducive to squirrels, their plague-carrying fleas, and the plague bacillus. Although isolated cases continue to occur, epidemics have not occurred and are quite unlikely since squirrels usually live in an environment somewhat separated from that of humans.

CHAIN OF CAUSATION

As our thinking about disease causation has grown more complex around the tripartite model of host, agent, and environment, epidemiologists have used the idea of a chain of causation (see Figure 9-3). The chain begins by identifying the *reservoir,* that is, where the causal agent can live and multiply. In plague, that reservoir may be other humans, rats, squirrels, and a few other animals. In malaria, humans are the major reservoir for the parasitic agents, although recent evidence has shown that certain primates also act as reservoirs (Burnet, 1962). Next, the agent must have a portal of exit from the reservoir as well as some mode of transmission. The next link in the chain of causation is the agent itself. Malaria, for example, actually consists of four distinct diseases caused by four kinds of protozoa, which are tiny microorganisms. These agents spend part of their life cycle in the body of the *Anopheles* mosquito, which acts as a mode of transmission. The mosquito bite provides a portal of exit as well as a portal of entry into the human host.

The circle surrounding this chain of causation in Figure 9-3 represents the environment, which can have a profound influence at almost any point along the chain. Consider the impact of environmental factors in the malaria epidemic of Ceylon in 1934–1935. Two or three million cases occurred, resulting

Figure 9-3
Chain of causation in infectious disease.

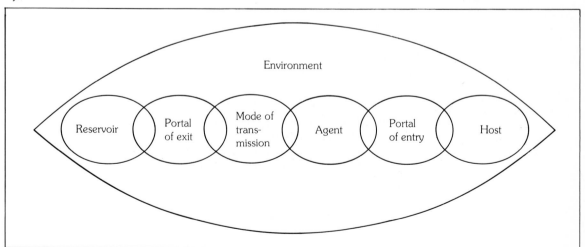

in eighty thousand deaths. Malaria occurred frequently in the dry northern area where sparse vegetation allowed pools of water to be exposed to the sun, providing excellent breeding grounds for the *Anopheles* mosquito. The more populous southwestern area had heavy monsoon rains and was relatively free from malaria. In 1934 a severe drought changed this environment drastically; rivers almost dried up, leaving stagnant pools of water for mosquito breeding. Widespread crop failure caused the population to become badly undernourished, which added to the conditions that would foster a malaria epidemic. The epidemic hit in October 1934 with devastating results for the population, and the environment must certainly be seen as a major part of the causal chain (Burnet, 1962).

MULTIPLE CAUSATION

Recently, a more advanced concept of multiple causation has emerged to explain the existence of health and illness states and to provide guiding principles for epidemiologic practice. Sometimes discussed as a "web of causation," this model attempts to identify all the possible influences on the health and illness processes (Friedman, 1987). Figure 9-4 shows the web of causation for myocardial infarction; such a health problem cannot be explained in single causal terms, even if that cause represents part of a larger chain. Recognition of multiple causes provides many points of intervention for prevention, health promotion, and treatment. For example, examination of Figure 9-4 suggests interventions such as directly attacking significant coronary atherosclerosis (bypass surgery), reducing the incidence of obesity, helping people quit smoking, developing an exercise program, and making dietary modifications.

Contemporary epidemiologists continue to explore new and more comprehensive ways of viewing health and illness. Life-style, behavior, environment, and stress of all kinds affect health states. In the model of host, agent, and environment, we can note a shifting emphasis over time. Early epidemiologists worked to identify and manage the causative agent; the focus of concern was disease states. The emphasis then shifted to the host. Who was susceptible? What characteristics led to susceptibility? Through immunization and health promotion, efforts were made to improve hosts' resistance. Increasingly, however, we have come to realize the limitations imposed on individual control of health. Even those in the best of health cannot withstand toxic agents in the workplace, nuclear wastes in the atmosphere from power plant accidents, or other debilitating conditions created by modern society. More and more, public health professionals are turning to a study of environmental conditions and looking for methods to change conditions that contribute to illness. Gradually we are becoming more aware of the need to deal with the complex multiple causation involved in health and illness.

Figure 9-4
Web of causation for myocardial infarction. (From G. D. Friedman, Primer of Epidemiology. New York: McGraw-Hill, 1987. Reprinted by permission.)

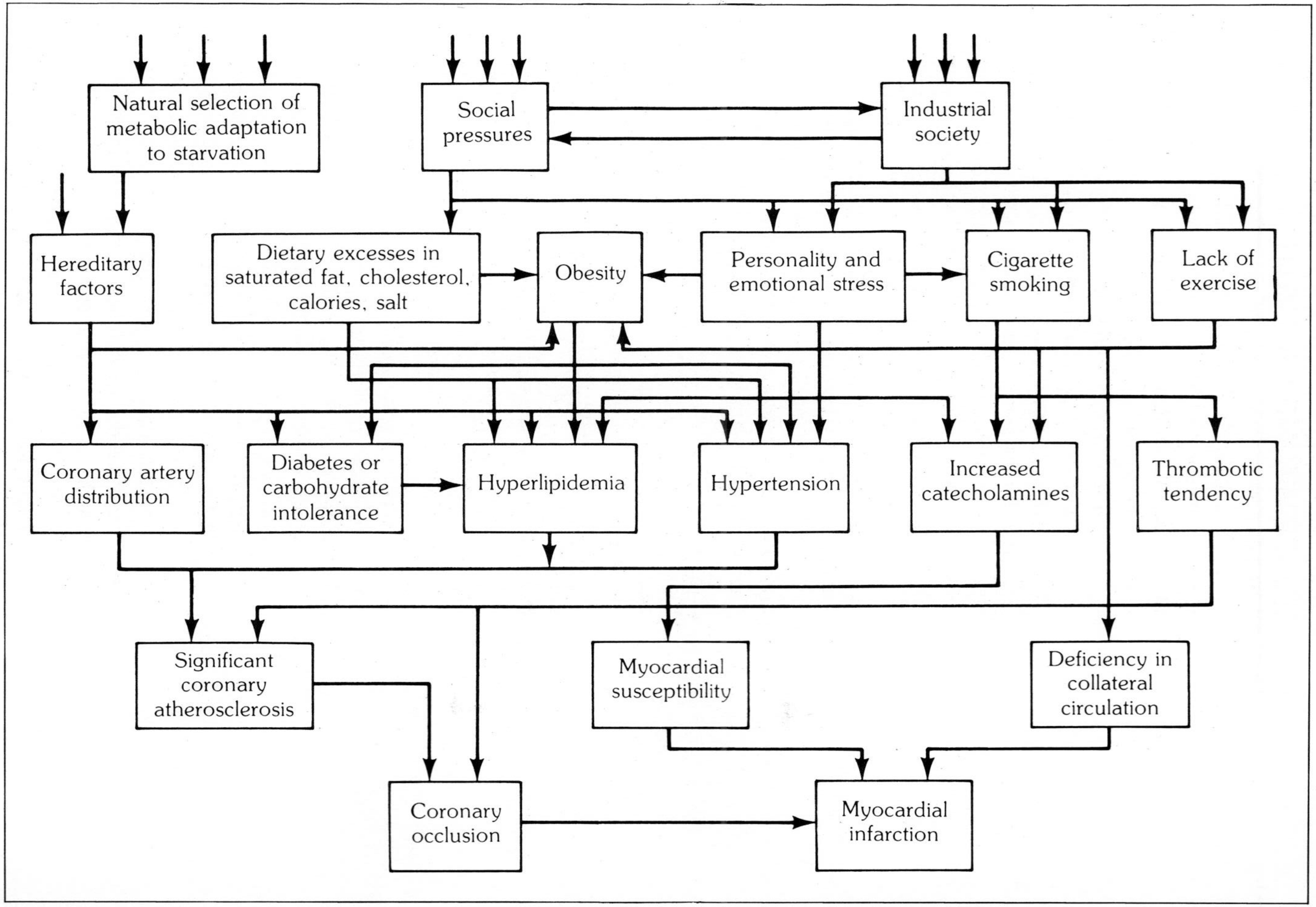

DETERMINING CAUSALITY IN EPIDEMIOLOGIC STUDY

One of the main challenges to epidemiology today is to identify causal relationships in disease and health conditions in populations. As we have suggested in the previous sections, the assessment of causality in human health is difficult at best; no single study is adequate to establish causality. Causal inference is based on consistent results obtained from many studies. Frequently the accumulation of evidence begins with a clinical observation or educated guess that a certain factor may be causally related to a health problem. Cross-sectional studies then show that the factor and problem coexist; retrospective studies allow a fairly quick assessment of whether or not an association exists. Nonepidemiologic animal studies may suggest a biologic mechanism whereby the factor could cause the disease or condition. At this point, prospective studies are crucial to assure that the presumed causal factor actually antedates the onset of the health problem. And finally, if ethically possible, the experimental approach is used to confirm the associations obtained from the observational studies. Thus, it often requires many years to accumulate enough evidence to provide adequate information for developing a health intervention strategy or for changing a current practice.

Epidemiologically, we accept that a causal relationship may exist when two major conditions are met: (1) the factor of interest (causal agent) is shown to increase the probability of occurrence of the disease or condition as observed in many studies in different populations; and (2) there is evidence that a reduction in the factor decreases the frequency of the given disease (Hennekens and Buring, 1987). The synthesis of data begins by selecting as many as possible of all the various types of epidemiologic studies on the problem. After discarding those studies that are not methodologically sound, the studies are reviewed. The better the data meet the following six criteria, the more likely the factor of interest will be one of several causes of the disease:

1. *Temporal relationship:* Exposure to the suspected factor must precede the onset of disease.
2. *Strength of the association:* This refers to the ratio of disease rates in those with and without the suspected causal factor. A strong association would be noted when disease rates are much higher in the group with the factor than in the group without it.
3. *Dose response relationship:* This relationship is demonstrated if, with increasing levels of exposure to the factor, there is a corresponding increase in occurrence of disease.
4. *Consistency:* Association is demonstrated in varying types of studies among diverse study groups.
5. *Biological plausibility and coherence of the evidence:* The hypothesized cause makes sense based on current biological knowledge.
6. *Lowering of disease risk:* Interventions that decrease the exposure or factor result in a lowering of disease risk (relative risk).

The goal of any epidemiologic investigation is to identify causal mechanisms which meet the above criteria and to develop measures for preventing illness and promoting health. The community health nurse may need to gather new data for this type of investigation, but should thoroughly examine existing, pertinent data before doing so. This type of information can be obtained by the community health nurse from a variety of sources.

SOURCES OF INFORMATION FOR EPIDEMIOLOGIC STUDY

Epidemiologic investigators may draw data from three major sources or a combination of these sources. They are (1) existing data, (2) informal investigations, and (3) scientific studies. The community health nurse will find all three sources useful in efforts to improve the health of populations.

Existing Data

A variety of information is available nationally, by states, and by sections, such as counties or urbanized areas. This information includes vital statistics, census data, and morbidity statistics on certain communicable or infectious diseases. Local health departments often can provide this data upon request. Community health nurses seeking information on their own communities may also find the health system agencies most helpful. These agencies work to collect health information for groups of counties within states and interact with health planning authorities at the state level. They have access to many types of information and can give advice on specific problems raised by nurses.

Vital Statistics.   Vital statistics is a term used for the information gathered from ongoing registration of "vital" events relating to births, deaths, adoptions, divorces, and marriages. Certification of births, deaths, and fetal deaths are the vital statistics most useful in epidemiologic study. The community health nurse can obtain blank copies of a state's birth and death certificates to become familiar with the information contained in each. It will become apparent that much more information is recorded than the fact and cause of death on the death certificate. Birth certificates also can provide helpful information. For example, the weights of babies and the amount of prenatal care received by their mothers have been used to identify high-risk mothers and babies.

Census Data.   Data from population censuses taken every ten years in many countries are the main source of population statistics. This information can be a valuable assessment tool for the community health nurse taking part in health planning for a community. These population statistics can be analyzed by age, sex, race, ethnic background, type of occupation, income gradient, marital status, or educational level, as well as by other standards, such as housing. Analysis of population statistics can provide the community health nurse with a better understanding of the community and help identify specific areas that may warrant further epidemiologic investigation.

Reportable Diseases. Each state has developed laws or regulations that require hospitals, clinics, and clinicians to report cases of certain communicable and infectious diseases that can be spread through the community. This reporting enables the health department to take the most appropriate and efficient action. All states require that the six diseases covered by international quarantine regulations be reported immediately. Among these are diseases unknown now in developed countries (plague, cholera) as well as "dead" diseases such as smallpox. (The World Health Organization announced the eradication of smallpox in 1979 after more than ten years of international cooperation and commitment [Henderson, 1980]. The disease remains listed because it may reappear and because the virus is being maintained in laboratories to ensure vaccine availability if needed.) The other reportable diseases (varying between 20 and 40 by state) are usually classified according to the speed with which the health department should be notified. Some should be reported by phone or telegraph, others by mailing information weekly. They vary in potential severity from chicken pox to rabies and include AIDS (acquired immune deficiency syndrome), encephalitis, syphilis, and toxic shock syndrome. Community health nurses should obtain the list of reportable diseases from their health department offices. Following up on occurrences of these diseases is a task frequently assigned to community nursing services.

Registries. In some areas or states there are disease registries or rosters for conditions with major public health impact. Tuberculosis and rheumatic fever registries were more common in past years when these diseases occurred more frequently. Cancer registries provide useful incidence, prevalence, and survival data and assist the community health nurse in monitoring cancer patterns within a community.

Environmental Monitoring. State governments, sometimes through health departments and sometimes through other agencies, have begun to monitor health hazards found in the environment. Pesticides, industrial wastes, radioactive or nuclear materials, chemical additives in food, and medicinal drugs have joined the list of pollutants. Concerned community members and leaders view these as risk factors that affect health at both the community and individual levels. Community health nurses can also obtain data from federal agencies such as the Food and Drug Administration, the Consumer Product Safety Commission, and the Environmental Protection Agency.

National Center for Health Statistics Health Surveys. On the national level (published data are frequently available also for regions), the National Center for Health Statistics (NCHS) furnishes valuable health prevalence data from surveys of Americans (Hanlon and Pickett, 1984). The Health Interview Survey includes interviews from approximately 40,000 households each year and provides information about the health status and needs of the entire country. The Health Examination Survey reports physical measurements on smaller samples of the population and augments the information provided by interviews. This survey provides prevalence information on injuries, diseases, and disabilities that appear frequently in the population. A third type of NCHS survey is of health records. This survey samples institutional records of hospitals and nursing homes, primarily. This survey provides information on those who are utilizing the service, along with diagnoses and other characteristics. Other NCHS surveys focus on fertility and family planning, follow-back studies on vital statistics events, and characteristics of ambulatory patients in physicians' community practices.

Each of these nationally sponsored efforts suggests ways in which community health nurses can examine health problems or concerns affecting their communities. Interviews, physical examinations of samples of community members, and surveillance of institutions, clinics, and private physicians' practices can be carried out locally when needs are identified and funds made available. Other sources may be found in data kept routinely but not centrally on the health problems of workers in local industry or health problems of school children, a key issue to many community health nurses. Existing epidemiologic data can be used to plan parent education programs, health promotion among students, and almost any other type of service. For example, the Division of Nursing of the National Institutes of Health, in cooperation with the Delaware State Department of Education, began a long-term epidemiologic study of school populations as a basis for changing school nursing practice (Basco et al., 1972). They found, for example, that parent-nurse contacts were most likely to occur among higher-income parents, both white and nonwhite, who worried about their children's health. They also found that parents varied in their reasons for keeping children home from school; a large proportion would send their children to school with symptoms of a communicable disease. This data suggests that community health nurses working with schools, at least in the state of Delaware, might seriously consider a parent education program regarding such parental decisions.

Informal Investigations

The second information source in epidemiologic study involves informal investigations. Almost every client encountered by the community health nurse can precipitate such a study. If you discover an abused child at a clinic, you might screen the clinic's records for possible additional cases of child abuse. If several cases of diabetes come to the attention of a nurse visiting homes on a Navaho reservation, she might conduct informal inquiries about the incidence and age of onset of this disease among the Native American population. A community health nurse working in a clinic may raise the question, "Why don't the people who need our services come to the clinic?" A single day spent collecting epidemiologic data in an informal manner can shed light on this question. Perhaps, as Selwyn found in Colombia, nonusers have less knowledge about health and health services (Selwyn, 1978). This information, complemented with existing data, could lead to a change in clinic activities that would increase communication with those who need services.

Consider an example of how one nurse used an informal epidemiologic study to improve health care within a city jail. In dealing with incarcerated habitual intoxicants, Katherine Chavigny observed that neither jail staff nor health professionals addressed chronic alcoholic patients by name. "When names were essential for communication with the latter group, diminutives, nicknames, or at best, first names were used" (Chavigny, 1976, p. 637). Chavigny hypothesized that a lack of respect for the patients in the jail threatened their health by creating barriers to services offered. She carried out an informal study by introducing a simple change: she began to say "Mr." when addressing each patient in every nursing contact. Within several months, eye contact with patients, which had been almost nonexistent, increased to an estimated 70 percent. Patients who were formerly withdrawn began to express needs for the services offered by the health care team. Epidemiology seeks to identify variables that affect the health of groups and larger populations. Although this experimental epidemiologic study was of an informal nature, the nurse was able to identify at least one important factor and introduce a change that affected health care delivery.

Scientific Studies

The third source of information used in epidemiologic inquiry involves carefully designed scientific studies. Nursing, as a profession, has recognized the need to develop a systematic body of knowledge on which to base nursing practice. In the future, systematic research will become an accepted part of the community health nurse's role. We have already noted Selwyn's study to determine the use patterns of health services for mothers with children under 5 years of age. Dozens of other epidemiologic research studies done by nurses could be cited. For example, three nurses in Salt Lake City collaborated on a study of women who chose home birth. They discovered that this group did not differ from the total population in age, marital, and socioeconomic status. However, nearly half of the women had planned to have home births as a result of reported hostility from health professionals (Cameron, Chase, and O'Neal, 1979). This study provides important information for community nurses working with women who plan to have home delivery. Following an outbreak of trichinosis in Illinois, two nurses became involved with other investigators in an epidemiologic study of the epidemic. They concluded that the medical expenses and lost wages from this epidemic could have been prevented by a program to control trichinosis in swine (Potter, 1976). Three other nurses in Houston wanted to prevent the battering of pregnant women. They conducted a scientific study and discovered that

36 percent of the study population (14,047 prenatal patients served by area clinics) had been battered or were at risk for battering and none had been assessed for abuse by their health care providers. The nurses started an educational program and successfully increased (to 75 percent) health care providers' knowledge of and routine assessment for abuse. Part of their study was a scientific evaluation of the outcomes of their nursing interventions (Helton et al., 1987). Systematic studies such as these, as well as informal studies and existing epidemiologic data, can provide the community health nurse with valuable information that can be used to positively affect the health of a community. We will now proceed to examine in more detail the investigative methods used to collect epidemiologic data.

METHODS OF EPIDEMIOLOGIC INVESTIGATION

The goal of epidemiologic investigation is to identify the causal mechanisms of health and illness states and to develop measures for preventing illness and promoting health. Epidemiologists employ two basic methods of investigation: observation and experimentation. Both methods have relevance for community health nursing.

OBSERVATIONAL METHOD

Observational studies can be either *descriptive* or *analytic*. As we shall see, the analytic studies always include descriptive data but go beyond it to search for causal relationships.

Descriptive Studies

Descriptive studies seek to describe health-related conditions as they naturally occur. For example, a community health nurse might try to discover how many children in a school have been immunized for measles, how many home births occur each year in the county, or how many cases of AIDS have occurred in the last month. Descriptive studies almost always involve some form of quantification and statistical analysis.

Counts.   The simplest measure of description is a count. For example, several health professionals did an epidemiologic study of rape to provide data for a rape treatment, detection, and prevention program offered by the City Health Department of Houston, Texas (Sanford et al., 1979). One of the first steps in their research was to make a simple count of the number of rapes that occurred. They gathered data from the Houston Police Department; in the two-year period from 1974–75, 875 rapes were reported and 258 rapes attempted. Obtaining a count of this type always depends on the definition of what you count. This count, for example, does not represent all rapes occurring, but only those reported to the police. As in most kinds of research, availability of data influenced the items counted in this case. Before making use of any statistics, whether from official state offices, the census bureau, or a health agency, it is necessary to determine what the information represents.

The count of reported rapes and attempted rapes describes two groups in Houston, but it does not describe all rape in the city. Only the number of persons who fall into the groups "reported being raped" and "reported an attempted rape" is known. If we want to use this count as a means of understanding a characteristic about the total city, it must be seen in proportion. That is, we have to divide it by the total population of this city. Consider the different meanings such counts would have if the population of Houston were 50,000 on the one hand, or 500,000 on the other.

Rates. In order to express a count as a proportion, or rate, you must first decide on the population you want to study. If you consider 875 reported rapes in relation to the total number of inhabitants, you will have one rate; if you consider them in relation to the total female population of Houston, you will have a different proportion. In epidemiology, the *population* represents the universe of people defined as the objects of your study. Because it is difficult, if not impossible, to study the entire population, most epidemiologic studies draw a sample to represent that group. For example, Beatrice Selwyn wanted to study "mothers with children under five years of age" in Cali, Colombia. She selected one barrio with 50,000 residents, and then drew a sample of 529 mothers for interviews (Selwyn, 1978). In the Houston study dealing with prevention of battering during pregnancy, the nurse investigators selected a random sample of 290 pregnant women to interview out of a population of 14,047 prenatal patients served by area clinics (Helton, et al., 1987). Sometimes it is important to seek a random sample; at other times, a sample of convenience is sufficient. In many small epidemiologic studies it may be possible to study nearly every person in the population, thus eliminating the need for a sample.

Several proportions have wide use in epidemiology. Those most important for the community health nurse to understand include prevalence rate, period prevalence rate, and incidence rate.

The *prevalence rate* describes a situation at one point in time (Friedman, 1987). If a nurse discovers 50 cases of measles in an elementary school, she has a simple count. If she divides that number by the number of students in the school, she has described the prevalence of measles. For instance, if the school has 500 students, the prevalence of measles on that day would be 10 percent (50 measles/500 population).

$$\text{Prevalence Rate} = \frac{\text{Number of Persons with a Characteristic}}{\text{Total Number in Population}}$$

In the study of reported rapes in Houston, on the other hand, the investigators had a count for a two-year period, 1974 to 1975. Rather than portraying only one day, this number covered an extended period of time. The two-year *period prevalence rate* was .08 percent of the total population of females in Houston.

$$\text{Period Prevalence Rate} = \frac{\text{Number of Persons with a Characteristic During a Period of Time}}{\text{Total Number in Population}}$$

Not everyone in a population is at risk for developing a disease, incurring an injury, or having some other health-illness characteristic. The *incidence rate* recognizes this fact; for example, some childhood diseases give lifelong immunity. The children in a school who have had such diseases would be removed from the total number of children at risk in the school population. The incidence rate, after three weeks of a measles epidemic in a school, was

$$\frac{200}{1000} \text{ or } \frac{200 \text{ New Cases}}{1000 \text{ Persons at Risk}}$$

during the three-week time period. The health literature is not always consistent in the use of the term *incidence;* sometimes this word is used synonymously with prevalence rates and the reader must take this into consideration.

$$\text{Incidence Rate} = \frac{\text{Number of Persons Developing a Disease}}{\text{Total Number at Risk}} \text{ per Unit of Time}$$

Computing Rates. In order to make comparisons between populations, such as those of San Francisco and Seattle, epidemiologists often use a common base population in computing rates. For example, instead of merely saying that the rate of an illness is 13 percent in one city and 25 percent in another, the comparison is made per 100,000 persons in the population. This population base can vary for different purposes from 1000 to 100,000. The following are some formulas for computing rates commonly used in community health:

$$\text{Mortality Rate} = \frac{\text{Number of Reported Deaths}}{\text{Estimated Population as of July 1 of Same Year}} \times 100,000$$

$$\text{Infant Mortality Rate} = \frac{\text{Number of Deaths Under 1 Year of Age for Given Year}}{\text{Number of Live Births Reported for Same Year}} \times 1000$$

$$\text{Case Fatality Rate} = \frac{\text{Number of Deaths from a Particular Disease}}{\text{Total Number with the Disease}}$$

The goal of descriptive studies is to identify the patterns of occurrence of any health-related condition. In a descriptive study of child abuse, for example, the investigator would note the age, sex, race or ethnic group, and physical and emotional conditions of the children affected. In addition, data would be collected that described the economic status and occupation of parents, the location and setting of abusive behavior, and the time and season of the year when abuse occurred. In the study on reported rape in Houston, the investigators described the age, sex, and ethnic background of victims and offenders, and other features such as location and time of the crime. Figure 9-5 shows two temporal characteristics—time of day and day of week—of the pattern of reported rape. Although this pattern does not identify the *cause* of

Figure 9-5
Distribution (by percent, scale 0 to 10) of reported rape by hour of day and day of week, in Houston, Texas, 1974–1975. (From J. Sanford et al., Patterns of reported rape in a tri-ethnic population: Houston, Texas, 1974–1975. Am. J. Public Health 69(5): 483, 1979). Reprinted by permission.

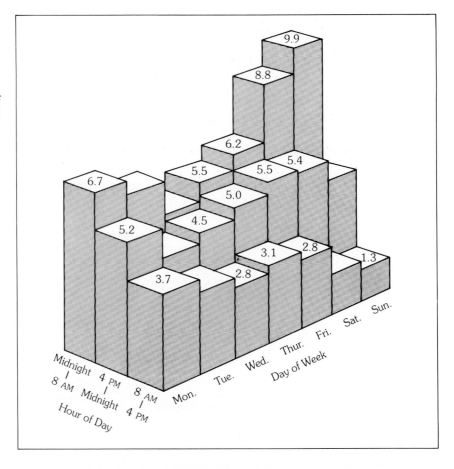

rape, it does describe facets of this health condition and suggest avenues for intervention or prevention.

Analytic Studies

The second kind of observational study is *analytic*. It differs from descriptive study only by its attempt to determine causal factors, or to explain the described phenomena. Analytic studies tend to be more specific than descriptive studies in their focus. They test hypotheses or seek to answer specific questions. For example, one nurse set out to test the hypothesis that "wife-battering is related to violence in the victim's childhood family of origin" (Parker and Schumacher, 1977). This study interviewed all the women who applied for legal assistance at a legal aid bureau in Baltimore, Maryland during a five-day period. Fifty women agreed to participate in an in-depth interview. The investigators described many characteristics of these women, 20 of whom were battered wives and 30 of whom were non-battered. No significant differences were found in variables such as age, race, education, and years of marriage. However, the hypothesis that those women beaten by their husbands had come from families where their mothers had been victims of the battered wife syndrome was confirmed. Like many analytic studies, this one gathered a great deal of descriptive data as well.

Analytic studies fall into three types—prevalence studies, case-control studies, and cohort studies. *Prevalence studies* describe patterns of occurrence, as in the study of reported rapes in Houston. They may examine causal factors, but these are always from the same point in time and the same population. Hypothesized causal factors are based on inferences from a single examination and most likely need further testing for validation.

Case-control studies make a comparison between persons with a health-illness condition (cases) and those who lack this condition (controls). These studies begin with disease (case) and look back over time for presence or absence of the suspected causal factor in both cases and controls. In the study of battered wives, the 20 women who had been beaten by their husbands represented the cases; the 30 who had not experienced violence were the controls. This study then reviewed the history of cases and controls for the presence of wife battering in the woman's nuclear family. In a case-control study, both groups should share as many characteristics as possible in order to isolate possible causes. Comparison between one group of women in their early twenties with another group in their late seventies would have invalidated the conclusion in the study of the battered wife syndrome.

Cohort studies, rather than measure the relationship of variables in existing conditions, study the development of a condition over time. A cohort study begins by selecting a group of persons who display certain defined characteristics before the onset of the condition being investigated. In studying a disease, the cohort might include individuals initially free of the disease but known to have been exposed to a particular factor. They would be followed over time to evaluate what variables were associated with the development or nondevelopment of the disease. In one school, several nurses studied two matched cohorts of children. One group received focused public health nursing attention; the other received routine school nursing services. These cohorts were studied over time to observe what differences may have occurred as a result of the different treatment. Decreased absenteeism was noted in the group that received focused nursing attention (Long et al., 1975).

RETROSPECTIVE AND PROSPECTIVE STUDIES

All of the various types of observational studies may be either retrospective or prospective. A retrospective study identifies cases and controls, and then goes back and reviews existing data. The study of reported rapes in Houston was a retrospective study, utilizing police department data that had been collected earlier. Prospective studies identify groups and exposure factors of interest, and then follow the groups and factors forward in time. These studies are concerned with current information and provide a direct measure of the variables in question.

In actual practice, the various types of studies just discussed are frequently mixed. A case-control study may include description and analysis with a retrospective focus; a cohort study may be conducted prospectively or retrospectively. Flexibility is essential to allow the investigator as much freedom as possible in choosing the most useful methodology.

EXPERIMENTAL METHOD

Experimental epidemiology, while used much less than the observational method, is valuable; it is used to study epidemics, the etiology of human disease, the value of preventive and therapeutic measures, and the evaluation of health services (Lilienfeld and Lilienfeld, 1980).

Experimental studies are carried out under controlled conditions. The investigator exposes one group (the experimental group) to some factor thought to cause disease, improve health, prevent disease, or influence health in some way. This exposure takes place under carefully controlled conditions and may involve animal or human populations. In human populations, experimental studies should almost always deal with disease prevention or health promotion; for obvious ethical reasons, studies that induce disease usually require an animal population. For instance, while humans can be used to test polio vaccine, experimental studies to test the cause of polio would not be done on humans. In addition to an experimental group, this method monitors a similar group (the control group) to see if any changes occur without the exposure.

Consider the following example of an experimental study in community health. Hypertension screening has been recognized as a valuable tool for identifying new hypertensive clients in the community. Many different strategies, from media advertising to setting up centers at local fire stations, have been used to motivate community members to have their blood pressure taken. One group of researchers wanted to find out what type of intervention would motivate the largest number of people to participate in the hypertension screening. They selected five target areas in an inner city and used a different form of experimental intervention with a sample of 200 households in four areas; the fifth area served as a control group. Intervention took forms such as home visits without prior notification by health workers offering to take blood pressures, letters inviting people to a clinic for blood pressure checks, and letters that offered gifts if people would come to the clinic. The results showed that the highest yield of new hypertensive clients came from home visits by community members trained to take blood pressure measurements. Even letters announcing the time and nature of the visit did not increase the number of new hypertensive clients (Stahl et al., 1977).

The community health nurse has many opportunities to conduct experimental studies in the course of working with groups. The study need not be elaborate; even without a control group, it can provide important data for future nursing practice. Several investigators associated with the Heart Disease Prevention Program at Stanford University carried out a small but valuable study. It involved a small sample size (eleven persons), used volunteers, and did not use a control group. The researchers reviewed the evidence that smoking by pregnant women significantly increases the incidence of perinatal deaths. Earlier studies had also shown that if women stopped smoking within the first trimester of pregnancy, the risk of perinatal death could be eliminated. A survey revealed that most intervention strategies used in this situation had been of short-term duration, such as admonishments from physicians. It was hypothesized that a longer, more intensive intervention strategy, that is, 6 two-hour classes over 7 weeks, would significantly increase the number of women who quit smoking during pregnancy. A group of eleven women volunteered, went through part or all of the course, and "the absolute level of abstinence achieved — both during the remaining period of pregnancy and postpartum — ranks well above other results reported in the literature" (Danaher et al., 1978, p. 897). Similar experimental studies could be done with almost any small group within the community health nurse's practice.

An expanding area of experimental epidemiology involves the use of computers to simulate epidemics. With mathematical models it is possible to determine the probability of various aspects of disease occurrence. This approach, called "theoretical epidemiology" by Lilienfeld, is making an increased contribution to our knowledge of etiology and prevention (Lilienfeld, 1980).

Occasionally, an experiment occurs naturally in which conditions offer the researcher the chance to make important discoveries. John Snow discovered such a "natural experiment" in London in 1854. In studying an epidemic of cholera, he observed one group that contracted the disease and another that did not. Closer inspection revealed that the major difference between these groups was their water supply. Eventually the spread of cholera was traced to the water supply of the group with high morbidity rate (sickness).

A community trial is a type of experimental study done at the population level (Hennekens and Buring, 1987). In this type of study communities are assigned to intervention (experimental) or non-intervention (control) groups and compared to determine whether the intervention produces a positive change in the community.

A well-known example of a community trial was done to test whether fluoridation of water significantly decreased the amount of dental caries in children. A community trial that is currently underway in the Minneapolis/St. Paul area is The Minnesota Heart Health Program. This study is comparing three sets of paired communities in the Upper Midwest. Each pair has one community in the intervention group and one in the non-intervention group. The intervention communities are receiving multiple intervention techniques such as dietary instruction, smoking cessation intervention, and risk factor instruction. Myocardial infarction, stroke, and mortality rates along with other measurements are being done at regular intervals to evaluate whether the interventions are improving health in the communities receiving them.

Community trials are extremely expensive and are not undertaken unless there is substantial evidence that the intervention will make a difference at the population level (Mittlemark et al., 1989).

THE INVESTIGATIVE PROCESS

The community health nurse who carries out an epidemiologic investigation becomes a detective. The nurse begins with a problem to solve, a puzzle to unravel, or a question to answer. Then she or he begins to search for basic information, clues that might help answer the question. But information is never self-explanatory and, like a detective, the nurse must analyze and interpret every additional clue. Slowly there is a narrowing of possible suspects until the nurse finally identifies the causes of a disease, the consequences of a prevention plan, or the results of treatment. On the basis of this investigation, the nurse can then draw further conclusions and make new applications to improve health services.

As discussed previously, epidemiologic studies are a type of research study. The steps outlined below are very similar to those that we will discuss later in the chapter on Research in Community Health Nursing. The epidemiologic investigative process involves six steps. Both an informal study in the course of nursing practice and the most comprehensive epidemiologic research project can be undertaken with these steps:

1. Identify the problem.
2. Review the literature.
3. Design the study.
4. Collect the data.
5. Analyze the findings.
6. Develop conclusions and applications.

We want to consider each of these steps in the context of a single health research project, a comprehensive clinic set up in a high school in St. Paul, Minnesota (Edwards, Steinman, and Hakanson, 1977).

IDENTIFY THE PROBLEM

Community health nurses are constantly confronted with threats to the health and well-being of the community. Almost daily, questions are raised, puzzles presented, and problems identified. Pregnant women who smoke or use cocaine threaten the health of their unborn children; what can be done to reduce this behavior? Rape is increasing; what can be done to bring aid to victims? Children are injured and die from bicycle accidents; why do these occur and how can they be prevented? Several farmers have been killed in tractor accidents; what can be done to prevent them? Any threat to the health of a group offers a fertile ground for epidemiologic investigation.

Health professionals in St. Paul began with a problem: inadequate delivery of health services to teenagers in the inner city. Evidence from the junior-senior high school population demonstrated a need for health services. The dropout rate was twice as great as the city's average; fertility rates were three to six times higher. The school dropout rate for girls who became pregnant was 45 percent. Testing for sexually transmitted disease, counseling regarding contraception, nutritional instruction, and other forms of health maintenance were needed.

REVIEW THE LITERATURE

All too often, after identifying a problem, health professionals rush to take immediate action. Every epidemiologic investigation should begin with a review of the literature. If you want to reduce the incidence of smoking among pregnant women, some other published study may suggest effective lines of action and research. If falls from windows have become a health problem in Chicago, the excellent study and prevention program developed in New York would be of great value (Spiegel and Lindaman, 1977). Even the discovery that little, if any, research has been done on the problem you select can be valuable information. Conversely, the fact that many studies already exist does not mean you should discard a project, but perhaps only narrow it into channels not previously investigated.

One of the most valuable sources in the literature is the "review article." For example, the team that set up the comprehensive clinic in St. Paul discovered an article in the *American Journal of Obstetrics and Gynecology* entitled "Medical and social factors affecting early teenage pregnancy: A literature review and summary of the findings of the Louisiana Infant Mortality Study" (Dott, 1976). Although not specifically about the delivery of health care to teenagers, it reviewed many articles that touched on this subject. A review of the literature often suggests hypotheses from discoveries made in other studies. For example, researchers in the clinic project found reports that pregnant students had a better chance of completing their education if they remained in their regular school. This finding became one hypothesis that could be tested by epidemiologic research. Even more important, the health care team used this finding as a basis for formulating a new hypothesis: that setting up a comprehensive clinic in the school would encourage pregnant students to complete their education (Edwards, Steinman, and Hakanson, 1977).

DESIGN THE STUDY

The first step in designing a study is to formulate a specific question to answer, and perhaps a hypothesis to test. Sometimes this hypothesis may emerge from the review of literature, as in the clinic project, but at other times it will have to be developed through your own analysis and hunches. It is a good idea to write out one or more hypotheses to test. We can rephrase the hypothesis implied by the clinic project as follows: The creation of a comprehensive clinic inside a public high school will improve the delivery of health services to teenagers.

In designing a study it is necessary to determine what type or combination of types will be used. Will an observational study or an experimental study best suit the goals of the research? Will the data be collected retrospectively from existing records or will new data be collected? Who will conduct interviews? What kinds of data will be needed to measure the outcomes of intervention?

Planning for the project in St. Paul began two full years before the clinic was established. Through the St. Paul-Ramsey Hospital, the Maternal and Infant Care Project No. 519 came into existence. The St. Paul public schools became involved, and a committee with representatives from students, parents, faculty, and other community agencies began work. This project involved an experimental study: the students at this junior-senior high school would be exposed to a new clinic. A specific control group in the form of another high school was not used; instead, data from the city as a whole would be used for comparative purposes.

It was decided that the health clinic would be led by a family-planning nurse clinician, assisted by a clinic attendant and a social worker. This team would offer services five mornings a week. In addition, numerous other health professionals, including a physician, a pediatric nurse associate, a nutritionist, and a maternity nurse clinician, would work part-time in the school. After the planning stage, the clinic opened in April, 1973.

COLLECT THE DATA

From the start of its program, the clinic staff began collecting data. They kept records on all clinic visits, the increase or decrease of utilization, and the characteristics of clinic users. For example, the clinic was used by nearly two-thirds of the senior class in 1975–1976, about equally by males and females. Records were kept on all sexually transmitted disease testing, requests for contraceptive information, fertility rates, and dropout rates among pregnant females.

Often it is useful to perform a pilot study that pretests an interview guide or questionnaire. If you want to interview women about battering during pregnancy, it might be useful to prepare a guide and interview one or two persons, then revise the guide on the basis of your experience. If you develop a questionnaire to assess the nutritional needs of elderly persons living alone, try out the survey on some volunteers to determine its clarity and relevance.

In community health nursing, data collection often can occur as part of ongoing practice. Unless the study has been carefully designed, however, you may collect data for months or years, only to discover that important questions have been omitted.

ANALYZE THE FINDINGS

In most epidemiologic studies, data analysis will consist of summarizing the findings, computing rates and ratios, and displaying the findings in tables and graphs. It is at this stage that the data is used to answer the original questions or test the original hypothesis. Does the data confirm or disprove the hypothesis? Summarized data can also generate more questions or indicate areas that warrant further investigation.

Consider the findings in a 54-bed nursing home in Florida. During a two-week period in November 1984 twelve patients died in this nursing home. Based on previous mortality patterns only 2.5 deaths would have been expected for the entire month. (See Figure 9-6.)

This data generated many questions and concerns. Numerous hypotheses were formulated, and although no definite cause for this increased death rate was found, many potential causes such as outbreak of infectious disease,

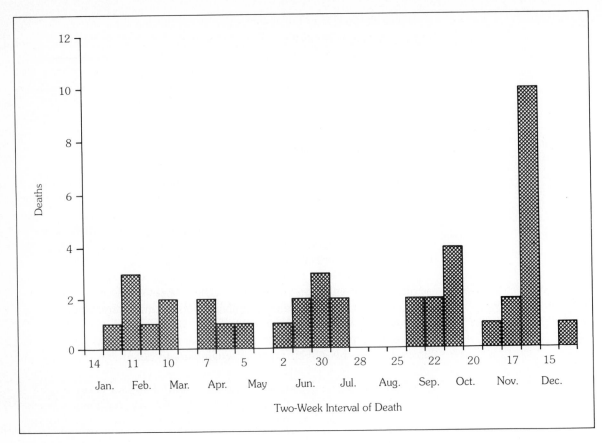

Figure 9-6
Bar graph depicting deaths
in a Florida nursing home
(Sacks, et al., 1988, p. 807).
Reprinted by permission.

change in client population, and change in environment were ruled out. Careful surveillance was continued in this facility (Sacks, et al., 1988).

Another recent study compiled findings from existing national data on leading causes of injury mortality in children ages 14 and under in the United States. (See Figure 9-7.) By compiling and categorizing this data, the researchers were able to identify geographic and subgroup injury problems that are often masked in larger, less specific categories. This identification increases the likelihood that specific injury problems will be targeted and given higher priority in prevention programs, eventually leading to a reduction in injury mortality (Waller, Baker, and Szocka, 1989, p. 315).

DEVELOP CONCLUSIONS AND APPLICATIONS

Stating conclusions is an outcome of analysis and interpretation. The investigator summarizes the results and their meaning for the purpose of sharing this information with others. Many times the research will have direct practi-

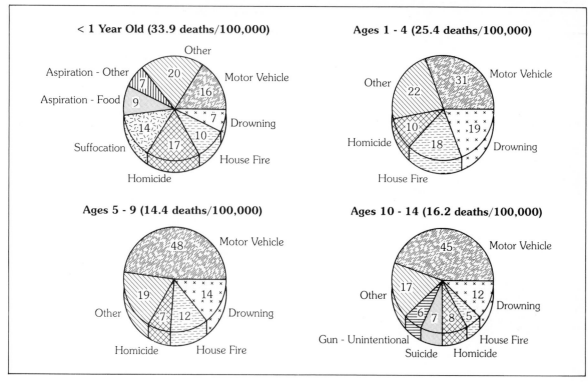

Figure 9-7
Pie charts showing percentages of childhood injury deaths by cause and age groups (Waller, Baker, and Szocka, 1989, p. 311). Reprinted by permission.

cal application for improving health services, continuing or discontinuing services, and conducting future research.

Many studies, as with the clinic project, combine research and intervention. For example, it was noted that each summer in New York City seemed to bring an epidemic of injured children who fell from unguarded windows. A study was conducted to determine the actual relationship of injuries to unguarded windows. As part of the study, community health nurses made follow-up visits to any home where an injury had occurred. This visit became a time for collecting data as well as educating family members in ways to prevent a recurrence of the injury. The New York City Health Department distributed free, easy-to-install window guards. Data collected during this project showed that falls had decreased significantly. The conclusions of the study were influential in a landmark decision by the New York City Board of Health to enact the first child accident prevention law in the United States. Passed in 1976, this law "requires owners of multiple dwellings to provide window guards where children ten years old and younger reside" (Spiegel and Lindaman, 1977).

After four years of operation and epidemiologic investigation, the clinic at the St. Paul junior-senior high school appeared to have proved its value. The investigators drew the following conclusions and offered recommendations for a direct application of the study (Edwards, Steinman, and Hakanson, 1977, p. 766):

> We feel that the measurable results to date as well as the positive response of the students themselves, justify the continuation and expansion of these services within the school system. We are convinced that this mechanism provides the best hope of reducing the incidence of the "unwed mother syndrome" by interrupting the vicious cycle of out-of-wedlock pregnancy, incomplete education, alienation from friends, family, and society, and repeat pregnancy, all of which may predetermine the futures of these young parents and their offspring.

Summary

Epidemiology is the study of the distribution and determinants of health and illness states in human population groups. It shares with community health nursing the common theme of the health of populations. Community health nurses can utilize three sources of information when conducting epidemiologic investigations: existing epidemiologic data, informal investigations, and carefully designed scientific studies.

Epidemiology uses a basic model of the interaction among host, agent, and environment. The community health nurse can intervene with any of these three factors to prevent the spread of disease or improve health in a population. Epidemiology is based on concepts regarding causal relationships among these three factors. Ideas about causation have changed from the early miasma theory, contagion theory, and germ theory of disease to an emphasis on multiple causation.

Epidemiology employs two basic methods of investigation: observation and experimentation. The observational method seeks to describe health-related conditions as they naturally occur. Although studies can be either retrospective or prospective, some merely describe existing conditions (descriptive studies) while others seek to explain causes (analytic studies). Epidemiologic studies of an experimental type actually intervene to expose a population of humans or animals to an illness or health condition. Observational studies can be of three types—prevalence, case-control, or cohort. In practice, all these types of studies often become combined in various ways. They also make use of quantitative concepts such as count, prevalence rate, incidence rate, mortality rate, and various types of morbidity (sickness) rates.

The investigative process of epidemiology in community health nursing includes six steps:

1. Identify the problem, which is usually some threat to the health of a population.
2. Review the literature to determine what other studies have found.
3. Carefully design the study. The investigator might decide to do an observational study or an experimental study. The methods of data collection are also identified during this step.

4. Collect the data.
5. Analyze the findings.
6. Develop conclusions and applications.

Thinking epidemiologically can significantly enhance community health nursing practice. Epidemiology provides both the body of knowledge — information on the distribution and determinants of health conditions — and methods for investigating health problems and evaluating services.

Study Questions

1. Define epidemiology. How is it like or unlike other types of research?
2. Explain the concept of the multiple causation theory of health or disease. How can this concept influence your practice as a community health nurse?
3. What is "risk"? What is "relative risk"? Why are these concepts important in community health practice?
4. Explain the difference between a prospective and a retrospective study. When is it appropriate to use a prospective study? A retrospective study?
5. Describe one community health situation in which you might use epidemiologic investigation for primary-level prevention.

Glossary of Terms

Agent: Refers to a putative cause of a health problem, particularly a biological infecting organism such as Hepatitis A virus.

Analytic studies: Investigations designed to identify associations between a particular human disease or health problem and its possible cause(s).

Association: Events are associated when they appear together more often than they would by chance alone. These events may include risk factors or other characteristics and disease or health states.

Attack rate: The proportion of a group or population that develops a disease among all those exposed to a particular risk. This term is used frequently in investigations of outbreaks of infectious diseases. See incidence rate.

Case series: A complete description of persons considered disease cases. No comparison group is present; no conclusion can be drawn.

Causal relationship/association: Inferred if the incidence of disease increases when the putative cause is present and decreases in the absence of this same putative cause or risk factor.

Cohort: A group of people who share a common experience in a specific time period.

Descriptive studies: Investigations describing groups of people with regard to certain characteristics (for example, time, place or person) as these relate to disease occurrence.

Endemic: "The habitual presence of a disease or infectious agent within a geographical area . . . or the usual prevalence of a given disease within such area" (Berenson, 1980).

Environment: Everything outside of human individuals — physical, chemical, biological, and social factors, including other people, social customs and codes, and so on.

Epidemic: Disease rates that clearly exceed normal or expected frequency in a community or region.

Epidemiology: The study of the distribution and determinants of health, health conditions, and disease in human population groups.

Experimental study: A study design in which the investigator actually controls or changes the factors suspected of causing the health condition under study and observes what happens to the health state. Experiments to test the cause of disease in human populations are rarely ethical. However, this approach can be used in trials to prevent disease or to treat established disease processes (clinical trials).

Host: An organism that harbors and provides nourishment for another organism.

Incidence: All new cases of a disease or other health conditions appearing during a given time.

Incidence rate: A proportion in which the numerator is all new cases appearing during a given time and the denominator is the population at risk during the same period of time.

Morbidity: The condition of being diseased; the ratio of number of sick individuals to the total population of a community.

Mortality: The condition or quality of liability to death; the death rate; the whole sum of deaths in a given population at a given time.

Pandemic: Epidemics that are worldwide in distribution.

Population at risk: Persons with one or more characteristics in common, to whom a health or disease event could have happened whether or not it did. The total number of persons in this group serves as the denominator for vital rates, and for incidence or prevalence rates. This population is sometimes called the referent population.

Prevalence: All people with a health condition existing in a given population at a given time. The condition may be new or have affected some persons for many years.

Prevalence rate: A proportion in which the numerator is all new and old cases of a health condition prevailing at a particular place and time, and the denominator is the total population for the same place and time.

Prospective study: (from the words "looking forward") The study group consists of persons free of the health condition in question (e.g., lung cancer). Persons are initially classified on the basis of their exposure characteristics (e.g., smoking vs. non-smoking), are followed longitudinally (forward over periods of time), and are observed for new development of the health condition or disease.

Rate: A statistical way of expressing the proportion of persons with a given health problem (or who develop a given health problem) among a population at risk. A rate is a quotient, or a fraction (e.g., prevalence rates, incidence rates, attack rates, and vital rates). A true rate exists when the numerator is a part of the denominator, and the denominator represents the entire population at risk. Compare with ratio.

Ratio: A statistical way of expressing the size or magnitude of one condition or occurrence in relation to the size of another. A ratio (e.g., sex ratio) need not be a rate.

Relative risk (RR): The comparison of disease occurrence in a group of people when a certain factor is present with the occurrence of the same disease in persons when that certain factor is absent.

Retrospective study: (From the words "looking back") A design whereby the investigator begins by identifying cases of a disease and controls without the disease, and looks backward in time to identify exposures or precursor factors.

Risk factor: When the presence of a particular factor increases the likelihood that a disease will occur, then for that disease the factor is a risk factor, and people with that factor are at high risk for that disease.

Sensitivity: Refers to a screening test or set of criteria that detects a very high percentage of persons with the specific disease or condition tested for — detects true positives. (Compare with "Specificity.")

Specificity: Refers to a screening test or set of criteria that accurately indicates a very high percentage of persons who do not have the disease or condition tested for — indicates true negatives. (Compare with "Sensitivity.")

References

Basco, D., S. Eyres, J. H. Glasser, and D. E. Roberts. (1972). Epidemiologic analysis in school populations as a basis for change in school-nursing practice. *American Journal of Public Health* 62: 491.

Benenson, A. S. (1985). *Control of communicable disease in man* (13th ed.). Washington, D.C.: American Public Health Association.

Burnet, MacFarlane. (1962). *Natural history of infectious diseases.* 3rd ed. Cambridge, England: Cambridge University Press.

Cameron, J., E. S. Chase, and S. O'Neal. (1979). Home birth in Salt Lake County, Utah. *American Journal of Public Health* 69: 716.

Chavigny, K. (1976). Self esteem for the alcoholic: An epidemiological approach. *Nursing Outlook* 24: 636.

Cohen, I. (1984). Florence Nightingale. *Scientific American* 250(3): 128–33.

Danaher, B. G., C. M. Shisslak, C. B. Thompson, and J. D. Ford. (1978). A smoking cessation program for pregnant women: An exploratory study. *American Journal of Public Health* 68: 896.

Dott, A. B. (1976). Medical and social factors affecting early teenage pregnancy: A literature review and summary of the findings of the Louisiana Infant Mortality Study. *American Journal of Obstetrics and Gynecology* 125: 532.

Edwards, L. E., M. E. Steinman, and E. Y. Hakanson. (1977). An experimental comprehensive high school clinic. *American Journal of Public Health* 67: 765.

Friedman, G. D. (1987). *Primer of epidemiology*. New York: McGraw-Hill.

Helton, A., J. McFarlane, and E. Anderson. (1987). Prevention of battering during pregnancy: Focus on behavioral change. *Public Health Nursing* 4(3): 166–74.

Henderson, D. A. (1980). Smallpox eradication. *Public Health Reports* 95: 422–26.

Hennekens, C. H., and J. E. Buring. (1987). *Epidemiology in medicine*. Boston: Little, Brown.

Lilienfeld, A. M., and D. E. Lilienfeld. (1980). *Foundations of epidemiology*. 2nd ed. New York: Oxford University Press.

Long, G., C. Whitman, M. Johansson, C. Williams, and R. Tuthill. (1975). Evaluation of a school health program directed to children with history of high absence. *American Journal of Public Health* 64: 388–93.

Mittlemark, M., R. Luepker, D. Jacobs, N. Bracht, R. Carlaw, R. Crow, J. Finnegan, R. Grimm, R. Jeffrey, G. Kline, R. Mullis, D. Murray, T. Pechacek, C. Perry, P. Pirie, and H. Blackburn. (1986). Prevention of cardiovascular disease: Education strategies of the Minnesota Heart Health Program. *Preventive Medicine* 15: 1–17.

Parker, B., and D. N. Schumacher. (1977). The battered wife syndrome and violence in the nuclear family of origin: A controlled pilot study. *American Journal of Public Health* 67: 760.

Potter, M. E., et al. (1976). A sausage-associated outbreak of trichinosis in Illinois. *American Journal of Public Health* 66: 1194.

Sacks, J., J. Herndon, S. Lieb, F. Sorhage, L. McCaig, and D. Withum. (1988). A cluster of unexplained deaths in a nursing home in Florida. *American Journal of Public Health* 78: 806–8.

Sanford, J., L. Cryer, B. L. Christensen, and K. L. Mattox. (1979). Patterns of reported rape in a tri-ethnic population: Houston, Texas, 1974–1975. *American Journal of Public Health* 69: 480.

Selwyn, B. J. (1978). An epidemiological approach to the study of users and nonusers of child health services. *American Journal of Public Health* 68: 231–35.

Spiegel, C. N., and F. C. Lindaman. (1977). Children can't fly: A program to prevent childhood morbidity and mortality from window falls. *American Journal of Public Health* 67: 1143.

Stahl, S. M., T. Laurie, P. Neill, and C. Kelley. (1977). Motivational intervention in community hypertension screening. *American Journal of Public Health* 67: 345.

Waller, A., S. Baker, and A. Szocka. (1989). Childhood injury deaths: National analysis and geographic variations. *American Journal of Public Health* 79: 310–15.

Selected Readings

Abramson, J. H. (1984). Application of epidemiology in community oriented primary care. *Public Health Reports* 99: 437–42.

Allen J. R., and J. W. Curran. (1988). Prevention of AIDS and HIV infection: Needs and priorities for epidemiologic research. *American Journal of Public Health* 78: 381–86.

Baker, S. P. (1975). Determinants of injury and opportunities for intervention. *American Journal of Epidemiology* 101: 98.

Barancik, J. I., B. F. Chatterjee, Y. C. Greene, E. M. Michenzi, and D. Fife. (1983). Northeastern Ohio trauma study: I. Magnitude of the problem. *American Journal of Public Health* 73: 746–51.

Barkauskas, V. H. (1983). Effectiveness of public health nurse home visits to primiparous mothers and their infants. *American Journal of Public Health* 73: 573–80.

Block, D. (1975). Evaluation of nursing care in terms of process and outcome: Issues in research and quality assurance. *Nursing Research* 24: 256–63.

Block, G. (1982). A review of validations of dietary assessment methods. *American Journal of Epidemiology* 115: 492–505.

Brady, M. T. (1986). Cytomegalovirus infections: Occupational risk for health professionals. *American Journal of Infection Control* 14: 197–203.

Branch, L. G., and A. M. Jette. (1981). The Framingham disability study: Social disability among the aging. *American Journal of Public Health* 71: 1202–10.

Broadhead, W. E., B. H. Kaplan, S. A. James, et al. (1983). The epidemiologic evidence for a relationship between social support and health. *American Journal of Epidemiology* 117: 521–37.

Brookbanks, M. (1987). Controlling an epidemic: Health visitors Margaret Brookbanks and Nancy Hampstead describe how they acted to stop the spread of an outbreak of Hepatitis B. *Nursing Times* 83: 38–39.

Butler, W. J., L. D. Ostrander, W. J. Carman, and D. E. Lamphiear. (1982). Diabetes mellitus in Tecumseh, Michigan: Prevalence, incidence, and associated conditions. *American Journal of Epidemiology* 116: 971–80.

Celentano, D. D. (1987). The epidemiology of alcohol consumption and hypertension with special reference to stroke. *Public Health Review* 15(2): 83–119.

Christenson, K., and J. A. Lingle. (1972). Evaluation of effectiveness of team and non-team public health nurses in health outcomes of patients with strokes or fractures. *American Journal of Public Health* 62: 483–90.

Corrigan, M., and L. Corcoran. (1961). *Epidemiology in nursing.* Washington: Catholic University of America Press.

Deolin, L. (1984). Epidemiology: The buzz word for the future. *Community Outlook* (October 10): 372.

Derschewitz, R. A., and J. W. Williamson. (1977). Prevention of childhood household injuries: A controlled clinical trial. *American Journal of Public Health* 67: 1148–53.

Dever, G. E. A. (1984). *Epidemiology in health services management.* Rockville, Md.: Aspen Systems.

Dever, G. E. A. (1980). *Community health analysis: A holistic approach.* Rockville, Md.: Aspen Systems.

Drotman, P. (1987). Now is the time to prevent AIDS. *American Journal of Public Health* 77: 143.

Duffy, M. E. (1988). Statistics: Friend or foe? *Nursing and Health Care* 9: 73–75.

Earp, J. A. L., M. G. Ory, and D. S. Strogatz. (1982). The effects of family involvement and practitioner home visits on the control of hypertension. *American Journal of Public Health* 72: 1146–54.

Frerichs, R. R., C. S. Aneshensel, and V. A. Clark. (1981). Prevalence of depression in Los Angeles County. *American Journal of Epidemiology* 113: 691–99.

Graitcer, P., and S. Thacker, (1986). The French connection. *American Journal of Public Health* 76: 1285–86.

Green, L., and C. L. Anderson. (1986). *Community Health.* St. Louis, Mo.: Times Mirror/Mosby.

Harter, L., F. Frost, G. Grunenfelder, K. Perkins-Jones, and J. Libby. (1984). Giardiasis in an infant and toddler swim class. *American Journal of Public Health* 74: 155–56.

Haynes, S. G., M. Feinleib, S. Levine, N. Scotch, and W. B. Kannel. (1978). The relationship of psychosocial factors to coronary heart disease in the Framingham study: II. Prevalence of coronary heart disease. *American Journal of Epidemiology.* 107: 384–402.

Helton, A., J. McFarlane, and E. Anderson. (1987). Prevention of battering during pregnancy: Focus on behavioral change. *Public Health Nursing* 4(3): 166–74.

Hennekens, C. E., and J. E. Buring. (1987). *Epidemiology in medicine.* Boston: Little, Brown.

Jensen, R. C. (1988). Epidemiology of work-related back pain. *Topics in Acute Care and Trauma Rehabilitation* 2: 1–15.

Johansson, S., A. Vedin, and C. Wilhelmsson. (1983). Myocardial infarction in women. *Epidemiologic Reviews* 5: 67–95.

Kark, S. L. (1974). *Epidemiology and community medicine.* New York: Appleton-Century-Crofts.

Kennedy, E. T., S. Gershoff, R. Reed, and J. E. Austion. (1982). Evaluation of the effect of WIC supplemental feeding on birth weight. *Journal of American Dietetic Association* 80: 220–27.

Langford. H. G. (ed.). (1982). Hypertension and obesity: Epidemiologic, physiologic and therapeutic considerations: Proceedings of a symposium. *Journal of Chronic Diseases* 35: 873–919.

Last, J. M. (1987). *Public health and human ecology.* East Norwalk, Conn.: Appleton and Lange.

Lauzon, R. (1977). An epidemiologic approach to health promotion. *Canadian Journal of Public Health* 68: 311.

Levinson, S. S., J. L. Bearfield, D. K. Ausbrook, et al. (1982). The Chicago Rheumatic Fever Program: A 20 plus-year history. *Journal of Chronic Diseases* 35: 199–206.

Lilienfeld, A. M. (ed.). (1980). *Times, places, and persons: Aspects of the history of epidemiology.* Baltimore, Md.: Johns Hopkins University Press.

Linn, S., S. C. Schoenbaum, R. R. Monson, R. Rosner, P. C. Stubblefield, and K. J. Ryan. (1983). The association of marijuana use with outcome of pregnancy. *American Journal of Public Health* 73: 1161–64.

MacMahon, B., and T. F. Pugh. (1970). Epidemiology: Principles and methods. Boston: Little, Brown.

Massanari, R. M. (1987). Risk management: An epidemiologic approach. *Infection Control* 8: 3–6.

Mauser, J. S., and S. Kramer. (1984). *Mauser and Bahn Epidemiology: An introductory text.* Philadelphia: W. B. Saunders.

McNeil, H. J., and S. S. Holland. (1972). A comparative study of public health nurse teaching in groups and in home visits. *American Journal of Public Health* 62: 1629–37.

Morton, R. F., and J. R. Hebel. (1979). *A study guide to epidemiology and biostatistics.* Baltimore, Md.: University Park Press.

Mullan, F. (1984). Community oriented primary care: Epidemiology's role in the future of primary care. *Public Health Reports* 99: 442–45.

Payne, S. M. C., and D. M. Strobino. (1984). Two methods of estimating target population for public maternity service programs. *American Journal of Public Health* 74: 164–66.

Quick, J. D., M. R. Greenlick, and K. J. Rothmann. (1981). Prenatal care and pregnancy outcome in an HMO and general population: A multivariate cohort analysis. *American Journal of Public Health* 71: 381–90.

Schoenbach, V. J., B. H. Kaplan, E. H. Wagner, R. C. Grimson, and F. T. Miller. (1983). Prevalence of self-reported depressive symptoms in young adolescents. *American Journal of Public Health* 73: 1281–87.

Shapiro, S., M. McCormick, B. Starfield, J. P. Krischer, and D. Bross. (1980). Relevance of correlates of infant mortality for significant morbidity at one year of age. *American Journal of Obstetrics and Gynecology* 136: 363–73.

Smith, D. P. (1986). Common day-care diseases: Patterns and prevention. *Pediatric Nursing* 12: 175–79.

Terris, M. (1975). Approaches to an epidemiology of health. *American Journal of Public Health* 65: 1037.

Thompson, S. E., and A. E. Washington. (1983). Epidemiology of sexually transmitted *Chlamydia trachomatis* infections. *Epidemiologic Reviews* 5: 96–118.

Turner, J. G., and K. H. Chavigny. (1988). *Community Health Nursing: An Epidemiologic Perspective.* Philadelphia: J. B. Lippincott Company.

Valanis, B. (1986). *Epidemiology in nursing and health care.* East Norwalk, Conn.: Appleton-Century-Crofts.

Valdieseiri, R. (1988). The immediate challenge of health planning for AIDS: An organizational model. *Family and Community Health* 10: 33–48.

Valleron, A. J., E. Bouvet, P. Garnerin, J. Menares, I. Heard, S. Letrait, and J. Lefaucheux. (1986). A computer network for the surveillance of communicable diseases: The French experiment. *American Journal of Public Health* 76: 1289–92.

Waller, J. A. (1985). The epidemiologic basis for injury prevention. *Public Health Reports* 100: 575–76.

Willet, W. C., C. H. Hennekens, C. Bain, B. Rosner, and F. E. Speizer. (1981). Cigarette smoking and non-fatal myocardial infarction in women. *American Journal of Epidemiology* 113: 575–82.

Winkelstein, W., Jr., E. J. Shillitoe, R. Brand, and K. K. Johnson. (1984). Further comments on cancer of the uterine cervix, smoking, and herpes virus infection. *American Journal of Epidemiology* 119: 1–8.

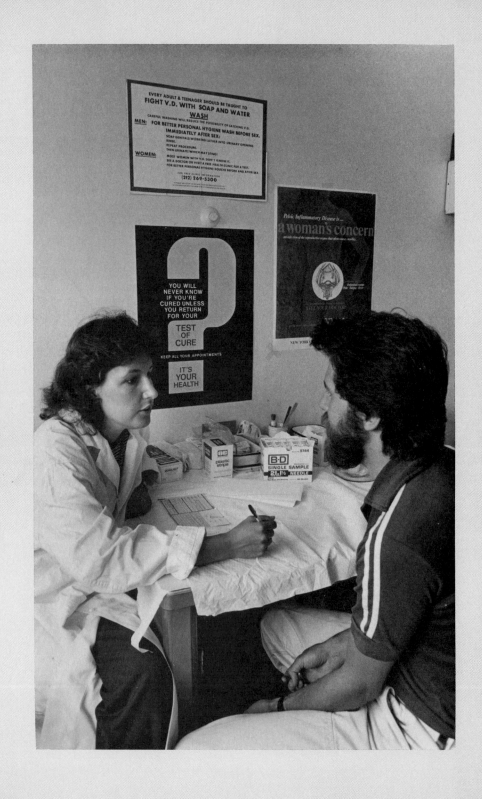

10 The Helping Relationship and Contracting

The helping relationship is a primary tool for community health nurses. It contributes both to the prevention of illness and to the promotion of client health. In order to use the helping relationship skillfully in community health practice, we must understand the meaning and value of a therapeutic relationship. Unlike ordinary social relationships, a helping relationship is based on mutual participation in establishing and carrying out goals. Clients and the nurse enter into a working agreement to meet specific client needs. The concept of contracting is closely tied to use of the helping relationship. In this chapter we examine both of these tools and discuss their integration into community health nursing practice.

THE HELPING RELATIONSHIP: A DEFINITION

The concept of a helping relationship has undergone a change in recent years. Traditionally, the term *helping* has implied that one individual gives help, and the other individual receives help. Viewed in this manner, the helping relationship inadvertently created a dependency relationship. It made clients dependent on the nurse, undermined their self-confidence, and undercut their self-respect. In short, it reduced the very characteristics that the nurse hoped to foster. This traditional view of the helping relationship reduced clients' motivation to participate in the health care process and detracted from their sense of responsibility for maintaining their health.

This traditional definition has another inherent problem. It implies that the helping relationship occurs only between two individuals, the nurse and a single patient or client. Even the community health nurse working with a family, for example, may think in terms of establishing a helping relationship only with the mother or some other individual, rather than with the family as a whole. In community health nursing, the client will range from a single individual to an entire community. For example, a single community health nurse might develop helping relationships with the following range of clients: (1) an elderly widower living alone in his own home, (2) an extended family of Cuban immigrants, (3) a parenting class of 15 mothers, (4) a lumber company with 95 employees seeking to develop a wellness program, (5) a cluster of elementary schools seeking to improve nutrition among students, and (6) an entire community conducting a self-survey about health practices. Throughout this book, the term *client* can refer to an individual or a group. In order to maximize the effectiveness of the helping relationship in promoting client health, we need to redefine the helping relationship to mean *purposeful interaction between nurse and clients based on mutual participation.* This definition highlights two basic features of the helping relationship: it has a goal, and it involves both parties in setting and achieving that goal.

CHARACTERISTICS OF THE HELPING RELATIONSHIP

In order to explore the meaning of the helping relationship in the context of community health nursing, we shall examine five characteristics that distinguish it from other types of interaction, which will be referred to as simply "social relationships."

Emphasis on Goals

First, the helping relationship in community health nursing is goal-directed. The nurse and client recognize specific reasons for entering into the relationship. For example, a large Thai family that recently immigrated wants to learn about food shopping in the United States; the community health nurse can provide that information. The client group and the nurse enter into the relationship with stated needs to be met and goals to accomplish. Other forms of social interaction, such as encounters between friends, often lack recognized goals.

Unilateral Benefits

Second, in community health nursing the helping relationship is unilateral; that is, it exists for the benefit of the clients. In developing a helping relationship with the Thai immigrant family concerned about adjusted eating patterns, the nurse may teach the family how to shop for food, cook, and eat in a new cultural setting. The direct benefits accrue to the family. Certainly the nurse gains satisfaction from the interaction, but the relationship is established to meet the needs of the clients. The nurse's satisfaction and growth are a side effect, not a stated objective. Many other social relationships, as among friends, business acquaintances, or professional colleagues, are bilateral. Both parties come to the relationship with an expectation of almost equivalent benefits.

Explicit Mutual Agreement

Third, in community health nursing the helping relationship involves explicit mutual agreement. When you interact with a friend, relative, salesperson, or neighbor, the relationship operates with tacit rules; you probably do not talk about the relationship or direct your energy toward seeking an explicit consensus. The helping relationship, on the other hand, involves a reciprocal exchange in which both parties discuss what their interaction will involve. The mother, father, and grandparents in the Thai family may express their desire to provide their children with nutritious food. They may be concerned about loss of traditional foods and feel overwhelmed when shopping in supermarkets. They want the nurse to assist them in achieving their goals. The nurse discusses her role in giving this assistance. The nurse-client relationship arises from an explicit, mutual agreement. Discussion of the goals and the nature of the relationship provides a channel within which the work of the relationship takes place.

Set Responsibilities

Fourth, in community health nursing the helping relationship assigns set responsibilities to each party. A well-defined relationship clearly states what the client will do and what the nurse will do to accomplish the identified goals. The nurse, for example, might agree to take several members of the Thai family on a shopping trip, help them prepare a balanced meal, and provide reading materials on infant nutrition. The family would agree to study the materials (perhaps through an older child who can interpret for the adults), ask questions, and follow the example and instructions of the nurse. Each party to the helping relationship develops an understanding of individual responsibilities based on realistic and honest expectations. This understanding may not come with the first visit, but as the relationship develops, the nurse works toward this division of responsibilities. Together with the client, the nurse explores necessary resources, assesses the capabilities of clients, and discovers their willingness to assume tasks. This structure of recognized responsibilities is often absent in other human relationships. Two friends can enjoy long years of companionship without ever saying, "You do this and I will do these other things." A local church committee, set up to help an immigrant family, may assume all the responsibility for helping provide food for the family rather than dividing the responsibility.

Set Boundaries

Fifth, the helping relationship in community health practice has set boundaries. Nearly every therapeutic relationship has a beginning and an end. A crucial part of defining the helping relationship is determining when and under what conditions to terminate it. The temporal boundaries are determined sometimes by progress toward the goal, sometimes by the number of

Table 10-1
Contrast between Helping and Social Relationships

Helping Relationship	Social Relationship
Goal-directed	No specific goals
Unilateral; benefits client	Bilateral; benefits both parties
Explicit mutual agreement	No consensus; casual interaction
Set responsibilities	Unstructured
Time-limited; set boundaries	Open-ended in length and frequency of contacts

nurse-client contacts, and often by setting a time limit. A nurse might set up eight sessions to help the Thai family with nutrition problems, or she might meet with the family weekly until the goal of adequate knowledge and skill was met. Social relationships, in contrast, are generally open-ended in length. A friendship may end because of misunderstanding, or a business relationship may stop when a partner moves to another city. Table 10-1 summarizes the characteristics that distinguish the helping relationship from social relationships.

CLIENT PARTICIPATION

In this text we have stressed that the helping relationship is based on mutual participation. The extent of that participation varies, however, depending on the client's readiness and ability to participate. The level of wellness at the time of initial nurse-client encounter directly influences participation. Some people are not physically or emotionally well enough to assume an active role in the relationship. Women recently discharged from the hospital following a mastectomy, for example, have many physical and emotional adjustments with which to cope. Their families, too, must expend additional energies to provide needed support and to cope with the temporary loss of each woman's usual role in the family. They may find it difficult to engage actively in identifying their needs and goals at the start of the relationship. The nurse may have to take stronger initial leadership; however, the goals of a helping relationship are not abandoned. Eventually, as the women's wellness levels improve, the nurse can encourage more active participation from the clients and their families.

Sometimes clients' previous experiences with health personnel limit participation in the helping relationship. Clients from poverty areas, from different cultural backgrounds, or with little education may need extensive encouragement to participate actively in the helping relationship. Working with a Thai family, recently immigrated to the United States, will be quite different from helping a group of suburban women with infant development. Clients previously regarded by health professionals as incapable of managing their own lives will also take a more passive role in the helping relationship. Even well-educated people with comfortable incomes often have learned to behave passively when dealing with physicians, nurses, or other health professionals. With all these people, unless the nurse persists in efforts to reduce the dependence of clients, the relationship can fall far short of the therapeutic goals.

The nurse's own view of the helping relationship will also influence the degree of client participation. Those nurses accustomed to relating to clients in an adult-to-child manner will restrict client involvement. If the nurse sees her position as more informed and the client's position as one of complete ignorance and need, a paternalistic relationship may develop. All clients have resources on which to build, and the community health nurse helps clients discover them.

Clients who initiate care, such as postpartum mothers who ask for home visits or families who request follow-up care after hospitalization, are frequently best able to assume an active participant role. They have already demonstrated a sense of responsibility for their health by identifying a need and asking for assistance. The nurse will still have to work carefully to build mutual participation, but its development is more likely to occur.

COMMUNICATION IN THE HELPING RELATIONSHIP

Communication is the lifeblood of the helping relationship. It provides the vitality and nourishment necessary to foster a healthy nurse-client relationship. For communication to take place, clients and nurses send and receive messages. As participants in the communication process, community health nurses play both roles — sender and receiver (Lancaster and Lancaster, 1982). The nurse working with an alcoholic housewife must learn to "read" the messages this woman sends. The nurse will also have to speak and act in ways that communicate effectively. Community health nursing requires two sets of communication skills: sending skills and receiving skills.

SENDING SKILLS

Sending skills enable nurses to communicate messages effectively. Through these skills nurses convey thoughts and feelings to clients. Two important considerations will influence clarity and effectiveness of message sending. First, the extent of the nurse's self-awareness will affect the communication. Does she feel anxious, angry, impatient, or concerned? Is she tired? Do certain clients irritate her? What motives and interests does she have for wanting to communicate with these clients? Second, her awareness of the receiver will influence the sending of messages. What do these clients seem to want or need? Is the message suited to their cultural background and level of understanding? Does the message have significance for them? How do clients respond as she sends the message?

Two main channels are used to send messages: nonverbal and verbal. Nonverbal messages, those conveyed without words, constitute nearly two-thirds of the messages transmitted in normal communication (Brill, 1973). We send messages nonverbally in many ways. Our personal appearance, dress, posture, and cleanliness all communicate messages about us. They may enhance or discredit what we say. Body language often speaks louder than words. Facial expressions convey acceptance or rejection, interest or boredom, and apprehension or confidence. Gestures and bodily movements such as hand clenching, finger tapping, or foot swinging all communicate strong messages to clients. Eye contact or lack of it carries additional meaning. Tone of voice and use of silence also will send nonverbal messages. Accepting food may communicate acceptance, while getting a chair for a client may say "I'm interested in your welfare."

Verbal messages communicate ideas, but they also convey attitudes and feelings (Veninga, 1982). Nurses cannot assume that the intent of their words is always understood by clients. Effective sending skills depend on asking for feedback to make certain that the receiver has understood the verbal message's intent. Communication can improve if speakers avoid jargon. Like all occupations, nursing has its own vocabulary. Often unfamiliar to clients, this jargon may carry different meanings or make the client feel inferior because he cannot speak that language. Mr. Jones did not know what to answer when the nurse asked if he had "voided." Mrs. Wendt felt confused when asked if she had noticed any expressions of "sibling rivalry" by her three-year-old child. When nursing jargon becomes part of everyday speech, only special effort will enable nurses to set it aside when interacting with clients. The basic rules for effective sending can be summarized in this manner: keep the message honest and uncomplicated; use as few words as possible to state it; and ask for reactions (feedback) to make certain that it is understood.

RECEIVING SKILLS

Receiving skills are as important to communication as sending skills. They enable nurses to receive accurate and complete messages. Receiving skills involve not only listening to what people say but also observing their behavior. If a client says, " I haven't been feeling well," the nurse needs to discover the context of this statement. What tone of voice did the client use? What was the meaning of the client's facial expressions? What gestures accompanied the statement? When did the client mention these feelings? Effective receiving skills require training to observe these kinds of details.

The other main source of receiving is active listening, the skill of assuming responsibility for understanding the meaning of the client's message (Wismer, 1978). Instead of requiring the client to make the nurse understand, the nurse should actively work to discover what a client means. Understanding the message from the client's perspective demands careful attention. It arises from a genuine interest in what the speaker has to say. Active listeners demonstrate their interest, perhaps by sitting forward, sustaining eye contact, nodding the head, and asking occasional questions for clarification. They concentrate in order to avoid daydreaming or the pretense of listening, both of which block communication.

Nurses can also listen actively by asking reflective questions. Such questions restate what the client has said:

> Client: "Quitting smoking is impossible."
> Nurse: "You feel you can't quit smoking?"

Reflective questions have a twofold purpose: to show a sincere attempt to understand clients' messages, and to make clear that the messages and the clients are important to the nurse.

Active listening will communicate acceptance and increase trust, especially when a negative evaluation of the message or the way it is delivered is withheld (Veninga, 1982). A critical response to the message cuts off communication. Active listening enables nurses to encourage clients to deliberate carefully and to develop problem-solving skills; it avoids the pitfall of telling them what to do.

INFLUENCES ON COMMUNICATION

Effective communication, both sending and receiving, is strongly influenced by three factors. First, the previous experiences of both sender and receiver influence their perceptions and the meanings they attach to messages. Requests for clarification will help verify that messages are being received as intended. Second, the respective cultures of sender and receiver influence understanding and acceptance of messages. A nervous laugh, appropriate as an outlet in one culture, may appear rude and disrespectful to someone from another culture. Silence may indicate patience and thoughtfulness to one group of people but weakness or indifference to another. With many clients, the nurse will have to communicate cross-culturally, which requires patience and constant effort to ensure accurate and inoffensive messages. Third, the relationships among participants during communication can significantly influence its effectiveness. Since much of community health nursing involves families and groups, communication patterns become quite complex. When a large number of people are involved, interaction requires skill in eliciting feedback from all members and in generating a common understanding among the group.

INTERPERSONAL SKILLS AND THE HELPING RELATIONSHIP

In addition to effective communication, the helping relationship also requires three other interpersonal skills: showing respect, empathizing, and developing trust. Each of these skills depends on effective communication but surpasses the mere exchange of messages.

SHOWING RESPECT

Showing respect means conveying the attitude that clients have importance, dignity, and worth. Community health nurses can express respect by helping clients feel that they have valuable ideas. Nurses can let them know that they want to understand the situation from the clients' points of view. Nurses show respect by the manner in which they address clients — for instance, by using the courtesy titles of "Mr." or "Mrs." until permission is granted to use first names. On a more subtle level, the tone of voice can either show respect or make people feel inferior and insignificant. Clients need to feel respected if they are to enter fully into the mutual exchange necessary for a true helping relationship.

EMPATHIZING

Empathizing is another important interpersonal skill. Empathy means the "ability to borrow another person's feelings...[and] to understand them while maintaining one's own identity" (Kalisch, 1973). Nurses empathize by reflecting the client's feelings. Empathy is best expressed in the client's language. The same terms and, if possible, the same tone of voice as the client's should be used. For example, the nurse can reflect sadness if the client seems sad. Empathy is best expressed provisionally, showing that the nurse is still attempting to ascertain the client's true feelings while allowing the client to validate each provisional expression. It counters any defensiveness or anxiety that the client may be feeling (Veninga, 1982). Empathy conveys the message, "This is the way it seems to me. Is that right?" It focuses attention on clients and their feelings. It shows that the nurse shares their concerns, and it makes clients feel important.

DEVELOPING TRUST

Developing trust is necessary for an effective helping relationship. Clients will not express their true feelings if they do not fully trust the nurse. Many times clients will say what they think the nurse wants to hear. They may agree to a plan of action simply because they do not want to displease the

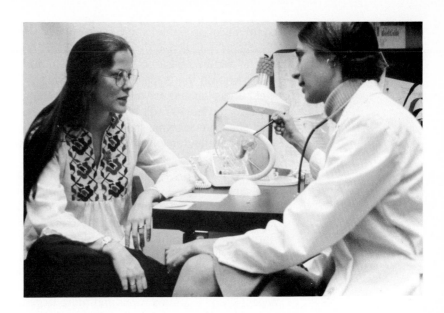

Figure 10-1
Development of trust is
crucial to an effective
helping relationship.

nurse. They may hide true feelings because they think that the nurse is eager for a decision. Nurses develop trust by showing that they truly accept clients, that they believe in them as people. Trust generates trust; as the nurse shows confidence in clients, they will respond in kind. Treating them as fully participating partners in the relationship shows clients that they are trustworthy with responsibilities. Trust is also developed through an open, honest, and patient approach with clients. Candid discussion in a flexible time frame encourages clients to share their real feelings and to move at their own pace. As trust develops, the relationship becomes a truly helping one, focused on client needs (see Figure 10-1).

STRUCTURE OF THE HELPING RELATIONSHIP

The skills that lead to an effective helping relationship are used within a particular structure. Awareness of this structure can greatly increase the nurse's ability to help clients. Because the relationship is bound by time, the structure involves several phases. The way nurses use their skills during the first and last phases of the helping relationship may contrast. It is useful to think of the helping relationship as following a sequential structure: (1) a beginning phase when the relationship is just being established; (2) a middle, working phase; and (3) a termination phase when the relationship ends (Brill, 1973). In the context of this process, the work of identifying and meeting client needs takes place.

The first phase is a period of establishing and defining the relationship. The nurse and clients are getting to know each other; they seek to establish communication patterns and develop trust. From these bases, they identify the clients' needs and determine the goals toward which they will work.

The middle phase occurs when nurse and clients start working together to accomplish the goals of the relationship. Their work may include assessment and planning as well as implementation and evaluation. The cycle of the nursing process will be repeated as needed during this working phase until goals are accomplished and no further goals identified.

The termination phase occurs when the need for nurse and clients to work together has ended. In many instances, clients can function on their own. When clients and nurse have grown close in the relationship, termination can be difficult. It often requires careful advance preparation to make certain that all parties understand when and why it is taking place. Termination helps to ensure a clear-cut end to the relationship. One nurse had made home visits to a refugee family for nearly a year. As the family's multiple needs declined, she decided to taper off her assistance. Two months before ending the relationship, she discussed termination with the family. At first the family members were frightened at the loss of help, but slowly they came to accept it and assumed more and more responsibility for their health needs. Had she announced the end of her visits more abruptly, without consulting with them, the family might easily have felt confused or rejected.

THE CONCEPT OF CONTRACTING

The primary goal of community health nursing is to promote the public's health through identifying and meeting people's needs. Success demands the active participation of clients. The helping relationship is "helping" only in the sense that nurses assist people in this process. Without mutual participation, clients cannot develop ability in self-care. Contracting makes the goal of self-care explicit.

The concept of self-care has a long history in community health nursing. Public health nursing, as Norris (1979) has shown, was founded on self-care concepts and originated self-care practice. More recently, self-care has come into its own through the growth of independent nursing practice. Kinlein (1977), for example, based her independent practice squarely on this concept. She found that clients had far more capability than was believed in achieving self-care. She believed that nursing meant helping clients choose the self-care practices best for them. Like the shopkeeper who expects his customers to make their own selections, the nurse treats clients as independent consumers, saying, "I believe in your ability to assume responsibility for your own health." By making self-care more explicit, contracting can become a powerful tool in community health nursing (Helgeson et al., 1985).

Contracting means negotiating a working agreement between two or more parties. They come to a shared understanding and then give consent to the purposes and terms of the transaction. Some kinds of contracts are familiar, such as a contract connected with buying a car. Other, less obvious agreements, such as paying tuition for an education, still involve a form of contracting. As a student, you agree with an educational institution on the purposes (their financial reimbursement, your degree) and terms of the contract (regular tuition payments, regular learning opportunities), even though a formal document is not signed.

In contrast to legal contracts that are written, binding agreements, the contract in a helping relationship is flexible and based on mutual understanding and trust. Sloan and Schommer (1982, p. 222) define the community nursing contract as "any working agreement, continuously renegotiable" between client and nurse. When viewed from this perspective, contracting becomes a valuable tool for community health nurses.

FEATURES OF CONTRACTING

The concept of contracting as used in the helping relationship incorporates four distinctive features: partnership, commitment, format, and negotiation.

Partnership

All aspects of contracting involve shared participation and agreement between client and nurse; they become partners in the relationship. For example, the Ericksons, an older couple who requested community health nursing visits at home, entered into a partnership with a nurse after the husband was discharged from the hospital with a colostomy. They came to an agreement on what the couple needed and what the nurse could provide. Together they developed goals, outlined methods to meet those goals, and explored resources to help achieve them. They defined the time limits for the contract as well as their separate responsibilities. The contract involved reciprocal negotiation and shared evaluation. A partnership means that both parties are responsible for setting up and carrying out the terms of the agreement.

Commitment

Second, every contract implies a commitment. Both parties make a decision that binds them to fulfilling the purpose of the contract. In the helping relationship, contracting does not mean making a binding agreement in the legal sense; rather, it is a pledge of trust and dedication. Accompanying that sense of dedication is a strong motivation to see the contract through to completion. Both parties feel responsible for keeping promises; both want to achieve the intended outcomes. When the nurse and the Ericksons identified their separate tasks, they committed themselves: "Yes, we will do thus and so. . . ."

Format

Format is the third distinctive feature of the concept of contracting. Unlike many nurse-client interactions, contracting defines the terms of the relationship. Thus both client and nurse obtain a clear idea of the purpose of the relationship, of their respective responsibilities, and of the specific limits within which they will work. In other words, contracting provides a framework for the relationship. Once the terms of the contract have been spelled out, there is no question about what has to be done, who is to do it, or within what time frame it is to be accomplished. This format helps to prevent a frequently recurring problem in community health nursing—the difficulty of terminating a long-term relationship. It also helps to prevent dependency relationships from developing.

Negotiation

Finally, contracting always involves negotiation. The nurse proposes to accept certain responsibilities, and then asks if the clients agree. The nurse might ask, "What do you feel you can do to achieve this goal?" A period of give-and-take occurs in which ideas are discussed and conclusions, which often represent compromises, are reached. A few weeks later, nurse and clients may find that terms they had agreed upon need modification. Perhaps clients have assumed more responsibility than they can realistically handle at that point in time. Perhaps the nurse does not feel comfortable teaching a complex technique and needs to utilize an outside resource. Negotiation during contracting allows for changes that facilitate the ultimate achievement of goals. It provides contracting with built-in flexibility and encourages ongoing communication between clients and nurse. Negotiation gives contracting a dynamic quality. (See Figure 10-2.) It becomes a complex process that moves through eight stages, each negotiated between the nurse and clients. This process will be considered later in the chapter.

VALUE OF CONTRACTING

The value of contracting has been demonstrated in many settings. Contracts have been used for many years in psychiatric nursing settings to promote client self-respect, problem-solving skills, autonomy, and motivation (Davis and Woodcock, 1971; Rosen, 1978). Other disciplines, such as social work, have used contracting as a tool in the helping relationship to enhance realistic planning and emphasize partnership (Sauer, 1973). Educational contracts between students and instructors have proven valuable for facilitating learning (Lindberg and Simms, 1974; Brown et al., 1987; Gross et al., 1986). Community health nursing also has used the concept of contracting for many

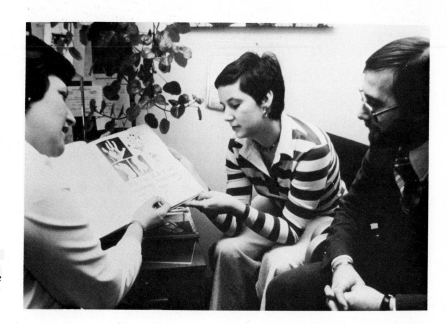

Figure 10-2
An important feature of contracting involves mutual agreement between the family and the nurse on the material they want to cover in their sessions together.

years. Without always labeling their work as such, community health nurses have contracted with clients who, for example, wanted to lose weight, mutually agreeing to certain exercise and eating patterns for clients and teaching and support responsibilities for the nurse. Often they have set a time limit, such as six months, within which to achieve the intended weight loss. Community health nurses have entered into contractual relationships with postpartum mothers, new diabetics, postsurgical patients, prenatal groups, and many others. In each case, a partnership developed, with agreement about the purpose of the relationship and the conditions under which it would be carried out. Nurses and clients were, in effect, contracting.

Recognition of contracting as a tool has come more recently. Blair (1971) described her developing awareness of the need for the nurse to encourage clients to act for themselves rather than to place them in a passive, dependent role. Using transactional analysis theory, she developed a professional treatment contract that she defined as "a mutual understanding of the reason for the service and the problems or areas that will be discussed during the [community nursing] visits" (1971, p. 588). Others have worked with the concept and refined it further. In one nursing education setting, students contracted with families and found that reaching a mutual agreement about the goals of service was beneficial to both clients and nurses (Sheridan and Smith, 1975). Nurses in many settings have recognized the value of the mutual participation model and used it to involve clients in the helping relationship and in use of the nursing process. Some suggest that contracting should be treated as a specific step in the helping process (Brill, 1973; Langford,

1978). As more and more nurses seek to promote client autonomy and self-care, contracting's wide applicability to nursing practice is being increasingly recognized (Brockenshire, 1987; Helgeson et al., 1985; Larson, 1987).

Emphasis on contracting as a *method* rather than a *concept* can create problems. If one's experiences with contracts have all been business agreements, it is possible to carry the stereotype of a cold, formal arrangement into the nursing practice setting. Some nurses fear that asking clients to negotiate a contract will place clients under stress, impede the development of trust, and negatively influence the helping relationship (Lindell, 1986). Others have found that some clients, who prefer to have the nurse make decisions for them, are not ready to enter into any kind of negotiation.

The concept of contracting, however, has much broader application than as a simple methodology. As a concept, contracting applies basic principles of adult education: self-direction, mutual negotiation, and mutual evaluation (Gustafson, 1977). These principles become both the means and the ends of contracting. To varying degrees, all clients are able to assess, plan, implement, and evaluate in contracting, yet the concept can be applied in a variety of ways. Sloan and Schommer (1982) demonstrate that contracting can be formal or informal, written or verbal, simple or detailed, and signed or unsigned by clients and nurse. Like all nursing tools, contracting will enhance client health only if adapted to each situation.

The advantages of contracting in community health nursing can now be summarized:

1. It involves clients in their own care.
2. It motivates clients to perform necessary tasks.
3. It individualizes care by focusing on clients' unique needs, whether the client is an individual or a group.
4. It increases the possibility of achieving health goals identified by clients and nurse.
5. It develops problem-solving skills of nurse and clients.
6. It fosters client participation in the decision-making process.
7. It promotes clients' autonomy and self-esteem as they learn self-care.
8. It makes nursing service more efficient and cost-effective.

THE PROCESS OF CONTRACTING

Because contracting is rather complex, some stages will occur before others. Without some kind of sequence, negotiation of a contract can become overwhelming. Consider the fact that this working agreement depends on knowing what clients want, agreeing on goals, identifying methods to achieve these goals, knowing the resources that the nurse and clients bring to the relationship, utilizing appropriate outside resources, setting limits, deciding on responsibilities, and providing for periodic reviews. Each of these tasks requires discussion between and decision making by nurse and clients.

These tasks are incorporated into the process of contracting in a sequence that provides a guide for nurses and their clients. Sloan and Schommer (1982) describe eight phases in the process:

1. *Exploration of needs:* Assessment of client's health, problems, and needs by client and nurse
2. *Establishment of goals:* Discussion and agreement between client and nurse on goals and objectives
3. *Exploration of resources:* Defining what client and nurse each have to offer to and expect from each other; identifying appropriate resources such as significant others, agencies, and other professionals
4. *Development of a plan:* Identifying methods and activities for achieving the stated goals
5. *Division of responsibilities:* Negotiating the activities for which client and nurse will each be responsible
6. *Agreement on time frame:* Setting limits for the contract in terms of length of time or number of visits
7. *Evaluation:* Periodic and final assessment of progress toward goals occurring at agreed-upon intervals
8. *Renegotiation or termination:* Agreement to modify, renegotiate, or terminate the contract.

As community health nurses use this process to negotiate a contract, they must adapt it to each situation. The exact sequence of phases may change and some steps may overlap. Nevertheless, the basic elements remain important considerations for successful contracting. (See Figure 10-3.)

To illustrate the process of contracting, we will consider the way one community health nurse used the contractual process. Eileen met the Nelsons through the agency's well-child clinic. Mrs. Nelson had been bringing 16-month-old Thor in for regular checkups and immunizations since they had moved to the city a year earlier. After becoming pregnant again, she approached Eileen about prenatal home visits to learn more about pregnancy and delivery. They made an appointment for Eileen's first visit.

EIGHT PHASES OF CONTRACTING

Exploration of Needs

Eileen explained the importance of focusing the visits on Mrs. Nelson's wants. She questioned Mrs. Nelson about her previous pregnancy, concerns, and interests and suggested possible topics for discussion. In Eileen's

Figure 10-3
The concept and process of contracting. Contracting is based on four distinctive features shown here as spokes that support a wheel. These features form the basis for a reciprocal relationship between nurse and clients. This relationship is not static; it is a dynamic process that moves through phases, represented here as the outer rim of the wheel. The relationship moves forward, focused on meeting clients' needs, and enables the nurse to facilitate ultimate achievement of clients' goals.

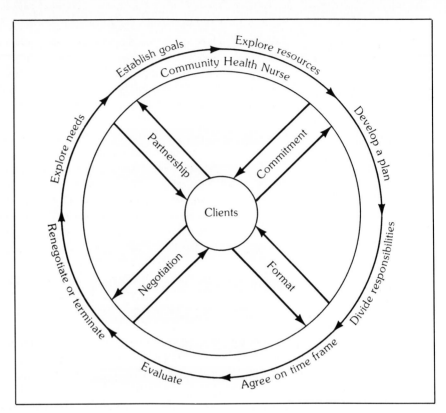

agency, the supervisor and staff had developed a prenatal catalog, a scrapbook of topics helpful to prospective mothers, which was illustrated with pictures from magazines. It was, in effect, a sales catalog that depicted many of the services the nurses could offer. Activities shown included teaching nutrition; demonstrating exercises; and discussing growth and development of the fetus, changes in the mother's body, the process of labor and delivery, postpartum developments, and care of the newborn. Eileen had found the catalog useful for helping clients to become aware of their choices and to select topics to cover in the contractual relationship. She offered to bring it on the second visit, and at that time, they would make some definite decisions about what Mrs. Nelson wanted.

Establishment of Goals

After examining and discussing the catalog items and exploring other potential health needs, Eileen and Mrs. Nelson agreed to focus on pregnancy, labor, and delivery. They agreed upon the goals of a comfortable pregnancy and a modified natural childbirth for Mrs. Nelson. To make these goals more workable, they broke them down into objectives. One, for example, was for the Nelsons to use Lamaze breathing techniques during childbirth. Another was for Mrs. Nelson to eat a well-balanced diet that would make her feel energetic and still keep her weight gain under 20 pounds.

Exploration of Resources

Eileen questioned further about the amount of time and energy Mrs. Nelson wanted to commit to this project. Could she spend half an hour a day, for instance, on exercises? They discussed what Mrs. Nelson was willing to do and what Eileen, given her time schedule, could realistically do. Mr. Nelson wanted to be present during teaching sessions. They also agreed that Mrs. Nelson would consult her obstetrician.

Development of a Plan

By the end of the second visit, Eileen and Mrs. Nelson had made a list of the specific, goal-related topics to cover in each session. Beside each topic they wrote down methods and activities. For example, on the next visit, Eileen would bring teaching tools and pamphlets and explain components of a well-balanced diet during pregnancy. Mrs. Nelson then would prepare a sample menu for her family that included a proper balance of the foods she needed. Since Mr. Nelson was to be part of the contract, they decided to have him look over the plan, make suggestions, and meet with them on the subsequent visits. The Nelsons both agreed to be present for each appointment. They changed the visit time to late afternoon when Mr. Nelson arrived home from work.

Division of Responsibilities

Eileen encouraged the Nelsons to take an active role in each visit. Mrs. Nelson agreed to practice the exercises half an hour daily and to keep a record of her diet. Mr. Nelson's responsibilities were to encourage his wife to stick to the diet and exercises and to practice the exercises with her when feasible. They agreed that Eileen would be responsible for presenting new material, demonstrating exercises and other techniques, and indicating whether or not the Nelsons were performing new activities correctly.

Agreement on Time Frame

Their list of topics helped Eileen and the Nelsons decide on the number of visits needed. They agreed on a schedule that spread visits throughout the pregnancy and six weeks postpartum. From the start, then, all parties agreed on a tentative termination date for the relationship.

Evaluation

A part of their plan was to do monthly evaluations to determine the satisfaction each felt with the plan and the progress being made. This built in the possibility of renegotiation; anyone could suggest needed changes at the evaluation times. At the conclusion of the contract period (six weeks postpartum), Eileen and the Nelsons agreed to discuss how well all the goals had been met.

Renegotiation or Termination

The Nelsons and Eileen agreed to renegotiate the time frame of the contract if new needs arose. Otherwise, they would terminate the service six weeks after the baby was born.

LEVELS OF CONTRACTING

Community health nurses conduct the contracting process at levels that range from formal to informal. The degree of formality depends in large measure on the nurse's comfort in using this tool and clients' readiness to assume responsibility for self-care. At the most formal level, the parties usually negotiate a written contract. It is drawn up by mutual agreement, each person signs it, and a third party may witness the signing. This form of contract has sometimes been used in mental health settings where the seriousness of the working agreement and the need to involve the client actively were important aspects of therapy (Davis and Woodcock, 1971). Less formal contracts, such as that with the Nelsons, are more commonly used. The nursing care plan becomes the written contract; thus no additional paperwork is required. In one suburban health department in Minnesota, community health nurses contract with clients of a hypertension clinic. Part of their written care plan is a list of the client's goals and methods for achieving them (see Figure 10-4). Under the column entitled "Responsibility," the nurse or client is listed as responsible for carrying out the activity.

Some situations lend themselves best to a modified use of contracting. For example, one nurse had been making regular visits to a man dying of cancer. After his death, she contracted informally with his wife to continue visits for the purpose of helping her work through the grieving process. They discussed and agreed on the goals, methods, and responsibilities each would have, but did not negotiate a formal contract. Another community mental health nurse formed a therapy group composed of her individual clients. She used modified contracting by discussing with clients the purpose of the group and the number of sessions needed, and by obtaining their agreement to attend all sessions.

CLIENT-NURSE CONTRACT

Date accomplished	Goals	Date begun	Date ended	Methods	Respon-sibility
	1. To understand hypertension			a. Explain physiology of hypertension	N
				b. Interpret pamphlet on hypertension	C
				c. List risk factors associated with hypertension	C
	2. To decrease stress at work			a. Identify coping skills	N-C
				b. Explore possibility of job change	C
				c. List ways to relieve stress on job	N-C
				d. Design plan to relieve stress at work	C
				e. Implement plan until blood pressure is down to 115/75	C
	3. To lose 10 lb within 2 months			a. Explain nutritional factors influencing hypertension	N
				b. Design a diet plan	N-C
				c. Prepare exercise plan	C
				d. Implement plans until weight goal achieved	C

Length of contract:

Fee determination:

Signatures: Client _____ Date _____

Nurse _____ Date _____

Figure 10-4
Part of a contract developed between a client (C) and a nurse (N) in a community hypertension clinic.

Informal contracting does involve some form of verbal agreement about relatively uncomplicated tasks: "You take your pills every day as prescribed, and I will get a homemaker for you" or "You come to the clinic each week, and I will show you how to plan your diabetic diet." Sometimes nurses use contracting informally without realizing it. They conclude a home visit by agreeing with the family about the purpose and time of the next appointment. Conscious use of contracting, however, is a more effective way to provide structure for the relationship and foster client involvement, regardless of the level at which it is applied.

The level of contracting may also change during the development of a helping relationship. Clients often need education about their options. Initially they may have difficulty in identifying needs and making choices. The nurse can work to promote their self-confidence and help them assume increasing responsibility for their own health (Larson et al., 1987). Through these efforts, contracting becomes a consciously recognized part of the relationship. Clients can then become fully participating partners.

Summary

The helping relationship is a tool for promoting client health and the ability to engage in self-care. It is goal-directed, unilateral in that it exists for the benefit of the client, and limited by time; it encourages mutual participation and involves clearly defined responsibilities.

Successful development of a helping relationship depends on the community health nurse's effective use of communication and interpersonal skills. To send and receive verbal or nonverbal messages well, nurses must be aware of themselves as well as of clients. They must be able to recognize variables that might influence a message's interpretation. Nurses can cultivate the following skills: active listening, seeking feedback, showing respect, empathizing, and developing trust.

The helping relationship moves through three phases. During the beginning phase, the relationship is established and defined. The middle phase is a working period focused on meeting identified goals. The termination phase occurs when clients and nurse no longer need to work together.

Contracting has four distinctive features. First, it involves partnership. Contracting utilizes shared participation and two-way agreement between client and nurse. Second, it involves commitment, a promise to carry out certain responsibilities. Third, contracting's format defines goals, methods, responsibilities, and time limits. Fourth, contracting involves negotiation between clients and nurse.

The process of contracting utilizes eight phases that may sometimes vary in sequence or overlap: (1) exploration of needs, (2) establishment of goals, (3) exploration of resources, (4) development of a plan, (5) division of responsibilities, (6) agreement on time frame, (7) evaluation, and (8) renegotiation or termination.

Community health nurses practice contracting at levels ranging from formal to informal. Choice of level depends on the skill of the nurse, readiness of the client, and demands of the situation. Clients may need assistance and instruction before they can assume the responsibilities of partners in contracting.

Study Questions

1. Describe the five characteristics of a helping relationship that distinguish it from other kinds of interactions. Discuss how you would apply these characteristics to working with a group of unwed adolescent mothers.
2. What is contracting? Discuss its four distinctive features and the advantages that contracting offers to the community health nurse.
3. Why is termination an important consideration for community health nursing practice? Describe how you would handle termination with a group of post-mastectomy women (or other group) as your client.

References

Blair, K. K. (1971). It's the patient's problem and decision. *Nursing Outlook* 19: 588–89.

Brill, N. I. (1973). *Working with people: The helping process.* Philadelphia: J. B. Lippincott.

Brockenshire, A. (1987). Therapeutic contracts: A nursing tool. *Perspectives* 11(1): 13–14.

Brown, S. T., et al. (1987). Contract learning: A leadership experience for the RN student in a BSN program. *Nurse Manager* 18(4): 66–68, 70.

Davis, R. C. and E. Woodcock. (1971). The nursing contract: An alternative in care. *Journal of Psychiatric Nursing* 9: 26–27.

Gross, J. W., et al. (1986). Modified contractual grading. *Nursing Outlook* 34(4): 184–87.

Gustafson, M. B. (1977). Let's broaden our horizons about the use of contracts. *International Nursing Review* 24(1): 18–19.

Helgeson, D. M., et al. (1985). Contracting: A method of health promotion...more clearly define a purpose for home visiting. *Journal of Community Health Nursing* 2(4): 199–207.

Kalisch, B. (1973). What is empathy? *American Journal of Nursing* 73: 1548–52.

Kinlein, M. L. (1977). *Independent nursing practice with clients.* Philadelphia: J. B. Lippincott.

Lancaster, J., and W. Lancaster. (1982). *Concepts for advanced nursing practice: The nurse as change agent.* St. Louis, Mo.: C. V. Mosby.

Langford, T. (1978). Establishing a nursing contract. *Nursing Outlook* 26: 386–88.

Larson, E., et al. (1987). Effect of a written nurse/patient contract on the practice of primary nursing. *Nurse Manager* 18(11): 113.

Lindberg, J. B., and L. M. Simms. (1974). Contract grading: Incentives and rewards. *Image* 7(1): 20–23.

Lindell, A. R. (1986). Clinical contractual agreements: Liability or blessing? *Journal of Professional Nursing* 2(3): 138.

Norris, C. M. (1979). Self-care. *American Journal of Nursing* 79: 486–89.

Rosen, B. (1978). Contract therapy. *Nursing Times* 74: 119–21.

Sauer, J. K. (1973). The process of contracting in the helping relationship. *Minnesota Welfare* (Summer): 12–14, 23.

Sheridan, A., and R. Smith. (1975). Student-family contracts. *Nursing Outlook* 23: 114–17.

Sloan, M., and B. T. Schommer. (1982). The process of contracting in community nursing. In B. W. Spradley (ed.), *Readings in community health nursing.* 2nd ed. (pp. 197–204). Boston: Little, Brown.

Veninga, R. (1982). *The human side of health administration.* Englewood Cliffs, N.J.: Prentice-Hall.

Wismer, J. (1978). Communication effectiveness: Active listening and sending feeling messages. In J. W. Pfeiffer and J. Jones (eds.), *The 1978 annual handbook for group facilitators.* La Jolla, Calif.: University Associates.

Selected Readings

Almore, M. G. (1979). Dyadic communication. *American Journal of Nursing* 79: 1076–78.

Brammer, L. M. (1973). *The helping relationship: Process and skills.* Englewood Cliffs, N.J.: Prentice-Hall.

Combs, A. W., D. Avila, and W. Purkey. (1978). *Helping relationship: Basic concepts for the helping professions.* 2nd ed. Boston: Allyn and Bacon.

Delaney, C., and V. Schoolcraft. (1977). Promoting autonomy: Clinical contracts. *Journal of Nursing Education* 16(9): 22–28.

Fay, P. (1986). Contracting: A collaborative approach. *Journal of Nursing Staff Development* 2(4): 157–61.

Gustafson, M. B. (1977). Let's broaden our horizons about the use of contracts. *International Nursing Review* 24(1): 18–19.

Hames, C., and D. H. Joseph. (1980). *Basic concepts of helping: A holistic approach.* New York: Appleton-Century-Crofts.

Hein, E. C. (1980). *Communication in nursing practice.* 2nd ed. Boston: Little, Brown.

Helgeson, D. M., et al. (1985). Contracting: A method of health promotion . . . more clearly define a purpose for home visiting. *Journal of Community Health Nursing* 2(4): 199–207.

Kinlein, M. L. (1977). *Independent nursing practice with clients.* Philadelphia: J. B. Lippincott.

Kjervik, D. K., et al. (1988). The legal meaning of consent in unequal power relationships. *Journal of Professional Nursing* 4(3): 192–204.

La Monica, E., and J. Karshmer. (1978). Empathy: Educating nurses in professional practice. *Journal of Nursing Education* 17(2): 3–11.

Langford, T. (1978). Establishing a nursing contract. *Nursing Outlook* 26: 386–88.

Larson, E., et al. (1987). Effect of a written nurse/patient contract on the practice of primary nursing. *Nurse Manager* 18(11): 113.

Levin, L. S., A. Katz, and E. Holst. (1976). *Self-care: Lay initiatives in health.* New York: Neale, Watson.

Lindell, A. R. (1986). Clinical contractual agreements: Liability or blessing? *Journal of Professional Nursing* 2(3): 138.

Loomis, M. (1979). The health care contract. In M. Loomis (ed.), *Group process for nurses* (pp. 59–69). St. Louis: C. V. Mosby.

Milio, N. (1977). Self-care in urban settings. *Health Education Monographs* 5: 136.

Murphy, S. (1977). Mutuality and the message: A conceptual model for nurse-client communication. *Oregon Nurse* 42: 10.

Norris, C. M. (1979). Self-care. *American Journal of Nursing* 79: 486–89.

O'Brien, M. (1978). *Communications and relationships in nursing.* St. Louis: C. V. Mosby.

Peplau, H. E. (1952). *Interpersonal relations in nursing.* New York: Putnam.

Petosa, R. (1984). Using behavioral contracts to promote health behavior change: Application in a college-level course. *Health Educator* 15(2): 22–26.

Price, J., and C. Braden. (1978). The reality in home visits. *American Journal of Nursing* 78: 1536–38.

Rosen, B. (1978). Contract therapy. *Nursing Times* 74: 119–21.

Sauer, J. K. (1973). The process of contracting in the helping relationship. *Minnesota Welfare* (Summer): pp. 12–14.

Seeger, P. A. (1977). Self-awareness and nursing. *Journal of Psychiatric Nursing* 15(Aug.): 24–26.

Sheridan, A., and R. Smith. (1975). Student-family contracts. *Nursing Outlook* 23: 114–17.

Sloan, M., and B. T. Schommer. (1982). The process of contracting in community nursing. In B. W. Spradley (ed.), *Readings in community health nursing.* 2nd ed. (pp. 197–204). Boston: Little, Brown.

Ulschak, F. L. (1978). Contracting: A process and a tool. In J. W. Pfeiffer and J. Jones (eds.), *The 1978 annual handbook for group facilitators.* La Jolla, Calif.: University Associates, 138–42.

Van Dersal, W. R. (1974). How to be a good communicator—and a better nurse. *Nursing '74,* 4(12): 57–64.

Veninga, R. (1982). *The human side of health administration.* Englewood Cliffs, N.J.: Prentice-Hall.

Wismer, J. (1978). Communication effectiveness: Active listening and sending feeling messages. In J. W. Pfeiffer and J. Jones (eds.), *The 1978 annual handbook for group facilitators.* La Jolla, Calif.: University Associates, 199–222.

Zangari, M., and P. Duffy. (1980). Contracting with patients in day-to-day practice. *American Journal of Nursing* 80: 451–55.

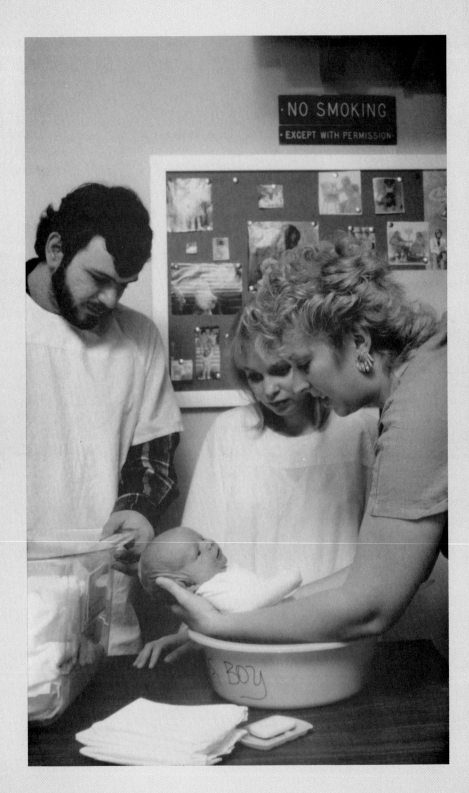

11 Community Health Education

Clients in community health nursing's sphere of practice have many educational needs. Families with newly diagnosed diabetic members need to understand and regulate the diabetic regimen. Young couples with their first babies want to learn aspects of infant care, such as bathing, feeding, diapering, breastfeeding, and formula preparation. Parents of young children form a group because they want to learn about parenting. A women's self-help group seeks to develop understanding of the female role and to acquire skills in assertiveness. Senior citizens adjusting to retirement search for increased understanding of the aging process and meaningful activities. Such situations present community health nurses with the opportunity and challenge to meet client needs through health education.

Educating represents a fundamental task in the nursing profession (Redman, 1980). "All nurses function as teachers. Nurses teach patients, families, ancillary personnel, and each other. Teaching is inherent in the nurse's role whether or not the nurse consciously cultivates and exhibits teacher behaviors" (Douglass and Bevis, 1974). Education is also a basic community health nursing intervention, as we discussed in Chapter 3. Identifying a need that is best met through health education raises a series of questions. How can nurses teach effectively? What content should they cover? What method of presentation will communicate most effectively? What pamphlets or other visual aids can nurses use as teaching devices? How do they know when the client has grasped the information or mastered the skills? In other words, what makes teaching effective, and how are teaching skills acquired? In this chapter we address these questions and discuss education as an intervention tool in community health nursing practice.

THE NATURE OF LEARNING

The goal of all teaching is learning. Learning involves far more than the simple sharing of information. We have all been presented with information that was not interesting, relevant to our needs, or comprehensible. In such situations, we found it difficult to learn. The nurse as a teacher seeks to transmit information in such a way that the learner understands and some change in behavior results. Effective teaching is a cause; learning becomes the effect. Nurses cannot assume that imparting knowledge will guarantee understanding or change client health practices. To teach effectively in community health, nurses must understand the nature of learning and learning theories. We will first consider three forms of learning: cognitive, affective, and psychomotor (Bloom, 1956). Then we will examine the teaching strategies that produce these kinds of learning.

LEARNING THEORIES

What is a learning theory? A learning theory is a "systematic, integrated outlook in regard to the nature of the process whereby people relate to their environments in such a way as to enhance their ability to use both themselves and their environments more effectively" (Bigge, 1982, p. 3). Since each of us, whether we know it or not, has a theory of learning and that theory, in turn, dictates the way we would teach, it is helpful to discover what our learning theory is and how it would affect our practice as health educators.

There are many ways to view the basic nature of the learning process. Historically this perspective has changed; the major learning theories, developed over time, fall into three categories. Let us briefly examine these categories and the specific theories residing in each.

Mental Discipline Theories

Before the twentieth century, several learning theories developed that continue to influence the way many teachers teach. This category of learning theories conceives of the learner, the person, as having a substantive mind, separate from the body. Various points of view developed about the nature of the human mind. One group saw the mind of the learner as being active but innately bad and in need of correction. This group used mental discipline—drilling, testing, and more drilling—to encourage learning. Strict discipline was seen as a way to promote perseverance and willpower. This learning theory was called "theistic mental discipline."

A second group viewed the mind of the learner as active but neutral and in need of exercise to cultivate the intellect. This approach, too, used mental training and discipline as a way to develop intrinsic mental power. It became known as the "humanistic mental discipline" theory.

A third group viewed the learner's mind as both active and good and believed that the learner's mind should unfold naturally. This theory promoted a permissive style of education that centered on feelings. It was known as the "natural unfoldment" or "self-actualization" theory.

The fourth was called "apperception" learning theory. Subscribers to this theory saw the learner's mind as passive and neutral. The mind, they said, takes in ideas from the outside world and stores them in the subconscious. Learning occurs when ideas are brought to the conscious level and assimilated with other conscious ideas. As Bigge (1982, p. 35) wrote, "Apperception is a process of new ideas associating themselves with old ones."

Stimulus-Response Conditioning Theories

This category of learning theories developed in the twentieth century and is derived from a behavioristic point of view. It says that learning is behavioral change—a response to certain stimuli. Thus the behavioristic teacher seeks to significantly change learners' behaviors through a series of selected stimuli.

Three specific theories are found in this category. The stimulus-response "bond" theory proposes that with conditioning, certain stimuli evoke certain response patterns. The causes (stimuli) are connected or "bonded" to the effects (responses). The teacher promotes acquisition of the desired stimulus-response connections so that transfer of learning can occur in another situation with the same stimulus-response elements present. Pavlov's early work with stimulus-response and involuntary reflex actions is perhaps the best-known application of this theory. Two other theories are conditioning with no reinforcement and conditioning through reinforcement. Both emphasize the promotion of desired responses but use different approaches. No-reinforcement theorists count on the learner's innate reflexive drives to accomplish the desired response after conditioning. The reinforcement theorists use successive, systematic changes in the learner's environment to enhance the probability of desired responses. B. F. Skinner's work with operant conditioning made a major contribution to stimulus-response theory (Hergenhahn, 1982).

Cognitive Theories

A third category of learning theories seeks to influence learners' understanding of problems and situations, in contrast to stimulus-response conditioning, which attempts to change their behaviors. These contemporary learning theories are known as the Gestalt-field family of cognitive theories. The Gestalt-field assumption is that people are neither good nor bad—they simply interact with their environment, and their learning is related to perception. Thus, this theory defines learning as a "reorganization of the learner's perceptual or psychological world—his psychological field" (Bigge, 1982, p. 57). *Gestalt,* the German noun, in this case refers to the total configuration or pattern of related psychological theories.

The first of three theories in the Gestalt-field family is called "insight" theory. This point of view regards learning as a process in which the learner develops new insights or changes old ones. Learners sense their way intuitively but intelligently through problems. The "insight" is useful only if the learner understands its significance. A second theory, called "goal-insight," is very similar to insight theory but goes beyond intuitive hunches to tested insights.

Teachers subscribing to this theory promote insightful learning but assist learners in developing higher-quality insights. In the third theory, known as "cognitive-field," the learner is seen as purposive and problem-centered. Teachers seek to help learners gain new insights and restructure their lives accordingly.

The progression in these three categories of learning theories reflects the trends in educational and psychological thinking. Current learning theorists generally subscribe more to the cognitive theories, but we see many evidences of the others still in practice (Hergenhahn, 1982). Our own learning experiences will influence the form and function of our health education. Moreover, awareness of our beliefs about learning and teaching provides a base for improving our practice.

TYPES OF LEARNING

Cognitive Learning

Cognitive learning involves the mind and thinking processes. It is mental knowledge. When we grasp the meaning and relationship of a series of facts, we experience cognitive learning. For example, acquisition of the following facts and relationships involves cognition: population groups have health needs; learning can meet some of those needs; community health nurses can foster learning among client populations; and effective teaching fosters learning. The cognitive domain deals with "the recall or recognition of knowledge and the development of intellectual abilities and skills" (Bloom, 1956). It is useful to consider six major categories or levels in the cognitive domain (Gronlund, 1970): knowledge, comprehension, application, analysis, synthesis, and evaluation.

Knowledge.   Knowledge, the lowest level of learning, involves recall. If students can remember material previously learned, they have acquired knowledge. Nurses purposely aim for this level in teaching with some clients, particularly those who have limited ability to grasp the rationale behind prescribed health measures. For example, it is entirely appropriate to teach elderly clients the symptoms of stroke. The nurse's goal may be for them to recall the facts about this illness rather than to understand underlying causes or treatment procedures. Clients may then remember that medication should be taken daily, that regular exercise will restore function, and that abstinence from alcohol is necessary, even though they may not grasp the reasons behind these measures.

Comprehension.   The second level of cognitive learning, comprehension, combines remembering with understanding. When possible, teaching aims at instilling at least minimum understanding. Nurses want clients to grasp the meaning and to recognize the importance of suggested health behaviors. At the first level of cognitive learning, a nurse can teach a hypertensive person to take medication daily, but comprehension will occur when this individual and his family understand how his medication and life-style affect blood pressure and how control of each factor can reduce the risk of stroke. Nurses can teach pregnant women the relationship between nutrition and fetal development to help them realize the importance of a healthy diet.

Application. Application is the third level of cognitive learning. Here the learner takes understood material and applies it to new and actual situations. A more desirable level than the first two, application approaches the possibility of self-care, in which clients use their knowledge for improvement of their own health. To encourage application, the nurse can design teaching plans that show clients how to put knowledge into practice. A sex education study using this approach resulted in decreased sexual activity among the adolescents taught (Furstenberg, 1985). One nurse suggested that a diabetic client write down his Clinitest readings on a sheet of paper to show her at the next visit. Another, after instructing adolescents in a weight-loss group about nutrition, asked each to keep a diet record for a week, draw up a diet plan, and share this plan with the group at the next meeting.

It is one thing to show a new mother how to bathe her infant; it is quite another to observe a return demonstration. The test of application is a transfer of understanding into practice. The pregnant woman who understands that her physical health and eating habits directly influence the health of her baby has not reached this level if she continues smoking and eating unbalanced meals. The diabetic who recognizes the high risk of infection has not applied this knowledge if he is careless with foot care. The construction worker who understands on-the-job hazards but seldom wears a protective hat in the work area has yet to transfer comprehension into practice.

Analysis. The fourth level of cognitive learning is analysis. At this level, the learner breaks material down into parts, distinguishes between elements, and understands the relationships among the parts. A mother, for example, analyzes when she seeks to determine the cause of an infant's crying. After viewing the total situation, she breaks it down into variables such as hunger, pain, loneliness, type of crying, and intensity of crying. She examines these parts and draws conclusions about their relationships. Analysis precedes problem solving in the same way that diagnosis precedes treatment. The learner carefully scrutinizes all the variables or elements and their relationships to each other in order to explain the situation. Similarly, analysis precedes identification of needs because we must first study all the assessment variables before we can draw conclusions about client needs. A family that studies its own communication patterns for the purpose of identifying sources of conflict is using analysis. This level of learning becomes a preliminary step toward problem solving. In health teaching, community health nurses foster clients' analytic skills by showing them how to isolate the parts in a situation and then encouraging them to do so themselves.

Synthesis.   Synthesis, a fifth level of cognitive learning, is the ability to form elements into a new whole. At this level of intellectual functioning, learners go beyond analyzing material to create something unique from it. Clients who achieve learning at this level will not only analyze their problems but also find solutions for them. For example, a nurse-teacher may assist mental health clients in a therapy group to analyze their frequent depression and then to generate their own plan for alleviating it. Synthesis combines all the earlier levels of cognitive learning to culminate in the production of a unique plan. A young couple who want to toilet train their two-year-old child learn the physiological and psychological dimensions of toilet training, analyze their own situation, and then develop strategies (their own unique plan) for training the child. Health teachers facilitate synthesis by assisting and encouraging clients to develop their own solutions with specific plans. When someone identifies a problem, they can ask clients, "What are some possible causes? Do you see anything we have overlooked about the problem?" But when the client asks for a solution after such analysis, the nurse can encourage synthesis by asking, "What are some possible solutions to this problem that you might carry out?"

Evaluation.   The highest level of cognitive learning is evaluation. For the learner, to evaluate means to judge the usefulness of new material compared with a stated purpose (Gronlund, 1970). Such a judgment requires specific criteria. Clients can learn to judge their own health behavior by comparing it with standards such as abstinence from smoking, maintenance of normal weight, or regular exercise. These are criteria established by others; however, clients may establish their own criteria. Parents may evaluate their parenting effectiveness when their parenting group sets up specific objectives as desired outcomes. The group, for example, could design activities to enhance parent-child communication, and members could then judge their performance by using the desired outcomes as evaluation criteria. When nurse-teachers aim for this level of client learning, they have made self-care a concrete objective. Evaluation, because it goes beyond attempts at problem solving, enables the client to judge the adequacy of solutions, to critique lifestyle and health-related behavior, and to anticipate needed improvements.

Cognitive learning at any of the levels described can be measured easily in terms of learner behaviors. Nurses know, for instance, that clients have achieved teaching objectives for application of knowledge when their behavior demonstrates actual use of the information taught. Client roles in cognitive learning range from relatively passive (at the knowledge level) to active (at the evaluation level). Conversely, as clients become more active, the nurse-teacher role becomes less directive. Table 11-1 illustrates client and nurse behaviors for each level.

Table 11-1
Cognitive Learning: Case Study in Controlling Diabetes

Level	Illustrative Client Behavior	Illustrative Nurse Behavior
Knowledge (recalls, knows)	States that insulin, if taken, will control own diabetes	Gives information
Comprehension (understands)	Describes insulin action and purpose	Explains information
Application (uses learning)	Adjusts insulin dosage daily to maintain proper blood sugar level	Suggests how to use learning
Analysis (examines, explains)	Discusses relationships between insulin, diet, activity, and diabetic control	Demonstrates and encourages analysis
Synthesis (integrates with other learning, generates new ideas)	Develops a plan, incorporating above learning, for controlling own diabetes	Promotes client formulation of own plan
Evaluation (judges according to a standard)	Compares degree of diabetic control (outcomes) with desired control (objectives)	Facilitates evaluation

Affective Learning

The second domain in which learning occurs involves emotion, feeling, or affect. This kind of learning deals with "changes in interest, attitudes, and values" (Bloom, 1956). Here teachers face the task of trying to influence what clients value and feel. Nurses want them to develop an ability to accept ideas that promote healthier behavior patterns even though those ideas may conflict with their own values.

Attitudes and values are learned (Bigge, 1982). They develop gradually over time as the way that an individual feels and responds is molded by family, peers, experiences, and societal influences. These feelings and responses are the result of imitation and conditioning. In this way, clients acquire their health-related beliefs and practices. Because attitudes and values become part of the person, they are difficult to change unless the nurse-teacher is aware of how they develop.

Affective learning occurs on several levels as learners respond with varying degrees of involvement and commitment. At the first level, learners are simply receptive. They are willing to listen, show awareness, and be attentive. The teacher aims at acquiring and focusing learners' attention (Gronlund, 1970). This limited goal may be all that clients are ready for at the early stages of the nurse-client relationship.

At the second level, learners become active participants by responding to the information in some way. At this level, clients show willingness to read educational material that nurses give them, participate in discussion, complete assignments such as keeping a diet record, or voluntarily seek out more information on their own.

At the third level, learners attach value to the information. Valuing ranges from simple acceptance through appreciation to commitment. For example, a nurse taught members of a therapy group a number of principles concerning group effectiveness. She explained the importance of a democratic group process and ways to improve group skills. Members showed acceptance when they acknowledged the importance of these ideas. They showed appreciation by starting to practice the ideas. Commitment came when they assumed responsiblity for having their group function well.

The final level of affective learning occurs when learners internalize an idea or value. The value system now controls learner behavior. Consistent practice is a crucial test at this level. Clients who know and respect the value of exercise but only occasionally play tennis or do calisthenics have not internalized the value. Even several weeks of enthusiastic jogging is not evidence of an internalized value. If the jogging continues for six months, a year, and longer, learning is probably internalized.

Affective learning often remains elusive, difficult to measure. Indeed, this quality may influence community health nurses to concentrate their efforts on cognitive learning goals. Yet client attitudes and values have a major effect on the outcome of cognitive learning—desired behavioral changes. For this reason, the two domains must remain linked in teaching; otherwise, results may quickly fade.

Attitudes and values can change in the same way they were first learned, that is, through imitation and conditioning (Redman, 1980). Role models, particularly those from the client's peer group who practice the desired health behaviors, can be a strong influence. Groups like mastectomy clubs or chemical dependency support groups can have a powerful effect. Attitudes often change when the nurse provides clients with a satisfying experience during the learning process. The nurse who recognizes clients' participation in a group, praises them for completing assignments, or commends them for sticking to diet plans will have more success than the nurse who only criticizes failures. Table 11-2 shows client and nurse behaviors for each level of affective learning.

To influence affective learning requires patience. Values and attitudes will seldom change overnight. Keep in mind that other forces will continue to reinforce former values. For example, a middle-aged housewife may value pursuing a career for self-fulfillment but cannot because her husband opposes an independent activity. Promoting cognitive learning by helping the client understand and try out positive health practices is also useful for influencing attitude change.

Psychomotor Learning

The psychomotor domain includes visible, demonstrable performance skills that require some kind of neuromuscular coordination. Community health

Table 11-2
Affective Learning: Case Study in Family Planning

Level	Illustrative Client Behavior	Illustrative Nurse Behavior
Receptive (listens, pays attention)	Attentive to family planning instruction	Directs client's attention
Responsive (participates, reacts)	Discusses pros and cons of various methods	Encourages client involvement
Valuing (accepts, appreciates, commits)	Selects a method for use	Respects client's right to decide
Internal consistency (organizes values to fit together)	Understands and accepts responsibility for limiting number of children	Brings client into contact with role models
Adoption (incorporates new values into life-style)	Consistently practices birth control	Positively reinforces healthy behaviors

clients need to learn skills such as infant bathing, range-of-motion exercises, catheter irrigation, crutch-walking, breast self-examination, temperature taking, special diet preparation, and prenatal breathing exercises.

For psychomotor learning to take place, three conditions must be met. First, learners must be capable of the skill. If a nurse attempts to teach an elderly diabetic man with tremulous hands and fading vision to give his own insulin injections, it could frustrate and possibly harm him. Some other person more physically capable should probably be enlisted and taught the skill. Clients' intellectual and emotional capabilities also influence their capacity to learn motor skills. No one should expect persons of limited intelligence to learn complex skills. The degree of complexity should match the learners' level of functioning. Developmental stage is another point to consider in determining whether a skill is appropriate to teach. For example, most children can put on some article of clothing at two years of age but are not ready to learn to fasten buttons until well past their third birthday.

Learners must also have a sensory image of how to perform the skill. This is a second condition for psychomotor learning. Through sight, hearing, touch, and sometimes taste or smell, clients gain a picture of the skill. They acquire this sensory image by means of demonstration. Our first image of how to drive a car, for instance, comes from watching someone else drive. We observe their eyes, hands, and feet; the coordination between clutch and gear shift; auto speed, and road conditions. Verbal explanations enhance our understanding of the mechanics of driving. In order to teach clients motor skills effectively, the nurse has to provide them with an adequate sensory image. The nurse-teacher must demonstrate and explain slowly, one point at a time, and repeatedly if needed, until they understand the proper sequence of actions necessary to achieve the skill.

The third necessary condition for psychomotor learning is practice. After acquiring a sensory image, learners can start to perform the skill. Mastery will

Table 11-3
Nurse Behaviors in Psychomotor Learning

Determining Capability	Providing Sensory Image	Encouraging Practice
Nurse assesses client's physical, intellectual, and emotional ability	Nurse demonstrates and explains	Nurse uses guidance and positive reinforcement

come over time as learners repeat the performance until it is smooth, coordinated, and unhesitating. During this process the teacher should be available to provide guidance and encouragement. In the early stages of practice the teacher may need to use hands-on guidance to give learners a sense of how the performance should feel. Similarly, a nurse demonstrates passive range-of-motion exercises on a client's wife to show her how they should feel before she learns to do them for her husband. During practice, feedback from the nurse will enable the learner to know if the skill is being performed correctly. When clients give a return demonstration, the teacher can make suggestions, give encouragement, and thereby maximize learning effectiveness.

The psychomotor domain, like the cognitive and affective domains, ranges from simple to complex levels of functioning. It is necessary to exercise judgment in assessing clients' ability to perform a skill. Even clients with limited ability can often move on to higher levels once they have mastered simple skills. Nurse behaviors that influence psychomotor learning are shown in Table 11-3.

EFFECTIVE TEACHING

A sixth-grade teacher recently announced to her class: "My job here is to teach; your job is to learn. I don't care whether you learn or not, but if you want to learn, that's your responsibility. I'm being paid to teach." This kind of noncaring message only creates confusion and consternation among students. Yet, without meaning to, nurses may convey a similar message to clients. "I'm here to teach you how to get healthy and stay healthy," they say in so many words. "Whether you do or not is up to you." It is almost as though, having carried out their teaching responsibility, they can wash their hands of the whole business. How often do nurses chart, "Patient taught colostomy care," "Diabetic teaching done," "Explained medication dosage and side effects," and "Baby bath and formula preparation demonstrated" with little awareness of whether and how much learning occurred?

Teaching lies at one end of a continuum. At the other end is learning. Without learning, teaching becomes useless in much the same way that communication does not occur unless a message is both sent and received (Lorig, 1985). The sixth-grade teacher was trying to point this out to her students when she pushed the entire responsibility for learning onto their shoulders. While we can question the effectiveness of her approach, her point remains valid. Learners must take responsibility for their own learning (Levin, 1978). Teachers obstruct that process if they assume complete responsibility for bringing about changed behavior. Clients can be led to the "water" of health knowledge, but without a thirst for health information, they will not participate in the learning process. Teaching, then, becomes a matter of facilitating both the thirst and the best conditions for satisfying it. Teaching in community health nursing means to influence, motivate, and act as a catalyst in the learning process. Nurses "bring knowledge and learner together and stimulate a reaction" (Douglass and Bevis, 1974). Nurses facilitate learning when they make it as easy as possible for clients to change. To do this, the nurse-educator needs to know seven basic principles underlying the teaching-learning process. Health education also requires the use of appropriate tools to influence learning. We will discuss both of these topics in the remainder of this chapter.

TEACHING-LEARNING PRINCIPLES

To maximize the amount of learning that takes place when community health nurses provide health education, they need to be familiar with the teaching-learning principles described in this section and summarized in Figure 11-1.

Figure 11-1
Seven principles for maximizing the teaching-learning process.

Teaching Principles	Learning Principles
1. Adapt teaching to clients' level of readiness.	1. The learning process makes use of clients' experience and is geared to their level of understanding.
2. Determine clients' perceptions about the subject matter before and during teaching.	2. Clients are given the opportunity to provide frequent feedback on their understanding of the material taught.
3. Create an environment that is conducive to learning.	3. The environment for learning is physically comfortable, offers an atmosphere of mutual helpfulness, trust, respect, and acceptance, and allows for free expression of ideas.
4. Involve clients throughout the learning process.	4. Clients actively participate. They assess their needs, establish goals, and evaluate learning progress.
5. Make subject matter relevant to clients' interest and use.	5. Clients feel motivated to learn.
6. Ensure client satisfaction during the teaching-learning process.	6. Clients sense progress toward their goals.
7. Provide opportunities for clients to apply material taught.	7. Clients integrate the learning through application.

Source: Adapted from Knowles (1980), pp. 57–58.

Client Readiness

Clients' readiness to learn influences teaching effectiveness (Miller, 1985). For instance, one community health nurse found that a young primipara was not ready for prenatal teaching on fetal growth and development. She had strong fears, the nurse discovered, that "losing her figure" would make her sexually unattractive to her husband. Until these anxieties had subsided, the teaching would remain ineffective. Clients' needs, interests, and concerns determine their readiness for learning. Another factor that influences readiness is educational background. If a group of women who never completed grade school meet to learn how to care for a sick person in the home, sessions should present material simply, factually, and in terms that they understand. To discuss complex concepts of health, illness, and scientific research would be above their level of readiness.

Maturational level also affects readiness. A one-year-old child is not ready to share his toys, but a five-year-old child has reached a level that makes him ready to learn these social skills. An adolescent mother who is still working on normal developmental tasks of her age group may not be ready to learn parenting skills. Readiness of the client will determine the amount of material presented in each teaching session (Figure 11-2). The pace or speed with which you present information must be manageable. A moderate amount

Figure 11-2
The boy in this family is old enough to help measure the ingredients for the cake. His younger sister helps to stir. Their maturational levels influence their readiness to learn new tasks.

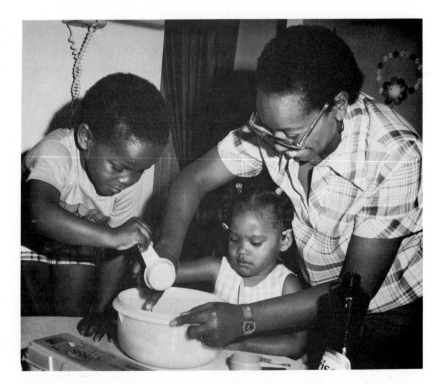

of anxiety will often increase client receptivity to learning; however, high or low levels of anxiety can have the opposite effect.

Client Perceptions

Clients' perceptions affect their learning. People's perceptions, the way they see the world, serve as a screening device through which all new information must pass (Marriner, 1979). Our perceptions help us to interpret and attach meaning to things. For example, one person views a piece of sculpture and exclaims over its beauty. Another person, seeing the same object, remarks on its ugliness and lack of coherence. These two people have different perceptions. In community health nursing, one client may view the experience of parenting as a positive, growth-producing relationship; another may see it as a conflict-ridden, unhappy experience to avoid. Each kind of perception has a different consequence for learning.

A wide range of variables affects human perception. These variables include values, past experiences, culture, religion, personality, developmental stage, educational and economic level, surrounding social forces, and the physical environment. Adolescent girls and boys who have been told to stop taking drugs will resist if they perceive this instruction as an affront to their identities and independence. They want to make decisions for themselves. The nurse-teacher, recognizing the forces at work, will try to work within the adolescents' frame of reference by presenting information in a way that still gives them options to make their own choices. Otherwise, their perception of the situation will limit their learning.

Frequently clients use selective perception. They screen out some statements and pay attention to those that fit their values or personal desires. A nurse was teaching a client the various risk factors in coronary disease; the individual screened out smoking and obesity, paying attention only to factors that would not require a drastic change in life-style. Nurses must know their clients, understand their backgrounds and values, and learn what their perceptions are before health teaching can influence their behavior.

Educational Environment

The setting in which the educational endeavor takes place has a significant impact on learning. Most of us have had the experience of sitting in a too-warm room and trying to stay awake during a lecture or of being distracted by noise, cold, uncomfortable seating, or some other nuisance. Ventilation, lighting, decor, room temperature, view of the speaker, smoking, whispering, and other physical conditions need to be controlled so as to provide the most comfortable learning environment possible.

Equally important for learning is an atmosphere of mutual respect and trust. The nurse-teacher needs to convey this attitude through both verbal and nonverbal means. The way learners are addressed, courtesies shown, and recognition given will make a considerable difference in establishing respect and trust. Both teacher and learners need to be mutually helpful and considerate of one another's needs and interests. All participants should feel free to express ideas, know that their views will be heard, and feel accepted despite differences of opinion and perspective. According to Knowles, this requires that the nurse-teacher refrain from seeming judgmental or inducing competitiveness among learners. Knowles adds that the teacher shares her or his own feelings and knowledge "as a colearner in the spirit of inquiry" (1980, p. 58).

Client Participation

The degree of client participation in the educational process directly influences the amount of client learning (Murray and Zentner, 1985). One nurse discovered this principle when working with a group of people nearing retirement. After talking to them about the changes they would face and receiving little response, she shifted to a different method of teaching. She distributed pamphlets and asked everyone to read each week and come prepared for discussion. Slowly the group began to participate in their own learning to a greater degree. Whenever the nurse works with clients in a learning context, one of the first questions to discuss is " What does the client want to learn?" As Carl Rogers (1969, p. 159) has said: "Learning is facilitated when the student participates responsibly in the learning process. When he chooses his own directions, helps to discover his own learning resources, formulates his own problems, decides his own course of action, lives with consequences of each of these choices, then significant learning is maximized."

The amount of learning is directly proportional to the learners' involvement. A group of senior citizens attended a class on nutrition and aging, yet still made almost no changes in diet or eating patterns. It was not until the members became actively involved in the class, encouraged by the nurse to present problems and solutions for food purchasing and preparation on limited budgets, that any significant behavioral changes occurred.

Contracting, discussed in Chapter 10, can contribute to the nurse's teaching goals. It directly involves the client in a partnership to determine goals, content, and time for learning. Contracting in the context of teaching can develop a great sense of accountability in clients for their own learning.

Subject's Relevance to Client

Subject matter that is relevant to the client is learned more readily and retained longer than information that is not meaningful. Learners gain the most from subject matter immediately useful to their own purposes. This is particularly true of adult learners. Some characteristics of adult learners are summarized below (Knowles, 1980).

1. They are more self-directed.
2. They have more life experiences to which to relate learning.
3. Developmentally, they are more ready to learn.
4. They are more present-oriented than future-oriented in learning.
5. They are more motivated to learn.
6. They tend to see the immediate relevance of material taught.

Consider two middle-management men taking a physical fitness course offered by their employer. One, the father of a cub scout, has agreed to co-lead his son's troop on a two-week backpacking trip in the mountains. He wants to get in shape. The second man is taking the course because it is required by the company. Its only relevance to his own purposes is that it keeps him from gaining his boss's disfavor. There can be little question about which man will learn and retain the most. The course has considerable relevance and meaning to the first man and almost none to the second.

Relevance influences the speed of learning. When a two-year-old child sees his little friend from down the street riding a tricycle, he quickly learns to pedal his own. It becomes very important to him to learn; therefore, he learns quickly. Diabetics who must give themselves daily injections of insulin learn that skill very quickly (Figure 11-3). A housewife and mother with a broken leg rapidly learns to manage crutch-walking. Each client sees considerable relevance in the learning and thus accomplishes it with great speed. According to Rogers (1969), "There is evidence that the time for learning various subjects would be cut to a fraction of the time currently allotted if the material were perceived by the learner as related to his own purposes. Probably one-third to one-fifth of the present time allotment would be sufficient."

When subject matter is relevant to the learner, there is also greater retention of knowledge. The learner, upon seeing the usefulness of the material, develops a strong motivation to acquire and utilize it and will be less likely to forget it. Even in instances when a previously learned motor skill has not been used for many years, it is often quickly recaptured under such conditions.

Client Satisfaction

Clients must derive satisfaction from learning to maintain motivation and increase self-direction (Redman, 1980). Learners need to feel a sense of steady progress in the learning process. Obstacles, frustations, and failures along the way discourage and impede learning. Many stroke patients with potential for rehabilitation give up trying to regain speech or move paralyzed limbs because they become too frustrated and dissatisfied in the process. On the other hand, clients who experience satisfaction and progress in their speech and muscle retraining maintain their motivation and work on exercises without prompting. Nurses can promote client satisfaction through support and encouragement.

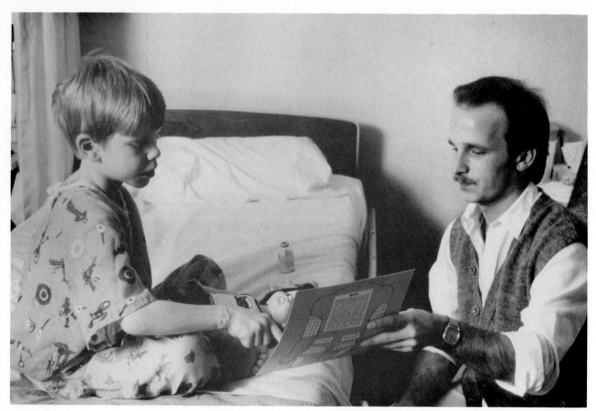

Figure 11-3
This young client learns to give himself daily insulin injections because he is
eager to function as normally as possible despite his diabetes.

Realistic goals contribute to learner satisfaction. Objectives should be set within the learner's ability, thereby avoiding the frustration that comes from a too-difficult task and the loss of interest that results from one too easy. Setting objectives requires agreement on goals, periodic reviews, and revision of goals if they become too easy or too difficult. Nurses further promote clients' learning satisfaction by designing tasks with rewards. One nurse led a class for obese adolescents, and together they set the goal of a weekly three-pound weight loss. The school nurse helped the group design a plan that included counting calories and a buddy system as ways to help bring about a behavior change. If each member in the group achieved the three-pound goal, the group went on a field trip or excursion of their choice as a reward. These students found this learning experience satisfying because goals were attainable and their progress was rewarded. Instead of competing with one another, the group set out to help each member achieve the goal. As a result, most kept the weight off after the class had finished.

Client Application

Learning is reinforced through application (Shropshire, 1981). The students in the weight-loss group began immediately to count calories. They could begin to apply their knowledge. Learners need as many opportunities as possible to apply the learning in daily life. If such opportunities arise during the teaching-learning process, clients can try out new knowledge and skills under supervision. Learners are given an opportunity to start integrating the learning into their daily lives at a time when the teacher is there to help reinforce that pattern.

Take a prenatal class as an example. The learning only begins with explanations of proper diet, exercise, breathing techniques, hygiene, avoidance of alcohol and tobacco, and so on. More learning occurs as the group members discuss these issues and apply them intellectually, exploring ways they could practice them at home. Additional reinforcement comes by demonstrating how to do these activities. Sample diets, demonstrations of exercises, display of posters, pamphlets, or models may be used. The group can begin application in the classroom by making diet plans, doing exercises, role playing parenting behavior, or engaging in group problem solving. Then the members can be encouraged to apply these activities on a daily basis at home and prepare to share their results at future sessions.

Frequent use of newly acquired information fosters transfer of learning to other situations. Our major goal of prevention and health promotion depends on such a transfer. For instance, mothers who learn and practice a well-balanced diet, free of nonnutritious snacks, can be encouraged to offer more nourishing foods to other family members. A family that practices asepsis and good hand-washing techniques when caring for a postsurgical wound can learn to transfer this same principle to prevention of infection in daily living.

TEACHING PROCESS

The process of teaching in community health nursing follows steps similar to those of the nursing process:

1. *Interaction:* Establish basic communication patterns between clients and nurse.
2. *Assessment and diagnosis:* Determine clients' present status and identify needs for teaching.
3. *Setting goals and objectives:* Analyze needed changes and prepare objectives that describe the desired learning outcomes.
4. *Planning:* Design a plan for the learning experience that meets the objectives; include the content to be covered, sequence of topics, best conditions for learning (place, kind of environment), methods, and

tools (visual aids, exercises, etc.). A written plan is best; it may or may not be part of the written nursing care plan.

5. *Teaching:* Implement the learning experience by carrying out the planned activities.

6. *Evaluation:* Determine whether learning objectives were met and if not, why not. Evaluation measures progress toward goals and can indicate future learning needs.

Interaction

Reciprocal communication must take place between the nurse-teacher and client-learners. It is essential in the helping relationship and requisite to effective use of the nursing process. Community health nurses need to develop good questioning techniques and listening skills to determine clients' learning needs and levels of readiness. (The concept of interaction has also been discussed in Chapter 8.)

Assessment and Diagnosis

Identifying clients' learning needs presents a challenge to the nurse-teacher. Too often teaching occurs based on the teacher's assumption of what the learner needs to know. In client education, we have a serious responsibility to tailor teaching to clients' real and perceived needs. Knowles (1980) describes educational needs as gaps between what people know and what they need to know to function effectively. He goes on to say that the potential learners, the sponsoring organization, and the community may all help determine the needs to be addressed in the teaching-learning situation.

Assessing educational needs may be accomplished in several ways. The nurse-teacher can use surveys, interviews, open forums, task forces that include representative clients as members, and many other methods. The important principle to keep in mind is that clients should be involved in identifying what they want to learn. When a "need" to learn something, such as ways to prevent HIV carriers from infecting other people, is identified by the nurse rather than clients, then the nurse may need to "sell" clients on the importance of the topic.

Setting Goals and Objectives

Once a need has been clearly identified, then teacher and learners can establish mutually agreed-upon goals and objectives. Goals are broad statements of intent, and objectives are more specific descriptions of intended outcome (Mager, 1975). Sometimes in a teaching situation a goal may be stated as a purpose. For example, the nurse-teacher may have identified a client group's need to stop smoking. The need and teaching goal (or purpose) might be stated thus:

Need
Group of smokers do not wish to be addicted to an unhealthy habit.

Goal (Purpose)
All members of the group will stop smoking within two months and remain off cigarettes for six months.

Objectives should be stated in measurable behavioral terms. That is, each statement of an objective should include a single idea that describes an outcome that can be measured. To accomplish the above-stated goal of smoking cessation, the educational objectives might include the following:

Objectives
All client learners will do the following things:
1. Describe three reasons why smoking is dangerous and/or objectionable.
2. Identify at least two factors that have influenced their addiction.
3. Plan a series of action steps that will lead to smoking cessation within two months.
4. Remain off cigarettes for six months following cessation.

Each of the above objectives can be readily measured, because each describes a specific outcome and specific learner behaviors. Well-written objectives meet these criteria and greatly enhance evaluating the success of the educational effort.

Planning

Teaching preparation can be done formally or informally. Generally, however, it is best to have a written plan that includes the following:

1. *Subject*
2. *Intended audience*
3. *Date(s), time, and place*
4. *Goal (purpose) statement*
5. *Activities:* After listing the objectives, the nurse-teacher will find it helpful to identify specific activities geared toward meeting each objective. For example, to meet Objective 1 above, the nurse may choose to show a film on the dangers of smoking and have participants list all the reasons they can think of to stop. They can then select their three strongest reasons and describe these to the class.
6. *Teaching-learning methods:* Identify how the content will be presented; using a variety of methods addresses unique needs of the learners and makes the teaching more interesting. Include and combine such methods as lectures, discussions, demonstrations, role playing, and films. (We discuss teaching-learning methods more thoroughly later in this chapter.)
7. *Assignments:* Readings, presentations, papers, practice experiences, and demonstrations are among many possible ways to reinforce and synthesize the learning.

8. *Course outline of topics and dates:* The nurse-teacher may abbreviate this to hand out to learners but will need a complete outline of notes to use in the teaching process.

9. *Evaluation method and criteria:* Results of pre- and post-testing, return demonstrations, learner behavior changes or actions taken, and other criteria can be used to determine whether objectives have been met (Windsor et al., 1985). Criteria need to be clearly defined to indicate satisfactory performance. For example, if breast self-examination is being taught, criteria for satisfactory performance might include a description of proper hand placement and a verbal explanation of what to feel for by the learner.

Teaching

The class or workshop should be conducted according to the plan prepared above. The nurse-teacher will find that a well-designed plan will greatly enhance the smoothness and effectiveness of the actual teaching situation.

Evaluation

This final step is a critical one in the teaching-learning process. It is at this point that the nurse-teacher determines whether the goals and objectives for the educational experience have been met, and if not, why not. Clear, measurable objectives will facilitate evaluation. For example, to measure Objective 3 in the stop-smoking program, "Plan a series of action steps that will lead to smoking cessation within two months," the nurse-teacher may ask group members to put their plan in writing and turn it in for the teacher's comments. To measure the fourth objective, not smoking for six months, would require follow-up contacts, perhaps regular laboratory testing for nicotine presence or at least regular self-reporting.

If objectives have not been met, or have been met only partially, this too requires attention. The nurse-teacher will wish to explore this outcome with the client learners to determine what hindered their completion and what remedial action, if any, might be indicated.

TEACHING METHODS AND TOOLS

Teaching occurs on many levels and incorporates various types of activities. It can be formal or informal, planned or unplanned. Formal presentations, such as lectures, are generally planned and fairly structured. Some teaching is less formal but still planned and relatively structured, as in group discussions in which questions stimulate exploration of ideas and guide thinking. Informal levels of teaching, such as counseling or anticipatory guidance, require background preparation but often no definite plan of presentation. All teachers, however, use one or a combination of methods and tools to facilitate the teaching-learning process. We will close this chapter by discussing four commonly used methods (lecture, discussion, demonstration, and role playing) and several teaching tools for community health nursing education with clients.

Lecture

There are times when the community health nurse will present information to a large group, such as a local PTA, a women's club, or a county board of commissioners. Under such circumstances, the lecture method, a formal kind of presentation, may be the most efficient means of communicating health information. However, lecturers tend to create a passive learning atmosphere for the audience unless they use strategies devised to involve the learners. Many individuals are visual rather than auditory learners. To capture their attention, slides, overhead projections, films, or videotapes can supplement the lecture. Allowing time for questions and discussion after a lecture will also involve the learners more actively.

Discussion

Two-way communication is an important feature of the learning process. Learners need an opportunity to raise questions, make comments, reason out loud, and receive feedback in order to develop understanding. When discussion is used in conjunction with other teaching methods such as demonstration, lecture, and role playing, it will improve their effectiveness. In group teaching, discussion enables clients to learn from one another as well as from the nurse. One difficulty that can arise is monopolization of the discussion by one person while others seldom express themselves. The nurse-teacher must exercise leadership in controlling and guiding the discussion so that learning opportunities are maximized. Prepared objectives and discussion organized around specific questions (Bavaro, 1980) or topics make the discussion most fruitful.

Demonstration

The demonstration method is often used for teaching motor skills and is best accompanied by explanation and discussion. It can give clients a clear sensory image of how to perform the skill. Because a demonstration should be within easy visual and auditory range of learners, it is best to demonstrate in front of small groups. Use the same kind of equipment that clients will use in order to show exactly how the skill should be performed, and provide them with ample opportunity to practice until the skill is perfected. Again, objectives, content, and sequence of learning activities should all be planned ahead of time.

Role Playing

There are times when having clients assume and act out roles maximizes learning (Wise, 1980). A parenting group, for example, found it helpful to place themselves in the role of their children; their feelings about various ways to respond became more apparent. Reversing roles can effectively teach spouses in conflict about better ways to communicate. In order to prevent role playing from becoming a game with little learning, plan the proposed drama with clear objectives in mind. What behavioral outcomes do you hope to achieve? Define the context, the "stage," clearly so that everyone shares in the situation. Then define each role ahead of time, making sure everyone understands his or her performance. Emphasize that no wrong or right performance exists, and that participants should merely behave the way people behave in everyday life. Avoid having people play themselves; it can embarrass them and make it difficult for them to achieve objectivity. After the drama has concluded, elicit discussion with carefully prepared questions.

Teaching Tools

Many different tools, often used in combination, are useful during the teaching process. Visual images — pictures, slides, films, posters, chalkboards, videotapes, bulletin boards, flash cards, pamphlets, and even gestures — can enhance almost any learning. Some tools such as sound films, record players, or tape recorders provide an auditory stimulus. Other tools, such as models or objects, allow clients both visual and tactile learning (Figure 11-4). Still others, such as programmed instruction or games, involve learners through reading and activity (Frantz, 1980).

The choice of teaching tools varies with clients' interests and abilities and with the demands of the situation. Teaching often occurs in casual conversations, spontaneously in situations in which clients raise unexpected questions, or when a crisis arises. In these instances, nurses draw on their background of knowledge and exercise professional judgment in their selection of content, methods, and tools. Finally, nurses teach by example: actions usually speak louder than words. If a nurse teaches the importance of a healthy lifestyle and then lights up a cigarette, the message of her actions will carry more impact than her words. The healthy nurse who exhibits healthy practices uses herself as a tool and serves as a role model as well as a health teacher.

Summary

A large part of community health nursing practice involves teaching. Far more than to simply give health information to clients, the purpose of teaching is to change client behavior to healthier practices.

Understanding the nature of learning contributes to the effectiveness of teaching in community health. Learning theories can be grouped into three

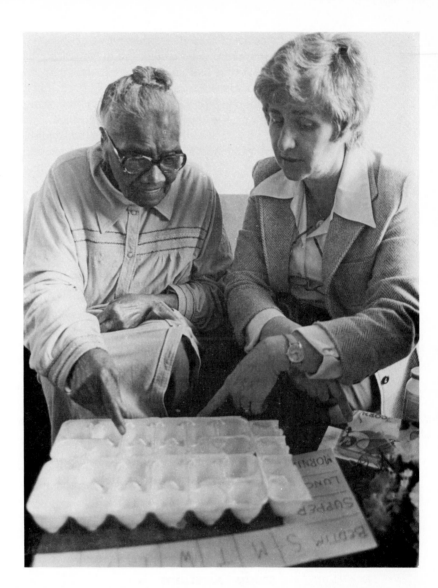

Figure 11-4
Teaching methods and tools vary with clients' learning needs. On this home visit the nurse uses an egg container with labels to help an elderly woman with limited vision devise a plan for taking her medications.

broad categories. The first group, consisting of mental discipline theories, views learning as the promotion of mental training, ranging from strict discipline, through natural unfolding of the learner's mind, to building on the learner's store of ideas. The second category, stimulus-response conditioning, views learning as a change in behavior (response to stimuli). Cognitive learning theories form the third category. These seek to influence learners' understanding of problems and situations through promoting their insights.

Learning occurs in three domains: cognitive, affective, and psychomotor. The cognitive domain refers to learning that takes place intellectually, through the mind. It ranges in levels of learner functioning from simple recall to complex evaluation. As learners move up the scale of cognitive learning, they become more self-directed; the nurse-teacher assumes a more facilitative role.

Affective learning means the changing of attitudes and values. Learners may experience several levels of affective involvement from simple listening to adopting the new value. Again, as the client-learner increases involvement, the nurse-teacher becomes less directive.

Psychomotor learning involves the acquisition of motor skills. Clients who learn psychomotor skills must meet three conditions: they must be capable of the skill; they must develop a sensory image of the skill; and they must practice the skill.

Teaching in community health nursing is the facilitation of learning that leads to behavioral change in the client. Thus teaching is a catalytic process based on the following teaching-learning principles:

1. Clients' readiness for learning influences teaching effectiveness.
2. Clients' perceptions affect their learning.
3. Learners' physical and emotional comfort within an educational setting influences learning.
4. The degree of client participation in the educational process directly influences the amount of client learning.
5. Subject matter that is relevant to the client is learned more readily and retained longer than information that is not meaningful.
6. The client must derive satisfaction from learning experiences to maintain motivation and increase self-direction.
7. Learning is reinforced through application.

The teaching process in community health nursing is similar to the nursing process. It includes interaction, assessment and diagnosis, goal setting, planning, teaching, and evaluation. The actual teaching may be formal or informal, planned or unplanned. Methods may range from structured lecture presentations to demonstration and role playing. Selection of a tool depends on how well it suits client-learners and helps to meet the desired objectives.

Study Questions

1. What learning theory or theories discussed in this chapter most closely reflect your own position? Discuss how you would apply it or them in your practice.
2. A children's day-care center is located in your service area. What populations in this setting could be potential recipients of health teaching? How would you assess each group's learning needs?
3. Your county health board often makes decisions that appear to reflect lack of knowledge regarding health and health care. How might you

"educate" them using the concepts and principles described in this chapter?

4. Discuss the differences between cognitive, affective, and psychomotor learning. Why do cognitive and affective learning need to be linked in health teaching?

5. Explore the possible use of role models as a teaching tool for community health nursing practice. What examples already exist in your community? What new ones might you develop?

References

Bavaro, J. A. (1980). Questioning: The key to learning. *Supervisor Nurse* 11(6): 26.

Bigge, M. L. (1982). *Learning theories for teachers.* 4th ed. New York: Harper & Row.

Bloom, B. (ed.). (1956). *Taxonomy of educational objectives: The classification of educational goals. Handbook I: Cognitive domain.* New York: Longman.

Douglass, L. M., and E. O. Bevis. (1974). *Nursing leadership in action: Principles and application to staff situations.* St. Louis: C. V. Mosby.

Frantz, R. A. (1980). Selecting media for patient education. *Topics in Clinical Nursing* 2(2): 77.

Furstenberg, F., K. Moore, and J. Peterson. (1985). Sex education and sexual experience among adolescents. *American Journal of Public Health* 75(11): 1331–32.

Gronlund, N. E. (1970). *Stating behavioral objectives for classroom instruction.* New York: Macmillan.

Hergenhahn, B. R. (1982). *An introduction to theories of learning.* 2nd ed. Englewood Cliffs, N.J.: Prentice-Hall.

Knowles, M. (1980). *The modern practice of adult education: Androgogy versus pedagogy.* 2nd ed. Chicago: Follett.

Levin, L. S. (1978). Patient education and self-care: How do they differ? *Nursing Outlook* 26: 170–75.

Lorig, K. (1985). Health education: Beyond health teaching. In S. Archer and R. Fleshman (eds.), *Community health nursing.* 3rd ed. Monterey, Calif.: Wadsworth.

Mager, R. F. (1975). *Preparing instructional objectives.* 2nd ed. Belmont, Calif.: Pitman Learning.

Marriner, A. (1979). Health teaching. In A. Marriner (ed.), *The nursing process.* 2nd ed. St. Louis: C. V. Mosby.

Miller, A. (1985). When is the time ripe for teaching? *American Journal of Nursing* 85(7): 801.

Murray, R., and J. Zentner. (1985). *Nursing concepts for health promotion.* 3rd ed. Englewood Cliffs, N.J.: Prentice-Hall.

Redman, B. K. (1980). *The process of patient teaching in nursing.* 4th ed. St. Louis: C. V. Mosby.

Rogers, C. (1969). *Freedom to learn.* Columbus, Ohio: Merrill.

Shropshire, C. D. (1981). Group experiential learning in adult education. *Journal of Continuing Education in Nursing* 12(6): 5.

Windsor, R., et al. (1985). The effectiveness of smoking cessation methods for smokers in public health maternity clinics: A randomized trial. *American Journal of Public Health* 75(12): 1389–92.

Wise, P. (1980). Methods of teaching—revisited. Character play and role play. *Journal of Continuing Education in Nursing* 11(1): 37.

Selected Readings

Bavaro, J. A. (1980). Questioning: The key to learning. *Supervisor Nurse* 11(6): 26.

Bigge, M. L. (1982). *Learning theories for teachers.* 4th ed. New York: Harper & Row.

Bloom, B. (ed.). (1956). *Taxonomy of educational objectives: The classification of educational goals. Handbook I: Cognitive domain.* New York: Longman.

Bryan, N. E. (1974). Every nurse a teacher. *Australian Nurses Journal* 4(1): 31–33.

Cooper, S. (1980). Methods of teaching—revisited. Role playing, part 10. *Journal of Continuing Education in Nursing* 11(1): 36.

Cooper, S. (1981). Methods of teaching—revisited. Films and videotapes. *Journal of Continuing Education in Nursing* 12(1): 34.

Cooper, S. (1981). Methods of teaching—revisited. The interview. *Journal of Continuing Education in Nursing* 12(4): 34.

Cooper, S. (1982). Methods of teaching—revisited. Open forum: buzz session. *Journal of Continuing Education in Nursing* 13(1): 38.

Cummings, K. M., R. Sciandr, and S. Markello. (1987). Impact of a newspaper-mediated quit smoking program. *American Journal of Public Health* 77(11): 1452–53.

Evans, L. K. (1980). Health education from a group perspective. *Topics in Clinical Nursing* 2(2): 45.

Flay, B. R. (1987). Mass media and smoking cessation: A critical review. *American Journal of Public Health* 77(2): 153–60.

Frantz, R. A. (1980). Selecting media for patient education. *Topics in Clinical Nursing* 2(2): 77.

Furstenberg, F., K. Moore, and J. Peterson. (1985). Sex education and sexual experience among adolescents. *American Journal of Public Health* 75(11): 1331–32.

Green, L. W. (1977). Evaluation and measurement: Some dilemmas for health education. *American Journal of Public Health* 67: 155–61.

Green, L., et al. (1980). Health Education Planning: A Diagnostic Approach. 2nd ed. Englewood Cliffs, N.J.: Prentice-Hall.

Gronlund, N. E. (1970). *Stating behavorial objectives for classroom instruction.* New York: Macmillan.

Hein, E. C. (1978). Teaching psychosocial wellness in family and community health nursing. *Nurse Educator* 3: 22–25.

Heit, P. (1978). Educating the nurse-community health educator to educate. *Journal of Nursing Education* 17(1): 21–23.

Hergenhahn, B. R. (1982). *An introduction to theories of learning.* 2nd ed. Englewood Cliffs, N.J.: Prentice-Hall.

Job, R. F. S. (1988). Effective and ineffective use of fear in health promotion campaigns. *American Journal of Public Health* 78(2): 163–67.

Jones, P., and W. Oertel. (1977). Developing patient teaching objectives and techniques: A self-instructional program. *Nurse Educator* 2(5): 3–18.

Knowles, M. (1975). *Self-directed learning: A guide for learners and teachers.* New York: Associated Press.

Knowles, M. (1980). *The modern practice of adult education: Androgogy versus pedagogy.* 2nd ed. Chicago: Follett.

Kopelke, C. E. (1975). Group education to reduce overweight . . . in a blue-collar community. *American Journal of Nursing* 75: 1993–95.

Levin, L. S. (1978). Patient education and self-care: How do they differ? *Nursing Outlook* 26: 170–75.

Lorig, K. (1985). Health education: Beyond health teaching. In S. Archer and R. Fleshman (eds.), *Community health nursing.* 3rd ed. Monterey, Calif.: Wadsworth.

Mager, R. F. (1975). *Preparing instructional objectives.* 2nd ed. Belmont, Calif.: Pitman Learning.

Marriner, A. (1979). Health teaching. In A. Marriner (ed.), *The nursing process*. 2nd ed. St. Louis: C. V. Mosby.

Milio, N. (1976). A broad perspective on health: A teaching-learning tool. *Nursing Outlook* 24: 160–63.

Milio, N. (1976). A framework for prevention: Changing health-damaging to health-generating life patterns. *American Journal of Public Health* 66: 435–39.

Miller, A. (1985). When is the time ripe for teaching? *American Journal of Nursing* 85(7): 801.

Murray, R., and J. Zentner. (1985). *Nursing concepts for health promotion*. 3rd ed. Englewood Cliffs, N.J.: Prentice-Hall.

Narrow, B. (1979). *Patient teaching in nursing practice: A patient and family-centered approach*. Somerset, N.J.: Wiley.

Rankin, S., and K. Duffy. (1983). *Patient Education: Issues, Principles, and Guidelines*. Philadelphia: J. B. Lippincott.

Redman, B. K. (1980). *The process of patient teaching in nursing*. 4th ed. St. Louis: C. V. Mosby.

Reilly, D. E. (ed.). (1978). *Teaching and evaluating the affective domain in nursing programs*. Thorofare, N.J.: Charles B. Slack.

Roberts, F. B. (1981). A model for parent education. *Image* 13: 86.

Robinson, G., and M. Filkins. (1964). Group teaching with outpatients. *American Journal of Nursing* 64: 110–12.

Rogers, C. R. (1969). *Freedom to learn*. Columbus, Ohio: Merrill.

Schweer, J. E., and K. M. Gebbie. (1976). *Creative teaching in clinical nursing*. St. Louis: C. V. Mosby.

Shropshire, C. D. (1981). Group experiential learning in adult education. *Journal of Continuing Education in Nursing* 12(6): 5.

Simmons, J. (ed.). (1975). Making health education work. *American Journal of Public Health* 65(Oct. Suppl.): 1–49.

Thompson, W. (1978). Health education: II. How do we communicate? *Nursing Times* 74: 1561–62.

Timmreck, T. C., et al. (1987). The health education and health promotion movement: A theoretical jungle. *Health Education* 18(5): 24–28.

Tones, B. K. (1986). Health education and the ideology of health promotion: A review of alternative approaches. *Health Education Research* 1(1): 3–12.

Veninga, K. A. (1983). How to establish a nutrition education program. *Occupational Health Nursing* 12: 34–38.

Warner, K. E. (1987). Television and health education: Stay tuned. *American Journal of Public Health* 77(2): 140–42.

Wilson, W., and C. Pratt. (1987). The impact of diabetes education and peer support upon weight and glycemic control of elderly persons with noninsulin-dependent diabetes mellitus (NIDDM). *American Journal of Public Health* 77(5): 634–35.

Windsor, R., et al. (1985). The effectiveness of smoking cessation methods for smokers in public health maternity clinics: A randomized trial. *American Journal of Public Health* 75(12): 1389–92.

Wise, P. (1980). Methods of teaching—revisited. Character play and role play. *Journal of Continuing Education in Nursing* 11(1): 37.

Wise, P. (1980). Adult teaching strategies. *Journal of Continuing Education in Nursing* 11(6): 15.

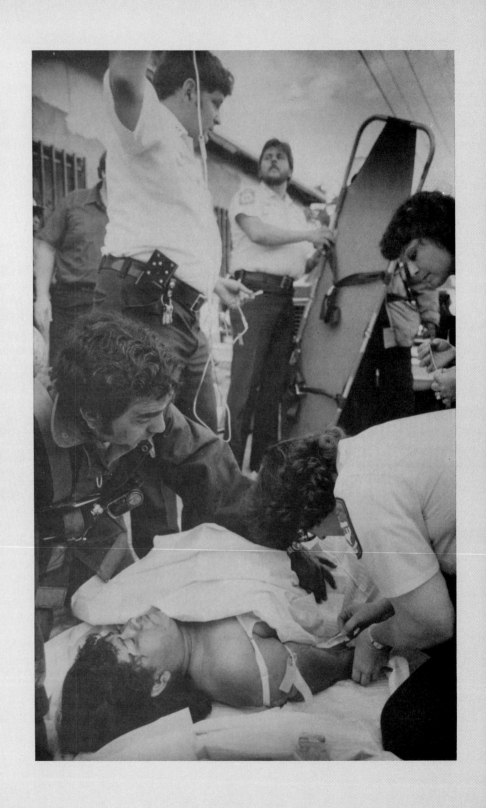

12 Community Crisis Prevention and Intervention

All human beings, individually and collectively, experience periods of upset, trouble, even danger. A teenager discovers she is pregnant. The father and breadwinner in a family loses his job. A beloved leader dies. A worker faces retirement. An accident at a nuclear power plant threatens a community. A woman has her first baby. These life experiences can produce stress and anxiety. Each event can cause changes in peoples' behavior; each can require days, weeks, or even months of adjustment and coping. When people need help in coping, they have entered a time of crisis.

People respond differently to a potential crisis. Some see the event as a challenge; others see it as adversity. What one person experiences as crisis, another treats as a normal occurrence. Some seek out the help they need and come through the experience unscathed, perhaps even stronger than before. Others, unable to cope, incur severe, sometimes permanent, damage.

Regardless of their responses, people in a crisis-producing situation need help. Equally important, they are receptive to help. Community health practitioners have a unique opportunity to provide assistance because they can see clients frequently and in a broad environmental context. Not only can they give assistance during a time of crisis, but more importantly, they can help people equip themselves with the tools needed for crisis management and prevention. In particular, community health practitioners are concerned about crises or potential crises at the aggregate level. When the Three Mile Island nuclear power plant accident occurred, for example, it created a crisis for families, groups, communities, and, indeed, society as a whole. Major professional challenges in community health are to prevent crises and to help people in crisis. In this chapter we examine how nurses can sharpen their knowledge and skills in the practice of crisis prevention and intervention for community health.

CRISIS THEORY

Our understanding about crises has grown considerably. At one time, we equated crisis only with disaster; it might have been natural (a hurricane), economic (a stock market crash), political (a presidential assassination), environmental (water polluted with chemicals), personal (death of a loved one), or another form of disaster. Researchers have studied the nature of crisis and have now developed a body of knowledge called *crisis theory*. Initially limited to the field of mental health, crisis theory now influences every field of health care (Lawler and Yount, 1987). We know, for example, that a crisis is not an event per se, but rather people's perception of the event. We know that different kinds of crises occur; we can explain why people respond the way they do in a crisis; we can predict the phases that people go through in a crisis of any kind. These are important aspects to understand before we can attempt to prevent, manage, or intervene in crises.

The Chinese character for the word *crisis* has a dual meaning: danger and opportunity. A crisis means danger in that it poses a threat to the people involved, but it also means an opportunity for overcoming difficulty and achieving growth.

DYNAMICS OF CRISIS

How does a crisis occur? People as living systems behave in certain ways, which are generally unconscious, in order to maintain relative equilibrium within themselves and in their relations with others. When some internal or external force disrupts the system's balance and alters its functioning, loss of equilibrium occurs. To restore equilibrium, people attempt to cope. They develop problem-solving behaviors that become habitual through repeated, although not always successful, use. Caplan (1964) points out that during the brief period before a problem is resolved, people experience tension. But the tension is manageable because they know from previous problem-solving successes that the outcomes will be positive. They have also learned techniques for handling the tension. For example, Sharon has a flat tire while driving her car. This event creates a brief period of tension. But as Sharon locates the spare and begins to jack up the car, her anxiety subsides. She uses her knowledge to solve the problem.

In a crisis, the dynamics change. The problem is unfamiliar and greater than usual. It calls for a dramatic alteration of people's accustomed roles, responsibilities, or both (Brownell, 1984). Tension develops. They try their customary problem-solving responses only to find them inadequate. It becomes impossible to restore equilibrium; anxiety mounts. If, instead of having a flat tire, Sharon is caught in a blizzard with blinding snow and driving winds obliterating her vision and making temperatures drop to levels that threaten her survival, she cannot use her past experience to solve the problem. Her anxiety may rise and a crisis ensue.

The problem persists and tension grows more apparent. People continue to apply their usual problem-solving techniques or direct their efforts toward handling the tension. Sharon, for example, may think about walking to the nearest farmhouse or tell herself, "No, I should stay with the car and try to keep warm until help comes." If these efforts fail to solve the problem, the feelings of anxiety and inadequacy will increase: "A person in this situation feels help-less — he is caught in a state of great emotional upset and feels unable to take action *on his own* to solve the problem" (Aguilera and Messick, 1986, p. 1).

Increased stress caused by a further rise in tension and anxiety serves as a catalyst for some people to resolve the problem. Realizing that they cannot solve it on their own with their usual coping mechanisms, they mobilize new internal resources, seek outside help, or both, or they define the problem in a new way that makes it manageable. Following a sudden spring storm, community residents in a Midwestern town faced a rapidly rising river and the threat of flood. After the initial shock and disorientation, they mobilized to form teams: one for rescue and first aid, one for sandbagging the river banks, and one to evacuate low-level area homes. As a result, no lives were lost and minimal property damage occurred. Their efforts were successful.

In other situations, the problem remains. Stimulated by the same tension, people may seek inappropriate solutions without success. The help they receive may not redefine their problem in a realistic and workable manner. They may choose to avoid the problem by resigning themselves to it or minimizing its importance. Tension and anxiety mount rapidly or gradually, but ultimately people reach a point beyond which they can no longer function. Drastic results can follow, such as suicide, mass hysteria, heart attacks, psychotic breaks, and family or group disintegration.

Caplan (1964) has summarized in four stages the effect of rising tension on the functioning of people in crisis:

1. Tension develops (as a result of precipitating event).

   People use customary problem-solving responses in order to restore equilibrium.

2. Tension increases.

   Failure to cope leads to feeling upset and ineffectual.

3. Tension rises further.

   Increased tension acts as a stimulus to mobilize internal and external resources. People try to redefine the situation and may solve the problem, in which case tension abates.

4. Tension reaches threshold.

   If problem continues unsolved (or avoided), the breaking point is reached, causing major disorganization both socially and individually.

Thus, in a crisis, a certain amount of tension or stress may promote problem resolution and restoration of equilibrium. However, stress that becomes too intense and is unrelieved will ultimately lead to system breakdown (Veninga and Spradley, 1981, p. 35).

DEFINITION OF CRISIS

Crisis is a temporary state of severe disequilibrium for persons who face a situation they find threatening that they can neither escape nor solve with their usual coping abilities (Caplan, 1964; Fink, 1967; Infante, 1982).

Let us look at several key characteristics of this definition in the context of a family in which the father is killed unexpectedly in a plane crash. Crisis begins with a sense that things are *out of balance*. It causes the awareness of being upset, a state of considerable disequilibrium with resulting tension. Crises create "sudden discontinuities in the functioning pattern" (Caplan, 1964, p. 39). The man's wife and three children feel shattered by the news. The rhythm of their family life comes to a halt. Bills go unpaid; someone else must prepare meals. The family has been pushed out of balance.

Crisis is a *temporary condition*. A system's strong need to regain homeostasis means that the disequilibrium of a crisis does not go on indefinitely. Most crises last from four to six weeks (Aguilera, 1986). In this family, as shocking as the loss might seem, life begins to return to a more regular pattern in a few weeks. Although the members will feel the loss of husband and father for years, the crisis will soon disappear.

A crisis involves *cognitive uncertainty*. Much stress comes from not understanding the situation and not knowing its outcome. Immediate questions about notifying friends and planning the funeral raise uncertainty for the family that has lost a father. Long-range questions about how they will adjust can plague every family member.

A crisis situation is *hazardous*. For the persons involved, crisis represents an actual loss (the death of a loved one), the threat of a loss (terminal illness), or an overwhelming challenge (the offer of an important job). With her husband dead, the wife faces sudden financial insecurity. She may have also lost her major source of emotional support.

Crisis brings on *psychophysiological symptoms*. People react somatically to the stress. They may experience appetite fluctuations, sleeplessness, body aches, nausea, muscle tension, perspiration, rapid pulse, and other signs of anxiety, as well as fear, shame, guilt, or excitement. The specific reaction depends on the nature of the situation, how it is perceived, and inherited tendencies. The children who have lost their father become irritable, cry, and may feel sick. The wife and mother may experience shortness of breath and exhaustion.

A crisis situation is *inescapable*. People face an unavoidable demand for change. The experience cannot be reversed or ignored. It requires some kind of action or response. When the head of a household dies suddenly, the other family members cannot escape the loss. Death brings inevitable changes for each of the remaining individuals.

Crisis often reveals *inadequate coping skills.* Habitual problem-solving resources do not work in this situation. The children have all known times when their father was absent from the family and have developed ways to cope with such temporary loss. But in this crisis situation, their father's death means permanent loss. They cannot deal with it in the same way.

Crisis creates a feeling of *helplessness.* The person feels overwhelmed, paralyzed, and unable to think or take action on his or her own. It is a time when the family members may ask others what to do. Sometimes helplessness takes the form of immobility; the wife may be unable to make even the simplest decisions.

Crisis elicits *exaggerated defense mechanisms.* Behaviors such as rationalizing excessively, compensating for losses, and blaming others are often evident. The wife may blame her husband's boss for overworking him and making him take the business trip that ended fatally.

Each crisis presents a unique problem, one too difficult for the person to solve alone with his normal coping mechanisms yet one too important to ignore. The problem represents a threat to the satisfaction of some basic need. An imbalance exists between supply and demand: the resources of the person are insufficient under the circumstances.

Every crisis constitutes a turning point. It presents people with an opportunity for growth toward a healthier state; it also brings the danger of increased vulnerability to illness. Growth occurs when we mature in the crisis and develop more effective problem-solving skills. Some persons, drawing on new resources, redefine the crisis of divorce, for instance, as a challenge to make a new life, to discover themselves and their potential, and to learn to establish healthier relationships with others. Those who engage in healthy adaptation during a crisis will emerge unharmed, even strengthened. They have become prepared to cope with similar events in the future.

Crises, however, present dangers as well as provide opportunities. The loss of homeostasis increases people's vulnerability to illness, whether mental or physical, and regression (Murray and Zentner, 1985). Some divorced persons, for instance, may not handle the crisis well; they may not accept or receive adequate help from others and may become bitter, withdrawn, and resentful. These individuals have moved toward an unhealthy outcome as a result of maladaptive behavior. Ways in which nurses can help clients handle crisis adaptively will be examined later.

KINDS OF CRISES

When acquired immune deficiency syndrome (AIDS) struck the city of San Francisco a few years ago, panic and fear spread quickly. Who would contract the rapidly developing symptoms next and perhaps die? The situation threatened the very lives of the community. An overwhelming feeling of helplessness arose as public health authorities and city officials struggled to control the disease and identify its cause. For many people the situation was clearly a crisis. In numerous other parts of the country that crisis has repeated itself.

Other less dramatic and less threatening events also can create anxiety and stress if they require coping skills beyond those regularly practiced by the persons involved. A young couple is overwhelmed at the responsibility of becoming parents. An elderly woman panics at the thought of moving to a nursing home. A deteriorating neighborhood is threatened by a rise in crime. Like the AIDS outbreak, these too are crises, but of a different magnitude.

There are two kinds of crises. The AIDS event exemplifies a situational (or accidental) crisis. The other kind is a maturational (or developmental) crisis.

MATURATIONAL CRISES

Maturational crises are periods of disruption that occur at transition points in normal growth and development. The people involved feel threatened by the demands placed on them. They have difficulty making the changes necessary to fit the new stage of development.

During the process of normal biopsychosocial growth, we go through a succession of life cycle stages. These begin with birth and continue through old age, each stage quite different from the previous one. As we leave one stage and enter a new one, we experience a transitional period characterized by changes in role expectations and behavior. It is a period of upset and disequilibrium. In recent years popular writers like Sheehy (1976), Levinson (1978), and Goodman (1979) have called these periods "passages," "transitions," and "turning points." They are the times when maturational crises occur (Figure 12-1).

Groups and communities, too, develop through successive stages that frequently parallel the birth-to-old-age pattern. Theorists have variously described the stages of group growth (Sampson and Marthas, 1977), which will be summarized in Chapter 14, as dependence, counterdependence, and interdependence. Community development may be less easily distinguished. Nonetheless, anthropologists, sociologists, philosophers, historians, and other social scientists down through the years have observed and recorded the birth, rise, decline, and sometimes renewal (Gardner, 1981) of societies, communities, and other aggregates of people. Groups and communities, like most living systems, encounter stages of growth with accompanying transitions that require adaptation and lead to what can be described as "maturational" crises. For example, a new community may find that its growing population of young children lacks adequate playgrounds and recreational activities. The community is experiencing a maturational transition that requires adaptation.

Most maturational crises begin with a gradual onset. The change is evolutionary rather than revolutionary. We can anticipate and even prepare to

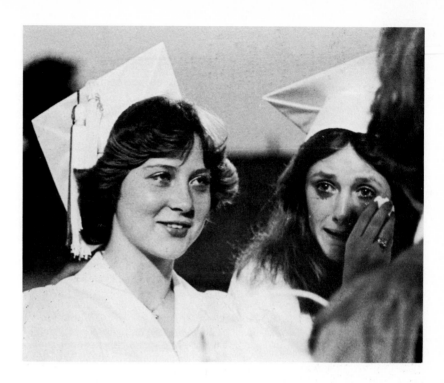

Figure 12-1
Graduation, like any
maturational transition,
is a time of mixed feelings.
Some individuals can take it
in stride. For others, it may
become a time of crisis.

start school, enter adolescence, leave home, get married, have a baby, retire, or die. People move into and through each transitional period knowing in advance that some kind of change will be required. So, too, with communities. A new town needs to develop its schools, businesses, city ordinances, recreational areas, hospitals, law enforcement, and churches. As it grows, the needs change to maintenance and controlled expansion. In many instances, we have already seen other people or communities of people experience these transitions. As a result, maturational crises have a degree of predictability. They offer the possibility of a period of time for anticipation and adjustment.

Maturational crises arise from both physical and social changes. Each new life stage confronts us with changed relationships, responsibilities, and roles. Consider the transition to parenthood, for example. It demands a change in role from caring for oneself and one's mate to include nurturing, caring for, and protecting a completely helpless child. Relationships with other adults, other children, and even one's own parents also change. Parenthood becomes an entrance into a previously unexperienced part of the adult world. New parents may fear the unknown. Will this infant develop normally? Can I give adequate care? Parents often feel anxiety over the responsibility of shaping this new person's life and satisfying society's expectations for their child's proper education and training. They may worry about the increased financial burden and struggle with mixed feelings about giving up a large measure of freedom. At the aggregate level, a community may find it lacks adequate resources to cope with increasing law enforcement demands, or a small town may struggle with its identity as it increases in size and loses its unique intimacy. These transitions put people under considerable stress, which contributes to tension build-up, feelings of helplessness, and resultant crisis. Some people adapt quickly; others cannot cope, probably because earlier maturational crises went unresolved. If people lack a repertoire of adaptive skills, a crisis can become major and disastrous. We can easily see how abused children become abusive parents when most, if not all, of their maturational crises have been detrimental rather than healthy.

Case Example

Marcia Sand is 39 years old. Married for 22 years, she has been a capable homemaker and mother of four children. Her husband, Lou, a construction worker for the past 20 years, thinks Marcia does a "super job at home." In the past, Marcia's time was filled with cooking, laundry, cleaning, shopping, and meeting the endless demands of the family. Their limited income prompted her to adopt many money-saving strategies. She made most of her own and the children's clothes, did all her own baking, and raised vegetables in her backyard garden. Now the youngest of the children, Tommy, has just left home to join the Navy. Her husband spends much of his spare time at the local bar with his friends, leaving Marcia alone. With a nearly empty house and little need for cooking, baking, and sewing, Marcia has lost her sense of usefulness. She thinks of taking a job, but knows her choices are limited because she has only a high school education. Marcia has not slept well in weeks; she wakes up tired and drags through the day barely able to manage the simplest task. She cries frequently but does not know why. Her hair, always neat and attractive in the past, looks bedraggled, and her shoulders slump. "I just can't seem to get on top of things anymore," she complains.

Marcia has entered a maturational crisis that is sometimes called the "empty nest syndrome." She faces a turning point in her life, a time when parenting has seemingly ended. Leaving her satisfying homemaker role, she faces a new life stage filled with unknowns, changes, and a seeming lack of purpose. The transition came about gradually, almost imperceptibly, but now she must deal with it. Yet she feels unable to cope and wishes to turn to someone who would understand and lend her strength. She can be helped, but her crisis could also have been prevented.

SITUATIONAL CRISES

A situational crisis is an acute state of disequilibrium precipitated by an unexpected external event perceived as hazardous. It requires behavioral changes and coping mechanisms beyond the abilities of the people involved.

Sudden events over which we have little or no control come in many forms (Figure 12-2). A flood destroys a family's home and all their possessions. Another family loses its young mother through cancer. A group of workers

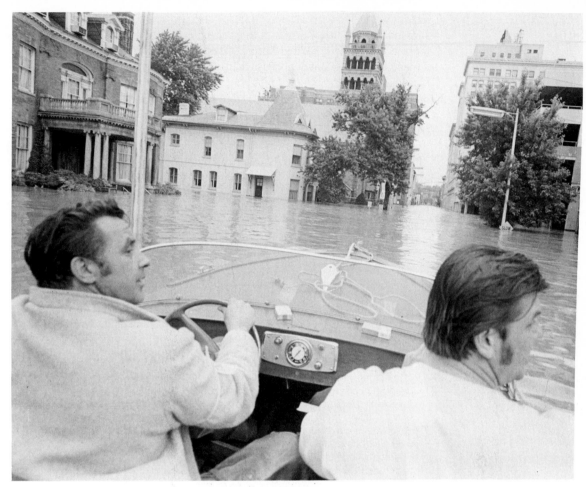

Figure 12-2
This flood in Wilkes-Barre, Penn., in July 1972 created a situational crisis for
that community. Here, Red Cross disaster workers search for victims in the
flood-inundated downtown area.

lose their jobs. After 25 years of marriage, a couple gets divorced. An epidemic of serious influenza strikes a city. These kinds of events, which involve loss or the threat of loss, represent life hazards to those affected. Some crisis-precipitating events can be positive, such as a significant job promotion or news of a large inheritance; however, they still make increased demands on individuals (Caplan, 1964). Integrity is threatened and equilibrium disrupted during these situational or accidental crises.

Situational crises arise from external sources, that is, events or conditions generally outside of people's normal life processes. They are extraordinary experiences. They create life changes and disrupt equilibrium by imposing stresses that are usually foreign to ordinary living. The result is overwhelming tension and incapacitation. Natural disasters, for example, are clearly an external cause of a situational crisis. Said one client, "I shall never forget my feelings when one of my high school classmates was killed instantly by lightning. Mel was a popular boy, and his death threw us all into crisis."

Community health nurses see an almost infinite variety of situational crises; included are debilitating disease, economic misfortune, unemployment, physical abuse, divorce, unwanted pregnancy, chemical abuse, sudden death of a loved one, tragic accidents such as mine explosions, and many others. In each situation, people feel overwhelmed and need help to cope. Skilled intervention can make the difference between a healthy or unhealthy outcome.

Case Example

The Cooper family eagerly anticipated the birth of their first child. When they first learned that Danny had a harelip and cleft palate, Jan and Frank were numb. They were overwhelmed by the shock of seeing their disfigured baby and worried about the possibility of other defects. Then came the first painful days adjusting to Danny's appearance and trying to feed and care for him. Jan and Frank alternated between feelings of guilt ("Perhaps we didn't do something right during pregnancy!") and resentment ("Why did this have to happen to us?"). Added to these anxieties was the specter of several corrective surgeries. Each operation threatened them with the risk to Danny, the stress of hospitalization, the struggle to stay with Danny while juggling jobs, the consequences to home life, and the impossible financial costs. How could they handle it all? They felt unable to cope.

As with most situational crises, this one took the Coopers completely by surprise. It upset their normal pattern of living and disrupted their equilibrium. The onset was sudden, precipitated by an event that they perceived as threatening to their well-being. Unlike maturational crises that are brought on by normal demands of growth, their child's congenital defect was externally imposed. Also, it required behavioral changes and adjustments that the Coopers' usual coping abilities were not equipped to handle. These abilities needed help too.

Maturational and situational crises share the general characteristics of crises described earlier. Their major differences are summarized in Table 12-1. Different kinds of crises can overlap in actual experience, compounding the stress

Table 12-1
Major Differences between Types of Crises

Maturational Crisis	Situational Crisis
Part of normal growth and development	Unexpected period of upset in normalcy
Precipitated by a life transition point	Precipitated by a hazardous event
Gradual onset	Sudden onset
Response to maturational demands and society's expectations	Externally imposed "accident"

felt by the persons involved. The Coopers, for example, experienced a maturational crisis (birth) and a situational crisis (birth defect) simultaneously; thus their stress was compounded. A maturational crisis of midlife may become complicated by situational crises such as divorce and job change occurring at the same time. The transition a child faces entering school may occur at the same time the family moves to a new neighborhood and a new infant joins the family. The child must share his parents' attention and affection with a new sibling at a time when all the resources the child can muster are needed. Individuals, such as members of a football team experiencing the group crisis of an unexpected and embarrassing defeat, may also be undergoing separate maturational or situational crises of their own. Research has shown that these accumulated stresses can lead to ill health (Holmes and Rahe, 1967). Those who might normally work through one crisis in a healthy way may find that compound events overwhelm them and cause disaster.

CRISIS PREVENTION

Many people unnecessarily go through crises that might have been prevented. Other crises could be shortened in length or diminished in intensity through preventive measures (Underwood and Fiedler, 1983). Because of the nature and philosophy of community health practice, nurses should place a high priority on crisis prevention. Community health nurses are in a unique position to prevent or detect crises early. They encounter clients or would-be clients in their natural settings where direct observation and discussion can occur. Also, through their participation in communities' communication networks, they can learn about potential family and community programs.

PRIMARY PREVENTION

We shall consider crisis prevention on three levels: primary, secondary, and tertiary. Primary crisis prevention means keeping the crisis from ever happening; action completely obstructs its occurrence. Both maturational and situational crises can, in many cases, be prevented altogether. Let us examine what this prevention involves.

A primary crisis prevention program in community health has two major goals (Caplan, 1964). The first objective is to make certain that people have adequate provision for basic needs. For the community health nurse, this goal involves health promotion. Any activity that fosters healthful practices and counteracts unhealthful influences can help prevent a crisis. For instance, nurses teach and encourage safety practices in the home and workplace. They work for stronger legislation and enforcement to keep drunk drivers off the roads. They promote improved nutrition for adolescents. Healthy people have less trouble coping with crises that occur than do those in poor health.

Health promotion should deal with physical, psychological, sociocultural, and spiritual needs. Like purchasing insurance or depositing money in an account, storing up reserves in these areas safeguards clients against stressful times.

The second goal of primary crisis prevention is anticipatory action. Because maturational crises are often predictable, community nurses can help clients prepare for them. Clients can discuss with the nurse the kinds of adjustments and role changes the next transition period will require. Marcia Sand could have avoided an empty nest midlife crisis through anticipatory planning. Knowing that the children would inevitably leave home and that they contributed to her primary satisfactions in life, Marcia could have made plans to start developing new relationships and new work outlets. Placing an aging parent in a nursing home is often very stressful for the entire family, an event that anticipatory planning can make less intense, averting a crisis. Even situational crises, like many "accidents," are often predictable. There may be a family history of myocardial infarctions, for example, but family members can change life-styles to prevent heart attacks in the living generations. Making changes in diet, exercise patterns, and job choices as well as learning coping skills may greatly reduce the risks.

Anticipatory work means experiencing some of the feelings of loss, tension, or anxiety before the crisis-precipitating event occurs (Lawler and Yount, 1987). It is much easier to do this at a time when energy and intellectual processes are at a high level of functioning. Anticipatory work dissipates the impact of the crisis event (Christensen and Harding, 1985). Grief work, for example, can begin before the terminally ill family member actually dies. If such preparations are made, a crisis of large proportions can thus be prevented.

SECONDARY PREVENTION

Secondary crisis prevention focuses on early detection and treatment. It seeks to reduce the intensity and duration of a crisis and to promote adaptive behavior. Community health nurses often encounter clients in the early stages of a crisis. A mobile home community, devastated by a tornado, can be provided with emergency assistance to prevent group disintegration and mental health problems.

During the course of normal practice, community health nurses can watch for signs that people may be entering a crisis. By considering suspect any event that might potentially provoke crisis, the nurse can monitor clients' responses. Several simultaneous or rapidly succeeding stress events may forecast impending crisis. One family appeared to handle a job loss well; family members coped adequately with the death of a grandparent a few weeks later. However, their crisis became full-blown when the mother of the family learned that she needed surgery. Nursing intervention at an early stage could have prevented the crisis from reaching major proportions and enabled the family to regain equilibrium sooner.

TERTIARY PREVENTION

Tertiary crisis prevention involves reducing the amount and degree of disability or damage resulting from crisis. Although it involves rehabilitative work, it can help clients' recovery and reduce the risk of future crises (McCombie, 1980). In this sense, it is a preventive measure. Clients can easily become caught in a web of maladaptive responses. For instance, workers laid off from their jobs may remain bitter and hostile, and reinforce one another's heavy drinking. A grieving widower continues for months or years to deny his wife's death, withdraws socially, and develops chronic physical problems. A person in the crisis of old age cannot accept her aging and adopts bizarre and offensive dress and mannerisms. Tertiary crisis prevention involves helping these clients to face the reality of their present situations and to develop improved coping skills. Working with individuals in groups is a particularly effective means of providing support, reality orientation, and the prevention of further disability.

PHASES OF A CRISIS

Regardless of the kind of crisis — situational or maturational — people follow a fairly predictable pattern when they respond to the event and seek to regain equilibrium. This pattern progresses in four phases — shock, withdrawal, acknowledgment, and resolution (Caplan, 1964; Fink, 1967; Murray and Zenter, 1985). (See Table 12-2.) These phases correspond in many respects to Kübler-Ross' stages of dying: shock, denial, anger, bargaining, and acceptance (Kübler-Ross, 1969).

Table 12-2
Phases of Crisis

Phase	1. Shock	2. Defensive Retreat	3. Acknowledgment	4. Adaptation
Duration	Hours	Days	Weeks	Months
Perception of reality	Momentarily clear, then clouded	Avoids or denies reality	Gradually faces reality	Tests reality
Emotional response	Numb, then anxious, helpless, overwhelmed	Indifferent, euphoric, or angry	Depressed (agitated, apathetic, or bitter)	Less anxious, more optimistic
Cognitive ability	Unable to plan, reason, or comprehend situation	Rigid, narrowly focused, resistant to change	Disorganized, begins redefinition and problem solving	Reorganized, effective reconstruction
Behavior	Disoriented, unable to cope	Fight or flight	Reoriented toward coping, purposeful	Mastery and stabilizing efforts

Source: Adapted from S. L. Fink (1967).

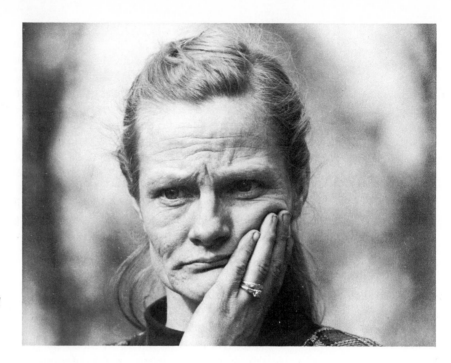

Figure 12-3
A crisis can throw people into severe disequilibrium. This woman waits for word of her coal-miner husband who is trapped in a mine accident in West Virginia.

SHOCK

The shock, or impact, phase occurs when clients encounter the crisis situation. For the first few moments or even hours, people are primarily aware of the event itself. Their homes are gone; their jobs have ended. However, the significance of that knowledge has not yet been absorbed. The impact of the shock leaves them feeling numb or indifferent, possibly even momentarily euphoric. Then a period of realization follows when panic sets in. They feel overwhelmed, anxious, and helpless (Figure 12-3). Their perception of reality becomes clouded, and it becomes difficult to make plans, think logically, or understand the situation. This stage is, in many respects, the same as Kübler-Ross' shock stage. During the shock phase, clients may try usual problem-solving means but without success. Self-esteem is threatened, and behavior is disorganized and disoriented. Clients at this point are usually receptive to suggestions and assistance. The entire shock phase generally lasts only a few hours, although in some instances it may extend into days.

DEFENSIVE RETREAT

As clients move into phase 2, defensive retreat, their chief efforts are aimed at reducing the stress of the moment. At first, they may directly confront the problem with previously effective strategies. Flood victims may say, "This is tough, but we've handled tough problems before. We can do it again." However, the demands of the situation are such that stress remains. They may unrealistically try to redefine the problem by saying, "We'll build again." Because they have not dealt with reality or their sense of loss and anxiety, the stress continues unabated. Out of necessity, like organisms under attack, clients respond with fight or flight. The fight response often expresses itself in attacking and blaming others for the situation. Avoidance of reality, wishful thinking, and denial represent typical attempts by people in this phase to escape the situation. The bereaved person may refuse to believe that the loved one is dead; patients with a new diagnosis of cancer will ignore it and avoid treatment. Emotional expressions in this phase fluctuate between indifference, apathy, euphoria, and anger. As though people wore blinders, there is a narrowing of focus, a progressive rigidity in thinking, and a strong resistance to viewing the situation in any other way.

Some people find it difficult to leave the defensive retreat phase of crisis. Corresponding to Kübler-Ross' second stage, their denial temporarily provides security behind which they can hide; they can avoid the harshness of reality. It also offers a brief respite, a time for recouping energy needed to regain equilibrium. In this sense, denial may be useful as a stepping stone toward healthy adaptation. People in defensive retreat may experience denial in the first part of this phase and move on to anger in the latter part of the phase. Again, much like Kübler-Ross' third stage, anger replaces denial. "Why did this happen to me?" they ask. "It isn't fair," they cry. Extended denial or anger, a maladaptive response, leads to poor physical, mental, spiritual, and psychological health.

ACKNOWLEDGMENT

The time comes when people working through a crisis must face reality. Phase 3 begins when the facts of the situation force themselves on the people involved. Gradual recognition and acceptance occur, with concomitant efforts to resolve the crisis. The people who have lost jobs, for example, can no longer deny that it has happened. There is recognition and gradual, albeit painful, acknowledgment of the loss. Assessing the situation's significance and planning for its management can now begin.

However, the harshness of reality frequently leads to depression expressed in apathy, agitation, remorse, or bitterness. Divorced persons may feel at fault or, conversely, that they have been treated unfairly. The pain of rejection, loss of relationships, and anxiety about how to cope with the present and future can all combine to create severe depression. The acknowledgment phase is a time of mourning, self-deprecation, and emotional decline. It may be marked by a period of bargaining—"If you'll help me, God, I promise to go to church regularly"—much like Kübler-Ross' fourth stage. From these feelings, however, and with outside help, a restructuring of coping abilities begins. People move from disorganized thinking to redefining and attempting to solve the problem. Their behavior becomes more purposeful, their planning more realistic. Tension, though still felt, is converted into a constructive energy force.

Again, maladaptive responses can occur when people retreat from this phase and continue to deny the problem. Some choose long-term nonreality or the more drastic escape of suicide. Most people, however, discover that the acknowledgment phase is often completed within a few weeks.

ADAPTATION

The final phase of crisis occurs as people engage in successful problem resolution and adaptation to a new life. They not only face and accept reality but test it by restructuring their lives to make them workable. The adaptation phase is marked by feelings of hope and a positive approach to problem solving. The level of anxiety diminishes as people gain a new sense of identity and self-worth. They can talk about the situation openly. They reorganize their thinking toward effective reconstruction, making the best use of their own and other available resources. Their behavior is directed toward mastering the situation and stabilizing the change. People who successfully complete the adaptation phase, which may last for weeks or months, have developed new coping abilities. They have grown stronger, more mature, and better equipped to deal with future crises. This period corresponds in many respects to Kübler-Ross' final stage of acceptance.

EMOTIONAL STAGES

It is helpful for the nurse to recognize the pattern that emotions follow throughout the crisis sequence. Emotions are initially high, then begin to decline rapidly during the shock phase as people feel overwhelmed and increasingly anxious. If it is a crisis for a group, anxiety seems to spread from one person to another. Emotional decline's lowest point occurs at the end of the defensive retreat phase, resulting in depression and exhaustion. In the acknowledgment phase, the emotional level begins to climb as people start to face and cope with reality. Finally, emotions are back to a normal level of functioning by the end of the adaptation phase (Hirschowitz, 1966).

In the crisis sequence, each succeeding phase lasts longer than the previous one; thus, an increasing amount of adaptive energy is required. Effective professional intervention may significantly reduce the length of time spent in each phase. Figure 12-4 depicts the emotional curve in relation to the varying lengths of each phase. As we mentioned previously, these phases parallel the Kübler-Ross (1969) stages of dying—shock, denial, anger, bargaining, depression, and acceptance. They have also been expressed as (1) Who, me? (2) Not me! (3) Why me? and (4) Yes, me. The latter sequence provides a colloquial but useful description of the crisis stages.

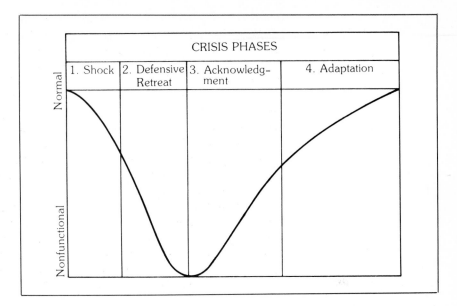

Figure 12-4
*Varying emotional levels
during crisis.*

CRISIS INTERVENTION

People in crisis need help. They often desperately want help. The crisis and its associated disequilibrium has a two-fold effect on the individuals involved. It renders them temporarily helpless, unable to cope on their own, and thus makes them especially receptive to outside influence. Also, this very desire for assistance triggers a helping response from the people nearby. Caplan (1964, p. 48) explains that "in crisis . . . , as the individual's tension rises to a climax, he begins not only to mobilize his own resources, but also to solicit help from others. The signs of his increasing tension appear to have a significant effect on others, so that they are stimulated to come to his assistance. This reciprocal pattern of seeking and offering help appears to have primitive biosocial roots; similar phenomena can be found in many social animals."

The significance of this phenomenon cannot be overemphasized. People in crisis will seek and generally receive some kind of help, but the nature of that help can rule in favor of or against a healthy outcome (Brownell, 1984). Clients' desires for assistance give the helping professional a prime opportunity to intervene; this opportunity also presents a challenge to make that intervention as effective as possible.

GOAL

The primary goal of crisis intervention is to reestablish equilibrium. Minimally that goal involves resolving the immediate crisis and restoring clients to their pre-crisis levels of functioning. Ultimately, however, intervention seeks to raise that functioning to a healthier, more mature level that will enable them to cope with and prevent future crises. As we discussed earlier, crises tend to be self-limiting, which causes intervention time to last from four to six weeks (Aguilera and Messick, 1986). The urgency of the situation and its time limitations require the prompt, focused attention of clients and nurse working together to achieve intervention goals.

METHODS

Crisis intervention in community health may utilize one or both of two approaches: generic and individual. For the majority of crisis encounters, the generic approach is more appropriate.

Generic Approach

The generic approach designs intervention to fit a particular type of crisis. That is, treatment focuses on the nature and course of the crisis, rather than on the psychodynamics of each client (Aguilera and Messick, 1986). Crisis intervention using the generic approach is tailored to a specific kind of crisis, situational or maturational, and includes four important elements: (1) direct encouragement of adaptive behavior, (2) general support, (3) environmental manipulation, and (4) anticipatory guidance (Jacobson, Strickler, and Morely, 1968). For example, the generic approach used with mastectomy clients encourages discussion and analysis of feelings, uses exercises to regain physical functioning, and creates a supportive, caring atmosphere. The nurse helps in fitting and use of prostheses, rebuilding of self-image, and strengthening of self-esteem through positive interpersonal relationships. The community nurse also prepares clients to handle future feelings of depression and anxiety related to bodily disfigurement and the possibility of metastasis.

The generic approach does not require advanced professional psychotherapy skills. More important for community health practice, it works well with families, groups, and even communities caught in crisis. The community health nurse may lead a group of cancer patients, grieving spouses, adolescents struggling with developmental crisis, or an entire community recovering from some natural disaster. The generic approach allows the nurse to intervene with any group of people who have a crisis in common. It offers a broad base of support, since such a group can offer resources for the members beyond those brought by the nurse. Whether a family or a group of divorcées, new ostomy patients, or new retirement home residents, clients can benefit from the generic approach in a time of crisis.

Individual Approach

The individual approach is used when clients do not respond to the generic approach or need special therapy. Individual crisis intervention should not be confused with individual psychotherapy. The latter tends to focus on clients' developmental past, although the extent of that focus depends on the type of psychotherapy. Crisis intervention, on the other hand, directs treatment toward the immediate state of disequilibrium, identifying its causes and developing coping mechanisms. Family members or significant others are included during the process of crisis resolution. An entire group may need this type of intervention. When this approach is needed, clients are usually referred to a professional with specialized training.

STEPS FOR INTERVENTION

Crisis intervention in community health assumes that clients have resources (Figure 12-5). If their potential for managing stressful events can be tapped, people in crisis will need minimal direct assistance. In accordance with the self-care concept, crisis intervention seeks to identify and build on client strengths. Aguilera and Messick (1986) outline a series of four steps for intervention during crisis: assessment, planning, intervention, and resolution.

Assessment

Initially, the nurse must assess the nature of the crisis and the clients' response to it. How severe is the problem, and what risks do the clients face? Are other people also at risk? Assessment must be rapid but thorough, focusing on some specific areas.

Figure 12-5
Many women minimize midlife crisis by returning to school and starting a new career after raising their children.

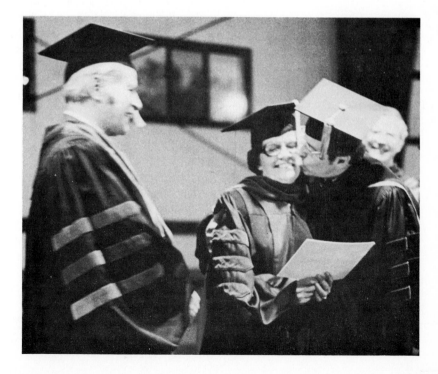

First, concentrate on the immediate problem in order to make an accurate diagnosis. Why have clients asked for help right now? How do they define the problem? What happened to precipitate the crisis? When did it occur? Was it a sudden accidental event or a slower developmental one?

Next, focus on the clients' perceptions of the event. What does the crisis mean to them, and how do they think it will affect their future? Are they viewing the situation realistically? When crisis occurs to a family or group, some members see the situation differently from others. During intervention, all should be encouraged to express themselves, to talk about the crisis, and to share their feelings about its meaning. Acceptance of the range of feelings is important.

Determine what persons are available for support. Consider family, friends, clergy, other professionals, community members, and agencies. To whom are clients close and whom do they trust? One advantage of group intervention is that the members provide some of this support for each other. In subsequent sessions, the *quality* of support should be evaluated. Sometimes a well-meaning individual may worsen the situation or deter clients from facing and coping with reality.

Next, assess the clients' coping abilities. Have they had similar kinds of experiences in the past? What techniques have they previously used to relieve tension and anxiety? Which ones have they tried in this situation, and if they have not worked, why not? Clients should be encouraged to think of other stress-relieving techniques, perhaps ones used formerly, and to try them.

Finally, and of crucial importance, find out if there is a possibility of suicide or homicide. Ask directly and specifically about any plans or hints of anyone to kill himself or anyone else. If plans are specific and the threat appears real, psychiatric referral is indicated. Do not discount threats as idle talk.

Planning Therapeutic Intervention

Several factors influence the extent of the clients' disequilibrium; try to determine them before making intervention plans. The major balancing factors — clients' perceptions of the event, situational supports, human resources, and clients' coping skills — have been assessed in the first step (Aguilera and Messick, 1986). While continuing to explore these, the nurse now also considers clients' general health status, age, past experiences with similar types of situations, sociocultural and religious influences, and the actual assets and liabilities of the situation. This additional assessment helps to clarify the situation and gives the nurse the opportunity to further encourage clients' participation in the resolution process. If clients remain in the defensive retreat phase of crisis, they can complete only simple tasks until they face reality and begin problem-solving.

The plan is based on the kind of crisis (situational or maturational, acute or chronically recurring), the crisis's effects on the clients (can they still work, go to school, keep house?), the phase of crisis the clients are in, the ways significant others are affected and respond, and the clients' strengths and available resources.

Using the problem-solving process, nurse and clients develop the plan. They review the event that precipitated the crisis, obvious symptoms, and the disruption in the clients' lives. The plan may focus on one or several areas. For instance, clients may need to grasp intellectually the meaning of the crisis, to engage in greater expression of feelings, or both. Part of the plan may be directed toward finding appropriate replacement, such as temporary housing, emergency financial aid, or physical care, for material losses. Another part may focus on helping clients to identify and use more effective coping techniques or locate supportive agencies and resource persons (McCombie, 1980). The plan will also include the development of realistic goals for the future.

Intervention

During intervention it is important for nurse and clients to continue to communicate. They should discuss what is happening, review the plan and the rationale behind its elements, and make appropriate changes in the plan when indicated. It is helpful to assign definite activities at the end of each session so that clients can try out different solutions and evaluate various coping behaviors.

The intervention step is enhanced by use of the guidelines below (Cadden, 1964; Morely, Messick, and Aguilera, 1967; Murray and Zentner, 1985).

1. *Demonstrate acceptance of clients.*
   A crisis will often shatter the ego. Clients need to feel the support of a positive, caring person who does not judge their feelings or behavior. Some negative expressions such as anger, withdrawal, and denial are normal aspects of the early phases of crisis. Accept them as normal.

2. *Help clients confront crisis.*
   Clients need to face and discuss the situation. Expressing their feelings reduces tension and improves reality perception. Recounting what has actually occurred may be painful, but it helps clients confront the crisis. Do not assume that once clients have told about the event, no further recounting is necessary. Each time the story is told, they come closer to dealing realistically with the crisis.

3. *Help clients find facts.*
   Distorted ideas and unknown factors of the situation create additional tension and may lead to maladaptive responses. For instance, it would help the Coopers to know that their son's cleft palate was unpreventable. Facts about surgical treatment and speech training would also be important for them to know.

4. *Help clients express feelings openly.*
   Suppressed feelings can be harmful. For instance, a widow may feel guilty that she is glad her husband is gone. Expression of these feelings helps reduce tension and gives clients an opportunity to deal with them.

5. *Do not offer false reassurance.*
   Clients need to face reality, not avoid it. A statement such as "Don't worry, it will all work out" is demeaning and meaningless. Rather, make positive statements about faith in their ability to cope: "It is a very difficult situation, but I believe you will be able to deal with it."

6. *Discourage clients from blaming others.*
   Clients often blame others as a way to avoid reality and the responsibility for problem solving. Withhold judgment when they blame others, but point out other causal factors and avenues for dealing with the situation.

7. *Help clients seek out coping mechanisms.*
   Explore and test old and new techniques to reduce stress and anxiety. Ask questions. What are all the things clients and nurse might do together to resolve the problem? What are the things that need to be done? What do clients think they can do? This assistance gives clients more adaptive energy to work toward resolution.

8. *Encourage clients to accept help.*
   Denial in the early phases of crisis cuts off help. Encouraging clients to acknowledge the problem is a first step toward acceptance of help. Often, however, clients fear the loss of their independence and the invasion of their privacy. They may state, "We ought to be able to handle this problem." At this point, the community nurse can assure clients that people in a crisis of this sort almost always need help. Preparing people to accept help will enable them to make the best use of what others have to offer.

9. *Promote development of new positive relationships.*
   Clients who have lost significant persons through death or divorce should be encouraged to find new people to fill the void and provide needed supports and satisfactions.

Resolution and Anticipatory Planning

In the final step, clients and nurse evaluate, stabilize, and plan for the future. First, evaluate the outcome of the intervention. Are clients using effective coping skills and exhibiting appropriate behavior? Are adequate resources and support persons available? Is the diagnosed problem solved, and have the desired results been acomplished? Analysis of these outcomes gives a greater understanding for coping with future crises.

To stabilize the change, identify and reinforce all the positive coping mechanisms and behaviors. Discuss why they are effective and explore ways to use them in future stressful situations. Summarize the crisis experience, emphasizing the clients' successes with coping in order to reconfirm progress and reinforce self-confidence. Point to evidence that they have reached their pre-crisis, or an even higher, level of functioning.

Clients' plans for the future should include setting realistic goals and means for implementing them. Review with clients how their handling of the present crisis can help them cope with, minimize, or preferably prevent future crises. A similar crisis intervention model based on Aguilera and Messick's work is proposed by Lawler and Yount (1987). They call the four stages (1) analysis, (2) design, (3) intervention, and (4) anticipatory guidance. Applied to an organizational setting, their model holds considerable potential value for community health nurses working with organizations and communities.

Summary

Crisis is a temporary state of severe disequilibrium for persons who face a threatening situation. It is a state that they can neither avoid nor solve with their usual coping abilities. A crisis occurs when some force disrupts normal functioning and thus causes a loss of equilibrium. A crisis creates tension; subsequently, efforts are made to solve the problem and reduce the tension. When such efforts meet with failure, people feel upset, redefine the situation, try other solutions, and, if failure continues, eventually reach the breaking point.

There are two kinds of crises: maturational and situational. Maturational crises are disruptions that occur during transitional periods in normal growth and development. They usually have a gradual onset and are often predictable. Situational crises, on the other hand, are precipitated by an unexpected external event. They have a sudden onset.

Crises can be prevented or their frequency and intensity can be diminished. Primary crisis prevention seeks to obstruct occurrence of crisis through promoting a high level of wellness and teaching people to anticipate and thus avoid possible crises. Secondary crisis prevention focuses on early detection and treatment. Tertiary crisis prevention seeks to reduce the degree of disability resulting from crisis.

Crises tend to progress through four stages: shock, defensive retreat, acknowledgment, and adaptation. People's perception of the crisis changes through these four stages, as do emotional response, cognitive ability, and behavior.

People in crisis both need and seek help. Crisis intervention builds on these two phenomena to achieve its primary goal — reestablishment of equilibrium. The two major methods for crisis intervention are the generic and individual approaches. The generic approach deals with a single type of crisis, such as rape, and often works with groups of people caught in the same crisis.

The individual approach is used when clients do not respond to the generic approach or need additional therapy. Crisis intervention begins with assessment of the situation; then a therapeutic intervention is planned. Next, the nurse carries out the intervention, building on the strengths and self-care ability of clients. Crisis intervention concludes with resolution and anticipatory planning to avert possible future crises.

Study Questions

1. What are the major differences between a maturational and a situational crisis? Give an example of each from your own experience.
2. Describe a maturational crisis experienced by a community known to you. What was this community's response? Describe some actions a community health nurse might have taken (alone or with a team) to help the community cope with the crisis.
3. Mobile home communities are frequent victims of tornadoes. What preventive actions could the community health nurse take? Design actions at each level of prevention.
4. Family violence is becoming an increasing public health problem. Assume that a battered wife becomes your client and you suspect there may be more women with this problem in the community. Describe how you might assist her using the crisis intervention steps. Then discuss how a three-level preventive program might be instituted in the community.

References

Aguilera, D. C., and J. M. Messick. (1986). *Crisis intervention: Theory and methodology.* 4th ed. St. Louis, Mo.: C. V. Mosby.

Brownell, M. J. (1984). The concept of crisis: Its utility for nursing. *Advances in Nursing Science* 6:10.

Cadden, V. (1964). Crisis in the family. In G. Caplan, *Principles of preventive psychiatry* (pp. 288–96). New York: Basic Books.

Caplan, G. (1964). *Principles of preventive psychiatry,* New York: Basic Books.

Christensen, S., and M. Harding. (1985). Integrating theories of crisis intervention into hospice home care teaching. *Nursing Clinics of North America* 20: 499.

Fink, S. L. (1967). Crisis and motivation: A theoretical model. *Archives of Physical Medicine and Rehabilitation* 48: 592.

Gardner, J. (1981). *Self-renewal: The individual and the innovative society* (rev. ed.). New York: Norton.

Goodman, E. (1970). *Turning points.* New York: Doubleday.

Hirschowitz, R. G. (1966). Crisis/transition sequence. In *Levinson Letter.* Cambridge, Mass.: Levinson Institute.

Holmes, T., and R. Rahe. (1967). The social readjustment rating scale. *Journal of Psychosomatic Research* 11: 213–17.

Infante, M. S. (1982). *Crisis theory: A framework for nursing practice.* Reston, Va.: Reston Publishing Co.

Jacobson, G., M. Strickler, and W. Morely. (1968). Generic and individual approaches to crisis intervention. *American Journal of Public Health* 58: 339–41.

Kübler-Ross, E. (1969). *On death and dying.* New York: Macmillan.

Lawler, T. G., and E. H. Yount. (1987). Managing crises effectively: An intervention model. *Journal of Nursing Administration* 17(11): 39–43.

Levinson, D. J. (1978). *The seasons of a man's life.* New York: Knopf.

McCombie, S. (ed.). (1980). *The rape crisis intervention handbook.* New York: Plenum Press.

Morely, W. E., J. M. Messick, and D. C. Aguilera. (1967). Crisis: Paradigms of intervention. *Journal of Psychiatric Nursing* 5: 537–40.

Murray, R., and J. Zentner. (1985). *Nursing concepts for health promotion.* 3rd ed. Englewood Cliffs, N.J.: Prentice-Hall.

Sampson, E., and M. Marthas. (1977). Theories of group development. In E. Sampson and M. Marthas (eds.), *Group process for the health professions.* New York: Wiley.

Sheehy, G. (1976). *Passages: Predictable crises of adult life.* New York: Dutton.

Underwood, M. M., and N. Fiedler. (1983). The crisis of rape: A community response. *Community Mental Health Journal* 19: 227–30.

Veninga, R., and J. Spradley. (1981). *The work-stress connection.* Boston: Little, Brown.

Selected Readings

Aguilera, D. C., and J. M. Messick. (1986). *Crisis intervention: Theory and methodology.* 4th ed. St. Louis: C. V. Mosby.

Brandon, S. (1970). Crisis theory and possibilities of therapeutic intervention. *British Journal of Psychiatry* 117: 541–45.

Brose, C. (1973). Theories of family crisis. In D. Hymovich and M. Barnard (eds.), *Family health care* (pp. 271–83). New York: McGraw-Hill.

Cadden, V. (1964). Crisis in the family. In G. Caplan, *Principles of preventive psychiatry* (pp. 288–96). New York: Basic Books.

Caplan, G. (1964). *Principles of preventive psychiatry.* New York: Basic Books.

Chandler, H. M. (1972). Family crisis intervention: Point and counterpoint in the psychosocial revolution. *Journal of the American Medical Association* 64: 211–15.

Christ, J. (1972). The adolescent crisis syndrome: Its clinical significance in the outpatient service. *Psychiatric Forum* 3(1): 25–32.

Clark, T. (1976). Counseling victims of rape. *American Journal of Nursing* 76: 1964–66.

Clark, T., and D. T. Jaffe. (1972). Change within youth crisis centers. *American Journal of Orthopsychiatry* 42: 675–79.

Cohen, A. (1982). Crisis management: How to turn disasters into advantages. *Management Review* 71: 27–40.

Collins, M. (1977). *Communication in health care: Understanding and implementing effective human relations.* St. Louis: C. V. Mosby.

Comstock, B., and M. McDermott. (1975). Group therapy for patients who attempt suicide. *International Journal of Group Psychotherapy* 25(1): 44–47.

Crow, G. (1977). *Crisis intervention.* New York: Association Press.

Dixon, S. (1979). *Working with people in crisis.* St. Louis, Mo.: C. V. Mosby.

Donner, G. J. (1972). Parenthood as a crisis. *Perspectives in Psychiatric Care* 10(2): 84–87.

Dzik, R. S. (1976). Transactional analysis in crisis intervention. *Journal of Gynecological Nursing* 5(1): 31–36.

Ebersole, P. P. (1976). Crisis intervention with the aged. In I. M. Burnside (ed.), *Nursing and the aged.* New York: McGraw-Hill.

Eisler, R., and M. Hersen. (1973). Behavioral techniques in family-oriented crisis intervention. *Archives of General Psychiatry* 28(1): 111–16.

Fallom, C. W. (1973). Providing relevant brief services to couples in marital crises. *American Journal of Orthopsychiatry* 43: 235–37.

Fink, S. L. (1967). Crisis and motivation: A theoretical model. *Archives of Physical Medicine and Rehabilitation* 48: 592–97.

Foreman, N. J., and J. V. Zerwekh. (1971). Drug crisis intervention. *American Journal of Nursing* 71: 1736–38.

Freudenberger, H. J. (1974). Crisis intervention, individual and group counseling, and the psychology of the counseling staff of a free clinic. *Journal of Social Issues* 30(1): 77–81.

Golan, N. (1969). When is a client in crisis? *Social Casework* 50: 389–91.

Goldstein, S., and J. Giddings. (1973). Multiple impact therapy: An approach to crisis intervention with families. In G. Specter (ed.), *Crisis intervention* (Behavioral Publications No. 210) (pp. 193–204). New York: Behavioral Publications.

Hall, J. E., and B. Weaver (eds.). (1974). *Nursing of families in crisis.* Philadelphia: Lippincott.

Hitchcock, J. M. (1973). Crisis intervention—The pebble in the pool. *American Journal of Nursing* 73: 1388–90.

Hoff, L. (1978). *People in crisis: Understanding and helping.* New York: Addison-Wesley.

Holstrom, L., and A. Burgess. (1975). Assessing trauma in the rape victim. *American Journal of Nursing* 75(8): 1288–90.

Hott, J. R. (1976). The crisis of expectant fatherhood. *American Journal of Nursing* 76: 1436–40.

Hott, J. R. (1977). Mobilizing family strengths in health maintenance and coping with illness. In A. Reinhardt and M. Quinn (eds.), *Current practice in family-centered community nursing.* St. Louis: C. V. Mosby.

Jacobson, G. (1974). Emergency services in community mental health: Problems and promise. *American Journal of Public Health* 64: 124–27.

Jacobson, G., M. Strickler, and W. Morely. (1968). Generic and individual approaches to crisis intervention. *American Journal of Public Health* 58: 339–41.

Kübler-Ross, E. (1969). *On death and dying.* New York: Macmillan.

Lavietes, R. L. (1974). Crisis intervention with ghetto children: Mythology and reality. *American Journal of Orthopsychiatry* 44: 241–45.

Lawler, T. G., and E. H. Yount. (1987). Managing crises effectively: An intervention model. *Journal of Nursing Administration* 17(11): 39–43.

Marks, M. J. (1976). The grieving patient and family. *American Journal of Nursing* 76: 1488–91.

Marmer, J. (1972). The crisis of middle age. In L. H. Schwartz and J. L. Schwartz (eds.), *The psychodynamics of patient care.* Englewood Cliffs, N.J.: Prentice-Hall.

McClellan, M. S. (1972). Crisis groups in special care areas. *Nursing Clinics of North America* 7: 363–71.

Messick, J. M. (1972). Crisis intervention concepts: Implications for nursing practices. *Journal of Psychiatric Nursing* 10(5): 3–7.

Morely, W. E., J. M. Messick, and D. C. Aguilera. (1967). Crisis: Paradigms of intervention. *Journal of Psychiatric Nursing* 5: 537–40.

Murray, R., and J. Zentner. (1985). *Nursing concepts for health promotion.* 3rd ed. Englewood Cliffs, N.J.: Prentice-Hall.

Nakushian, J. (1976). Restoring parents' equilibrium after sudden infant death. *American Journal of Nursing* 76: 1600–1604.

O'Brien, M. J. (1978). *Communication and relationship in nursing.* 2nd ed. St. Louis: C. V. Mosby.

Parad, H. J. (ed.). (1965). *Crisis intervention.* New York: Family Service Association of America.

Price, J. L., and C. Braden. (1978). The reality in home visits. *American Journal of Nursing* 78: 1536–38.

Rapoport, R. (1963). Normal crises, family structure, and mental health. *Family Process* 2: 68–76.

Selkin, J. (1975, January). Rape. *Psychology Today,* pp. 71–76.

Specter, G. (1973). *Crisis intervention* (Behavioral Publications No. 210). New York: Behavioral Publications.

Strickler, M., and B. LaSor. (1970). The concept of loss in crisis intervention. *Mental Hygiene* 54: 301–3.

Van Antwerp, M. (1970). Primary prevention: A challenge to mental health associations. *Mental Hygiene* 54: 453–57.

Williams, F. (1971). Intervention in maturational crises. *Perspectives in Psychiatric Care* 9: 240–42.

Woehning, M., and I. Martinson. (1975). Family nursing during death and dying. In B. W. Spradley (ed.), *Contemporary community nursing* (pp. 405–411). Boston: Little, Brown.

Zelbach, J. Z. (1971). Crisis in chronic problem families: Psychiatric care of the underprivileged. *International Psychiatry Clinics* 8(2): 101–5.

THREE Care of Communities

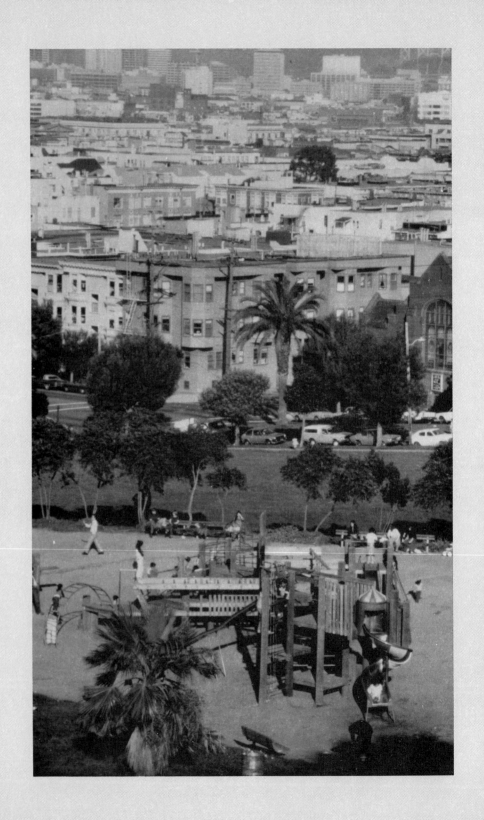

13 The Community: Assessment and Planning

A central theme of this book has been community health nursing's involvement in promoting the health of aggregates of people. This idea has been emphasized because, in both subtle and direct ways, our culture works against it. The value of individualism is one of the greatest barriers to carrying out the mission of community health nursing.

INDIVIDUALISM AND COMMUNITY HEALTH

Every society has a small number of core values that give meaning to life. In the United States, for example, we value success and material rewards. Such values provide motivation for millions of people. They uphold the work ethic; they become the measures by which we elevate successful and wealthy people to the status of popular heroes. The very existence of our society and its way of life depends on a deep commitment to such values. We learn them early in life and come to take them for granted as the way things ought to be. One value that most Americans hold as God-given, a value that profoundly influences the entire practice of nursing, is individualism.

Nearly every social observer who has written about American society has identified this value. A cornerstone of our civilization, this basic premise underlies most of our institutions. "Protect the rights of the individual"; "Equal justice for all under the law"; "Life, liberty, and the pursuit of happiness for all individuals" are familiar cries. More than 50 years ago, the sociologist Robert Lynd described this value: "Individualism, 'the survival of the fittest,' is the law of nature and the secret of America's greatness; and restrictions on individual freedom are un-American and kill initiative" (Lynd, 1939, p. 60).

We reward individual effort in the school and in the workplace. Our criminal justice system punishes individual crimes far more harshly than corporate crimes. A woman who steals five dollars in a southern state serves several years in prison; a large oil company that steals millions by overcharging customers pays a relatively small fine or suffers no punishment at all. Health care in our society is dominated by a commitment to the treatment of individuals. The vast majority of our research, personnel, and health care institutions engage in the care of individual illness rather than promote community health.

How does this value of individualism affect community health nursing? All nurses are first educated and trained in the individualistic perspective of clinical nursing. The individual patient is the focus of nursing service. Moreover, this early education is supported by powerful cultural premises; together, they create a mind-set that nurses bring into community health nursing. Unless nurses become aware of this mind-set and consciously set it aside, clients will remain individuals instead of families, groups, organizations, populations, and communities (*Redesigning Nursing Education,* 1973; Campbell, 1988).

MYTHS PERPETUATED BY AN INDIVIDUALISTIC FOCUS

The mind-set described above is influenced by three pervasive myths, all touched on in earlier chapters.

The Location Myth

Community health nursing, this myth says, is only clinical nursing outside the hospital setting. This myth silently influences nurses to think of their task as simply nursing *in* the community. Community health nursing, from this perspective, seems to have the merit of reducing hospital costs. It is *easy* to think that patients do not have to spend so much time in the hospital; health professionals can treat them and care for them in their homes. Instead, community health nursing is practice *to* and *with* the community. It may include the hospital.

The location myth defines community health nursing in terms of *where* it is practiced—a setting-based focus. On the contrary, as we discussed in Chapter 3, community health nursing focuses on assessing and treating the health needs of population groups or aggregates (Williams, 1981, 1985).

The Skills Myth

This myth states that community health nurses employ only the skills of clinical nursing when working with community clients. This myth leads many nurses to assume that their clinical skills are completely adequate for population-focused practice. It can lead them to overlook a large and sophisticated body of knowledge required for effective community health nursing.

Clinical skills that prepare nurses for decision making with individuals are very different from those required for defining problems and developing solutions for populations (Williams, 1985). To assess and manage decisions regarding a community's health status, the nurse needs skills drawn from the public health sciences in measurement and analysis (epidemiology and biostatistics), skills in social policy based on the history and philosophy of public health, and skills in management and organization for public health (Milbank, 1976). At the baccalaureate level, nurses can begin to build these skills; they can strengthen and refine them at the masters and doctoral levels.

The Client Myth

Community health nursing involves working with populations, but this myth says that the primary client is the individual within a family context. Nurses who believe in this myth are prevented from taking a broad perspective that sees the health of groups, subpopulations, communities, and populations as central to community health nursing practice. In reality, it is its population-focused practice that distinguishes community health nursing from other nursing specialties (Williams, 1985; APHA, 1981). In order to escape the constricting influence of this final myth, it is helpful to think of the scope of community health nursing practice by envisioning six levels of clients ranging from individuals to communities.

LEVELS OF COMMUNITY HEALTH NURSING PRACTICE

On a typical day as a community health nurse, you might work with clients at six different levels: individuals, families, groups, subpopulations, populations, and communities. In a city such as Atlanta, Georgia, as a community health nurse, you might leave an agency to visit an unmarried adolescent in the last trimester of her pregnancy. As you offer service to this individual, you will also assess her family as a group and seek to promote the health of that family. You might invite this young woman to a group of expectant mothers with whom you will meet that evening. Before noon, let us say that you stop by The Family Tree on Selby Avenue to meet with the staff for a discussion of how to reach the subpopulation of teenage girls in the neighborhood. In the early afternoon you meet with other staff at your agency to discuss assessing the population of unmarried, pregnant adolescents in the city of Atlanta. Before you finish your day's work, you might testify at a city council hearing on a local ordinance regarding abortion, or you might prepare a written statement for a committee hearing in the Georgia state legislature on the use of state funds for abortion by women on welfare. These last two activities involve nursing practice at the community level.

Table 13-1 summarizes some of the major differences among the various levels of practice within community health nursing. In Chapters 4 and 15 we describe the family as client, the characteristics of a healthy family, and ways to provide nursing service to families. In Chapter 14 we examine the nature of groups, what causes groups to function effectively, and how community

Table 13-1
Variations in Scope of Community Health Nursing Practice

	Client	Example	Characteristics	Health Assessment	Nursing Involvement
Individual	Individual	Kim Murphy	One person with various needs	Individual health assessment	A dyad; interaction with the individual
	Family	Murphy family (seven members)	A small group based on kin ties; specific roles	Family health assessment	Family visits; interaction with members as a group
	Group	Parenting group; Alanon club	Two or more people; face-to-face communication; interdependency	Assessment of group effectiveness in fulfilling its functions	Group participation; having a role in meetings
	Subpopulation	Unmarried pregnant adolescents in a school district	Large group sharing one or more characteristics (subset of a larger group)	Assessment of collective health problems and needs	Study of and planning for meeting specific health needs
Aggregate	Population	Homeless people in Chicago	An aggregate of people who share one or more personal or environmental characteristics	Study of health needs and vital statistics	Membership in organizations such as a health planning council
	Community	East Harlem; New York City; gay community in the United States	A large aggregate sharing geographic location or special interests	Study of community health characteristics and competence	Researching the community; planning and setting up services

health nurses can work with groups. In Chapter 14, we also discuss working with populations and subpopulations. In this chapter we focus our attention on the community as an aggregate.

Although community health nurses work at all six levels of practice, working with communities is a primary mission and is of considerable significance for two important reasons. First, the community is a collection of people who share one or more environmental characteristics, and as such, it directly influences the health of individuals, families, groups, subpopulations, and populations. When the city of Los Angeles failed to take aggressive action to stop air pollution, this failure affected the health of millions of people. Similarly, when the gay community in one city assisted health officials to identify AIDS carriers, this action affected the health of people at all the other levels. Second, working with communities is important because it is at this level that most health service provision occurs. Community agencies develop specific health programs and disseminate health information to many types of groups and populations.

The community health nurse, then, must deal with the community as the client (Anderson et al., 1986; Hanchett, 1988). Understanding the community is a prerequisite for effective service at every level of community nursing practice.

THE COMMUNITY AS CLIENT

Community is a term that we use in many different ways. Some people talk about the "community of professional nurses," those nurses who are trained and work in the field. On a small college campus in the south, students and faculty talk about the "college community." You probably think of your hometown or city as a "community." On occasion, the president of the United States will refer to the "American community." In England and France, people talk about the "European Economic Community," and representatives of the United Nations refer to the "world community."

In Chapter 1, we defined a community as having three features: (1) a location, (2) a population, and (3) a social system (Lynd, 1939). This three-dimensional view, which is similarly expressed in other writings (Wellman and Leighton, 1979; Shamansky and Pesznecker, 1981; Goeppinger et al., 1982), is represented in Figure 13-1 and especially suits our idea of a local community. The size of a local community can vary by expanding or constricting the geographic boundary. The community of Seattle, for example, may refer to the city as defined by all the people within the city limits. But we also speak of "greater Seattle," a community composed of the city, its suburbs, and many other small towns located near Seattle. For purposes of service or study, a community health nurse might want to restrict the size of the community within Seattle to the Wallingford district. If you worked in the Washington State Health Department in Olympia, you would probably think of your community as the entire state. However, all these communities still share the three common denominators of an identified location, population, and social system.

Think of these three dimensions of every community as a rough map you can follow whether you are working in a rural town of 250 people or in the city of Chicago. This concept of community is a useful tool for assessing needs or planning for service provision, whether the particular community is a refugee camp in Cambodia or the state of New Hampshire. As we consider each dimension, we will pay particular attention to the questions that must be asked to assess the health of a community.

LOCATION

Every community carries out its daily existence in a specific geographic location. The health of a community is affected by this location, by the location of health services, the geographic features, climate, plants, animals, and the

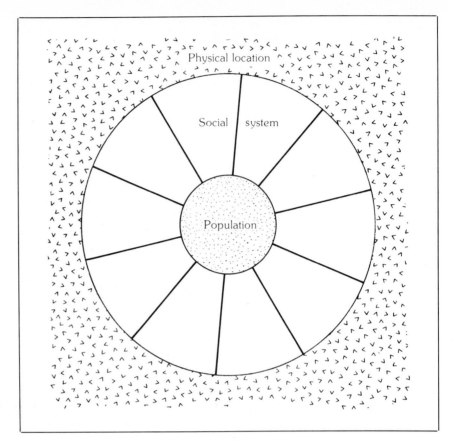

Figure 13-1
A community has (1) a physical location, represented here by the square boundary; (2) a population, shown here by the central circle; and (3) a social system, divided here into subsystems.

human-made environment (Allor, 1983). The community health nurse will want to become aware of all these location variables and their implications for community health.

The location of a community places it in an environment that offers resources and also poses threats (Neuman, 1982; Anderson et al., 1986; West, 1984). The healthy community is one that makes wise use of its resources and is prepared to meet threats and dangers. In assessing the health of any community, it is necessary to collect information not only about these location variables, but also about how the community relates to them. Do groups cooperate to identify threats? Do health agencies cooperate to prepare for an emergency such as flood or earthquake? Does the community make sure that its members are given available information about resources and dangers?

Guiding the nurse in assessing the health of any community is a Community Profile Inventory (Tables 13-2 to 13-4). It is divided into three parts — location, population, and social system — in order to conform to our definition of

Table 13-2
Community Profile Inventory: Location Perspective

Location Variables	Community Health Implications	Community Assessment Questions	Information Sources
Boundary of community	Community boundaries serve as basis for measuring incidence of wellness and illness, and for determining spread of disease.	Where is the community located? What is its boundary? Is it a part of a larger community? What smaller communities does it include?	Atlas State maps County maps City maps Telephone book City directory Public library
Location of health services	Use of health services depends on availability and accessibility.	Where are the major health institutions located? What necessary health institutions are outside the community? Where are they?	Telephone book Chamber of commerce State health department County or local health departments Maps Public library
Geographic features	Injury, death, and destruction may be caused by floods, earthquakes, volcanoes, tornadoes, or hurricanes. Recreational opportunities at lakes, seashore, mountains promote health and fitness.	What major landforms are in or near the community? What geographic features pose possible threats? What geographic features offer opportunities for healthful activities?	Atlas Chamber of commerce Maps State health department Public library
Climate	Extremes of heat and cold affect health and illness. Extremes of temperature and precipitation may tax community's coping ability.	What are the average temperature and precipitation? What are the extremes? What climatic features affect health and illness? Is the community prepared to cope with emergencies?	Weather atlas Chamber of commerce State health department Maps Local government Weather bureau Public library
Flora and fauna	Poisonous plants and disease-carrying animals can affect community health. Plants and animals offer resources as well as dangers.	What plants and animals pose possible threats to health?	State health department Poison control center Police department Emergency rooms Encyclopedia Public library
Human-made environment	All human influences on environment (housing, dams, farming, type of industry, chemical waste, air pollution, etc.) can influence levels of community wellness.	What are the major industries? How have air, land, and water been affected by humans? What is the quality of housing? Do highways allow access to health institutions?	Chamber of commerce Local government City directory State health department University research reports Public library

a community. Although not exhaustive, it suggests the implications for community health of each variable, provides a set of community assessment questions, and gives some information sources. Let us consider the six location variables that define, in part, every human community.

Table 13-3
Community Profile Inventory: Population Perspective

Population Variables	Community Health Implications	Community Assessment Questions	Information Sources
Size	The number of people influences number and size of health care institutions. Size affects homogeneity of the population and its needs.	What is the population of the community? Is it an urban, suburban, or rural community?	State health department Census data Maps City or town officials Chamber of commerce
Density	Increased density may increase stress. High and low density often affect the availability of health services.	What is the density of the population per square mile?	Census data State health department
Composition	Composition of the population often determines types of health needs.	What is the age composition of the community? What is the sex composition of the community? What is the marital status of community members? What occupations are represented and in what percentages?	Census data State health department Chamber of commerce U.S. Department of Labor Statistics
Rate of growth or decline	Rapidly growing communities may place excessive demands on health services. Marked decline in population may signal a poorly functioning community.	How has population size changed over the past two decades? What are the health implications of this change?	Census data State health department
Cultural differences	Health needs vary among sub-cultural and ethnic populations. Utilization of health services varies with culture. Health practices and extent of knowledge are affected by culture.	What is the ethnic breakdown of the population? What racial groups are represented? What subcultural populations exist in the community? Do any of the subcultural groups have unique health needs and practices? Are different ethnic and cultural groups included in health planning?	Census data State health department Social and cultural research reports Human rights commission City government Health planning boards
Social class	Class differences influence the utilization of health services. Class composition influences cost of public health services.	What percentage of the population falls into each social class? What do class differences suggest for health needs and services?	State health department Census data Sociological reports
Mobility	Mobility of the population affects continuity of care. Mobility affects availability of service to highly mobile population.	How frequently do members move into and out of the community? How frequently do members move within the community? Are there any specific populations, such as migrant workers, that are highly mobile? How does the pattern of mobility affect the health of the community? Is the community organized to meet the health needs of mobile groups?	State health department Census data Health agencies serving migrant workers Farm labor offices Programs serving transients and the homeless

Table 13-4
Community Profile Inventory: Social System Perspective

Social System Variables	Community Health Implications	Community Assessment Questions	Information Sources
Health system Family system Economic system Educational system Religious system Welfare system Political system Recreational system Legal system Communication system	Each system must fulfill its functions for a healthy community. Collaboration among the systems to identify goals and problems affects health of community. Undue influence of one system on another may lower the health of the community. Agreement on the means to achieve community goals affects community health. Communication among organizations in each system affects community health.	What are the functions of each major system? What are the major subsystems of each system? What are the major organizations in each subsystem? How well do the various organizations function? Are the subsystems in each major system in conflict? Is there adequate communication among the major systems? Is there agreement on community goals? Are there mechanisms for resolving conflict? Do any parts of the total system dominate the others? What community needs are not being met?	Chamber of commerce Telephone book City directory Organizational literature Officials in organizations Community self-study Community survey Local library Key informants

Boundary of Community

In order to talk about the community in any sense, one must first discover its boundary (Shamansky and Pesznecker, 1981). All measurements of wellness and illness within the community depend on knowing the unit under consideration. All communities are also related to other communities, however, and it is important to know about such locations. If nurses are working in a small community of 5,000 persons, they need to know whether it is part of a huge metropolis or an isolated rural town.

Location of Health Services

If the members of a town must travel 300 miles to the nearest clinic or dental office, the health of the community will be affected. When assessing a community, the community health nurse will want to identify the major health institutions and know where they are located. In one city, for example, the alcoholism treatment center for skid row alcoholics was located 30 miles outside of the city. This location profoundly affected who volunteered for treatment and how long they remained at the center. The location of services may be restricted from some members who have transportation problems. If a well-baby clinic is located on the edge of a high-crime district, parents may avoid using it. It is often enlightening to place the major health institutions, both inside and outside the community, on a map that shows their proximity and relation to the community as a whole.

Geographic Features

Communities have been constructed in every conceivable physical environment. Mountain communities face problems that are foreign to a desert town. A healthy community takes into consideration the geography of its location, identifies the possible problems and likely resources, and responds in an adaptive fashion (Neuman, 1982).

In Anchorage, Alaska, the community is set in the midst of mountains and almost on top of a geologic fault line. The same is true for San Francisco, where in 1906 a massive earthquake destroyed many buildings and fire swept through the city. Seven hundred persons died. In such places, the health of the community is partly determined by its preparedness for an earthquake and its ability to cope when such a crisis occurred.

A geographic feature such as a lake offers food supplies for community members. A healthy community uses such a local resource in many ways: as a source of food, recreation, or water supply. The same resource, however, can also present a public health danger if drownings or contamination of fish occur. Sometimes the contamination comes from far distant communities; for example, "over 90 percent of the acid rain falling in Minnesota originates outside the state" (Northern States Power, 1987). In Ontario, Canada, a series of lakes called the Lac la Croix is a valuable resource for the Ojibway Indian communities. They depend on fish from the lakes for their livelihood. In recent years, however, acid rain has begun to affect the lakes and the fish. Coal-burning power plants in the United States and Canada emit large amounts of sulfur dioxide that rise high in the air and are then blown by strong winds over the Lac la Croix chain of lakes. In the atmosphere, the sulfur dioxide reacts with water vapor to form sulfuric acid, which then falls to earth in the rain and snow, eventually finding its way into the lakes. As the acidity of lakes rises, the egg-producing ability of the fish drops. More immediately, the acid in the water changes mercury in the lake sediment into methyl mercury, which is easily absorbed by the fish. A major food supply has thus become contaminated for the Ojibway Indian communities.

Climate

The climate also has a direct influence on the health of a community (Green and Anderson, 1986). When Buffalo, New York, is blanketed with deep winter snows, members of this community are sometimes immobilized for days. Deaths from coronary occlusions increase as people attempt to shovel their walks and uncover their cars. The intense summer heat of another location, such as Phoenix, Arizona, can create other health problems. Skin cancer, for example, is highest in states that constitute the Sun Belt. A healthy community will encourage physical activity among its members, but the climate, in turn, affects this activity. Although long cold winters can restrict activity, one community, St. Paul, Minnesota, holds an annual Winter Carnival, which includes sporting events. Parades, ice sailing, dogsledding, a treasure hunt, and hot air balloon races bring thousands of people outdoors at a time when they might otherwise be confined by the weather.

Flora and Fauna

Plant and animal populations in a community are often determined by location. The way a community responds to these populations, whether wild or domesticated, can affect the health of the community. In Covina, California, black widow spiders make up part of the local insect population. The poison from a single bite may cause injury and death. In Seattle, Washington, a bushy, attractive plant, known as Deadly Nightshade, grows in yards and vacant lots. It has an appealing black berry that appears edible. However, it contains the drug belladonna, and people have died from ingesting the berries. The community health nurse will want to know about the major sources of danger from plants and animals in the community. Are there community agencies that provide educational information about these dangers? Does the populace understand their significance? Are emergency services, such as a poison control center, available to community members?

Human-Made Environment

Every community is located in the midst of an environment created and transformed by human ingenuity. We build houses and other buildings; we dump wastes into streams or vacant lots; we fill the air with gasses; we build dams to control streams. All these human alterations of the environment have important implications for community health (Blumenthal, 1985).

A community health nurse might improve the health of a community by working for legislation to prevent disposing of waste chemicals into water or landfills. Had such legislation been passed years ago, the disaster at New York's Love Canal, where toxic wastes are still seeping into the homes and yards of victimized citizens, might have been prevented.

One way in which we alter the environment is through agricultural activity. Southern Wisconsin is in the heart of midwestern farm country. The rich harvests attract thousands of seasonal workers, farm migrants, every year. Because of their nomadic life-style and their rural location, the health of migrants suffers. Community assessment in this area would include a careful examination of the migrant population, the health services available to them, their housing accommodations, and the community's economic resources.

Every community exists in some physical location. This fact has important implications for the community's health and any plans to assess or improve it. Table 13-2 shows the first part of a provisional assessment tool, the Community Profile Inventory. It will help the nurse sense the health implications of geographic location as well as give some direction for assessing the health of any community.

POPULATION

When we consider the community as the client, the second dimension to examine is the population of the total community. As we will discuss in Chapter 14, one level of practice in community health nursing is working with special population groups. These population groups may be within a community or cut across many communities (Anderson et al., 1986). For example, health care for the elderly population may be carried out in a city such as Des Moines, Iowa, or in the entire state of Iowa. From the perspective of the community itself, however, the population consists not of a specialized aggregate, but of all the diverse people who live within the boundaries of the community. As Sanders and Brownlee (1979, p. 413) have said, "A community can be viewed as a population, as a collection of people. Health authorities conduct demographic analyses in order to determine the extent of maternity, morbidity, and mortality within a community."

The health of any community is greatly influenced by the population that lives in it. Different features of the population suggest health needs and provide a basis for health planning (Dever, 1980). A healthy community has leaders who are aware of the population's characteristics, know its different needs, and respond to those needs. Community health nurses can better understand any community by knowing about population size, density, composition, rate of growth or decline, cultural differences, social class, and mobility (Figures 13-2 and 13-3). Let us consider each of these population variables briefly.

Size

The town of Dover, Delaware, with less than 10,000 people, and the city of Los Angeles, California, have radically different health problems. If a single case of salmonella poisoning occurred in Dover, health officials would likely learn of it. It would be relatively easy to trace the course, check the few restaurants in town, and interview people about sanitation practices. However, many cases might occur in Los Angeles without the health department's knowledge. Moreover, if these cases were discovered, tracing the source of contamination might involve a long and complicated search. This is only one small way in which population size might affect the health of a community, but it also would influence the presence of slums, heterogeneity of the population, and almost every conceivable area of health need and service. One of the first things community health nurses need to know about a community is its size.

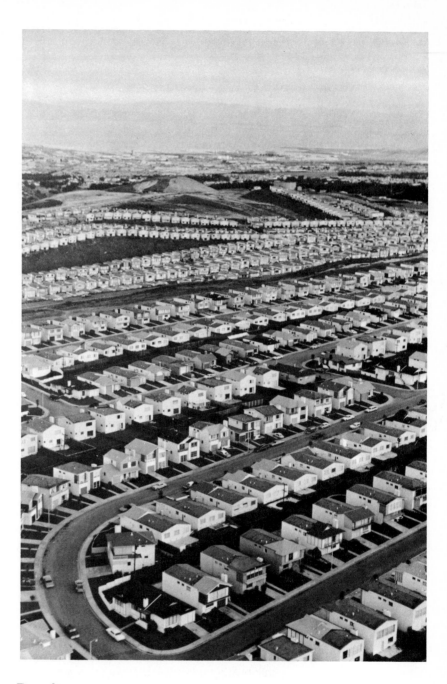

Figure 13-2
Many factors affect a
community's health. Urban
sprawl, shown here in this
San Francisco suburb,
influences commuting
distance to work, pressures
to conform to neighborhood
standards, and many other
variables affecting life-style
and health.

Density

In some communities, thousands of people are crowded into high-rise housing. In others, such as farm communities, people live at great distances from
one another. We do not yet know the full impact of living in high-density com-

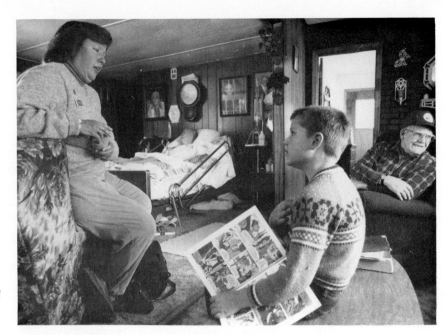

Figure 13-3
A community's resources, including its available services, profoundly affect its health. Here a homebound client's husband and grandson discuss care needs with the nurse.

munities, but some research has already shown that crowding affects individual and community health. A study of Ohio farmers, living in low-density communities, suggested that the absence of stress from crowding may have contributed to their reduced rate of coronary artery disease (Nagi, 1959).

A low-density community may have other problems. When people are spread out, health care provision may become difficult. There may not be enough resources in the form of taxes to support public health services. Rural communities often suffer from inadequate supplies of health care personnel, ranging from private physicians to community health nurses. A healthy community will take into consideration the density of its population. It will organize in ways to meet the differing needs created by its density levels; for example, it will recognize differences in density between the inner city and the suburbs and allocate services accordingly.

Composition

Communities differ in the types of people who live within their boundaries. A retirement community in Florida whose members are mostly over 65 years of age has one set of problems. A city with a large number of women in the childbearing years will have another set of problems. A healthy community is one that takes full account of, and provides for, differences in age, sex, educational level, and occupation of its members.

Occupations may be diversified among many industries or concentrated in a single field. In a town where 75 percent of the workers are employed by a textile mill, the community lives under the threat of brown lung disease, caused by cotton dust. Some textile mill communities ignored this danger, did nothing to inform workers of the dangers they faced, and provided little help for older workers who were laid off as a result of contracting this disease. A community nurse working to improve the health of this type of community would need to visit the textile mill, check on safety precautions such as face masks, and work to instigate regular lung examinations for all workers. Community leaders would have to be made aware of the problem. Such a nurse might find it necessary to become an advocate for workers and to encourage their organizing to negotiate with the textile mill managers for improved conditions in the mill. Understanding a community's composition is an important early step in determining its level of health.

Rate of Growth or Decline

Community populations change over time. Some grow rapidly, thus placing extreme demands on the provision of health services. Others, because of economic change, may decline. Any significant fluctuation in population size can affect the health of the community. As people leave to find new employment or better living conditions, overall consumption of goods and services drops. Community morale may suffer, and community leadership may decline. Even a stable community may have problems; for instance, members may resist needed change because they see little fluctuation in their population.

Cultural Differences

A community may be composed of a single cultural group. A Pennsylvania farming town may share a common commitment to its traditional Pennsylvania Dutch heritage. An Indian reserve in Washington state may reflect a single cultural tradition of Snohomish Indians. In many communities, however, several cultures or subcultures may be present. If a city has a large Hispanic population, a cluster of Native Americans who live in the inner city, and a scattering of Vietnamese refugees, the cultural differences among these members will influence the health of the community. These differences, for example, can create conflicting or competing demands for resources and services or create intergroup hostility. A university town in a southern state had a large influx of students from Iran, Iraq, Greece, Turkey, Saudi Arabia, and other Middle Eastern countries. When Iranian militants in Teheran held American citizens hostage, their action had a direct effect on the university town. A healthy community is aware of such cultural differences and moves quickly to promote understanding between subcultural groups.

Social Class

Social class refers to the ranking of groups within society by income, education, occupation, prestige, or a combination of these indexes (Goode, 1977). Upper-class people are generally rich, educated, and in the most powerful positions. Lower-class people tend to be uneducated, poor, held in low esteem, living on subsistence incomes or less, and powerless. In between is the group that makes up the majority of the population—the middle class. Professionals and white-collar workers form a large portion of this group. Further class distinctions are used to designate people who fall along the wide range within the middle-class category. For instance, "lower-middle" describes people with less prestigious occupations who are less affluent and sometimes less educated than most middle-class people but not truly "poor." There is no absolute agreement on the income amounts used to designate each category other than the government formula used to compute poverty level. Nor is there agreement on other indexes; consequently, the labeling tends to be very subjective. Although class distinctions are arbitrary, class rankings by such indexes as occupation or wealth (income plus assets) correlate with many different social patterns and are used frequently as research measures. Occupational level, in particular, has proven a reliable measure with extraordinarily similar rankings among all societies for which there are data. The reason for this, Goode (1977, p. 272) points out, is that "people at higher occupational levels enjoy higher incomes; typically they have more education; they have more political influence; and they receive more esteem from others."

Educational level, which is closely associated with social class, "is the most powerful determinant . . . with regard to influence on health-related behavior" (Green and Anderson, 1986, p. 35). People with higher educational attainment tend to be healthier, respond more readily to health professionals' interventions, and are more likely to modify their behavior in positive, health-enhancing ways. These modifications may include smoking cessation, weight control, exercise, dental care, and use of immunizations. Persons in the lower strata of society frequently have the worst health and are more difficult to reach with health information; they also tend to have a higher incidence of communicable diseases. "In general, preventive health services and health promotion activities are most needed by members of low-income groups and individuals of less educational attainment, but all people in a community will benefit from an overall community health program" (Green and Anderson, 1986, p. 35).

Some communities appear to be primarily middle class; others have large numbers of lower-class members. Still other communities may have a sprinkling of each social class. We know that social classes have different health problems, resources for coping with illness, and ways of using health services (Freeman, Levine, and Reeder, 1979). A healthy community recognizes these differences and creates health care services to meet these varied needs.

Mobility

American people are a mobile population. We move to go to college, take new jobs, or seek new climates upon retirement. This mobility has a direct effect on the health of communities. If the population turnover is extensive, continuity of care may suffer. Leadership for improving the health of the community may change so frequently that concerted action becomes difficult. High turnover may require special attention to health education about local conditions.

Population groups may arrive and depart in seasonal swings; migrant farm workers, tourists, and college students can affect a community. The community health nurse will want to identify those populations that are seasonally mobile. They not only present special health needs, but may place an added burden on a community. If a town of 3,000 people has an annual influx of 10,000 students who disappear in the summer, members must prepare to meet this population change. A healthy community neither ignores nor over-reacts to this kind of mobility. Rather, it identifies the nature of population change, determines the needs created by such change, and organizes to meet those needs.

As community nurses consider the population dimensions of the community, they will take a long step toward uncovering the true character of the community. Each of the variables related to population will suggest clues to the relative health of the community itself. Table 13-3 presents the second part of the Community Profile Inventory. It identifies seven population variables, suggests some implications for community health, and provides several community assessment questions as well as possible sources of information.

SOCIAL SYSTEM

In addition to location and population, every community has a third dimension: a social system. A social system consists of parts, such as the local government, churches, families, and hospitals, that are linked together (Anderson et al., 1986). The parts interact with and influence each other. Whether assessing a community's health, developing new services for the elderly within the community, or promoting the health of several families, the community health nurse needs to understand the community as a social system. A community health nurse working in a tiny village in Alaska needs to grasp the social system of that village no less than a nurse working in Washington, D.C., needs to understand the social system of our country's capital.

Case Study of One Community

A social system is an abstraction. For this reason, it can be elusive and difficult to grasp. Let us start with a specific example of a community of 20,000 people, which we will call Centerville. If you visited Centerville, you would not see the social system. It does not exist as a concrete reality, something that you can see, touch, or smell. What you would observe in Centerville is people. They would be walking, talking, playing, paying bills, performing surgery, saying prayers, water skiing, voting, and doing all the other things common in a community. Where, then, is the social system of Centerville? We can see how social scientists conceive of a community's social system by focusing briefly on a single individual.

Consider Marian Branch, mother of four children, director of the Centerville Public Health Nursing Agency. If you followed Marian Branch around for a few days, you would notice that she repeats certain activities. She prepares breakfast for her family each morning; she meets with her staff each day at the agency; she shops for food and clothes. If you expanded your observation to several weeks or months, other patterns of behavior, such as church attendance, participation in a subcommittee of the Centerville City Council, and theater patronage, would appear.

From a social system perspective, these patterns of activities make up the roles that Marian Branch enacts in the course of her daily life. She acts in the capacity of mother, agency director, store customer, church member, and Centerville City Council subcommittee member. When we take specific actions of a person and group them into patterns, we have identified social roles. Keep in mind, however, that these roles are only abstractions from observable, concrete actions.

We can also look for patterns among roles, such as those enacted by Marian and the people whom she encounters. In doing so, we quickly discover that certain roles are closely connected: interaction occurs between mother and daughter, nursing supervisor and staff nurse, customer and sales clerk, and church member and clergyman. These new patterns that emerge among roles form the basis of *organizations*. Some organizations, such as the Branch family, are informal; others, such as the Centerville City Council subcommittee, are formal. However, all organizations are constructed from roles that are enacted by individual citizens. You can see that by discussing organizations we have moved another rung up the ladder of abstraction.

Patterns of similarity can also be found among organizations. As people move in and out of organizations, playing out their roles, they connect with people from other organizations. When a group of organizations are thus linked and when they have similar functions, we can begin to refer to community systems and subsystems. For example, as a patron of the theater in Centerville, Marian Branch participates in the recreational system of the community. The Centerville Public Health Nursing Agency is linked to the Centerville Health Department, Centerville Hospital, Centerville Nursing Home, and other organizations that make up the health system of this community. The city council is part of the political system; Marian's church is part of the religious system. These systems all interact because people, in their various roles, move into and out of organizations, connecting with other people from still other organizations.

As a rough map of a community's social system, Figure 13-4 shows the ten major systems common to all communities. The people (or population) are represented by the circle at the center. They become part of the social system by virtue of the roles they enact, roles that form organizations and ultimately one or another major community system.

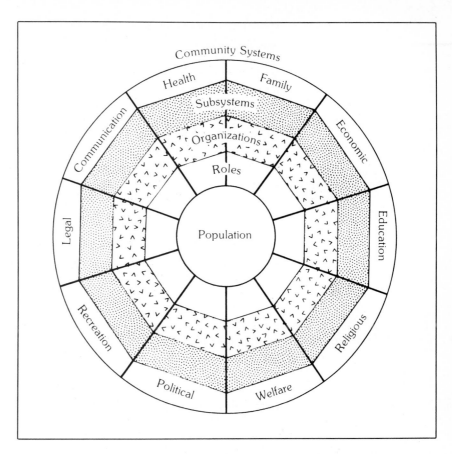

Figure 13-4
The community as a social system. Each of the ten major systems of a community includes a number of subsystems that are made up of organizations. Members of the community occupy roles in these organizations.

You may ask why it is important to understand Centerville, or any other community, as a social system. Perhaps you consider a social system as merely an abstract idea about a community. It may be abstract, but it reflects an important reality: the various community systems have a profound influence on one another. Because this interaction among parts determines the health of the whole, it is the total system that concerns community health nurses.

Let us consider one aspect of the health of Centerville. The city's department of health reported more than 75 pregnancies among teenage girls, a large number for the size of this community. This situation has placed a marked strain on the families of these girls as well as caused increased demands for services from the health system. Because the vast majority of these pregnancies are unwanted, they present a problem for the unwed teenage parents, their families, and eventually, the community. What will happen to the babies of these girls? Evidence from research suggests that, in the future, the girls are likely to have larger families, depend more frequently on the welfare system, and have a higher number of health problems than women who were not teenage mothers (Hanlon and Pickett, 1984). How is the community responding to this situation? Its response gives us clues to the overall health of Centerville.

For one thing, the problem has been ignored, a sign of defense rather than adaptation. When it does come to public attention, it divides various groups. Families blame the schools; school officials in turn blame the changing sexual mores represented in motion pictures. Some members of the health system asked Planned Parenthood to set up an office and clinic in Centerville in an effort to resolve the problem. Almost immediately, however, the religious system entered the picture with groups forming to picket Planned Parenthood facilities because of the association's stand on abortion. Planned Parenthood set up its office in an old restaurant on the edge of one business district in Centerville. Individuals from the religious and economic system (local businessmen) joined to file suit to prevent Planned Parenthood from occupying the old building. Within months, every major system of this community was involved in the problem, yet it was as far from solution as ever. Indeed, the original problem had almost fallen by the wayside as community members fought over the issues of abortion and the Planned Parenthood headquarters. Vandals set several fires that destroyed part of the building. Pickets daily called attention to this unwanted health agency. Moreover, in the midst of the trouble, more teenagers, some with parents who were deeply involved in the conflict, became pregnant.

Community health nurses work in such community situations. Their goal is to assess the community's level of health, identify needs, set priorities, and then work with community members to raise the level of health. It is a complex and challenging task. All the ways to assess the community as a social system cannot be described within the scope of this chapter, but the last part of the Community Profile Inventory (Table 13-4) suggests some of the health implications for the major systems. It also offers some suggestions for making an assessment of each system. Hanchett's (1988) discussion of nursing frameworks for community assessment provides information for further study.

The Health System as Part of a Community

Although community health nurses must have some understanding of all the systems in a community and how they interact, the health system is of particular importance. Let us compare community assessment, for a moment, with individual health assessment. Then we can examine the health system in greater depth, as an example of how a community health nurse might conduct a more detailed study of a community.

Initial assessment of individuals begins with a survey of major systems. One does not begin by minutely examining the health of each cell, but concentrates instead on the overall condition of the individual. This survey usually involves a head-to-toe examination during which one looks for indications of wellness and illness in the respiratory, musculoskeletal, glandular, skin, and circulatory systems, among others.

Initial assessment of a community also begins with a survey of major systems. Instead of asking, "Is the traffic policeman doing his job?" or "Is the mayor an effective leader?" one would inquire about the political system as a whole. What are its constituent parts? Are there any signs of health or illness?

When beginning an examination of a single person, the nurse asks whether the major body systems are functioning well or poorly. Pulse rate and blood pressure checks provide information about the level of functioning in the circulatory system. In order to answer questions about a system's level of functioning, one must first know its function — that is, the job it has to do as part of the larger system, the body.

The same holds true for community assessment. The nurse might ask, for example, "How well does the communication system keep citizens informed about important matters?" This question implies that this system has a basic function, information dissemination. The nurse might also ask, "Does the educational system offer equal education to all children of the community?", which implies that this system's function is to offer learning opportunities to everyone in a particular age group.

Each of the major systems in Figure 13-4 has developed over time in a community to meet the needs of its members. The major function of the health system is to promote the health of the community. Community assessment does not merely ask if, but also how well, the system is functioning. What is the level of health promotion as carried out by the health system of a community? In order to answer this question, which can be applied to any system, one needs a clear notion about the subsystems, organizations, and roles that make up the system.

Let us say that in examining an individual patient, you have surveyed all the general systems of the body and discovered that the person has an elevated blood pressure. You will now want to move from your initial survey to a more detailed examination of the circulatory system or other parts of the body. Any evidence of inadequate functioning becomes a warning signal for more careful assessment.

The same rule should be followed in community assessment. The rate of teenage pregnancies in Centerville signals inadequate functioning of some systems; perhaps the family, educational, religious, health, or all these systems need improvement. Thus, you want to take a closer look. What community values influence sexual behavior among adolescents? What sex education programs are available to this population? Does the health system provide information and counseling? Like high blood pressure in a single person, this sign in Centerville may quickly lead to discovery of many other underlying problems. They might require care as simple as regular exercise or as complicated as major surgery, each solution translated into community terms.

What are the components of the health system? Figure 13-5 abstracts one segment from our illustration of the community social system — the health system. It is composed of eight major subsystems, each with one or more organizations. Although the community health nurse must be aware of all

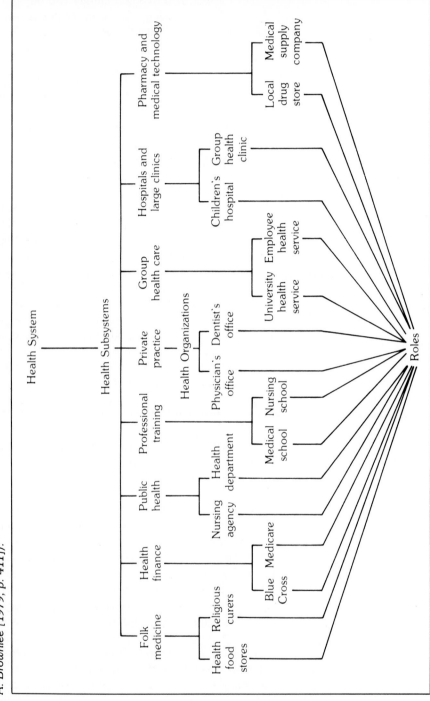

Figure 13-5
Components of the health system. (For a detailed discussion of the health system with slightly different categories of subsystems, see I. T. Sanders and A. Brownlee [1979, p. 411]).

the systems in a community, the health system is of central importance. Figure 13-5 shows some representative types of organizations for each of the major subsystems. Keep in mind that each of these organizations also has members with many different roles, and that the health of the entire system depends, in part, on how well these roles are carried out.

COMMUNITY DYNAMICS

Our discussion to this point may have suggested that the community is a rigid structure composed of a geographic location, a population, and a social system. Yet every community has a dynamic quality. Think of the diagram in Figure 13-4 as a wheel that turns rather than as a static structure. Two factors in particular affect community dynamics: citizen participation in community health programs and the power and decision-making structure of the community (Lynd, 1939; Green and Anderson, 1986).

In some communities, citizens show little concern about public health issues. They expect health officials to take the entire responsibility: "That's what we pay them to do." When apathy abounds, community health nurses will probably have to work on community education and awareness. In other communities, participation may be widespread but either uninformed or obstructive. The example of the Planned Parenthood Clinic in Centerville suggests that citizens can block the development of some programs or at least hamper them. It is much more difficult to work in a community where groups have become polarized by issues such as abortion and fluoridation. Assessing the type and extent of citizen participation will be a necessary first step in community work.

The goal of encouraging responsible participation touches on the concept of self-care discussed in earlier chapters. One goal of community nurses when working with families or groups is to encourage people to take responsibility for their own health care. They have the right to make decisions, to have adequate information, and to consult widely about their own health. The nurse's role is to encourage the full development of a self-care attitude. On a community level, self-care occurs when citizens become committed to the goal of a healthy community (Figure 13-6). Such a commitment includes responsible involvement in assessing, planning, and carrying out programs to meet community needs (Kinlein, 1978). Community self-care is community health nursing's goal.

The second factor, the power and decision-making structure, is a central concern to anyone wishing to bring about change. The description of the community as social system may suggest that power and decision making reside primarily in the political system, but that is not the case. Sanders and Brownlee (1979, p. 421) have argued against oversimplifying the decision-making process: "In its naïvest, simplest terms this [oversimplification] blandly

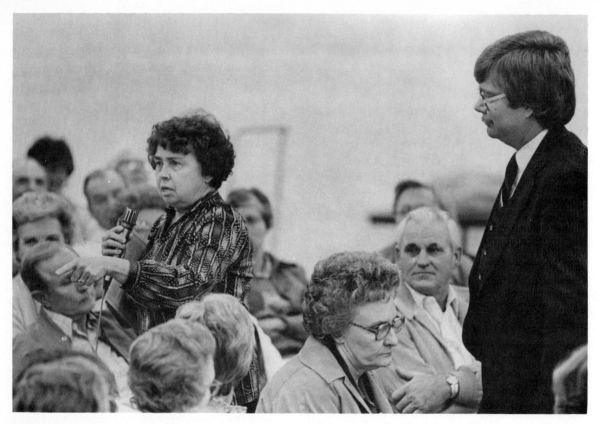

Figure 13-6
A healthy community encourages its citizens to participate in decision making.

states that (1) every community has an identifiable power clique and (2) that if you get the members on your side, all of your problems will be solved."

Decision making in any community is much more complex than this description. Sanders and Brownlee (1979) suggest that power is distributed unevenly among members of organizations in various community systems. A *key leader* may have influence in more than one system, but that power will be diffuse. Seldom does a public health official have power in the religious system or a clergyman in the legal system. A *dominant leader* is one who has specific power, but only within a single community system. An *organizational leader* will have power, but only within a single organization, not in the entire system. Sanders and Brownlee also say that key and dominant leaders will often work through other, less powerful leaders, which they call *functionaries, issue leaders,* and *spokesmen.* We will return to the topic of leadership and the types of leaders in Chapter 20.

Although power and decision making in any community are complex, Sanders and Brownlee (1979) do suggest several propositions to use as general guidelines for understanding this aspect of a community's dynamics.

1. Because communities differ widely in their power structures, do not assume that what you know about one community will be true of another.
2. The leaders within the health system have different degrees of power and varying spheres of influence; a knowledge of these differences is prerequisite to effective community work.
3. Those leaders whose power is limited to the health system or organizations often have a network of contacts with similar leaders in other systems. Many of the decisions are made informally through this network.
4. Power does not automatically flow through the established bureaucratic channels. Locate the informal patterns of power and decision making.
5. Beware of leaders who speak authoritatively on issues outside their sphere of power. Their power may be more apparent than real.
6. Leaders from the health system may become key leaders with power that extends far beyond the health system.
7. Learn to distinguish between political, economic, and social power; then use the appropriate combination needed to promote community health issues.
8. Do not overestimate the support of key leaders or power cliques; their support may be helpful but still leave much organizational work to be done.
9. Try to encourage participation in the decision-making process at every level, from average citizen to key leader.
10. You can assume that leaders in one part of a community are ignorant of needs and problems in other parts of the system. When you contact such leaders, recognize that you will have to educate them in community health issues.

TYPES OF COMMUNITY ASSESSMENT

When dealing with an individual patient, it is important to know whether to record temperature and check all vital signs or recommend a complete physical examination with thorough laboratory analysis. The same is true for community assessment. In some situations, an extensive community study becomes the first priority. In others, all that is needed is a study of one system or even one organization. At other times community health nurses may need to familiarize themselves with an entire community without going into any depth—in other words, to perform a cursory examination. The type of assessment will depend on variables such as the needs that exist, the goals to be achieved, and the resources available for carrying out the study. Although it is impossible to make such a decision ahead of time, it will be much easier if the nurse beginning a study understands the several different types of community assessment.

COMPREHENSIVE ASSESSMENT

The comprehensive assessment seeks to discover all relevant community health information. It begins with a review of existing studies and all the data presently available on the community. A survey would compile all the demographic information on the population, such as its size, density, and composition. Key informants would be interviewed in every major system — educational, health, religious, economic, and others (Neuber et al., 1980). Then more detailed surveys and intensive interviews would yield information on organizations and the various roles in each organization. A comprehensive assessment would not only describe the systems of a community but also how power was distributed throughout the system, how decisions were made, and how change occurred (Green and Anderson, 1986; Hanchett, 1988).

Because comprehensive assessment is an expensive, time-consuming process, it is seldom performed. Indeed, in many cases such a thorough research plan might be a waste of resources and repeat, in part, many other studies. Performing a more focused study based on prior knowledge of needs is often a better strategy. Yet knowing how to conduct a comprehensive assessment has an important influence over the approach to a more focused study.

FAMILIARIZATION

The second kind of community assessment is also the most necessary. Familiarization involves studying data already available on a community, and probably gathering a certain amount of firsthand data, in order to gain a working knowledge of the community. Such an approach has been used in nursing students' community survey courses (Flynn et al., 1978; Ruybal, Bauwens, and Fasla, 1975; Campbell, 1988). This type of assessment is needed whenever the community health nurse works with families, groups, organizations, or populations. It provides a knowledge of the context in which these other aggregates exist.

Consider use of community familiarization when the initial concern is a single family. Let us say that you, as the community health nurse, visit the Angelo family on the edge of Philadelphia. During your first few visits, you gather information, learning that the family is Italian-American and that there are four children. The father has been out of work for six months; the oldest boy has been in trouble with the juvenile authorities; a younger child is deaf; their house appears run-down to you. You assess this family, trying to determine its coping ability, its level of health. Furthermore, because community health nursing is population-focused, your concern is not only for the Angelo family but for the population of families with similar problems that this family represents.

However, your assessment is almost impossible without further knowledge of the community. Is theirs an Italian-American neighborhood with specific cultural influences? What is the extent of unemployment in this city? What are the services for the deaf? Are all the houses in this part of town old and in need of repair? Once you begin working with the family, familiarity with the community becomes even more imperative. You discover that as a result of the Angelos' low income, family conflicts are intense. The family members seldom get out; they make almost no use of the community's recreational system. Before you can help them make use of it, however, you must find out what resources are available. As you familiarize yourself with the community, you discover a group called "Friends of the Deaf," which sponsors a group for parents of deaf children. You can now help Mr. and Mrs. Angelo become part of that group. A quick survey of the religious system in the community reveals two job transition support groups, one of which will welcome Mr. Angelo. In the meantime, you will want to find out about the welfare system and how this family and other similar families can benefit from its services. Even your own attitude will change as you study the community. For instance, if you discover that a strike closed down the plant where Mr. Angelo worked for 20 years, you can then view his and others' unemployment from a broader perspective.

However, familiarization will go beyond connecting families to the community and its resources. Whatever role nurses play in community health promotion, they will want to be making a continuous study, an ongoing assessment. Whether nurses become client advocates, working with the local government, or operate from a nursing agency serving the elderly, this kind of assessment is a prerequisite for their work.

PROBLEM-ORIENTED ASSESSMENT

The third kind of assessment begins with a single problem and then assesses the community in terms of that problem. Assume that when you check around for services available for the Angelos' deaf child, you discover that there are none. Confronted with this problem, one family with one deaf child, you could make a problem-oriented community assessment. Your first step would be to seek to discover the incidence of childhood deafness, both in the community and in the state. Second, you might begin interviewing officials in the schools and health institutions to find out what has been done in the past with such problems. You could check the local library to find out what resources are available on the subject of deafness. Do they subscribe to *The Deaf American?* Are there interpreters available for adults who use sign language? How do hospitals and courts approach deafness? Are there any clubs or other organizations for deaf adults? Is there a state school for the deaf and where is it located?

The problem-oriented assessment is commonly used when familiarization is not sufficient and a comprehensive assessment is too expensive. It is the type of assessment that responds to a particular need. The data you collected will be useful in any kind of planning for a community response to the problem.

COMMUNITY SUBSYSTEM ASSESSMENT

In the community subsystem assessment, the community health nurse focuses on a single dimension of community life. For example, the nurse might decide to survey churches and religious organizations to discover their roles in the community. What kinds of needs do the leaders in these organizations believe exist? What services do these organizations offer? To what extent are services coordinated within the religious system and between it and other systems in the community?

The community subsystem assessment can be a useful way for a team to conduct a more thorough community assessment. If five members of a nursing agency divided up the ten systems in the community, and each person did an assessment of two systems, they could then share their findings and create a more comprehensive picture of the community and its needs.

COMMUNITY ASSESSMENT METHODS

Community health needs may be assessed through a variety of methods. We will discuss two. Surveys, among the most commonly used, provide a broad range of data and are helpful when used in conjunction with other sources or when other sources are not available. According to Dever (1980, p. 147), "The basic objective of planning and conducting community health surveys is to determine the occurrence and distribution of selected environmental, socioeconomic, and behavioral conditions important to disease control and wellness promotion." Thus, the nurse may choose to conduct a survey to determine such things as health care utilization patterns, immunization levels, demographic characteristics, or health beliefs and practices. The survey method involves nine steps needed to ensure an adequate design and appropriate collection of data (Dever, 1980, p. 147):

1. *Determine the objectives.*
   a. What information is needed?
   b. Why is it needed?
   c. How accurate does it need to be?

2. *Define the study population.*
    a. What groups will be studied?
    b. What are their distinguishing characteristics (i.e., age, occupation, location)?
3. *Determine data to be collected.*
    a. What specific data will be collected (i.e., behavior, opinions, beliefs)?
    b. What sources will provide this data (i.e., records, people)?
    c. How will you measure this data?
4. *Select sampling unit.*
    a. Will it be an individual, a household, a city block?
    b. What sample size is needed?
    c. What sampling method is most appropriate and feasible?
5. *Select contact method.*
    a. What will the data gathering method/instrument be (i.e., interviews, telephone calls, questionnaires)?
    b. Will you exclude any types of organizations or facilities (i.e., omit interviews in businesses)?
6. *Develop the instrument* (i.e., construct questionnaire or interview guide).
7. *Organize and conduct the survey.*
    a. Identify and train data collectors (i.e., interviewers).
    b. Pretest and adjust instrument.
    c. Supervise actual collection.
    d. Plan for nonresponses or refusals.
8. *Process and analyze data.*
    a. Code, keypunch, tabulate?
    b. Apply appropriate statistical methods, as indicated.
    c. Determine relationships and significance.
9. *Report the results.*
    Include implications and recommendations.

A descriptive epidemiological study is another important methodology applied particularly to problem-oriented needs assessment. Its design and use are detailed in Chapter 9. Choice of assessment method varies depending upon the reasons for data collection, goals and objectives of the study, and available resources. It also varies with the theoretical framework the nurse uses to view the community (Hanchett, 1988). That is, the community health nurse's theoretical basis for approaching community assessment will influence her or his purposes and selection of methodology in conducting the assessment. For example, Neuman's health care systems model forms the basis for the "community-as-client" assessment model developed by Anderson, McFarlane, and Helton (1986). You will find additional methodology resources for assessing community health (particularly Goeppinger and Baglioni, 1986; Hamilton, 1985; Muecke, 1984; Rogers, 1984; and Ruffing-Rahel, 1985) in the list of selected readings at the close of this chapter.

THE HEALTHY COMMUNITY

Throughout this chapter, we have emphasized that community health nursing's role is to promote the health of the entire community. Included in our discussion were suggestions about the characteristics of a healthy community. But what *is* a healthy community? If health practitioners are going to assess a community, set goals for community health, plan to improve the health of a community, and work toward goals, they require some criteria of wellness, health, and competence.

To begin, there is no such thing as a perfectly healthy community. All aggregates exist in a relative state of health. New needs emerge every day; the system is threatened or weakened and must respond to maintain equilibrium. Thus, whatever the concept of a healthy community is, it will be a relative idea.

Because of their complexity, criteria for healthy communities must be discussed cautiously. At present, there is not wide agreement on such criteria. We can begin with a classic article, "The Competent Community," by Leonard Cottrell, Jr. (1976). His concept of competence is close to current ideas of wellness expressed in this text. It is important to keep in mind that this discussion of community competence refers to the collective functioning of the total community unit, not to its various parts, such as single agencies, families, or individuals (Goeppinger, Lassiter, and Wilcox, 1982). Cottrell argues that a competent community is one whose various systems have four important characteristics:

1. They can collaborate effectively in identifying community needs and problems.
2. They can achieve a working consensus on goals and priorities.
3. They can agree on ways and means to implement the agreed-upon goals.
4. They can collaborate effectively in the required actions.

These general requirements take us closer to an understanding of a healthy community. However, we must still determine the factors that enable a community's systems to work together in these ways. Cottrell (1976) suggests several essential conditions for community competence: (1) commitment of members, (2) self-awareness and awareness of others among groups, (3) clarity of situational (positional) definitions, (4) articulateness of various subgroups, (5) effective communication, (6) conflict containment and accommodation, (7) participation (community involvement), (8) management of relations with the larger society, and (9) machinery for effective decision making. Drawing from this list and other sources (Goeppinger and Baglioni, 1986; Muecke, 1984; Klein, 1986), we can use the following list as a guide for assessing a healthy community:

1. A healthy community is one in which members have a high degree of awareness that "we are a community."
2. A healthy community uses its natural resources while taking steps to conserve them for future generations.
3. A healthy community openly recognizes the existence of subgroups and welcomes their participation in community affairs.
4. A healthy community is prepared to meet crises.
5. A healthy community is a problem-solving community; it identifies, analyzes, and organizes to meet its own needs.
6. A healthy community has open channels of communication that allow information to flow among all subgroups of citizens in all directions.
7. A healthy community seeks to make each of its systems' resources available to all members of the community.
8. A healthy community has legitimate and effective ways to settle disputes that arise within the community.
9. A healthy community encourages maximum citizen participation in decision making.
10. A healthy community promotes a high level of wellness among all its members.

PLANNING FOR THE HEALTH OF A COMMUNITY

Planning for community health is based on assessment of the community. Once community health nurses have this essential information, they can determine needs, rank them, establish goals and objectives, and develop a plan of action. The nursing process, detailed in Chapter 8, again becomes an important tool to facilitate nursing practice, this time with the community as the client. The health planning process reflects most planning methods. Nutt (1984) describes five stages for developing a health program.

1. *Formulation stage*
   Define the problem and assess the need.
2. *Conceptualization stage*
   Identify and explore possible solutions.
3. *Detailing stage*
   Analyze and compare pros and cons of various solutions.
4. *Evaluation stage*
   Examine costs and benefits of each alternative solution.
   Select best plan.
5. *Implementation stage*
   Present plan to sponsoring group or agency.
   Obtain acceptance (and funding).

Throughout this chapter, we have discussed elements to consider in planning for community health. We have examined characteristics of a healthy community (one characteristic is illustrated in Figure 13-7) as a guide to assessing the health of the community that community health nurses seek to serve. Nurses also need to understand what a healthy community is in order to establish planning objectives; in other words, they need to know what to aim for. A health subsystem with deficient communication patterns, for instance, will require intervention if health care services in the community are to function effectively.

Aggregate-level nursing practice requires teamwork. The job of planning for the health of an entire community or a community subsystem requires

Figure 13-7
Healthy communities provide needed resources for all their citizens. This city park in Austin, Texas, offers scenic beauty as well as opportunities for exercise and fun.

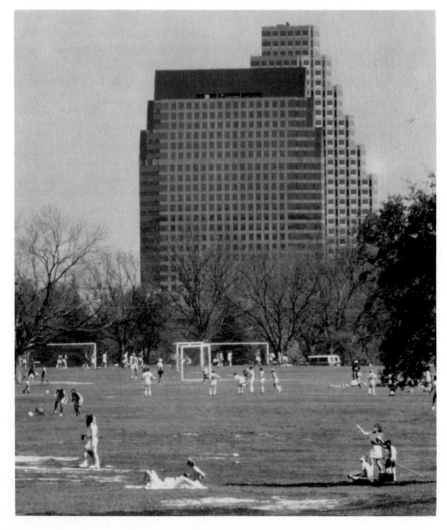

grams require, above all, more planning and coordination than do small-scale programs" (Green and Anderson, 1986, p. 40). Working with a health board task force to recommend methods for improved communication between health care agencies is one way the nurse works as a team member in serving the community as the client. All sound public health practice depends on pooling resources, including people, in ways that will best serve the public. Whether health service is aimed at the individual, family, group, subpopulation, population, or community, the consumer of that service is an equally important member of the team. In planning for a community's health, the community (represented by appropriate individuals and agencies) must be involved. Community health nurses cannot lose sight of the need for client involvement at all levels and in all stages of community health practice.

Summary

A major mission of community health nursing practice is to promote the health of aggregates of people. A strong value of individualism in the United States distracts nurses from a broad focus. It has led to three pervading myths: (1) community health nursing is only clinical nursing outside the hospital setting; (2) community health nursing employs only the skills of basic nursing when working with community clients; and (3) the primary client in community health nursing is the individual in a family context. Rather, community health nursing is practice with and to the community. It employs basic nursing expertise but adds many important concepts and skills from public health. Moreover, its practice focuses primarily on promoting the health of populations and aggregates.

Any geographic community has three important dimensions to consider when assessing its health needs: location, population, and social system. The effect of a community's location may be further analyzed by considering such variables as its boundary, location of health service, geographic features, climate, flora and fauna, and human-made environment. The health of a community is also influenced by its population. Knowledge of features, such as the population size, density, composition, rate of growth or decline, cultural differences, social class, and mobility, helps the community health nurse to better understand the community. The third dimension of a community, its social system, includes ten major systems (including the health system) and many subsystems. Each subsystem is composed of organizations whose members assume various roles. A Community Profile Inventory details the community health implications of each dimension, poses assessment questions for the nurse to ask, and suggests sources of information.

Initial assessment of a community begins with a survey of the major systems to determine how well they are functioning. Evidence of malfunctioning in any part becomes a stimulus for further and more detailed analysis.

Community dynamics, the driving forces that govern a community's functioning, also must be considered when assessing community health. Two factors, in particular, affect community dynamics: citizen participation in community health programs, and the power and decision-making structure. Community health nurses need to encourage community self-care by promoting the community's involvement in, commitment to, and responsibility for, its own health. Nurses also need to recognize the sources of community influence in order to use the system effectively to promote community health.

There are different types of community assessment. A comprehensive assessment surveys the entire community in depth, gathering thorough, original data. A familiarization assessment studies available data, perhaps adding some firsthand data, to gain a general understanding of the community. Problem-oriented assessment focuses on a single problem and studies the community in terms of that problem. Community subsystem assessment examines a single facet of community life. There are many methods for assessing a community's health. Two important ones are surveys and descriptive epidemiologic studies.

A healthy community has a number of characteristics that health practitioners look for when assessing its health. Among them are a sense of unity, ability to collaborate and communicate effectively, a problem-solving orientation, ability to utilize yet conserve resources, and ability to handle crises and conflict.

Planning for community health draws on a thorough assessment and utilizes the nursing process. Five health planning stages include (1) formulation, (2) conceptualization, (3) detailing, (4) evaluation, and (5) implementation. It involves a team effort by professionals and community personnel.

Study Questions

1. Why is it important to understand and work with the community as a total entity?
2. How does defining the total community as the client change the community health nurse's practice? List some specific examples of how this concept might be applied.
3. If you were part of a health planning team concerned about the health needs of the elderly in your community, what are some location, population, and social system variables you would want to assess? Name some of the sources from which you might collect the data.
4. Under what circumstances might you choose to conduct a problem-oriented community health assessment? What method would you consider using to conduct this assessment, and how would you carry it out?

References

Allor, M. T. (1983). The "community profile." *Journal of Nursing Education* 22(1): 12–17.

American Public Health Association. (1981). *The definition and role of public health nursing in the delivery of health care: A statement of the Public Health Nursing Section.* Washington, D.C.: The Association.

Anderson, E., J. McFarlane, and A. Helton. (1986). Community-as-client: A model for practice. *Nursing Outlook* 34(5): 220–24.

Blumenthal, D. (1985). *Introduction to environmental health.* New York: Springer Publishing.

Campbell, B. F. (1988). Program attunes students to population-focused care. *Nursing and Health Care* 9(1): 42–45.

Cottrell, L. S., Jr. (1976). The competent community. In B. H. Kaplan, R. N. Wilson, and A. H. Leighton (eds.), *Further explorations in social psychiatry* (pp. 195–209). New York: Basic Books.

Dever, G. E. A. (1980). *Community health analysis: A holistic approach.* Germantown, Md.: Aspen Systems.

Flynn, B., J. Gottschalk, D. Ray, and E. Selmanoff. (1978). One masters curriculum in community health nursing. *Nursing Outlook* 26: 633–37.

Freeman, H. E., S. Levine, and L. G. Reeder. (eds.). (1979). *Handbook of medical sociology.* 3rd ed. Englewood Cliffs, N.J.: Prentice-Hall.

Goeppinger, J., P. Lassiter, and B. Wilcox. (1982). Community health is community competence. *Nursing Outlook* 30: 464–67.

Goeppinger, J., and A. J. Baglioni, Jr. (1986). Community competence: A positive approach to needs assessment. *American Journal of Community Psychology* 13: 507–23.

Goode, W. J. (1977). *Principles of sociology.* New York: McGraw-Hill.

Green, L., and C. L. Anderson. (1986). *Community Health.* St. Louis, Mo.: Times Mirror/Mosby.

Hamilton, P. (1985). Community nursing diagnosis. *Advances in Nursing Science* 5: 21–36.

Hanchett, E. S. (1988). *Nursing frameworks and community as client: Bridging the gap.* East Norwalk, Conn.: Appleton and Lange.

Hanlon, J., and G. Pickett. (1984). *Public health: Administration and practice.* St. Louis, Mo.: Times Mirror/Mosby.

Kinlein, L. (1978). Nursing and family and community health. *Family and Community Health* 1(1): 57–68.

Klein, D. C. (1986). Assessing community characteristics. In B. Spradley, ed., *Readings in community health nursing.* 3rd ed. Boston: Little, Brown.

Lynd, R. (1939). *Knowledge for what? The place of social science in American culture.* Princeton: Princeton University Press.

Milbank Memorial Fund Commission. (1976). *Higher education for public health: A report.* New York: Prodist.

Muecke, M. A. (1984). Community health diagnosis in nursing. *Public Health Nursing* 1: 23–33.

Nagi, S. Z. (1959, October). Factors related to heart disease among Ohio farmers. *Ohio Agricultural Experiment Station Research Bulletin,* p. 842.

Neuber, K. A., W. T. Atkins, J. A. Jacobson, and N. A. Reuterman. (1980). *Needs assessment: A model for community planning.* Beverly Hills, Calif.: Sage.

Neuman, B. (1982). *The Neuman systems model: Application to nursing education and practice.* Norwalk, Conn.: Appleton-Century-Crofts.

Northern States Power. (1987). Acid rain? NSP is helping solve the problem. *Scene* 12(9): 3.

Nutt, P. (1984). *Planning methods for health and related organizations.* New York: Wiley.

Redesigning nursing education for public health: Report of the conference (Pub. No. 75-75). (1973). Bethesda, Md.: U.S. Department of Health, Education and Welfare.

Rogers, S. (1984). Community as client: A multivariate model for analysis of community aggregate health risk. *Public Health Nursing* 1: 210–22.

Ruffing-Rahel, M. A. (1985). Qualitative methods in community analysis. *Public Health Nursing* 2: 130–37.

Ruybal, S. E., E. Bauwens, and M. Fasla. (1975). Community assessment: An epidemiological approach. *Nursing Outlook* 23: 365–68.

Sanders, I. T., and A. Brownlee. (1979). Health in the community. In H. E. Freeman, S. Levine, and L. G. Reeder (eds.), *Handbook of medical sociology.* 3rd ed. (pp. 412–33). Englewood Cliffs, N.J.: Prentice-Hall.

Shamansky, S., and B. Pesznecker. (1981). A community is... *Nursing Outlook* 29: 182–85.

Wellman, B., and B. Leighton. (1979). Networks, neighborhoods, and communities: Approaches to the study of the community question. *Urban Affairs* 14: 363–90.

West, M. (1984). Community health assessment: The man-environment interaction. *Journal of Community Health Nursing* 1(2): 89–97.

Williams, C. A. (1981). Nursing leadership in community health: A neglected issue. In J. C. McCloskey and H. K. Grace (eds.), *Current issues in nursing.* Oxford, England: Blackwell Scientific Publications, Ltd.

Williams, C. A. (1985). Population-focused community health nursing and nursing administration: A new synthesis. In J. C. McCloskey and H. K. Grace (eds.), *Current issues in nursing.* 2nd ed. Boston: Blackwell Scientific Publications, Ltd.

Selected Readings

Allor, M. T. (1983). The "community profile." *Journal of Nursing Education* 22(1): 12–17.

Anderson, E., J. McFarlane, and A. Helton. (1986). Community-as-client: A model for practice. *Nursing Outlook* 34(5): 220–24.

Aneshensel, C., R. Frerichs, V. Clark, and P. Yokopenic. (1982). Telephone versus in-person surveys of community health status. *American Journal of Public Health* 72: 1017–21.

Archer, S. E., C. D. Kelly, and S. A. Bisch. (1984). *Implementing change in communities: A collaborative process.* St. Louis, Mo.: C. V. Mosby.

Blum, H. L. (1981). *Planning for health: Generics for the eighties.* 2nd ed. New York: Behavioral Publications.

Boyle, J. S. (1973). Community assessment. In A. Reinhardt and M. Quinn (eds.), *Family-centered community nursing.* St. Louis: C. V. Mosby.

Burke, E. M. (1979). *A participatory approach to urban planning.* New York: Human Sciences Press.

Campbell, B. F. (1988). Program attunes students to population-focused care. *Nursing and Health Care* 9(1): 42–45.

Cottrell, L. S., Jr. (1976). The competent community. In B. H. Kaplan, R. N. Wilson, and A. H. Leighton (eds.), *Further explorations in social psychiatry* (pp. 195–209). New York: Basic Books.

Dever, G. E. A. (1980). *Community health analysis: A holistic approach.* Germantown, Md.: Aspen Systems.

Flynn, B., J. Gottschalk, D. Ray, and E. Selmanoff. (1978). One masters curriculum in community health nursing. *Nursing Outlook* 26: 633–37.

Freeman, H. E., S. Levine, and L. G. Reeder. (eds.). (1979). *Handbook of medical sociology.* 3rd ed. Englewood Cliffs, N.J.: Prentice-Hall.

Fuerstein, M. T. (1980). Participatory evaluation—An appropriate technology for community health programmes. *Contact* 55: 1–8.

Goeppinger, J., P. Lassiter, and B. Wilcox. (1982). Community health is community competence. *Nursing Outlook* 30: 464–67.

Goeppinger, M., and A. J. Baglioni, Jr. (1986). Community competence: A positive approach to needs assessment. *American Journal of Community Psychology* 13: 507–23.

Gordon, M. (1982). *Nursing diagnosis: Process and application.* New York: McGraw-Hill.

Hamilton, P. (1985). Community nursing diagnosis. *Advances in Nursing Science* 5: 21–36.

Hanchett, E. (1979). *Community health assessment: A conceptual tool kit.* New York: Wiley.

Hanchett, E. (1988). *Nursing frameworks and community as client: Bridging the gap.* East Norwalk, Conn.: Appleton and Lange.

Hays, B., and N. R. Mockelstrom. (1977). Consumer survey: An approach to teaching consumer participation in community health. *Journal of Nursing Education* 16: 30–33.

Kark, S. L.. (1981). *The practice of community-oriented primary health care.* New York: Appleton-Century-Crofts.

Klein, D. C. (1986). Assessing community characteristics. In B. Spradley, ed., *Readings in community health nursing.* 3rd ed. Boston: Little, Brown.

MacStravic, R. (1978). *Determining health needs.* Ann Arbor, Mich.: Health Administration Press.

Milio, N. (1975). *The care of health in communities: Access for outcasts.* New York: Macmillan.

Moe, E. V. (1977). Nature of today's community. In A. Reinhardt and M. Quinn (eds.), *Current practice in family-centered community nursing.* St. Louis: C. V. Mosby.

Muecke, M. A. (1984). Community health diagnosis in nursing. *Public Health Nursing* 1: 23–33.

Neuber, K., W. T. Atkins, J. A. Jacobson, and N. A. Reuterman. (1980). *Needs assessment: A model for community planning.* Beverly Hills, Calif.: Sage.

Neuman, B. (1982). *The Neuman systems model: Application to nursing education and practice.* East Norwalk, Conn.: Appleton-Century-Crofts.

Nutt, P. (1984). Planning methods for health and related organizations. New York: Wiley.

Redesigning nursing education for public health: Report of the conference (Pub. No. 75-75). (1973). Bethesda, Md.: U.S. Department of Health, Education and Welfare.

Rogers, S. (1984). Community as client: A multivariate model for analysis of community aggregate health risk. *Public Health Nursing* 1: 210–22.

Ruffing-Rahel, M. A. (1985). Qualitative methods in community analysis. *Public Health Nursing* 2: 130–37.

Ruybal, S. E. (1978). Community health planning. *Family and Community Health* 1(1): 9–18.

Ruybal, S. E., E. Bauwens, and M. Fasla. (1975). Community assessment: An epidemiological approach. *Nursing Outlook* 23: 365–68.

Sanders, I. T., and A. Brownlee. (1979). Health in the community. In H. E. Freeman, S. Levine, and L. G. Reeder (eds.), *Handbook of medical sociology.* 3rd ed. (pp. 412–433). Englewood Cliffs, N.J.: Prentice-Hall.

Shamansky, S., and B. Pesznecker. (1981). A community is ... *Nursing Outlook* 29: 182–85.

Sheahan, S. L., and P. R. Aaron. (1983). Community assessment: An essential component of practice. *Health Values: Achieving High Level Wellness* 7(5): 12–15.

Sills, G. M., and J. Goeppinger. (1985). The community as a field of inquiry in nursing. In H. H. Werley and J. J. Fitzpatrick (eds.), *Annual review of nursing research.* New York: Springer Publishing.

Simmons, H. J. (1974). Community health planning—With or without nursing. *Nursing Outlook* 22: 260–64.

Stokinger, M., and J. Wallinder. (1979). A graduate practicum in health planning. *Nursing Outlook* 27: 202–5.

Weeks, M., R. Kulka, J. Lessler, and R. Whitmore. (1983). Personal versus telephone surveys for collecting household health data at the local level. *American Journal of Public Health* 73: 1389–94.

West, M. (1984). Community health assessment: The man-environment interaction. *Journal of Community Health Nursing* 1(2): 89–97.

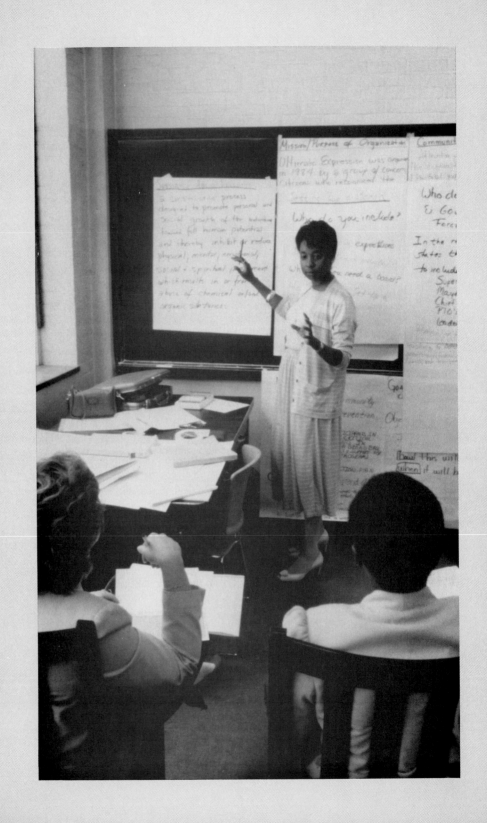

14 Working with Groups and Populations

Community health nursing offers us a considerable challenge: to promote the health of groups and populations. Outside public health, no other health care discipline has populations or aggregates as its primary concern or the entire community's health as its trust. For the community health nurse, then, the challenge lies in adopting an aggregate orientation for practice.

That orientation raises an important question. How do we work with aggregates? The purpose of this chapter is to explore how the community health nurse works with populations and groups of all sizes. Because small groups are more familiar, we shall begin by examining how to work with them. Then we shall apply our knowledge of groups to subpopulations and larger aggregates in the community.

UNDERSTANDING AND WORKING WITH SMALL GROUPS

Small groups are an important part of community health nursing service. Nurses meet the collective needs of many elements of the community population through work with groups. Each collection of people—a parenting group, a mastectomy club, a group of Southeast Asian refugees learning a new culture, a school health committee, or a group of discharged mental patients—has different needs. Some groups function for the purpose of problem solving; others for sharing, support, learning, or therapy. Whatever the reason for the group and regardless of whether the nurse serves as leader or member, basic knowledge and skill with groups enables the nurse to facilitate group process and outcomes.

All of us have had experience with groups. Our first group encounter is with the family, which is known as a primary group because it is one of several basic, informal social groups to which we belong during our lifetime (Sampson and Marthas, 1981). As we grow, our primary groups extend to include our childhood peer group, associations with our neighbors, friendship groups, and other social affiliations. Informal and generally social in nature, primary groups function with spontaneous and unstructured communication.

In addition to primary groups, we also experience secondary, or formal, group relationships (Sampson and Marthas, 1981). These groups usually exist for a specific purpose and include professional associations, therapeutic groups, work-related relationships, educational gatherings, and community affiliations. Examples are a student council, an exercise group, a patients' rights committee, and an assertiveness training class. These groups emphasize completing a job and accomplishing specific goals.

Although we spend much of our adult lives participating in formal and informal groups, how well do we understand such groups and how they function? With an increasing number of the community health nurse's activities taking place in and for groups—client groups, community groups, work groups, and others—the nurse's need for group skills becomes ever more important. Before we consider groups and ways in which nurses can work more effectively with them, we need to understand what a group is.

DEFINITION OF A GROUP

In this book, we will define a *group* as a collection of persons who engage in repeated, face-to-face communication, identify with each other, are interdependent, and share a common purpose or purposes. This definition suggests several characteristics of groups. A group must consist of at least two people, but it can never be so large that members cannot maintain direct communication with one another (Veninga, 1982). Because their collective social interaction influences the way they think, members assume similar values and norms and establish a sense of belonging to each other. Konopka (1954) refers to this characteristic as the development of "bonds," the links that connect individuals and create a group from a mass of loosely related people. Furthermore, the members of a group are interdependent; that is, they need and help each other. As Konopka points out (1954, p. 22), human beings need to belong to groups: "group life . . . gives the individual security and nourishment so that he can fulfill his greatest promise while helping others to fulfill theirs too." At the same time, the group molds its members' behavior and attitudes, thus developing its own personality, or identity (Veninga, 1982). Finally, group members share one or more common purposes. They have a reason for being a group. Whether a group forms to lobby for new playground equipment, to support persons experiencing a crisis, to exercise together, or to promote parenting skills, its members share a common purpose. We will explore this characteristic when we discuss types of groups.

Let us look at some examples of how these group characteristics influence the health of clients. Steve discovered when he was 15 years of age that he had epilepsy. The fact was difficult to accept, particularly because he had just been elected captain of his swim team. He was told that epilepsy meant an end to his future in swimming. After a seizure at work, his boss fired him. A period of several months of bitterness and frustration followed, and then he was invited to attend an epilepsy club recently formed in his high school. This group knew what it was like to be epileptic. Many of them had undergone experiences similar to Steve's and could truly empathize with him. The sense of belonging that developed for Steve soon erased his feelings of loneliness and gave him a new sense of hope. The attitudes and behavior of the group gradually shaped his own feelings to the point that he could accept his diagnosis and start developing constructive plans for his life.

A group of elderly persons started a bridge club in their retirement building. Although conversation covered many topics, several members initially were reluctant to discuss the future. "I have no future," one said. "I'm just biding my time until I die." Group camaraderie and influence gradually changed this attitude to fit the group norm of having a good time together and looking forward to living a long time.

Not all groups influence people positively. Take the case of Tommy, 13 years of age, who has gone from petty theft to armed robbery as a result of gang pressure. Or consider Nancy, once a promising student, now a hard drug user. Her friends made fun of anyone who did well in school and, instead, promoted drug taking as a condition for group membership.

Groups are powerful. Although groups meet basic individual needs for belonging, security, safety, and the opportunity to help others, they also shape their members' thinking and behavior through internal processes of acceptance and rejection (Figure 14-1). We have seen that they can be either a

Figure 14-1
Adolescents feel strong pressure to conform to their group's standards. Acting tough and laughing at each other's jokes are some of the ways this group influences its members' behavior.

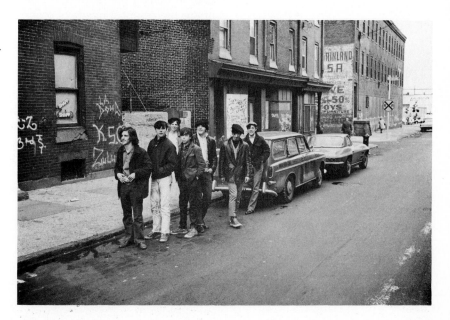

constructive or destructive force in people's lives. Our concern in community health is to facilitate their constructive use for client health.

Now that we have examined the definition of a group, we will explore the ways that community health nurses can work more effectively with groups. The framework for our discussion involves the major processes in which a community health nurse will be involved while working with small groups:

1. *Preparing for small-group work* occurs before the group begins, but may continue after the group forms. Preparation involves knowing the nature of groups, types of groups, and their functions and needs.
2. *Starting a group* involves specific activities to help the group begin work.
3. *Building group cohesiveness* is essential during the early growth of a group.
4. *Working with a group* involves recognizing its developmental phases, assuming appropriate leader and member roles, and solving various sorts of problems that arise.
5. *Terminating a group* begins early in the group's life and requires specific interventions.
6. *Evaluating a group* occurs in two dimensions: we examine group process as well as the outcomes of the group's work.

PREPARING FOR SMALL-GROUP WORK

As the nurse prepares to work with a group, she or he will need to know the answers to three important questions. First, what types of groups are there? Second, what are the essential needs of groups? Third, what are the major functions of a group?

Types of Groups

Community health nurses work with many different kinds of small groups. Since each group forms for some purpose, we shall categorize them according to their primary goals. There are five types of small groups with which community health nurses work: learning groups, support groups, socialization groups, psychotherapy groups, and task-oriented groups.

Learning Groups.   The primary goal of a learning group is to have its members gain understanding in order to effect behavioral change in some specified area of need. Many community health nurses lead prenatal groups. The parents-to-be have many practices to learn, such as exercises, diet, breathing techniques, and what to do during labor and delivery. For each topic, nurses leading these groups make certain that the needed information is covered and, when appropriate, they demonstrate its application. The parents-to-be practice their new skills regularly at home, and the nurse-leader may ask them to display their understanding by demonstrating what they have learned to the group. This learning group will have met its goals when the members have assimilated knowledge to the point that it changes their behavior (Figure 14-2).

A class can be a learning group, but the two are not necessarily the same. No doubt you have sat in many classes where, other than a brief conversation or two with a neighbor, you have had little interaction with the other class members. That class is not a true group. The members of a group have repeated, face-to-face communication. They identify with each other and are interdependent. These characteristics typify a learning group, whose function is to utilize the benefits of group identity and interaction to accomplish learning and behavioral change. Classes and learning groups share a common advantage of transmitting information more efficiently to a number of people than a one-to-one basis allows. However, learning groups, in contrast to most classes, use group commitment and reinforcement to produce desired behavior changes. Group members may actually practice natural childbirth, control hypertension, or maintain a postcoronary diet and exercise program. Individuals in these groups not only learn what to do and how to do it (the limit of most classes), but also have the advantage of group influence to promote and stabilize their practices at a healthier level.

The composition of a learning group varies with each situation and depends upon the group's goals. When a group goal is to teach assertiveness to females, for example, the membership would most likely be limited to women. A group goal aimed at preparing people for retirement would probably include members at midlife or approaching retirement. The composition of many learning groups, such as those concerned with weight loss, leadership training, or learning how to manage diabetes, is determined by its members' shared interest in the topic. The chief common denominator of most learning groups, however, is that the members are people who desire to gain information about some subject and to better themselves as a result (Sweeney, 1975).

Figure 14-2
This childbirth education class enables couples to practice techniques that will facilitate the birth experience.

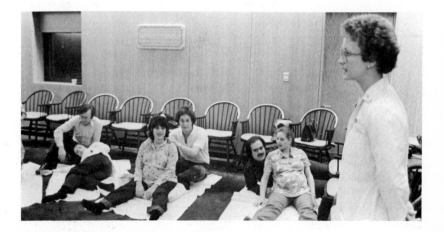

The nurse may start some learning groups; others, particularly self-help groups such as Weight Watchers or Alanon groups, will not require this kind of initiative. The nurse's role, therefore, will vary depending upon whether she initiates and leads the group, participates as a member, or participates as an outside consultant. Nevertheless, the nurse's role in any learning group includes providing some degree of structure and focus to the group's activities. The nurse also utilizes the basic teaching-learning principles described in Chapter 11 to encourage client interest in, and application of, the information presented.

Support Groups.   The primary goal of an emotional support group is to promote healthy behaviors and prevent maladaptive coping patterns among its members (Loomis, 1979). In community health, nurses encounter many people who already have good health practices but who need help during times of stress. The support of other people enables them to adapt and preserve their healthy behaviors (Pesznecker and Zahlis, 1986). Support groups meet this need. For example, a woman alone found adjustment to the ordeal of a mastectomy painfully difficult. Feelings of loss, disfigurement, changed body image, and fear of the cancer returning, in addition to her physical weakness and discomfort, were almost more than she could handle. A single woman, she was convinced that no man would ever want to touch her. She was invited to join a mastectomy club and, through this group, found the comfort and courage that she needed to face her situation. The other members had also had mastectomies. They shared a common experience and could empathize with her feelings. The support and acceptance of the group gave her the strength to put her life back together again.

Support groups, also called therapeutic groups (Marram, 1978), are composed primarily of emotionally healthy people (not needing psychiatric help) caught in some change or crisis. A laryngectomy club or a divorce support group, for example, contains people involved in situational crises who need therapeutic reinforcement. A developmental crisis, such as entering parenthood, may prompt others to form a parenting group for the purpose of reassurance and reinforcement of personal resources (Kagey et al., 1981). The need for support during adaptation to job change prompted one church to form its Job Transition Support Group for members and others in the community. So great was the need and so successful the group that, in 1989, the group, with an evolving membership, celebrated its twelfth anniversary. Groups such as this often have secondary learning goals. For instance, one week the Job Transition Support Group heard a lecture on the interview process, but its primary goal remained emotional support. The support group provides members with comfort and courage to face the difficulties of their present situation. It seeks to maintain and utilize their existing strengths; it helps them cope successfully and regain their equilibrium (Figure 14-3).

Support groups sometimes serve an advocacy role as well. They can plead the cause of their members whose physical and emotional health, job secu-

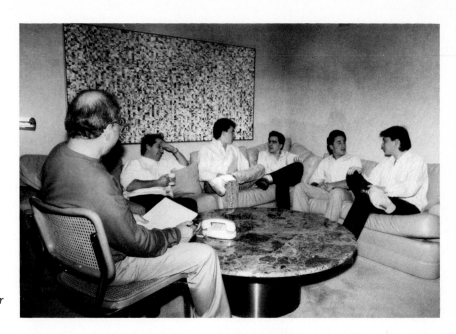

Figure 14-3
Members of this support
group listen and share their
feelings with one another.

rity, or social status may be threatened because of their current problem. Alcoholics Anonymous, while primarily a support group, represents a strong social force working in favor of its members' rehabilitation and constructive participation in the community. The Gray Panthers, a senior citizens' lobbying group, promotes the causes of the elderly while providing them with a group with which they can identify and from which they can derive sustenance. A support group for epileptics rallied around a member who had been fired from her job when her boss discovered her diagnosis. The nurse-leader of the group, accompanied by two of the group members, met with the boss, explained epilepsy, and convinced him that the woman's condition was under control. She kept her job.

Nurses working with support groups aim to facilitate group interactions, but their most important role is to model acceptance and caring. Demonstrating a warm, understanding attitude with, for example, a smoking cessation group or a group of individuals grieving the loss of spouses encourages members to assume these same caring feelings and to create a supportive climate. This approach energizes individuals to resume responsible, healthy behaviors.

Socialization Groups.   Occasionally nurses encounter clients from another culture or subculture who must learn new social roles in order to achieve a positive level of health. Their old patterns of behavior are inappropriate, nonfunctional, sometimes detrimental, or at least a source of uneasiness in the larger society. Some Native Americans, accustomed to living on a remote reservation, have difficulty adjusting to urban living. Southeast Asian refugees, flocking to American cities in increasing numbers, experience even greater culture shock. Contrasting patterns of eating, living, rearing children, and health practices, as well as language barriers and value differences, all call for adaptation in order for these clients to function in the new culture. Even armed services veterans returning from overseas experience some degree of culture shock upon re-entry to the United States. They must adjust to new values, clothing styles, social relationships, and political and economic changes. Some individuals in our society have lived in a confined subculture, such as a mental hospital, a prison, or a school for the deaf, and upon discharge must learn new ways of behaving. All of these individuals can benefit from a socialization group.

The primary goal of a socialization group is to help its members learn new social roles. A socialization group must not be confused with a purely social group. Nurses will want to be aware of social groups and their functions. For example, lonely, isolated individuals may benefit greatly from joining a bridge club, bowling league, or bird-watching group. Such groups offer friends, enjoyable activities and support. The elderly, for instance, may need information about an activities group in their area and encouragement, even assistance, to participate. However, in this chapter we are concerned with groups in which the community health nurse works. Socialization groups bring together people who are adapting to a new culture or subculture. They offer the nurse an opportunity to capitalize on the benefits of group influence to help people learn new social skills that will promote their physical and emotional health.

The nurse's role in a socialization group is first to demonstrate caring and acceptance of the group's members, to respect their present values and behaviors. The nurse also provides structure and focus to the group process. For example, with discharged mental patients or a refugee enculturation group, the nurse can encourage members to share their experiences and help them learn ways of coping with their new life-style. The mental patients may discuss how to interview for a job, how to meet people, or how to behave at parties. Topics such as shopping in a supermarket, how to ride a bus, or what to expect when one goes to a health clinic might be discussed in the refugee group. The nurse uses group support to give these people courage to give up their familiar practices and group influence to help them learn new roles.

Psychotherapy Groups.   Psychotherapy groups are formed for people who need treatment of an emotional disturbance. Many clients in community health have emotional problems ranging from minor neuroses to severe maladjustments. Psychotherapy groups can serve the needs of families in which child abuse or parent abuse occurs, married couples in conflict, chemically dependent persons, and those with suicidal impulses. These individuals may be referred by a family member, neighbor, professional worker, or agency. They may also refer themselves. Some receive group therapy following individual counseling; others are able to gain all the help they need from a psychotherapy group alone.

The primary goal of psychotherapy groups is to provide members insight into themselves and to help them change their behavior (Loomis, 1979). The group focuses on how its members relate to themselves and to each other; it becomes a "social microcosm" (Loomis, 1979, p. 10). That is, the group serves as a minisociety, allowing members to display their negative feelings and behaviors in an accepting and corrective milieu. An occasional group member may not be ready or willing to participate in self-change and may need to be counseled in some other setting.

Some nurses in community health have advanced training and experience in group psychotherapy and serve as therapists for these groups. More often, the community health nurse is a cotherapist working with a psychiatrist, psychologist, or psychiatric social worker. For example, a nurse and psychiatric social worker co-led a psychotherapy group for delinquent adolescent girls. They considered many behaviors, but they focused on the girls' tendency to "run away," to avoid anything perceived as unpleasant. The nurse's role included demonstrating acceptance and caring, encouraging the girls to share their feelings, helping them to understand the reasons behind their feelings and behavior, and providing structure and focus to the group process.

Task-Oriented Groups. A final category of small groups with which community health nurses work includes all those groups whose primary goal is to accomplish some predetermined task. In community health there are many complex problems to solve, decisions to make, and tasks to accomplish that require a collaborative effort (Callahan, 1980). Nursing staff in a public health agency disagree over the proper method for supervising home health aides. A day-care center needs new health and safety policies. Community residents are concerned about a rising incidence of vandalism in their area and want to develop a constructive program to keep children and teenagers busy. A local elementary school wants help in planning a health fair. Mothers attending a well-child clinic would like to make the waiting room more pleasant and interesting. Each of these tasks can be accomplished by people contributing their unique perspectives and skills and working together as a group. Community health nurses play a significant part in this process.

Membership in task-oriented groups varies but generally encompasses clients, community residents, and health-related professionals. Client task-oriented groups often form spontaneously out of a desire to improve an existing situation. With minimal assistance from their community health nurse, several elderly clients, feeling lonely and useless, established a foster grandparents program. Volunteering their services through local churches and clubs, these retirees soon had more requests than they could handle. As foster grandparents, they met real needs of children in the community and also contributed to their own enjoyment and satisfaction. The community health nurse may work with a group of clients whose goal is to accomplish some task but whose collaboration also serves other health-related functions. One such group was made up of mothers who wanted to redecorate the waiting room of a well-child clinic. The nurse helped them plan and implement a fund-raising rummage sale and worked as a group member during the redecoration. Group cohesiveness developed as a result of the many hours spent together, and the nurse was able to form an ongoing mothers' support group with these women.

Community residents frequently initiate task-oriented groups in which community health nurses participate. A school nurse was asked to lead an elementary school's task force in planning a health fair. Two community health nurses served on a local community council's planning committee to develop a hypertension screening program. In contrast, a nurse may initiate a task-oriented group involving community residents. A community health nurse influenced some concerned Native Americans to form a committee to raise the health consciousness of the people on their reservation. She met with the committee weekly for three months and accompanied its chairman when he presented the committee's recommendations to the tribal council. She assisted a woman who started a weekly health column, one element of the committee's health-consciousness-raising plan, for the tribal newspaper. In another instance, a community health nurse initiated a task-oriented group in order to develop a friendly visitor program for elderly shut-ins.

Professional task-oriented groups are a frequent part of community health nursing practice (Figure 14-4). They might include an agency team meeting, a state nursing association subcommittee, a state health planning commission, or an environmental safety task force. In these groups, the nurse, whether leader or member, works with other health-related professionals to accomplish specific tasks. For example, a community health nurse in St. Paul, Minnesota, chaired a subcommittee of the Metropolitan Health Board to study

Figure 14-4
Health planning groups, such as this Visiting Nurse Association directors' meeting, form a vital link in the provision of community health services.

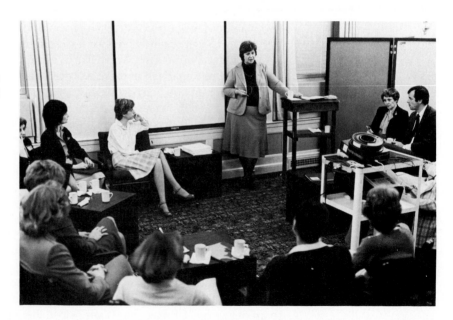

ways and means of facilitating greater collaboration between health care agencies. In addition to consumer members, the committee included health care administrators from public and private agencies, nurses, physicians, and health planners.

The nurse's role in task-oriented groups varies depending upon whether the nurse is the leader or a member of the group. Later in this chapter we will examine group leader and member roles in more detail. In either case, however, the nurse works to facilitate group progress toward goal achievement.

In Table 14-1 we summarize the five types of small groups with which community health nurses work by listing each type's primary goal, membership, and nurse's role.

Essential Group Needs

Group needs differ from individual needs. We are all familiar with various definitions of individual needs, such as those outlined in Maslow's classic hierarchy of needs (1954) or Erikson's eight ages of man (1963). These needs include belonging, recognition, generativity, and self-actualization. For individuals to achieve a maximum level of functioning, their basic needs must be met. A group, as an entity, has a different set of needs that must be satisfied and maintained in order to allow optimal group functioning. Four essential small-group needs are shared goals, consistent norms, motivation, and communication (Veninga, 1982; Sampson and Marthas, 1981).

Table 14-1
Types of Small Groups in Community Health

Type of Group	Primary Goal	Membership	Nurse's Role
Learning	Develop and apply knowledge	People desiring information and improvement in their lives	Provide structure and focus for group process
Support	Maintain healthy behavior and prevent maladaptive coping	Emotionally healthy people needing support during change or crisis	Present role model of acceptance and caring Facilitate group interaction
Socialization	Learn new social roles	People adapting to a new culture or subculture	Offer acceptance and caring Provide structure and focus for group process
Psychotherapy	Gain insight into self and change behavior	People needing treatment of an emotional disturbance	Offer acceptance and caring Encourage sharing of feelings Help members understand the reasons behind their feelings and behavior Provide structure and focus for group process
Task-oriented	Accomplish task	People assigned to or volunteering to complete a job	Facilitate progress toward goal achievement

Shared Goals. First, a group needs an agreed-upon goal and a shared understanding about the means for its achievement. No purposeful small group can function for long if its members have different ideas about what it is trying to accomplish. A group learning about family planning, for instance, can make little progress if some members define it as a sex education class, others join to help influence people against abortion, and some use it as a social outlet. The group must be solidly behind its stated goals if members are to work together and accomplish desired results.

Consistent Norms. Second, a group needs consistency in its norms. That is, there must be some continuity and stability in the internal rules and policies, spoken and unspoken, that govern the group's actions (Loomis, 1979; Veninga, 1982). Every group has to establish ground rules for operating. These rules govern areas such as membership eligibility, attendance requirements, whether or not new members can join after the group is in progress, what kind of participation is expected of each member, and what is expected of the leader. If rules and policies are ignored or frequently broken, the structure of the group is weakened, members do not feel secure, and the group eventually is unable to function.

Motivation. Third, a group needs members motivated to do their various jobs. Many variables influence motivation; among them are leader power and charisma, degree of member commitment to group goals and group success, how well individual needs are being met, group cohesiveness, and members' sense of belonging. Group goals can be accomplished only through collaborative effort; unless members do their share of the work, the job does not get done. Nor can the group function if members are lazy or morale is low. Each member has a unique role to play and, as for any system, the group's viability depends on the proper functioning of all its parts.

Communication. Fourth, every group needs stable communication channels among the members (Veninga, 1982). No group can function without a dependable system for giving and receiving information. The effectiveness of a divorce support group depends on members' ability to share their feelings of anger, rejection, or loneliness freely and to receive accepting, understanding responses in return. The work of a committee to study safety hazards in a summer camp cannot be done without an active exchange of ideas. Were it not for demonstrated acceptance and caring and constant two-way communication to help members gain insight into their feelings and behavior, a psychotherapy group would have minimal success. In order to function, all groups require viable lines of communication.

Group Functions

Every small group serves two types of functions: a task-related function and a group maintenance function (Sampson and Marthas, 1981; Veninga,

1982). The task function focuses on completing the job, while the maintenance function deals with how members are interacting. The former is goal-related and instrumental; the latter member-related and interpersonal.

Consider how a student council operates. Part of the group's focus will be on the task dimension. Members will explore ideas, make plans, decide on jobs to be done, keep discussions on target, and make certain that members have done their delegated tasks. The other part of the group's concentration is on the maintenance dimension, which includes responsibilities such as keeping up group morale, making certain that individual members' needs are met, encouraging and praising members' accomplishments, and mediating conflicts.

A well-functioning group emphasizes both task and maintenance concerns (Guthrie and Miller, 1978). You may have experienced membership in a group that focused so heavily on tasks that the interpersonal dimension was neglected. This situation happens most often in task-oriented groups, such as committees, where the job to be done becomes so important that it is accomplished at the expense of members' feelings. Internal dissatisfaction develops, resulting in poor attendance, disruptive behavior, or withdrawal. Everyone expects and needs to get something from group membership; if they do not, they will either drop out or possibly disrupt the group in some way. On the other hand, a group that concentrates too heavily on the interpersonal dimension may have happy members but not accomplish its goals. An appropriate balance between task and maintenance functions is needed.

STARTING A GROUP

When any group is about to be formed, certain questions must be answered. First, does a group need or wish to form, and who initiates that process? In some instances, several people may get together because they have identified a reason for meeting. Their common concern prompts the group's formation. Sometimes an outside person or agency, such as Alcoholics Anonymous, starts a new group in the community. On other occasions, a nurse, having identified a need, may be the initiator. For example, a community health nurse with several postpartum clients in her caseload may suggest that they meet as a group for mutual support and shared information. Or a nurse may contact several local churches and offer to form a group of interested volunteers who would begin making friendly visits to shut-ins. Initial formation of a group is based on identifying a need — determining a reason or reasons for people to get together — then convening the group. Once the decision is made to form the group, other questions must be addressed. Who should the members be? What is the best size for this group? What are the group's needs, and what should its goals be? Where should it meet, and what type of physical arrangements would best suit its purpose? How can members be oriented to facilitate effective group development and group process? We shall consider the answers to each of these questions separately.

Selecting Members

A group's membership is determined by several factors. One is the group's general purpose. If it is task-oriented, its members should be people who have expertise or skills pertinent to accomplishing the task. If its purpose is support, the members will be people who are experiencing change or crisis and need emotional reinforcement. In other words, the members should have something in common that relates to the group's primary goal.

Members should also exhibit similarities relative to the group's specific goals. Sometimes age- or sex-specific membership is necessary. For example, a support group for men in midlife crisis would limit its membership to middle-aged men. A preschoolers' mothers' group aiming to understand early childhood growth and development and learn appropriate mothering responses would limit its membership to young mothers. In other groups, the members may be very dissimilar in age, sex, or social role, but have some other common denominator. A weight-loss group, for instance, might be composed of members of a variety of ages and both sexes since obesity is their shared concern. The epileptic support group mentioned earlier included young people from grade school through high school. Their variant ages and sexes gave a broader range of perspectives to group discussion and further enhanced the group's value. Their common denominator was epilepsy.

Members should choose to be part of the group. Any group member who does not participate willingly is not likely to benefit from or contribute positively to the group. If, for example, a client is coerced into a psychotherapy group or a professional is drafted reluctantly to serve on a health committee, they may be passive or absent, cause conflict, or disrupt the group process.

One should also select members on the basis of their commitment to the group's success. People who are genuinely interested in the group's goals and motivated to work for their accomplishment will gain more from the group experience and make a greater contribution to its process and outcomes. We see strong evidence of this contribution particularly in self-help groups (Lipson, 1980), such as Alcoholics Anonymous, where group loyalty and commitment accomplish significant results.

Finally, leaders are helped by selecting members with whom they enjoy working and are more likely to be effective. Some leaders enjoy working with challenging groups, such as drug addicts, while groups with a strong commitment to change may be more satisfying for others. As Loomis (1979, p. 52) points out, "Therapists should be encouraged to become familiar with their own personal characteristics and preferences in the selection of clients." This factor clearly affects a group's success.

Determining Group Size

Not long ago a community health nurse and seven other professionals formed a task force to study service delivery problems and make recommendations to a county board. The group met for several months and formed a good working relationship. However, its final product, a set of recommendations, met with resistance from county agencies not represented on the original task force. They insisted on expanding the task force and restudying the problems. Later, composed of 22 members, the group met frequently but made almost no progress. Most of the leader's energy was spent resolving conflicts and attempting to pacify a few vocal members who dominated the discussion with lengthy diatribes defending their agencies' territory. Many members could not or chose not to participate. Attendance began to drop. As the deadline drew near, the leader, in desperation, appointed a subcommittee of five members to draft a proposal to which the larger group could respond. The draft, with minor changes, was approved, and the task force limped to its final conclusion with participation from about half of the original group.

Why was the first task force so successful and the second not? Because group size affects performance (Veninga, 1982). The larger the group, the longer it takes to reach decisions, especially if consensus is required. In addition, the subgroups that almost always develop within larger groups can polarize interests, create conflicts, and impede group progress.

Group size also influences satisfaction. We have known for many years that as a group expands, the individual member's satisfaction declines (Sampson and Marthas, 1981). The larger the group, the less likely is the opportunity for all members to participate. In a large group, a few people usually do most of the talking while the rest are either intimidated, bored, or dissatisfied to the point of choosing not to participate.

Large groups do exist; examples are professional nursing groups, parent-teacher-student associations, student bodies, and older adults' clubs. In order to meet specific group needs, however, formal, purposeful groups must divide into smaller units of workable size. Loomis (1979, p. 61) emphasizes: "It is not good clinical practice to remain with too large a group simply because there are not enough funds available to start a second group. Client needs and group task should be the primary consideration in determining group size."

The ideal number of members in a group varies, depending upon the situation and the group goals. To allow an appropriate mix of members and enough people to promote good interaction, a group should have at least five or six members. Ten to twelve members is considered the maximum size before subgroups start to form. The optimal size for any talk-oriented group that aims at problem solving, support, learning, insight, or behavior change is six to ten members (Loomis, 1979; Veninga, 1982). The choice of seven members is often preferred for providing the best balance of variety of ideas with opportunity for all members to participate.

Setting Group Goals

We set goals and objectives on the basis of needs. That important step in the nursing process, assessment, must be taken. A community health nurse, working with an interpreter, started a socialization group for deaf high school students. These young people attended a state residential school for the deaf and would soon be graduating. The nurse's assessment showed that they were concerned about functioning in a hearing world, about getting jobs, developing a social life, applying to colleges, and planning careers. They had needs. On the basis of these needs, the group established its goals and objectives.

Every group must identify its needs before setting goals. The process involves collecting and interpreting data, and then making a diagnosis and developing a plan for making needed changes. A detailed discussion of needs assessment, diagnosis, and goal setting is provided in Chapter 8. In order to set goals and objectives with a nursing leadership training group, for instance, a leader may ask the members what they think they need and then evaluate their leadership knowledge and skills. On the basis of this data the leader determines this group's specific needs, such as how to make decisions, how to plan, and how to delegate. Then the goals and objectives can be established.

Setting goals is a group activity involving all members. Unless members participate in this process, it is possible that their expectations for the group will differ (Callahan, 1980). Members and leader together need to agree on the group's major goals and its specific objectives, the activities that will ensure the desired outcomes. It is often helpful to negotiate a group contract in which the nurse-leader and members mutually agree on their expectations for the group and the manner in which the outcomes will be achieved. Negotiating a fee for service with some groups is an important element in the contract and contributes to group commitment (Loomis, 1979).

Making Physical Arrangements

Where, how, and when a group meets influences its productivity significantly. The meeting place must be conveniently located, perhaps near a bus line, in order to be accessible to members. It must also have appropriate facilities, such as wheelchair access or parking space, to accommodate members' needs.

Space is another consideration. Some groups, such as an exercise group or a first-aid demonstration class, need a larger meeting area in order to accomplish their goals. Other groups function best in a more intimate setting that is conducive to sharing and expressing feelings; for them, a smaller room works best.

Seating arrangements can influence group process. If chairs are set in classroom style, there is a tendency for members to direct their comments only to the leader. Many task-oriented groups, such as committees, work around long tables. It is difficult for members along the sides of the tables to have eye contact with others along the same side. As a result, communication is inhibited and group cohesiveness is slower to develop. A circular seating pattern in which every member can see every other member facilitates communication in all directions.

A comfortable atmosphere, compatible with group goals, is important. A group dealing with feelings may find softer chairs or even sitting on the floor relaxing, informal, and conducive to free expression, while a "think" group may need firmer seating. Background noise, a room that echoes, distracting posters, or distasteful decorations may often detract from group productivity.

Finally, the time when a group meets is also important. Dates and times should fit members' schedules so that all can attend, and length and frequency of meetings should enhance group goals. A support group, for instance, may find it most helpful to meet weekly to receive frequent reinforcement. Other groups, such as some learning or task groups, may need more time between sessions to practice new skills or research a problem.

Orienting Group Members

Three conditions must be met to ensure smooth functioning as a group starts. First, members must agree on the group's goals. Members should agree as early as possible in the life of the group to erase misconceptions and to help solidify the group behind its purpose.

Second, new group members need to know how the group will function; they must begin to establish its structure and rules for operating. Structure refers to the way a group defines and regulates its members' behavior in terms of roles, communication patterns, and power relationships within the group (Sampson and Marthas, 1981). It must be clear from the beginning of any group who, if anyone, is leader and what that person is expected to do. Expectations for the members should be clearly spelled out, and special roles, such as a timekeeper in a discussion group or a referee for debates, should be assigned. More specific leader and member roles will emerge during the life of the group; we will discuss these shortly. Communication patterns evolve as group members work together, but awareness from the start of how members communicate is important. The interaction networks tend to be most effective in groups whose members are all free to communicate with each other as well as with the nurse-leader (Veninga, 1982).

Power structure in informal groups often fluctuates, depending upon which members have the most influence, while formal groups, such as an agency's nursing organization, generally have a stable, clear-cut structure of power, influence, and authority. In any group, however, decisions can be made to designate who has power to do what. For example, the leader of a learning group may have absolute power over all decisions, or the group may choose a completely democratic format with decision-making power distributed among the members. Rules governing group action also need to be established early. The group must decide on matters such as attendance, physical arrangements, and whether smoking will be permitted.

Third, members need to hold the same expectations for the group's outcomes. The anticipated final product of the group can be restated and discussed to make certain that everyone understands and agrees that this is the desired outcome. Part of this discussion should include how the group members will evaluate the group's final product. How will they know when their goals have been met? Some groups will find evaluation easier than others will. A smoking cessation group or a weight-loss group, for instance, will have clear standards for measuring success. An assertiveness training group for women may decide that its outcome is the ability of every member to assert herself appropriately in public and will evaluate this outcome by having each member describe one such experience. A divorce support group may have more difficulty agreeing on outcomes but perhaps will choose to measure them in terms of each member's satisfaction, feelings of comfort, or self-confidence.

BUILDING GROUP COHESIVENESS

Group cohesiveness is the sum of all the forces that influence members to stay in a group. These forces include whether (1) members' needs can be met in the group, (2) group goals are consistent with members' needs, (3) members expect the group to benefit them, and (4) members actually perceive that the group is benefitting them (Loomis, 1979; Veninga, 1982). These are positive forces that attract members toward the group. In some instances, negative outside pressures may also promote group cohesiveness.

Cohesive groups display certain characteristics that begin early in the group's development and increase over time. There is an attraction of members to the group and a sense of pride in membership, which intensifies as the group becomes more successful. Pride is usually accompanied by an emotional commitment of the members to the group and manifests itself in increasing loyalty and high morale. The members feel good about one another and their group identification. They are loyal to each other and to the group's goals and values and, in some instances, may talk, dress, or act in similar ways. They work well together and enjoy spending time together, even outside of the regular group meetings.

During the life of every group there are times of internal problems and external threats. Group cohesiveness helps a group to weather these times (Kagey, 1981). When the members of a parenting group disagreed among themselves over ways to discipline children, their closeness and unity as a group helped them over this period of conflict and prevented the group from disintegrating. The members of a chemical dependency group discovered that their funding source had been cut off and that there would be no more money for medications or consultation. Because of the members' commitment to remaining together, they sought and found new resources and continued working on their goals.

Group cohesiveness is as important to the group as the nurse-patient relationship is to individual therapy (Yalom, 1975). Research demonstrates that there is a positive correlation between group cohesiveness and positive group therapy outcomes (Loomis, 1979). Thus it becomes essential to foster group cohesiveness in the small groups with which nurses work.

Nurse-leaders build cohesiveness in a group by making certain that its four basic needs are met. First, there must be agreement among all members on the group's goals and the means by which these goals will be achieved. No group will be cohesive if members disagree on or misunderstand the goals. To avoid misunderstanding, members need to know exactly what the goals mean, have a clear (preferably written) statement of them, agree on the methods and actions to use in implementing them, and have a sense of hope that they are attainable. Second, group norms, the standards for acceptable behavior in the group, must be continuous and stable to help the group function (Veninga, 1982). These norms are developed through discussion between leader and members about what is expected and acceptable behavior. Formal groups tend to define norms at the start. Norms often develop more gradually in informal groups. Third, there must be group motivation. Clarity and feasibility of goals can help members feel that working for the group is worthwhile. The leader can be a strong motivator by giving individual members recognition and positive reinforcement and by promoting each member's participation and sense of belonging. Fourth, communication channels within the group must remain viable. It is often up to the leader to monitor communication networks and make certain that they function effectively. Members, too, can help to facilitate a good exchange of information and feelings, but the group may need an outside process observer to make objective recommendations for improving its communication patterns.

Several factors can block group cohesiveness from developing or remaining (Loomis, 1979; Veninga, 1982). Open membership, particularly with an unlimited number of sessions, sometimes makes it difficult for a group to stabilize its norms. Some groups, such as Alcoholics Anonymous or Weight Watchers, overcome this difficulty by having established goals and norms for the group that essentially do not change as new members join. In a less formal group with open membership, such as an ostomy club, the nurse-leader can help the founding members to develop a charter or written statement describing the group's general purpose and policies. Then, as new members enter and old ones leave, there can be some flexibility within this structure to allow specific goals and norms to reflect the changing membership's needs. That is, both goals and norms would have to be renegotiated depending on the rate of member turnover. When members move into and out of a group very rapidly, it is almost impossible to establish cohesiveness. In general, the more stable the membership, the more likely is the achievement of group cohesiveness.

Other blocks to group cohesiveness include members who do not conform to norms or agree with goals, the formation of competitive subgroups, or a leader-centered group. Deviant members can sometimes be persuaded to change their behavior or perhaps to leave the group. Strong group agreement on goals and norms prevents competition and allows the formation of positive subgroups that enhance cohesiveness. One can also minimize splintering by keeping the subgroups task-specific and time-limited. Responsible group leadership focuses on uniting the group behind its goals and maximizing its potential to meet client needs.

Some groups need cohesiveness more than others. Without a close working relationship, a support group, for example, will probably not be able to function while a learning group may be able to accomplish its goals; however, the learning group's full potential cannot be realized without group cohesiveness.

WORKING WITH A GROUP

Let us say you have prepared for a group by gaining an understanding of the types of small groups and their needs. Then you actually started a group and worked to build cohesiveness. The group appears to be moving along well. Between this initial period of establishing a group and the final period of terminating it, you will be working with an ongoing group. This work requires an understanding of the phases of group development, the different roles that leader and members can play, and the ways problems can be resolved.

Phases of Group Development

Groups, like individuals, go through predictable growth phases. It is easiest to observe these phases in groups whose membership is constant; it is more difficult to distinguish the phases in groups whose membership or goals frequently change. The phases are dependence, counterdependence, and interdependence (Guthrie and Miller, 1978).

Dependence.   During this first phase, members depend on the leader for guidance and direction. They are still sorting out why they are there and what their roles will be. They do not question the leader's authority. It is during this phase that members are most concerned with inclusion in the group (Schutz, 1966). It is a time of personal contact and encounter. Members want to be part of the group but still feel some conflict in giving up their personal identity. Dependence has been called the "childhood" stage of group development (Guthrie and Miller, 1978).

Counterdependence.   As members become more comfortable in their roles, they also become more assertive. Conflict and power struggles develop, and acceptance of the leader's authority diminishes. The major issue in the counterdependent phase is control. Who has power and authority? Who will influence and control? Who will be controlled? This is an "adolescent" stage of group development.

Interdependence.   Finally, group members learn to work out their relationships. They make decisions together, engage in open communication, manage conflict sucessfully, and experience satisfaction in the entire group's accomplishments. During this phase, the issues revolve around communicating and meeting individual needs to express and receive affection. Subgroups develop and members pair to handle intimacy needs. Interdependence is a "mature" phase of group development that may take weeks, months, or even years for a group to reach, depending on the stability of the membership. Some groups never achieve interdependence.

While monitoring a group's development, leaders notice that as each new issue arises the group will again progress through the developmental phases with regard to that issue. According to Sampson and Marthas (1981, p. 196), "A particular developmental stage . . . is never fully completed for all time; rather, as circumstances change, the same developmental [stage] may crop up again and again." For example, a nursing team in a community health agency has been working on solving case problems. During the past five months the team members have worked through their dependence on the team leader and their conflicts over different ways to manage family problems; now they are communicating well and assuring everyone the opportunity to express ideas. They are experiencing the interdependent phase on this issue. Recently the team was told that it would have to redistribute members' geographic work boundaries. Feeling insecure and uncertain about how to accomplish this task, members initially looked to the team leader for suggestions (dependent phase). Soon they recognized advantages and disadvantages of various proposals for redefining work boundaries, ignored the leader, and began arguing among themselves over how to decide. Power struggles signal that they are currently in the counterdependent phase on this issue.

Knowing the phases of group development helps us recognize at what stage a group is and what to expect from the members. Groups must be allowed to progress through each phase at their own pace; this progress can be greatly enhanced by an understanding and facilitative leader.

Leader's Role

The group leader has a specific responsibility: to help the group achieve its goals. Sometimes a formal, designated leader assumes this role; at other times, an informal leader emerges to help focus the group's energy on its business. The nurse may be either a formal leader, an informal leader, or simply a member. All the members, including the leader, must be committed to working together to accomplish the group's goals. Leadership style influences this task. Whether the leader should assume an autocratic (leader-centered, persuasive) style, a democratic (member-centered, problem-solving) style, or a laissez-faire (noncentered) style depends on the group's needs. Each style has advantages as well as disadvantages, although the democratic style works best in most situations. Leadership styles are presented in more detail in Chapter 22. During the group process, the leader exercises some unique functions and employs certain techniques.

Functions. A leader performs a variety of activities designed to strengthen the group's ability to achieve its purpose. Important ones are the following (Sampson and Marthas, 1981):

1. Obtain and receive information
2. Help diagnose group goals, obstacles, and consequences of decisions
3. Facilitate communication
4. Help integrate varying perspectives and alternate possibilities for action
5. Test and evaluate proposals and decisions

Techniques. To carry out these functions, the leader needs skill in the use of certain techniques or leader interventions (Sampson and Marthas, 1981):

1. *Support* means to create an encouraging climate that reinforces positive behaviors and makes members feel secure and accepted. A leader could use this technique by telling the group, "You have made real progress today. Several people shared feelings as well as ideas, and you have all listened attentively and accepted these comments without judging them."
2. *Confrontation* is a technique that counters negative behavior through constructive feedback. The leader may direct it toward an individual member or the group as a whole. It consists of making direct, honest, reflective statements about how behaviors appear to us. People do not always want to hear these statements, but they may be necessary to facilitate group progress. It is helpful to combine support with confrontation.
3. *Advice and suggestions* can be offered when leader expertise or perspective is needed. Leaders should be careful to use it only when members are unable to solve problems for themselves.
4. *Summarizing* means providing the group with a concise, descriptive review. The leader may wish to summarize the group's actions to date, its progress in relationship to goals, its unresolved issues, and other areas of functioning. The value of this technique is to refocus group attention for future planning.
5. *Clarification* is used to prevent confusion or distortion of ideas. A leader could use this technique by saying, "From the comments I've heard, it seems to me that the group would like to switch to Tuesdays. Is that correct?"
6. *Questioning* is a useful technique for gaining information and greater understanding. By asking questions, leaders help members explore ideas in greater depth.
7. *Reflection* can be used to mirror people's ideas, feelings, or behaviors. To reflect ideas, leaders repeat, paraphrase, or highlight comments in order to facilitate communication. For example, when a member says, "I don't agree," a reflective response is, "You don't agree?"; thereby

the person receives an opportunity to discuss the idea further. Reflecting feelings means restating to the group or member the feelings the leader thinks are being conveyed. If a learning group complains, "We've never had to do anything like this before," the leader may reflect back, "You seem to be a little frightened of doing this." To reflect behavior, leaders simply describe the behavior they see, thus allowing the group to clarify the meaning. The leader can say to the group, "I notice that you've become silent since I made that last suggestion."

8. *Interpretation and analysis* may be used as a technique to uncover the underlying meaning of group comments and behaviors. In using this technique, leaders summarize observations of the group and then offer an analysis of the behavior's deeper meaning or reason. The leader might say, "I notice that several of you who are usually active have not participated in the past two sessions. I wonder if the decisions about this issue seem to be a foregone conclusion, and you feel it's useless to say anything?"

9. *Listening* attentively shows the group that the leader is interested in them and what they have to say. It also provides a positive model for group members to use with each other. Attentive listening helps sharpen the focus of the conversation by allowing specific responses to the comments being made.

Members' Roles

A new mothers' group has been meeting weekly now for a month and a half. As their leader, you notice that each person's behavior is unique in some way. Susan, for instance asks many questions and also tends to agree with whoever is speaking. Diane, on the other hand, is full of ideas and frequently offers suggestions or proposes some new plan of action. Then there is Maureen. Her friendly, warm responses seem to make the others feel better, in contrast to Fran's constant complaining. Verona has been especially helpful to you by keeping the group on track, helping to smooth out differences, and encouraging others to participate in the discussion. Each of the five women has assumed different group member roles.

Every group needs its members to perform specific roles. Member roles serve one of two basic functions necessary for a viable group—task or maintenance functions. Some roles are task-related: they help the group do its work. Diane, for instance, is an initiator of ideas, and Susan is both an information seeker and follower. Verona orients the group to its goals (keeps it on track). These are task roles. Other roles are maintenance-related: they deal with group members' participation. Maureen encourages members by showing acceptance and support, and Verona serves as gatekeeper, keeping communication channels open and facilitating member involvement. Both women play maintenance roles.

Task Roles.   These are behaviors that assist the group toward accomplishment of its goals. (See Table 14-2.) Two types of task roles are process roles and content roles (Kelly et al., 1989). *Process roles* include activities such as setting agendas, keeping records, leading the group, coordinating activities, delegating tasks, and managing information needed for and resulting from group decisions. *Content roles* include behaviors that contribute to the group's decision making, such as offering opinions, providing new information, summarizing discussions, or disagreeing with ideas.

Table 14-2
Roles and Functions of Group Members

Type of Role	Role	Functions Perfomed
Task Roles	Initiator	Proposes tasks, goals, or actions; defines group problems; suggests procedures
	Information Seeker	Asks for factual clarification; requests facts pertinent to the discussion
	Opinion Seeker	Asks for a clarification of the values pertinent to the topic under discussion; questions values involved in alternative suggestions
	Informer	Offers facts; expresses feelings; gives opinions
	Clarifier	Interprets ideas or suggestions; defines terms; clarifies issues before the group; clears up confusion
	Summarizer	Pulls together related ideas; restates suggestions; offers a decision or conclusion for the group to consider
	Reality Tester	Makes a critical analysis of an idea; tests an idea against some data to see if the idea would work
	Orienter	Defines the position of the group with respect to its goals; points to departures from agreed-upon directions or goals; raises questions about directions that the group discussion is taking
	Follower	Goes along with movement of group; passively accepts ideas of others; serves as audience in group discussion and decision
Maintenance Roles	Harmonizer	Attempts to reconcile disagreements; reduces tension; gets people to explore differences
	Gatekeeper	Helps to keep communication channels open; facilitates the participation of others; suggests procedures that permit sharing remarks
	Consensus Taker	Asks to see if the group is nearing a decision; sends up a trial balloon to test a possible solution
	Encourager	Is friendly, warm, and responsive to others; indicates by facial expression or remark the acceptance of others' contributions
	Compromiser	Offers a compromise that yields status when his own idea is involved in a conflict; modifies in the interest of group cohesion or growth
	Standard Setter	Expresses standards for the group to attempt to achieve; applies standards in evaluating the quality of a group process

Maintenance Roles. These are behaviors that promote a climate of co-hesiveness and effective working relationships among group members. Maintenance roles include activities such as encouraging other members, providing supportive comments, and mediating conflicts. (See Table 14-2.)

Functional and Dysfunctional Roles. The most common roles of group members are listed in Table 14-2 (Mill and Porter, 1976; Kelly et al., 1989). All of these roles are needed for a group to function effectively (Kelly et al., 1989). Some members will play several overlapping roles; others will play only one or two. A leader can determine the roles the group's members are playing by having an outside observer evaluate the group or by using one of various member participation checklists (Bradford, Stock, and Horwitz, 1976; Hill, 1977). Should a vital role, such as gatekeeper, be missing from a group, the leader and the group may wish to ask someone to assume this role.

Some roles are dysfunctional; they hinder the group from reaching its goals. Fran's constant complaining is an example of a dysfunctional role that inhibits communication and demoralizes the group. Other behaviors, such as being aggressive, blocking, dominating, distracting, or seeking recognition or sympathy, are also dysfunctional. These roles cannot be ignored. The group must identify and deal with them. If someone disrupts the group meeting, the leader may redirect the focus back to the topic by saying, for example, "I'd like to hear other people's ideas, too." When disruptive behavior is persis-tent, a technique such as reflection or interpretation and analysis may be a constructive way to deal with it. Confrontation should be used with discre-tion, particularly in front of the group, since it may be too threatening and counterproductive.

Solving Group Problems

Many difficulties arise during the life of a group. We have dealt with a few, such as how to start the group, avoid blocks to group cohesiveness, and deal with dysfunctional behavior. Three group problems in particular are worthy of further discussion. They are interpersonal conflict, dominance, and nonparticipation.

Resolving Conflicts. Conflict, by itself, is neither good nor bad. It is a form of tension frequently found in groups that may be used constructively by broadening the group's outlook and sharpening its problem-solving skills, or destructively by dissolving group cohesiveness.

Conflict arises when one or more members take sides against others in the group. There is sharp disagreement, arguing, tension, and impatience. Con-flict may occur because one or more members is seeking special status or mak-ing a power play, because some members have vested interests in or loyalty to another conflicting organization, or because members have overinvested in the group's productivity (Bradford et al., 1976).

Managing conflict means taking neither the extreme of flight (avoidance) or of fight (head-on confrontation), but rather a realistic attitude aimed at maximum gain for all those concerned. It is called a Win/Win approach (Guthrie and Miller, 1978; Veninga, 1982):

Lose/Lose   (you lose/I lose)
Win/Lose   (you win/I lose)
Lose/Win   (you lose/I win)
Win/Win   (you win/I win)

Using the Win/Win approach encourages people to work together to benefit all parties. Group members examine all the issues at stake and maximize the opportunity for everyone to satisfy at least some of their desires. Win/Win refocuses energy into problem solving instead of competition.

There are four steps to take to resolve conflicts. First, acknowledge that there is a conflict and reach agreement on its definition in the group. People may not be arguing different points, after all. Second, identify possible areas of agreement. There are nearly always some points that are not mutually exclusive. Third, determine the changes each party in the dispute must make to resolve the problem satisfactorily. Fourth, keep the focus of the conflict on issues rather than people. Personal attack will stalemate any attempt at resolution and may even strengthen the conflict (Veninga, 1982).

Dealing with Excessive Participation or Nonparticipation. Most groups need a relative equality of member participation for group work to be effective. To allow a full diversity of views, to foster cohesiveness through members' self-expression, and to make best use of the group's time, each member should have a fair share of the group's attention. Either nonparticipation or excessive participation will disrupt the group.

Excessive participation of members in the form of monopolizing conversation can produce feelings of anger and frustration for the leader and the group. Dominant members may be trying to cover up anxiety or seeking attention, recognition, and approval. However, their compulsive talking and apparent insensitivity to others in the group create dislike and disrespect. Other members feel cheated out of their share of the group's time. The group cannot benefit from a complete range of member contributions.

The leader copes with a dominant member by first trying supportive interruption: "Your point is well taken, but, in the interest of time, we need to allow others to express their views." If the member is not responsive to this approach, the leader may try another technique, such as reflection: "You seem to be doing most of the talking today." The leader might offer an interpretation: "I wonder if you are talking so much because you feel a little anxious about something, perhaps about how the group sees you?" Even confrontation may be necessary. It is also possible that the group is permitting the dominant member to monopolize as a way of avoiding its own responsibility. In that case, confrontation of the group may be needed.

A member may refuse to participate as a result of apathy, lack of commitment to the group's goals, anger, fear of ridicule, timidity, or poor self-image. When other members do not know why this person is quiet, they begin to feel uncomfortable (is this person judging us, ridiculing us, or not liking us?) and resentful (it is unfair of members not to carry their share of the group's work). The silence of several members may indicate an angry reaction to a few who are dominating or discomfort in the presence of conflict. When the entire group is silent or apathetic, they may be responding to the leader's style or the current task, which may seem unimportant or too difficult.

Nonparticipation must be diagnosed before the leader can intervene. Diagnosis can be made by offering a reflective or interpretive statement such as, "I've noticed that there is very little participation in the group today. Are people uncomfortable with this topic or perhaps with the way I'm leading the group?" or "Susan, you haven't said much in the last few sessions. Are the rest of us not giving you a chance?" From member responses and discussion, the leader learns the reasons behind the nonparticipation and then can take appropriate action. Nonintervention is sometimes best if it appears that too much group time and energy will be spent on the problem or if nonparticipation is infrequent. Occasional silence, particularly in one individual, may only be temporary. As the group becomes increasingly supportive and accepting, such individuals may gradually feel secure enough to start participating on their own.

TERMINATING A GROUP

Termination is an extremely important phase in the life of a small group (Loomis, 1979). Like any ending, including death, termination involves a mixed set of feelings that the group must face, explore, and resolve. Members must cope with feelings of loss and grief at leaving people to whom they have become attached. They must deal with a sense of success or failure, depending on whether their goals were met. They must recognize that they will no longer experience the group's support and other benefits. Termination is important because it is a time in the group's life when members have an opportunity to analyze the meaning of the group experience, which they can build on when planning for the future. Successful termination creates a sense of completion and a positive attitude toward future group experiences.

Termination is an issue that must be dealt with in every group. Most health care groups mark a beginning to their work and an ending when that work is complete. For these groups, the entire group will terminate. Other groups have an open-ended membership; thus the group (e.g., an ongoing support group) remains while members come and go. In these instances, the individual member terminates. Leaders, too, sometimes leave a group, perhaps for health reasons or a job change. Whether it is the entire group or an individual who is terminating, all the group members are affected. Positive leader intervention can make the difference in whether or not a group terminates successfully.

Preparing for Termination

Ideally, criteria for termination are established at the onset of the group. If the criteria are built into individual and group goals, clients know that, upon completion of their goals, it will be time to terminate. A failure on the part of many leaders, however, is not to explain these criteria fully to clients. The subject of termination is even avoided by some leaders, which suggests they may be denying its reality because they do not want to face the pain of separation. Part of the leader's responsibility, as early as possible in the life of the group, is to clarify with the group the exact conditions and date for termination.

Termination may be defined in terms of time (number of sessions or specific target date), behavior (when specific behavior changes have occurred), or circumstances (moving, job change, health). For example, a parenting group may choose to meet for 12 sessions and then terminate. If additional needs are identified at the end of that period, the group can renegotiate for more time. The members of a psychotherapy group will most likely decide that termination is appropriate when they see the desired changes in their behavior. Circumstances, such as moving or job change, are usually known far enough in advance to allow the group time to prepare adequately for termination.

Working Through Termination

When facing termination, group members may experience a mixture of feelings, such as sadness, anger, joy, or fear. They may deny the possibility of termination altogether. Members' behavior gives the leader clues about their reactions to termination. For instance, members who were formerly open in sharing feelings may become defensive and superficial. Others may appear angry and upset for no apparent reason. People may start to make plans for getting together beyond the termination date. Some may withdraw, come late, or act as if the group were no longer important to them. Most of these are unhealthy responses and require intervention.

Leader intervention during the termination process includes the following. First, the leader helps the group to identify and acknowledge that termination is occurring. Members must accept its reality. Second, the leader assists group members in finding appropriate alternatives for meeting the needs that the group has met. Fear of having to function without the group drives some members to return to old, unhealthy behaviors such as smoking or overeating after not having smoked or gone off their diets for months. Instead, the leader should encourage members to assess what the group has been providing for them and identify other ways to meet these needs outside of the group. For instance, one woman who was leaving an assertiveness training group decided to meet weekly with a friend for continued reinforcement of her new behaviors. The leader should allow enough time before termination for members to accomplish this task. Third, the leader gives group members an opportunity to express and deal with their feelings, which need to be worked through until the group senses that its business is finished. Finally, the leader facilitates termination by having the group evaluate its progress. "Here is where we were when we started. Look how far we have come" is a message that helps people leave with a sense of accomplishment and a positive outlook on the future.

EVALUATING A GROUP

Group evaluation includes two important areas, process measurement and outcomes measurement. The first examines ongoing group interaction, and the second looks at the group's final product.

Process Evaluation

It is important for groups to conduct periodic self-examinations. Leaders and members both need to hear reactions to their performances. Are they conducting their roles effectively? Are they making progress toward their goals? This information is vital to making improvements in the way members work together.

Process evaluation can be done in several ways. One useful method is to have an outside observer sit in on the group, watch for specific behaviors, and then give reactions to the group. The observer can use one of several guides available for this purpose (Bradford et al., 1976; Sampson and Marthas, 1981). Another method is to have a group member act as an impartial observer during a session in which the member only observes and refrains from participating. The group itself may diagnose its health by periodically or even regularly using some form of checklist or questionnaire, followed by discussion (Bradford et al., 1976; Guthrie and Miller, 1978; Hill, 1977). The kinds of behaviors to observe will vary with each group; generally, however, a group needs to examine all of the roles listed earlier and ask questions pertaining to areas such as communication skills and patterns, responses to leadership style, group climate, stage of group development, and progress on group objectives. Sweeney (1975) has developed a useful set of criteria that appraise the strength and effectiveness of groups in terms of their physical, interpersonal, intrapersonal, and community dimensions.

Measuring Group Outcomes

Determining the effectiveness of any group means measuring its outcomes. Did the group accomplish its objectives? Are the group members different now from how they were when the group started? Clear goals and specific objectives are the keys to unlocking the answers to these questions. Goals spell out the overall purpose of the group; objectives narrow goals down into specific behaviors that we can measure. For example, the group's goal may be to learn the techniques of natural childbirth. Objectives should describe separate behaviors, such as specific breathing techniques or exercises, that demonstrate the accomplishment of the goal. Thus, objectives that describe outcome behaviors are criteria for measuring the group's performance. If members can and do demonstrate ability in the breathing techniques and the exercises (or any other behaviors outlined in the objectives), then we can say that the group goal has been accomplished.

Some groups' goals are more difficult to evaluate than others, but all can be measured to some degree. A group of women with mastectomies may have a goal of learning to accept their own bodies. They can identify specific behaviors that will tell them when they have met this goal. The behaviors may include looking in the mirror without wincing, admitting to having undergone a mastectomy to another person outside the group, or wearing form-fitting clothing and not feeling overly self-conscious.

The group should participate equally with the leader in the evaluation process. Group members' own observations, insights, and feedback are essential to collecting the necessary data for evaluating the objectives. If specific behavior changes, such as staying on a special diet or exercising daily at home, are part of the objectives, then further supporting data can be solicited from family members or friends.

WORKING WITH POPULATIONS

Concern for populations or aggregates is a basic public health value but one that tends to be foreign to our individualistic, or even small-group, orientation and customary provision of health care. Enlarging that view requires adopting a new mind set, a new way of perceiving community health needs. Let us begin that process by hearing from a nurse who described her experience of broadening her focus to include these larger aggregates. She was employed by an agency we will call Wilford County Public Health Nursing Service.

> I received a referral to see a family whose 15-year-old daughter, Mary Jo, had run away from home for the third time. She was obese (215 pounds) and flunking out of school. There were so many problems in that family—unemployment, poor diet, stress, family conflict, another daughter's recent delivery of a sick illegiti-

mate baby, and the obesity of the mother and all three daughters—that I hardly knew where to begin, but the parents were willing to work with me. We discussed their concerns and started with their biggest worry—the running away of Mary Jo. We finally found her. She and another girl who was also flunking out of school had hitchhiked to the city to find jobs but had no luck and ended up at the YWCA. When they got home, we had some long talks, and she agreed to stay and give it another try.

Up to this point, I felt some success in working with this family, and Mary Jo in particular. Then, an offhand comment made by Mary Jo shifted my attention to a larger aggregate.

"I know a lot of other girls at school in the same boat as me," she said. I asked her what she meant. "Well, there's a lot of others who don't give a damn about school and feel that life is pretty worthless." I should have followed up on that remark right away, but I didn't. Then a girl committed suicide in that same school, one of *my* schools. I felt terrible. If some kind of effort had been made to reach those kids who were hurting emotionally, maybe that girl would be alive today. I had spent a lot of time with Mary Jo and her family, but it wasn't too late to work with other girls. We started to look at the needs of the whole population of adolescent girls. Then we went into both of my schools and started working with their organizations. We did something about those other students and, would you believe, we now have 35 girls coming to our Teen Topics meetings after classes on Tuesdays in one school and Thursdays in the other.

Because nurses have traditionally worked with individuals and families, it was not surprising that this nurse focused on Mary Jo. Here was a family that needed and, in fact, asked for help. The nurse understandably gave care where a need had been clearly identified. In contrast, a whole population of girls appeared to be an amorphous mass of people, too indistinct to be assessed, too nebulous to treat as a whole, and too large for one nurse to serve. But was it? Belatedly, this nurse discovered that she could assess and meet the needs of aggregates. In this case, the aggregate was a subpopulation of high school girls.

Identifying Populations

What is a population? A population is a large, unorganized collection of people grouped by one or more common demographic features. In contrast to a small group, a population is a loose collection of people. As a whole they do not have direct, face-to-face contact. They may or (more often) may not be aware of common problems or share similar goals. Members share a set of defining criteria but do not participate in a structure. That is, when we designate a special population, we identify one or more environmental or personal characteristics that the group of people have in common (Williams, 1977; Shamansky and Pesznecker, 1981). They might share the feature of age, as in a pediatric population or a population group of the elderly. The defining characteristic might involve language; consider the Spanish-, Italian-,

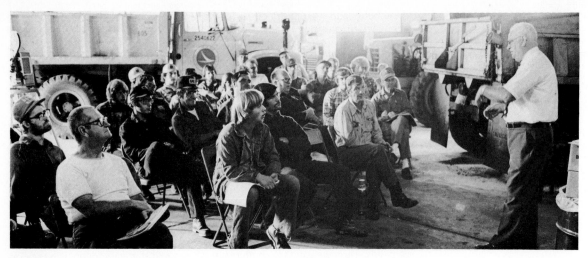

Figure 14-5
These farm workers constitute a population group. Here they meet to learn in an agricultural training session.

French-, Polish-, or Vietnamese-speaking populations within our country. Some population groups, such as blue-collar, pink-collar, and migrant workers, are defined in terms of their common type of employment (Figure 14-5). Other aggregates share a common diagnosis. We may speak of the diabetic population, or the populations of stroke or automobile accident victims. We often define aggregates in terms of their potential vulnerability to health problems; for instance, we identify populations at risk for coronary heart disease, home accidents, or family abuse. The special population groups of unwed teenage mothers in a city, managers demonstrating stress symptoms in a specific corporation, and farm workers in the state who have experienced accidents with machinery in the past year all share a clear set of defining criteria. These criteria describe the population group.

The purpose for designating a population group arises from some special need residing in that collection of people. When a number of school children in the same school district contract measles, the nurse may study all the children of that district as a population group to determine immunization levels and institute preventive immunization programs. There may be a large group of elderly people living alone in a community who are at risk of developing physical and emotional health problems because they do not utilize available resources. A significant number of employees with hypertension in an organization may attempt to function with their problem unrecognized and untreated. Community health professionals, therefore, single out population groups for the purpose of meeting health needs. The larger groups themselves become units for study and service.

STRATEGIES FOR WORKING WITH POPULATIONS

Aggregates, by definition, are quite different from small groups and require new approaches on the part of the community health nurse. Still, knowledge of the dynamics of groups, discussed earlier in this chapter, offers insights and strategies applicable to working with populations.

Assessment and Diagnosis

Aggregates as clients in community health have needs that are just as real as those identified for families or small groups (McGrath, 1986). The community health nurse assesses those needs through a combination of various methods. Four are especially useful.

Observation can provide valid information about aggregates. It is often one of the best ways to begin any assessment (Spradley, 1980). In the course of daily practice, nurses can watch for evidence of existing or potential problems. For example, after a community health nurse noticed symptoms of malnutrition in some migrant children, she broadened her observations to include the entire migrant community. Many of these hard-working people showed evidence of being undernourished. A nurse at an automobile manufacturing plant observed that several workers acted tense and fatigued. She began to pay attention to these symptoms when she walked through the plant.

Interviewing, a second assessment strategy, can offer detailed information about a population group (Spradley, 1979). The nurse working with migrants prepared a set of questions about diet and eating practices. She interviewed several families in their shacks and discovered they ate no meat or dairy products, but only white bread, potatoes, and occasional vegetable scraps stolen from the fields. Their income was too meager to allow purchase of better foods. At the automobile plant, the nurse interviewed several selected workers and discovered that they had frequent headaches and nausea. These symptoms were most evident at the end of the day after long hours of exposure to the chemicals they were using in their work.

The nurse concerned about migrant nutrition took her initial findings to the state health department. With a team of professionals, she helped design an *epidemiologic survey,* a third assessment strategy (Dever, 1980). In an organization such as the automobile manufacturing plant mentioned earlier, it is also possible to conduct an epidemiologic survey. In her role as part of the company's middle management, the nurse pointed out the symptoms among workers on this unit. Others agreed that they had noticed them, too, and had seen them in workers in other units as well. She then helped develop a study to determine the plant's chemical hazards and their impact on employees' health. (Epidemiologic research as an aggregate assessment tool was discussed in Chapter 9.)

A fourth assessment strategy uses *existing data.* Nurses can learn a great deal about a population group by examining information that has already been collected for other purposes. Census records, community demographic data, or surveys done by other community organizations can often provide needed information for assessment and health planning for population groups. Statistics on infant morbidity and mortality from automobile accidents, for example, as well as records describing infant car seat use could assist in a study of the safety of the infant car-riding population. Other sources of existing data are described in Chapters 8 and 9.

Thorough needs assessment at the aggregate level usually requires an interdisciplinary team effort to ensure proper data collection and analysis. Community-wide needs assessment is discussed in Chapter 13.

The determination of health problems among population groups, then, depends on careful analysis and interpretation of this collected data. At the aggregate level diagnosis becomes a more complex task, and the community health nurse seldom does it alone. As during needs assessment, the nurse requires the expertise and collaborative input of other public health professionals, such as epidemiologists, statisticians, health planners, and environmentalists. There must be a clear and accurate diagnosis of the problem to be addressed.

Planning and Implementation

Interventions at the aggregate level are on a larger scale and generally more complex than working with small groups. They are often what we know as community health programs. Nonetheless, many group principles apply. A clear goal and set of objectives are needed (Blum, 1981). There must be agreement among the planning team members (Nutt, 1984). Nurses cannot easily communicate with an entire aggregate to gain each person's input and cooperation; therefore, they ask representatives of that population to serve on the planning team along with an appropriate mix of health professionals. Because the planning is done by a team, the nurse can apply principles of small-group interaction to enhance the group's functioning. Health planning and implementation for aggregates follow the same general process as any kind of nursing care planning. For population groups, however, health planners must also be concerned about factors in the external environment, such as health policy, economic conditions, legislation, other programs competing for service to the same population, or funding, that may influence planning decisions. A family planning education program for Southeast Asian refugees, for example, was being considered by a local public health nursing agency. However, state funding for refugees' programs was drying up, and the nurses had to seek other sources of financial backing before the program could be implemented.

Evaluation

Most often we evaluate aggregate-level health care in terms of four types of results depending on our goals. They are outputs, outcomes, impact, and efficiency (Churgin, 1981). *Outputs* are measured in terms of quantity. That is, if a family planning program aims to teach a certain number of people in the population, then the evaluation effort measures how many people were served. *Outcomes* are a quality measure and refer to the consequences of the program. Were the desired end results accomplished? For example, did the family planning program accomplish fewer unwanted pregnancies? *Impact* evaluation looks beyond the immediate results of the intervention and asks what effect it had on the rest of the community. Did this program meet the needs of one subpopulation but overlook other populations' needs? Should more extensive programs be developed? Finally, *efficiency* evaluation asks if the resources (costs in money, time, and personnel) were used as effectively as possible, or if the resources produced as much as could reasonably be expected (Churgin, 1981).

Evaluation of community health programs follows five steps (Churgin, 1981). First, the planning group must develop a list of criteria to be used to determine successful completion of the objectives. This is best done during the planning stage. Second, it must devise ways to measure these criteria. The measures should be objective, reliable, and valid. For example, if the group is evaluating a child health promotion program, one criterion may be fewer school absence days, measured in number of days missed. Third is data collection, and fourth is analysis and interpretation of the data. Finally, the findings are presented to relevant groups or organizations for future planning decisions.

Evaluation may be formative or summative. Formative evaluation is conducted to give feedback during the development of the health program. It examines the program while it is forming, as one might wish to do with a new health education effort. Is the program process working effectively? Is the program generating the desired outcomes as it goes along? Summative evaluation is conducted after the program is complete. It is the sum of the program's final product.

SIMILARITIES IN WORKING WITH POPULATIONS AND GROUPS

As we have seen, populations, in contrast to small groups, require a different orientation and set of strategies for use by community health nurses. Despite the differences, however, there are many similarities in the approaches the nurse can apply. Let us summarize both.

Work with populations still employs the nursing process, but its application is on a larger scale. The nurse may work alone with a small group; aggregate work involves the expertise and input of a collaborating interdisciplinary team of which the nurse is a part. With small groups, every member is expected to participate to accomplish group goals. Work with populations should also involve people in the decisions that affect them, but that involvement, of necessity, means that representatives of the group speak for the rest. We recognize that small groups have a collective identity or personality, as do population groups, and we respect each group's uniqueness. Even as small groups go through stages of development, so do population groups' needs change over time. Both require ongoing assessment. We employ different tools, such as epidemiologic research, in working with aggregates to facilitate systematic assessment and health planning on a larger scale. Finally, external determinants of health, such as social, biological, organizational, and environmental factors, must be considered in working with groups of any size. Their significance in the context of the total community is greater, however, when applied to work with populations.

Summary

Groups of all sizes are an important focus for community health nursing service. A small group consists of a collection of persons who engage in repeated, face-to-face communication, identify with each other, are interdependent, and share a common purpose or purposes.

In preparing to work with small groups, the community health nurse must understand their different types, their essential needs, and their primary functions. There are five major types of small groups encountered by community health nurses:

1. Learning groups, whose primary goal is to gain understanding in order to change behavior in some specified area
2. Support groups, which aim to provide emotional reassurance and maintain healthy behaviors
3. Socialization groups, which help members to learn new social roles and skills
4. Psychotherapy groups, formed for people who need treatment of an emotional disturbance.
5. Task-oriented groups, whose primary goal is to accomplish some predetermined task

Individuals have needs; so do groups. The small groups with which community health nurses work need clear, shared goals and an agreement about how to reach those goals. They need consistent group norms and members who are motivated to participate in the group. Finally, every group needs stable communication channels among the members. Groups have two primary types of functions: task-related functions and group maintenance functions.

Starting a small group involves determining the criteria for membership and then selecting people who are committed to the goals of the group. It is important to determine the optimal size of the group, set clear group goals, make physical arrangements for the group, and orient the members.

Every small group varies in terms of the degree of cohesiveness experienced by members. The community health nurse can build a cohesive group by assuring that its four basic needs are met and avoiding certain barriers such as open membership. Building group cohesiveness must be an ongoing process in any group.

Working with a small group is enhanced by recognizing the phases of group development: dependence, counterdependence, and interdependence. The group leader has specific functions and ways to carry out those functions. Every group also needs its members to carry out specific roles such as initiator, information seeker, informer, and clarifier. Many difficulties arise during the life of a group. In particular, the community health nurse must be alert to resolving conflicts, dealing with those who monopolize the group, and handling members who do not participate.

Every small group must deal with the issue of termination, the last phase in the life of a group. It is important to prepare members for termination early in the life of a group and to work through the feelings generated by termination.

Group evaluation involves assessing the ongoing group interaction as well as the final outcome. Periodic self-evaluations are useful strategies for evaluating the process of group experience. Measuring the outcomes determines to what extent the group's goals were achieved. The entire evaluation process should involve both the leader and group members.

Working with aggregates involves a different orientation and some different strategies from those employed for small-group work. An aggregate, or population group, is a large, unorganized collection of people who share one or more demographic features in common, such as age, ethnic background, or vulnerability to a health problem.

Assessment strategies for working with population groups include observation, interviewing, conducting epidemiologic surveys, and use of existing data. The community health nurse works collaboratively with other public health professionals to assess needs, diagnose, and plan for, implement, and evaluate interventions on behalf of population groups. Evaluation efforts address four primary types of results: outputs, outcomes, impact, and efficiency.

Work with aggregates shares similarities as well as differences with small-group work. Community health nurses utilize the nursing process on a larger scale in work with aggregates. They work on a team. They seek input from population group representatives. They respect the group's unique features and recognize that its needs change. They employ epidemiologic research and other assessment and planning tools applicable for macro-level use. They consider the impact of external health determinants on the health of population groups.

Study Questions

1. Select a small group (not social) of which you are currently or have recently been a member. Which of the three phases of group development is it in? Would you describe this group as a healthily functioning one? Why or why not?

2.   Compare and contrast a socialization group with a social group. Is socialization a health-promoting activity? What are the reasons for your answer?

3.   Normally in groups we each tend to play certain typical roles. Analyze your own role behavior in groups. What roles do you commonly play as a member, and are they task- or maintenance-focused?

4.   Imagine yourself to be the community health nurse in the case study of the Wilford County Public Health Nursing Service. You have just become a member of a planning team newly formed to assess and plan for the needs of these adolescent girls. What are some assessment strategies you could use and suggest to the group? Discuss some specific actions you might take to begin the assessment.

References

Blum, H. L. (1981). *Planning for health: Generics for the eighties.* 2nd ed. New York: Human Sciences Press.

Bradford, L., D. Stock, and M. Horwitz. (1976). How to diagnose group problems. In S. Stone, et al. (eds.), *Management for nurses* (pp. 133–46). St. Louis, Mo.: C. V. Mosby.

Callahan, J., et al. (1980). Processing a task group: A continuing education committee at work planning a conference. *Journal of Continuing Education in Nursing* 11: 8.

Churgin, S. (1981). Evaluation. In H. L. Blum (ed.), Planning for health: Generics for the eighties. 2nd ed. (pp. 270–99). New York: Human Sciences Press.

Dever, G. E. A. (1980). *Community health analysis.* Germantown, Md.: Aspen Systems.

Erikson, E. (1963). *Childhood and society.* 2nd ed. New York: W. W. Norton.

Guthrie, E., and S. Miller. (1978). *Making change: A guide to effectiveness in groups.* Minneapolis, Minn.: Interpersonal Communication Programs.

Hill, W. F. (1977). *Learning through discussion: Guide for leaders and members of discussion groups.* Beverly Hills, Calif.: Sage.

Kagey, J. R., et al. (1981). Mental health primary prevention: The role of parent mutual support groups. *American Journal of Public Health* 71: 166.

Kelly, L., L. C. Lederman, and G. M. Phillips. (1989). *Communicating in the workplace: A guide to business and professional speaking.* New York: Harper & Row.

Konopka, G. (1954). *Group work in the institution.* New York: Whiteside.

Lipson, J. G. (1980). Consumer activism in two women's self-help groups. *Western Journal of Nursing Research* 2: 393.

Loomis, M. E. (1979). *Group process for nurses.* St. Louis: C. V. Mosby.

Marram, G. D. (1978). *The group approach in nursing practice.* 2nd ed. St. Louis, Mo.: C. V. Mosby.

Maslow, A. (1954). *Motivation and personality.* New York: Harper & Row.

McGrath, B. B. (1986). The social networks of terminally ill skid row residents: An analysis. *Public Health Nursing* 3: 192.

Mill, C. R., and L. C. Porter. (1976). What to observe in a group. In C. Mill and L. Porter (eds.), *Reading book for human relations training* (pp. 28–30). Washington, D.C.: National Training Laboratories Institute for Applied Behavioral Science.

Nutt, P. C. (1984). *Planning methods for health and related organizations.* New York: Wiley.

Pesznecker, B., and E. Zahlis. (1986). Establishing mutual-help groups for family-member caregivers: A new role for community health nurses. *Public Health Nursing* 3: 29.

Sampson, E., and M. Marthas. (1981). *Group process for the health professions.* Somerset, N.J.: Wiley.

Schutz, D. (1966). *The interpersonal underworld.* Palo Alto, Calif.: Science and Behavior Books.

Shamansky, S., and B. Pesznecker. (1981). A community is... *Nursing Outlook 29:* 182.

Spradley, J. (1979). *The ethnographic interview.* New York: Holt, Rinehart, and Winston.

Spradley, J. (1980). *Participant observation.* New York: Holt, Rinehart, and Winston.

Sweeney B. (1975). Learning groups: Survival level, growth level. *Journal of Nursing Education 14*(3): 20–26.

Veninga, R. (1982). *The human side of health administration: A guide for hospital, nursing, and public health administrators.* Englewood Cliffs, N.J.: Prentice-Hall.

Williams, C. (1977). Community health nursing—What is it? *Nursing Outlook 25:* 250–53.

Yalom, I. D. (1975). *The theory and practice of group psychotherapy.* New York: Basic Books.

Selected Readings

Abramson, J. H. (1974). *Survey methods in community medicine.* Edinburgh: Churchill Livingstone.

Berne, E. (1963). *The structure and dynamics of organizations and groups.* New York: Lippincott.

Blum, H. L. (1981). *Planning for health: Generics for the eighties.* 2nd ed. New York: Human Sciences Press.

Bormann, E. G., and N. C. Bormann. (1976). *Effective small group communication.* 2nd ed. Minneapolis, Minn.: Burgess.

Bradford, L., D. Stock, and M. Horwitz. (1976). How to diagnose group problems. In S. Stone, et al. (eds.), *Management for nurses* (pp. 133–46). St. Louis, Mo.: C. V. Mosby.

Bruhn, J. G. (1973). Planning for social change: Dilemmas for health planning. *American Journal of Public Health 63:* 602–5.

Burnside, I. M. (1978). *Working with the elderly: Group processes and techniques.* North Scituate, Mass.: Duxbury Press.

Callahan, J., et al. (1980). Processing a task group: A continuing education committee at work planning a conference. *Journal of Continuing Education in Nursing 11:*8.

Cathart, R. S., and L. A. Samovar, (eds.). (1974). *Small group communication: A reader.* 2nd ed. Dubuque, Ia.: Wm. C. Brown.

Chopra, A. (1973). Motivation in task-oriented groups. *Journal of Nursing Administration 3*(1): 15.

Cohen, P. (1982). Community health planning from an interorganizational perspective. *American Journal of Public Health 72:* 717–21.

Corbin, D. E. (1983). Self-help groups: What the health educator should know. *Health Values 7:* 10.

Dever, G. E. A. (1980). *Community health analysis.* Germantown, Md.: Aspen Systems.

Dombeck, M. T. (1986). Faculty peer review in a group setting. *Nursing Outlook 34:* 188.

Dyer, W. G. (1973). Working with groups. In A. Reinhardt and M. Quinn (eds.), *Family-centered community nursing: A sociocultural framework.* St. Louis, Mo.: C. V. Mosby.

Forsyth, D. M., et al. (1981). Preventing and alleviating staff burnout through a group. *Psychosocial Nursing and Mental Health Services 35:* 8.

Green L. (1980). *Health education planning: A diagnostic approach.* Palo Alto, Calif.: Mayfield Publishing.

Guthrie, E., and S. Miller. (1978). *Making change: A guide to effectiveness in groups.* Minneapolis, Minn.: Interpersonal Communication Programs.

Henkel, B. L. (1970). Solving health problems through small-group action. In B. Henkel (ed.), *Community health.* 2nd ed. (pp. 338–47). Boston: Allyn and Bacon.

Hill, W. F. (1962). *Learning through discussion: Guide for leaders and members of discussion groups.* Beverly Hills, Calif.: Sage.

Hogan, R. (1986). Gaining community support for group homes. *Community Mental Health Journal* 22: 117.

Hyman, H. H. (1981). *Health planning—A systematic approach.* 2nd ed. Germantown, Md.: Aspen Systems.

Kagey, J. R., et al. (1981). Mental health primary prevention: The role of parent mutual support groups. *American Journal of Public Health* 71: 166.

Kraegel, J. (ed.). (1980). *Organization-environment relationships.* Wakefield, Mass.: Nursing Resources.

Larson, M., and R. Williams. (1978). How to become a better group leader? Learn to recognize the strange things that happen to some people in groups. *Nursing '78,* 8(8): 65.

Lipson, J. G. (1980). Consumer activism in two women's self-help groups. *Western Journal of Nursing Research* 2: 393.

Loomis, M. E. (1979). *Group process for nurses.* St. Louis, Mo.: C. V. Mosby.

Mallick, M. J. (1985). A community-based support group for families and patients with acute coronary disease. *Public Health Nursing* 2: 43.

Marram, G. D. (1978). *The group approach in nursing practice.* 2nd ed. St. Louis, Mo.: C. V. Mosby.

McGrath, B. B. (1986). The social networks of terminally ill skid row residents: An analysis. *Public Health Nursing* 3: 192.

McLaughlin, J. (1982). Toward a theoretical model for community health programs. *Advances in Nursing Science* 5(2): 7–28.

McLemore, M. K. M. (1980). Nurses as health planners. *Journal of Nursing Administration* 1(9): 13–17.

Michael, M. M., et al. (1980). Symposium on the self-care concept of nursing: Use of the adolescent peer group to increase the self-care agency of adolescent alcohol abusers. *Nursing Clinics of North America* 15: 157.

Milio, N. (1975). *The care of health in communities.* New York: Macmillan.

Mill, C. R., and L. C. Porter. (1976). What to observe in a group. In C. Mill and L. Porter (eds.), *Reading book* (pp. 28–30). Washington, D.C.: National Training Laboratories Institute for Applied Behavioral Science.

Neuber, K. A. (1980). *Needs assessment: A model for community planning.* Beverly Hills, Calif.: Sage.

Nutt, P. C. (1984). *Planning methods for health and related organizations.* New York: Wiley.

Ohlsen, M. M. (1977). *Group counseling.* 2nd ed. New York: Holt, Rinehart and Winston.

Pesznecker, B., and E. Zahlis. (1986). Establishing mutual-help groups for family-member caregivers: A new role for community health nurses. *Public Health Nursing* 3: 29.

Reinhardt, A., and E. Chatlin. (1977). Assessment of health needs in a community: The basis for program planning. In A. Reinhardt and M. Quinn (eds.), *Current practice in family-centered community nursing* (pp. 138–87). St. Louis: C. V. Mosby.

Rossi, P., and H. Freeman. (1982). *Evaluation: A systematic approach.* 2nd ed. Beverly Hills, Calif.: Sage.

Sampson, E., and M. Marthas. (1977). *Group process for the health professions.* Somerset, N.J.: Wiley.

Shamansky, S., and B. Pesznecker. (1981). A community is... *Nursing Outlook 29*: 182.

Shaw, M. E. (1971). *Group dynamics: The psychology of small-group behavior.* New York: McGraw-Hill.

Shortell, S., and W. Richardson. (1978). *Health program evaluation.* St. Louis, Mo.: C. V. Mosby.

Smith, L. L. (1980). Finding your leadership style in groups. *American Journal of Nursing 80*: 1301.

Spradley, J. (1979). *The ethnographic interview.* New York: Holt, Rinehart, and Winston.

Spradley, J. (1980). *Participant observation.* New York: Holt, Rinehart, and Winston.

Sweeney, B. (1975). Learning groups: Survival level, growth level. *Journal of Nursing Education* 14(3): 20–26.

Tubbs, S. L., and S. Moss. (1974). The small group: Therapeutic communication. In S. Tubbs and S. Moss (eds.), *Human communication: An interpersonal perspective* (pp. 231–57). New York: Random House.

Veninga, R. (1973). The management of conflict. *Journal of Nursing Administration* 3(4): 12–16.

Veninga, R. (1982). *The human side of health administration: A guide for hospital, nursing, and public health administrators.* Englewood Cliffs, N.J.: Prentice-Hall.

Warheit, G., R. Bell, and J. Schwab. (1977). *Needs assessment approaches: Concepts and methods* (Pub. No. [ADM] 79-472). Washington, D.C.: National Institute of Mental Health.

Yalom, I. D. (1975). *The theory and practice of group psychotherapy.* New York: Basic Books.

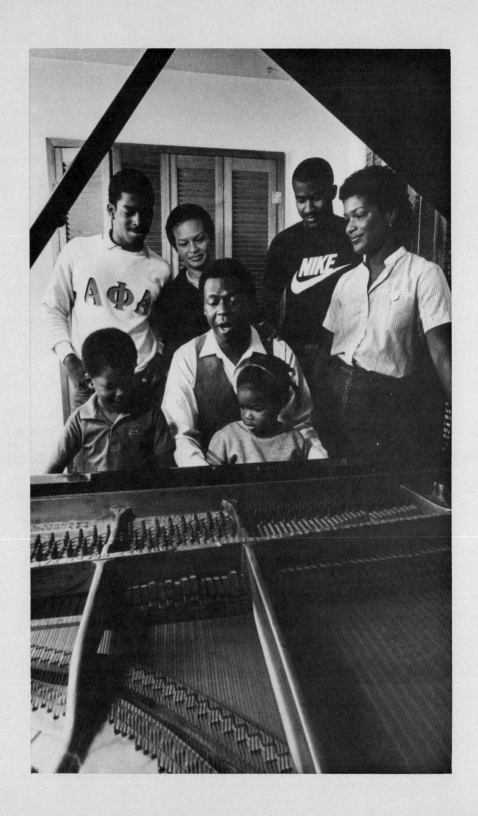

15 Family Health: Assessment and Practice

Community health nursing has a long history of concern for family health. During the nineteenth century, public health nurses became aware through home visits of the significant influence that the family had on individual health and on the health of the larger community. For example, many of the sick poor failed to recover because they lacked resources and support from their families, and these needy families, in turn, drained existing community resources. Nurses began to view client care from the more holistic perspective of family care. Nursing educators, as early as 1919, were introducing concepts of family care into curricula (Ford, 1973). By 1932, the National Organization of Public Health Nursing strongly declared that *family* health was the cardinal concern of all public health nursing practice.

Although nursing continues to emphasize the family as a unit of service, a gap exists between theory and practice (Freeman and Heinrich, 1981). The problem derives in part from a health care system that fosters an individualistic orientation, often to the exclusion of the family. We have a proliferation of programs geared to individuals in specific age groups or with specific health problems. Many third-party payers and reimbursement policies impose limits on the kinds of services funded, most of which are for individuals. Even public health agencies tend to organize their services around individuals. Often in response to governmental requirements, they must keep statistical records on specific disease or service categories, thus reflecting an individual, rather than family or population, orientation. Although community health nurses may subscribe to the value of a family and community orientation, their experience with acute care based on the medical model often leads them to practice individualistic nursing rather than taking an aggregate-based approach.

IMPORTANCE OF FAMILY HEALTH

Despite the obstacles just discussed, family nursing persists. Three major reasons underlie its continuing importance for community health. First, the family as a unit is a target for service. Second, family health and individual

435

health strongly influence each other. And third, family health affects community health. Let us examine each of these ideas more closely.

THE FAMILY AS AN ENTITY FOR SERVICE

Much research has demonstrated that families behave as units and need to be viewed in totality for therapy to be effective (Whall, 1987). The family does not simply provide the context for understanding and giving care to individuals. As we saw in Chapter 4, it is a separate entity with its own structure, functions, and needs. The total family can be viewed as the client. In every society throughout history, the family is the most basic unit; so too in community health (Pratt, 1976). It is the family, more than any other societal institution, that nurtures and shapes a society's members. Since community health practice serves population groups, we now focus on this basic societal unit, one in a series of increasingly larger communities.

EFFECT OF FAMILY HEALTH ON INDIVIDUAL HEALTH

The health of each family member affects the other members and contributes to the total family's level of health. Following her husband's stroke, for example, a woman may successfully cope with the resulting physical and emotional demands of his care but have inadequate reserves to effectively meet the needs of her children. The level at which a family functions — how well it is able to solve problems and help its members reach their potential — significantly affects the individual's level of health (Loveland-Cherry, 1984). A healthy family will foster individual growth and resistance to ill health and sustain its members during times of crisis (McCubbin et al., 1982). On the other hand, a family with limited capacity for problem solving and self-management is often unable to promote the potential of its members or assist them in times of need. Consider a family with an abused child. That family's level of functioning is generally very low, and the physical, emotional, and social health of each member suffers as a result.

Family health standards influence members' health practices. For instance, many individuals, even as adults, adhere to family patterns of eating, exercise, and communication. Family values influence decisions about health services such as whether or not a child receives immunizations or the mother uses birth control. Family decisions determine the kind of health care a member receives. For example, will sick members only receive care at home or will the family seek professional help? If professional advice is received, to what degree will the family carry it out? Is is clear that individuals influence family health and that the family can either obstruct or facilitate individual health. The family, then, becomes an important focus for community health nursing assessment and intervention.

EFFECT OF FAMILY HEALTH ON COMMUNITY HEALTH

Rarely do families live in isolation from one another. Even in the most uncommunicative of neighborhoods, one family's noisy children, another family's trash-littered yard, and another's barking dog all have an impact on the surrounding families. The level at which each family functions determines whether or not it can promote a healthier community and support other families and groups rather than merely remain a liability (Crooks et al., 1987).

Healthy families influence community health positively. Some families, for example, have temporarily housed Southeast Asian or Cuban refugees and assisted them in finding employment. Others have formed community groups to encourage neighborhood safety and beautification. Many families are regularly involved in church, scouting programs, parent-teacher-student associations, or other civic activities that promote the common good.

Conversely, families with a low level of health have a negative influence on community health. Because they lack the resources to manage their own affairs, they frequently create problems and even health hazards for others. Garbage left to accumulate in a backyard, for example, attracts rats; abandoned appliances may become death traps for playing children. Regardless of socioeconomic level, a poorly functioning family becomes a drain on community resources and a threat to community health. Consider the large proportion of tax dollars and private funds that go into remedial programs for children with learning and behavior difficulties caused by problems at home, for adults with mental health problems, for the chemically dependent, and for victims of family violence—groups significantly influenced by unhealthy families. Since family health affects the health of other families, groups, and communities, nurses who help families develop and maintain positive health patterns and practices are also promoting community health.

TWO FAMILY CASE STUDIES

You ring the doorbell and wait. Soon someone opens the door and ushers you into the living room. You explain, in response to their quizzical expressions, that you are here to help this family sustain or raise its level of health. Of course you do not say it quite that way. Perhaps you say, "I understand you have a new baby. I'm the community nurse, and I would like to assist you in any way that I can." Or you may say, "I have come to see how you are getting along since your surgery." However, your job extends far beyond simply teaching infant care or postsurgical rehabilitation. This is a family, an interdependent group of people who function as a unit. That individual, the precipitating cause of the referral, is only one part of the total group upon whom you should focus. How can you sustain or raise this family's level of health? How do you determine that level?

From our discussion in Chapter 4, we learned that families, to be healthy, must accomplish certain basic functions that they must adapt to their unique structure, environment, and needs (Hanson, 1984). To develop a clearer frame of reference for understanding family health, let us consider two families in particular.

The Murphys live in a modest two-story house that is clean, comfortable, and homey. There are seven of them: Jack, Bev, and their five children. Jack, now 43 years of age, has worked with the local Ford agency since high school, starting out as a mechanic and moving up to his present position of shop foreman. Bev, 41 years old, stayed home to care for the children until all were in school and then took a job as checker at a nearby supermarket. Because Bev had new responsibilities, Jack and the children took over many of the housekeeping tasks. As the Murphy children grew up, each assumed additional chores around the house and also found jobs in the community. Two children now have paper routes, one baby-sits, one does yard work, and the oldest boy bags groceries at the market where his mother works. Each family member feels encouraged toward independence; at the same time, each member also feels supported and loved.

As a family, the Murphys do many things together. When the children were younger, they had "family night" every Friday; they played games, ate homemade goodies, and went on outings together. Church activities, baseball, and PTA functions now involve the family as a unit. Trips to the grandparents' farm in the neighboring state are delightful ways to spend the holidays or part of a summer vacation. Harmony does not always prevail with the Murphys, however. There are many disagreements over family rules, financial decisions, and other areas of family life. However, since they are accustomed to talking things over, they resolve these conflicts without difficulty. Jack and Bev together usually make the major family decisions, such as whether to buy a new car or where to go on vacation. Frequently they involve the children in making decisions and encourage them to think for themselves. Around the dinner table, the Murphys often discuss current events, report on their activities, or debate various issues.

On the whole, they have had very few illnesses. There were some childhood diseases, a scattering of colds and flu, and a few broken bones over the years. Until Bev's cholecystectomy three years ago, none of them had undergone surgery. The family belongs to a prepaid health care plan through Jack's job and therefore is able to visit a clinic for regular checkups, immunizations, and early treatment of problems without feeling undue financial stress from health care costs. At home the Murphys eat well, and most of them are involved in some kind of exercise; even Bev, who has to watch her weight, swims regularly at the YWCA with a group of her friends from church.

The Stone family lives in the same town as the Murphys. Their sprawling rambler house in the suburbs is the center of much activity. John, 44 years old, is a professor at the community college located four blocks away. Because his office is so close, John often eats lunch, studies, and holds some of his classes in his home. Students also drop by frequently. Shirley, 45 years of age, became a social worker three years ago after going back to school. She has a heavy caseload and takes her clients' problems so much to heart that many of her evenings are spent on the phone or making extra visits. The Stones have two daughters and one son. Their 19-year-old daughter attends the community college and continues to live at home. Now the proud owner of his own car, the 17-year-old son, a junior in high school, has turned the family driveway into an auto repair shop where he and his friends spend hours tinkering with their cars. The youngest girl, a 14-year-old cheerleader in her junior high school, has a frenetic social life. The family's pets, two German shepherds and three cats, run unrestrictedly, creating occasional chaos.

John has always believed that the father is the head of the house and that his responsibility is to make the rules. He expects Shirley to enforce them. Shirley, however, is disorganized and unable to discipline herself or the children; thus, assigned tasks are not done, rules are not observed, meals are almost never eaten together, and the house is never clean. John retreats to his study while Shirley spends longer hours on the job and the children go their separate ways, unconcerned about helping at home. Communication among them is infrequent. In earlier years John and Shirley were close even though Shirley always had difficulty managing the home. Since she returned to school and then to work, Shirley has been unable to keep up with the dual demands of career and homemaking. The family still expects her to do all the shopping, cooking, cleaning, and laundry. John is supportive of her professional efforts as long as they do not require him to make any adjustments in his routine and life-style. Shirley has a cleaning woman come once a week, but the house quickly resumes its perpetual disarray.

The Stones spend very little time together as a family, and consequently know almost nothing about each other's activities, interests, or needs. John, frustrated at not getting a promotion this year, has become more reclusive and has begun to drink heavily. Feeling inadequate about her inability to manage her life, Shirley has stepped up her work activities, drinks coffee excessively, and takes two or three Valium each day. Their son, kicked off the football squad for violating training rules, uses his car as an outlet for aggression and to attract attention. Unbeknownst to her parents, the younger daughter has been experimenting with drugs for the past six months.

Some families, like the Murphys, are healthy. Others, like the Stones, are not. Still others are somewhere in between. In fact, family health, like individual health, ranges along a continuum from wellness to illness. A family may be at one point on that continuum now and at a much different point six months from now. Family health refers to the health status of a given family at a given point in time (Baranowski and Nader, 1985). What is it that tells us the Murphys are a healthy family and the Stones are not?

A cursory view shows that the Murphys are accomplishing their basic functions. We see indications of a loving, nurturing climate (affection). The family provides consistently for its members' physical and emotional needs (security). Each member appears to be growing in independence and successfully adding new roles (identity). The family is close and utilizes effective communication patterns (affiliation). Members' behavior appears consistent with family values (socialization), and division of tasks and use of resources are flexible and adapted to changing family needs (controls).

The Stones, on the other hand, are not accomplishing these functions. At an earlier stage, they were a close, loving family, but now the members have drifted apart. There is little evidence of an affectional climate. Physical and emotional needs are met only minimally, if at all, which contributes to lack of security and inadequate identity development. Communication patterns are poor; there is little sense of affiliation. Because guidance of values and behavior is almost nonexistent now, the family has little influence on members' socialization or social control. At this point in time, we see a poorly functioning, unhealthy family.

CHARACTERISTICS OF HEALTHY FAMILIES

How does the community health nurse determine family health status? Analysis of a family in terms of how it meets its basic functions does not give us a satisfactory picture of its health status. More definitive criteria are needed. Over the years, research on families, and particularly on family health behavior, gives us a growing body of data with which to assess family health.

One means of viewing family health is by examining family strengths. Olson and Associates (1983) identify seven major family strengths important for family functioning and coping with crises: family pride, family support, cohesion, adaptability, communication, religious orientation, and social support. This list builds on work done by earlier family researchers who saw family strengths as important and untapped resources. Otto (1963) emphasized the following family abilities:

To provide a sense of family unity, loyalty, and interfamily cooperation
To provide support and security
To perform roles flexibly
To maintain constructive relationships with the community

Other researchers have identified various characteristics, such as good communication patterns (Baranowski et al., 1982), spending time together, having a strong religious orientation, dealing with crises positively (McCubbin et al., 1982), having a sense of unity and commitment to one another (Peitze, 1984), and showing respect and appreciation for one another (Stinnett, 1981; Stinnett and Saur, 1977). Results from the White House Conference on Families survey defined "strong" families as (1) families that highly value their relationships and (2) families whose members support each other through good and bad times (Tanner-Nelson and Banonis, 1981). The literature on families describes healthy families as having six important characteristics (Duffy, 1988; Duvall and Miller, 1985; Friedman, 1986; Olson, McCubbin, and Associates, 1983; Otto, 1973):

1. There is a facilitative process of interaction among family members.
2. They enhance individual member development.
3. Their role relationships are structured effectively.
4. They actively attempt to cope with problems.
5. They have a healthy home environment and life-style.
6. They establish regular links with the broader community.

Let us examine these characteristics of healthy families more closely.

FACILITATIVE INTERACTION AMONG MEMBERS

Healthy families communicate. Their patterns of interaction are regular, varied, and supportive. Adults communicate with adults, children with children, and adults with children. These interactions are frequent and assume many forms. Healthy families use frequent verbal communication. Like the Murphys, they discuss problems, confront each other when angry, share ideas and concerns, and write or call each other when separated. They also communicate frequently through nonverbal means, particularly those families from cultural or subcultural groups that are less verbal. There are innumerable ways—smiling encouragingly, embracing warmly, frowning disapprovingly, being available, withdrawing for privacy, doing an unsolicited favor, serving tea, giving a gift—to convey feelings and thoughts without words. The family that has learned to communicate effectively has members who are sensitive to each other. They watch for cues and verify messages in order to assure understanding. This kind of family recognizes and deals with conflicts as they arise. Its members have learned to share and to work collaboratively with each other (Figure 15-1).

Effective communication is necessary for a family to carry out its basic functions. To demonstrate affection and acceptance, to promote identity and affiliation, and to guide behavior through socialization and social controls, family members must communicate. Like the correlation between a high degree of communication and a high degree of effectiveness in organizational functioning, families' facilitative communication patterns promote the health and development of their members (Friedman, 1986).

ENHANCEMENT OF INDIVIDUAL DEVELOPMENT

Healthy families are responsive to their individual members' needs and provide the freedom and support necessary to promote each member's growth: "The level of health will be greater in families which support their members'

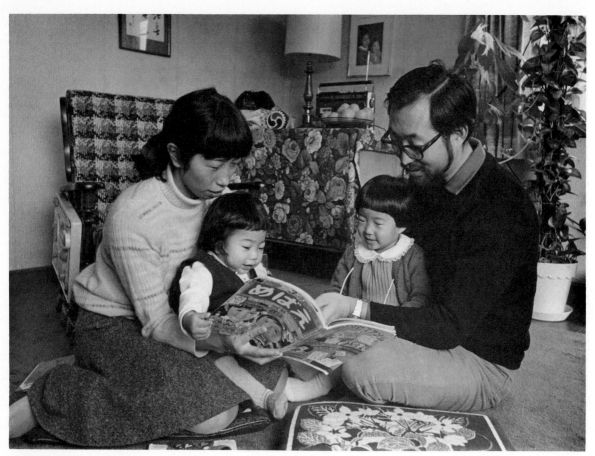

Figure 15-1
Healthy families have fun together and engage in activities that promote their members' growth.

personal needs and interests, assist the members' efforts to cope and function, and tolerate and encourage members' moves toward self-actualization" (Pratt, 1976, p. 125). If a father in a healthy family loses his job, his family will work to support his ego and help him use his energy constructively to adjust and find new work. The healthy family recognizes the growing child's need for independence, which it fosters through increasing opportunities for the child to try new things alone. This kind of family can tolerate differences of opinion or life-style. It is able to accept each member unconditionally and respect each one's right to be his or her own self. Within an appropriate framework of stability and structure, the healthy family encourages freedom and autonomy for its members (Friedman, 1986). Patterns for promoting individual member development will vary from one family to another, depending on its cultural orientation. The way autonomy is expressed in an Italian-American family will differ from its expression in a Chippewa Indian family, yet each family can promote freedom and autonomy. The result of promoting individuality is an increase in competence, self-reliance, social skills, intellectual growth, and overall capacity for self-management among family members (Clements and Roberts, 1983).

EFFECTIVE STRUCTURING OF RELATIONSHIPS

Healthy families structure their role relationships to meet changing family needs over time (Holman, 1983). In a stable social context, some families may establish member roles and tasks, such as breadwinner, primary decision maker, and homemaker, which are maintained as workable patterns throughout the life of the family. Families in rural areas, isolated communities, or religious and subcultural groups are more likely than others to retain role consistency because they face few, if any, external pressures or needs to change. The Amish communities in the midwest have maintained marked differentiation in family roles for more than 100 years.

In a technologically advanced industrial society such as ours, however, most families must adapt their roles to be consistent with changing family needs created by external forces. As women enter the work force, for instance, family roles, relationships, and tasks must change to meet the demands of the new situation (Hanson, 1986). Many husbands assume more homemaking responsibilities; fathers engage in child rearing; children, along with the adults in their families, assume shared decision making and a more equal distribution of power. The latter may be essential for the survival of a single-parent family in which the children must assume adult responsibilities while the parent is working to support the family (Mendes, 1979; Hanson, 1986).

Changing life cycle stages require alterations in the structuring of relationships (Olson, McCubbin, and Associates, 1983). The healthy family recognizes its members' changing developmental needs and adapts parenting roles, family tasks, and controls to fit each stage. Household chores of increasing complexity and responsibility are assigned as children become capable of handling them. Rules of conduct relax as members learn to govern their own behavior.

ACTIVE COPING EFFORT

Healthy families actively attempt to overcome life's problems and issues. When faced with change, they assume responsibility for coping and seek energetically and creatively to meet the demands of the situation (Olson, McCubbin, and Associates, 1983). One family dealt with the increased cost of food, for example, by raising all its own vegetables, doing home canning and freezing, cutting down on meat, substituting other protein foods, and eating at restaurants less. The result was a 25 percent decrease in overall food expenses. Healthy families are open to innovation. Their coping ability is enhanced by receptivity to new ideas and means for solving problems (Figure 15-2). The family that responds to gas shortages and increased gas prices by deciding to cut down on daily travel may only be adding to their difficulties. On the

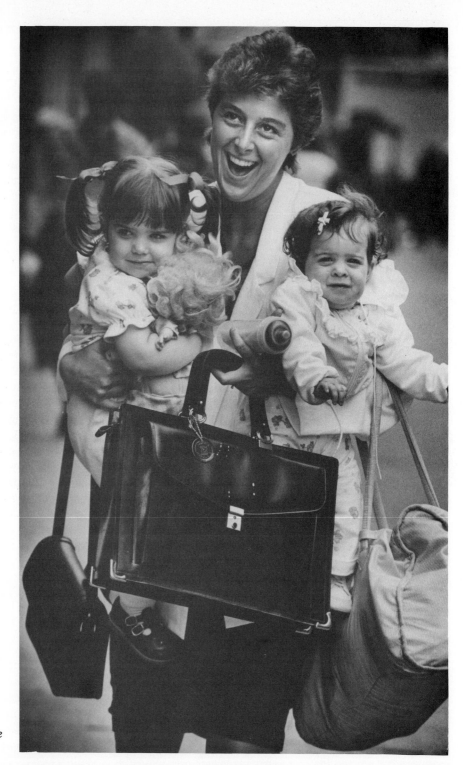

Figure 15-2
Many women today learn to creatively juggle family and career responsibilities. This mother is on her way to a day-care center before going to work.

other hand, a family facing the same problem may solve it by exploring new ways to reach destinations. These might include increased use of public transportation and car pools; walking, bicycling, or skiing to school or work; rearranged schedules to avoid frequency of trips to regular destinations; and shopping ahead to avoid last-minute trips to stores. In contrast to those who passively and fatalistically limit themselves to working with only the most obvious aids, healthy families actively seek and use a variety of resources to solve problems. They may discover these resources within the family or they may find them externally; they engage in self-care. For example, a professional couple who were faced with the expense of daytime baby-sitting arranged their schedules so that they could take turns staying home with the baby. Later, they joined a cooperative preschool that allowed their child to attend daily but required parental participation only one day a week. After having additional children, the parents, more financially able, hired live-in help. They were able to help themselves as well as accept outside help.

HEALTHY ENVIRONMENT AND LIFE-STYLE

Another sign of a healthy family is a healthy home environment and life-style. Healthy families create safe and hygienic living conditions for their members. For instance, the healthy young family removes the potential hazards of exposed electric outlets and cleaning solvents from the reach of crawling infants. Older families recognize a greater potential for falls, resulting from poor eyesight and coordination; they install good lighting and sturdy railings. These same families are concerned about cleanliness as a means of reducing infections and the spread of disease-causing organisms. Healthy families promote a healthy family life-style by encouraging an appropriate balance of activity and rest; they foster a nutritionally sound diet and promote regular exercise. The emotional climate of a healthy family is positive and supportive of member growth (Figure 15-3). Contributing to this healthy emotional climate is a strong sense of shared values, often combined with a strong religious orientation (Olson, McCubbin, and Associates, 1983). Such a family, like the Murphys, demonstrates caring, encourages and accepts expression of feelings, and respects divergent ideas. Members can express their individuality in the way they dress or decorate their rooms. The home environment makes family members feel welcome and accepted. As a result of all these emphases, individual members in a healthy family engage in positive personal health practices that range from regular toothbrushing all the way to coping effectively with a death in the family.

REGULAR LINKS WITH THE BROADER COMMUNITY

Healthy families maintain dynamic ties with the broader community (Pesznecker and Zahlis, 1986). They participate regularly in external groups and activities, often in a leadership capacity. We may see them join in local poli-

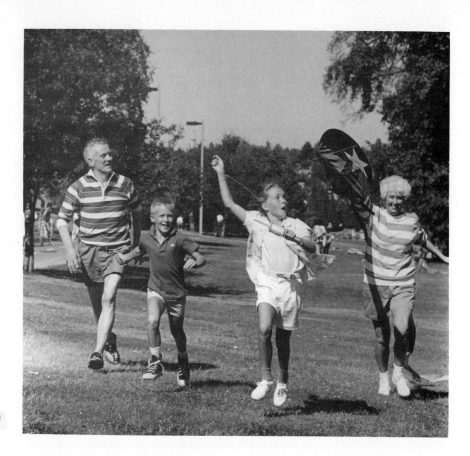

Figure 15-3
A positive, supportive emotional climate is a sign of a healthy family.

tics, participate in a church bazaar, or promote the school's paper drive to raise money for science equipment. They use external resources suited to their family's needs (Figure 15-4). For example, a farm family with teenagers, recognizing the importance of peer group influence on adolescents, became very active in the local 4-H club. Another family, in which the father was out of work, joined a job transition support group. The Murphys chose a health care plan that met their family's health care needs. Healthy families also know what is going on in the world around them. They show an interest in current events and attempt to understand significant social, economic, and political issues. This ever-broadening outreach gives families knowledge of external forces that might influence their lives. It exposes them to a wider range of alternatives and a variety of contacts, which increases their options for finding resources and strengthens their coping skills.

FAMILY HEALTH ASSESSMENT

A family's level of health may be elusive unless the nurse has some means for assessment. As with the Stones and the Murphys, the community health nurse may have a general idea or intuitive sense about whether or not a family

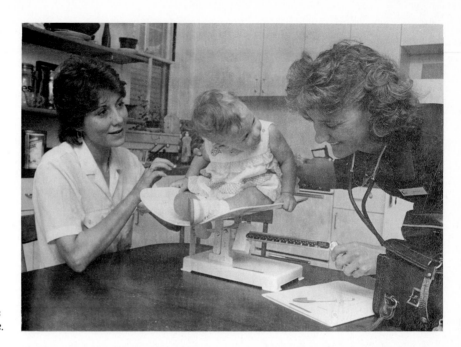

Figure 15-4
Healthy families seek out
and use external resources
such as regular health care.

is healthy. More difficult is knowing *how* healthy. What is that family's level of health? Assessing family health in a systematic fashion requires three tools: (1) a conceptual framework upon which to base the assessment, (2) a clearly defined set of assessment categories for data collection, and (3) a method for measuring a family's level of functioning.

CONCEPTUAL FRAMEWORKS

Several conceptual frameworks have been used historically to study families (Broderick, 1967; Christensen, 1964; Hill and Hansen, 1960). Three, in particular, continue to be used today: interactional, structural-functional, and developmental. The *interactional framework* describes the family as a unity of interacting personalities. It emphasizes communication, roles, conflict, coping patterns, and decision-making processes — all internal relationships — but neglects the family's interaction with the external environment.

The *structural-functional framework* describes the family as a social system relating to other social systems in the external environment, such as church, school, work, and health care system. This framework examines the interacting functions of society and the family, looks at family structures, and analyzes how families' structures affect their functioning.

The *developmental framework* studies families from a life-cycle perspective by examining members' changing roles and tasks in each progressive life cycle stage. This framework incorporates elements from the interactional and structural-functional approaches so that family structure, function, and interaction are viewed in the context of the environment through each stage of family development. Duvall and Miller (1985) use this conceptual framework.

Others have combined these concepts in various ways to design family assessment and intervention models. For example, one model emphasizes Rogers' human-environmental interactions (Johnston, 1987). Another, using interactional and structural-functional frameworks, incorporates self-care theory (Chin, 1985). Neuman's model (1983) combines interactional and structural-functional views to assess families' perceptions of and responses to stressors and then incorporates developmental considerations into the assessment and intervention process (Ross and Helmer, 1988). Still other writers utilize a developmental framework (Edelman and Mandle, 1986; Lancaster et al., 1987; Turk and Kerns, 1985).

The six characteristics discussed in the previous section provide us with a description of healthy families that serves as a beginning framework for assessing family health using interactional, structural-functional, and developmental concepts.

DATA COLLECTION CATEGORIES

Within a conceptual framework for assessing family health, the community health nurse selects specific categories for data collection. The amount of data that one can collect about any given family may be voluminous, perhaps more than necessary for the purposes of the assessment. Certain basic information is needed, however, to determine a family's health status and design appropriate nursing interventions. From many sources in the family health literature, particularly from Edelman and Mandle (1986), Friedman (1986), Turk and Kerns (1985), and Whall (1987), we have summarized a list of twelve data collection categories.

As the nurse gathers information about each category, she or he can divide it into three data sets corresponding with the following questions: (1) What are the family's strengths and self-care capabilities? (2) What are the family's stresses and problems? and (3) What are the family's resources? In Table 15-1 we list the twelve categories and illustrate how data can be grouped in response to the three questions. We define the family health assessment categories more fully here.

1. *Family demographics* refers to such things as a family's composition, socioeconomic status, and the ages, education, occupation, ethnicity, and religious affiliations of its members.
2. *Physical environment* data describe geography, climate, housing, space, social and political structures, food availability and dietary patterns, and any other elements in the internal or external physical environment that influence a family's health status.
3. *Psychological and spiritual environment* refers to information such as affectional relationships, mutual respect, support, promotion of

Table 15-1
Categories of data collection for family health assessment.

Assessment Categories	Family strengths and self-care abilities	Family stresses and problems	Family resources
1. Family demographics			
2. Physical environment			
3. Psychological and spiritual environment			
4. Family structure/roles			
5. Family functions			
6. Family values and beliefs			
7. Family communication patterns			
8. Family decision-making patterns			
9. Family problem-solving patterns			
10. Family coping patterns			
11. Family health behavior			
12. Family social and cultural patterns			

members' self-esteem and spiritual development, and family members' life satisfaction and goals.

4. *Family structure and roles* includes family organization, socialization processes, division of labor, and allocation and use of authority and power.

5. *Family functions* refers to a family's ability to carry out appropriate developmental tasks and provide for its members' needs.

6. *Family values and beliefs* influence all aspects of family life. Values and beliefs might deal with raising children, making and spending money, education, religion, work, health, and community involvement.

7. *Family communication patterns* include the frequency and quality of communication within a family and between the family and its environment.

8. *Family decision-making patterns* refer to how decisions are made in a family, by whom they are made, and how they are implemented.

9. *Family problem-solving patterns* describe how a family handles its problems, who deals with them, the flexibility of a family's approaches to problem solving, and the nature of its solutions.

10. *Family coping patterns* encompass how a family handles conflict and life changes, the nature and quality of family support systems, and family perceptions and responses to stressors.

11. *Family health behavior* refers to familial health history, current physical health status of family members, family use of health resources, and family health beliefs.

12. *Family social and cultural patterns* comprises family discipline and limit-setting practices; promotion of members' initiative, creativity, and leadership; family goal setting; family culture; cultural adaptations to present circumstances; and development of meaningful relationships within and outside the family.

ASSESSMENT METHODS

Many different methods are used to assess families. These methods serve to generate information about selected aspects of family structure and function; thus the methods must match the purpose for assessment.

Three well-known tools are the ecomap, the genogram, and the family sculpture (Holman, 1983). The ecomap is a diagram of the connections between a family and the other systems in its ecological environment. It could be used, for instance, to examine the various factors present (and possibly contributing to) a child abuse situation. Developed by Dr. Ann Hartman in 1975 to help child welfare workers study family needs, the tool visually depicts the dynamic family-environment interactions. The nurse involves family members in the map's development. They draw a center circle representing the family and then smaller circles on the periphery to represent people and systems, such as school or work, whose relationships with the family are significant. The map is used to discuss and analyze these relationships (Hartman, 1978; Holman, 1983). Figure 15-5 displays an ecomap.

The genogram provides information about a family's history over a period of time, usually three or more generations. It diagrams family relationships by listing the family genealogy accompanied by significant life events (birth, death, marriage, divorce, illness), identifying characteristics (race, religion, social class), occupations, and places of family residence (Holman, 1983). Again, this tool is used jointly with the family. It encourages family expression and sheds light on family behavior and problems. Figure 15-6 shows a sample genogram.

Family sculpture is a dynamic process that engages the family in creating a live family portrait (Holman, 1983). Family members assume postures and spatial relationships that represent their behaviors and feelings toward one another and their environment. Various members serve as sculptor, "molding" the family into the picture that they perceive as reality. The nurse uses this tool to help the family understand its relationships and to form a basis for nursing care planning and intervention.

Community health nurses also use a variety of family assessment instruments to gather data on family structure, functions, development, or combinations of all three (Kandzari, Howard, and Rock, 1981). Public health nursing agencies generally develop their own tools, often in the form of questionnaires, checklists, or interview guides. The format varies to fit organizational needs. For example, many agencies are changing to computerized information management systems and are adjusting data collection to be technologically compatible. Two sample assessment tools (Figures 15-7 and 15-8) are presented in this chapter.

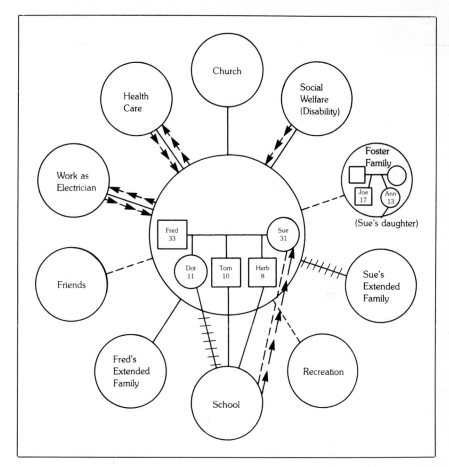

*Figure 15-5
Ecomap of a family's
relationship to its
environment. Lines indicate
types of connections: solid
lines, strong; dotted lines,
tenuous; lines with cross
bars, stressful. Arrows
signify energy or resource
flow, and absence of lines
indicates no connection.*

Other methods, such as videotaping family interaction, structured observation, or analysis of life-changing events using the Holmes-Rahe scale (Holmes and Rahe, 1967) are all useful adjuncts. Tools are often used in combination to enhance breadth of data collection and understanding of the family.

GUIDELINES FOR FAMILY HEALTH ASSESSMENT

An assessment of family health will be most accurate if it incorporates the following five guidelines.

1. Focus on the family as a total unit.
2. Ask goal-directed questions.
3. Collect data over time.
4. Combine quantitative and qualitative data.
5. Exercise professional judgment.

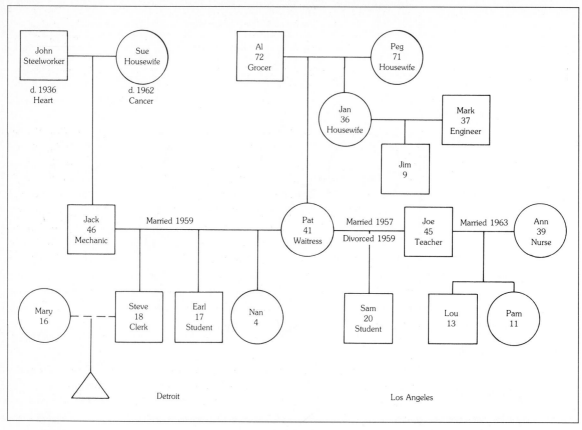

Figure 15-6
A genogram depicting three generations of family history.

FOCUS ON THE FAMILY, NOT THE MEMBER

Family health is more than the sum of its individual members' health. If we were to rate the health of each person in a family and then combine those scores, we still would not know how healthy that family was. To assess a family's health, we must consider that family as a single entity and appraise its aggregate behavior (Whall, 1987). As we consider each criterion in the assessment process, we ask, "Is this typical of the family as a whole?" Assume that you are assessing the communication patterns of a family. You notice that there is supportive interaction between two members in the family. What about the others? Further observation shows good communication among all but one member. You may decide that, in spite of that one person, the family as a whole has good communication. When individual member behavior deviates from the aggregate picture, you will want to note these differences. They can influence total family functioning and will need to be considered in nursing care planning.

UTILIZE GOAL-DIRECTED QUESTIONS

The activities of any investigator, if fruitful, are guided by goal-directed questions. When solving a crime, a detective has many specific questions in mind. So, too, does the physician attempting a diagnosis, the teacher trying to discern a student's knowledge level, or the mechanic repairing a car. Similarly, the nurse determining a family's level of health has specific questions in mind. It is not enough to make family visits and merely ask members how they are. If relevant data are to be gathered, relevant questions must be asked. Figure 15-7 provides a sample set of questions that community health nurses may use to assess a family's health. Built upon the framework of the characteristics of a healthy family, these questions guide thinking and observations. They direct attention to specific aspects of family behavior in order that the goal of discovering a family's level of health can be achieved. Consider the characteristic, "active coping effort." When visiting a family as the community health nurse, you watch for signs of their response to change and their problem-solving ability. You ask yourself, "Does this family recognize when it needs to make a change?" or "How does it respond when a change is imposed?" Perhaps a health problem has arisen: for instance, the baby has diarrhea. Does the family assume responsibility for dealing with the problem? Do family members consider a variety of ways to solve it? How do they respond to your suggestions? Do they seek out resources on their own, such as by reading about causes of infant diarrhea or consulting with you, their doctor, or a clinic? How well do they use resources, once identified? Do they take a problem, try creative methods for solving it, and see it through to resolution? As you focus on these behaviors, you are asking yourself goal-directed questions aimed at finding out the family's coping skills. This investigation will be one part of your assessment of the family's total health picture.

The set of questions presented in Figure 15-7 is one useful way to appraise family health. Another more open-ended format is used by some community health nursing agencies. This approach, displayed in Figure 15-8, proposes assessment categories as a stimulus for nursing questions. When exploring family support systems, for example, you will ask, "What internal resources or strengths does this family have?" "Who, outside of the family, can they and do they turn to for help?" "What agencies, such as churches, clubs, or community services, do they use?" The open-ended style of this assessment tool allows you to raise a variety of questions aimed at determining family health.

ALLOW ADEQUATE TIME FOR DATA COLLECTION

Accurate family assessment takes time. An appraisal done on the first or second visit will most likely give only a partial picture of how a family is functioning. You need time to accumulate observations, make notes, and see all

Family Assessment

Family Name _____

Family Constellation

Member	Birth Date	Sex	Marital Status	Education	Occupation	Community Involvement

Financial Status _____

Using the following scale, score the family based on your professional observations and judgment:

0 = Never   3 = Frequently
1 = Seldom   4 = Most of the time
2 = Occasionally   N = Not observed

	score	date	score	date	score	date	score	date

Facilitative Interaction among Members
    a. Is there frequent communication among all members?
    b. Do conflicts get resolved?
    c. Are relationships supportive?
    d. Are love and caring shown among members?
    e. Do members work collaboratively?

Comments _____

_____

                          Totals

Enhancement of Individual Development
    a. Does family respond appropriately to members' developmental needs?
    b. Does it tolerate disagreement?
    c. Does it accept members as they are?
    d. Does it promote member autonomy?

Comments _____

_____

                          Totals

	score	date	score	date	score	date	score	date

Effective Structuring of Relationships
   a. Is decision making allocated to appropriate members?
   b. Do member roles meet family needs?
   c. Is there flexible distribution of tasks?
   d. Are controls appropriate for family stage of development?

Comments _____

_____

Totals

Active Coping Effort
   a. Is family aware when there is a need for change?
   b. Is it receptive to new ideas?
   c. Does it actively seek resources?
   d. Does it make good use of resources?
   e. Does it creatively solve problems?

Comments _____

_____

Totals

Healthy Environment and Life-style
   a. Is family life-style health promoting?
   b. Are living conditions safe and hygienic?
   c. Is emotional climate conducive to good health?
   d. Do members practice good health measures?

Comments _____

_____

Totals

Regular Links with Broader Community
   a. Is family involved regularly in the community?
   b. Does it select and use external resources?
   c. Is it aware of external affairs?
   d. Does it attempt to understand external issues?

Comments _____

_____

Totals

Figure 15-7
Family assessment using questions based on characteristics of healthy families.

FAMILY ASSESSMENT

Family Name

Family Constellation

| Member names | Occupation | Educational background |

Significant change in family life

Coping ability of family

Energy level

Decision-making process within the family

Parenting skills

Support systems of the family

Use of health care (include plans for emergencies)

Financial status

Other impressions

Signature of Nurse _____ Date _____

Figure 15-8
Open-ended family assessment.

the family members interacting together in order to make a thorough assessment. To appraise family communication patterns, for instance, you will want to observe the family as a group, perhaps at mealtime or during some family activity. They will need to feel comfortable in your presence in order to respond freely; it takes time and patience for such an ambience to develop.

Consider one nurse's experience. Joe Burns had talked with the Olson family twice, first in the clinic and then at home. Since Mr. Olson had not been present either time, Joe asked to see the family together and arranged an evening visit. The Olsons were receiving nursing service for health promotion. They were particularly interested in discussing discipline of their young children and contracted with Joe for six weekly visits to be held in the late afternoon when Mr. Olson was home from work. Joe's assessment began on his first contact with the Olsons. He made notes on their chart and, guided by questions similar to those in Figure 15-7, he kept a brief log. After the fourth visit, he filled in an assessment form to keep as a part of the family record. It was not until then that Joe felt he had enough data collected to make valid judgments about this family's level of health.

COMBINE QUANTITATIVE WITH QUALITATIVE DATA

Any appraisal of family health must be qualitative. That is, you must determine the presence or absence of essential characteristics in order to have a data base for planning nursing action. To guide planning more specifically, you can also determine degrees of the presence or absence of these signs of health. This is a quantitative measure. You are not just asking whether a family does or does not engage in some behaviors, you are asking how often. Is this behavior fairly typical of the family, or does it occur infrequently? Figure 15-7 demonstrates one way to measure family health quantitatively. If you were to use this tool to assess the Murphy family's ability to enhance individuality, for example, you could score their behavior on a scale from zero to four, zero meaning never and four meaning most of the time. After several observations, you would probably conclude that they responded appropriately to the members' developmental needs (*a.* under "Enhancement of Individual Development") most of the time. Opposite *a.* on the assessment form, you would place the numeral 4 and the date of assessment.

The value of developing a quantitative measure is to have some basis for comparison. You can assess a family's progress or regression by comparing its present score with its previous scores. Had you conducted a family health assessment six months ago on the Stones, for instance, and compared it with their present level of health, you would probably have discovered a drop in their scores in several areas. Many of their communication patterns, role relationships, and coping skills, in particular, would show signs of deterioration. A scored assessment gives you a vivid picture of exactly which areas need intervention. For this reason, it is useful to conduct periodic assessments. Some have suggested that assessments be conducted every three months (Hott, 1977). In this manner, you can monitor the progress of high-risk families through the early introduction of particular preventive measures, should you see a trend or regressive behavior in some area. Periodic quantitative assessments also provide a means of evaluating the effectiveness of nursing action. You can point to documented signs of growth.

Quantitative data serve another useful purpose. You can compare one family's health status with that of another family in your caseload as a basis for priority setting and nursing care planning. The difference in the levels of health between the Stones and the Murphys tells you that the Stones need considerably more attention right now.

EXERCISE PROFESSIONAL JUDGMENT

Although nurses seek to validate data, their assessment of families is still based primarily on their own professional judgment. Assessment tools can guide observations and even quantify those judgments, but ultimately any assessment is subjective. Even though you observe that the Murphys make good use of their prepaid health plan, your decision that the use of this external resource is contributing to their health is still a subjective one. This decision is not bad. Indeed, effective health care practice depends on sound professional judgment. However, nurses must, at the same time, be cautious about overemphasizing the value of an assessment tool. It is not infallible. It is only a tool and should be used as a guide for planning, not as an absolute and irrevocable statement about a family's health status. This caution is particularly important when dealing with quantitative scores, which may seem to be objective.

Ordinarily, it is best to conduct assessment of a family unobtrusively. The tool is not a questionnaire to be filled out in the family's presence; its purpose is to guide observations and judgments. Before going into a family's home, the community health nurse may wish to review the questions while sitting in the car. The nurse may find it helpful to keep the assessment tool in a briefcase for easy reference during the visit. Depending upon the nurse's relationship with a family, notes may be made during or immediately after the encounter. Like Joe, the nurse may choose to keep a short log—an accumulation of notes—until enough data has been collected to complete the assessment form.

Occasionally, a family with high self-care capability may be involved in the assessment. The nurse will want to introduce the idea carefully and use professional judgment to determine when the family is ready to engage in this kind of self-examination.

FAMILY HEALTH PRACTICE GUIDELINES

Family nursing is a kind of nursing practice in which the family is the unit of service (Friedman, 1986). It is "not merely a family-oriented approach in which family concerns that affect the health of the individual are taken into account" (Robischon and Smith, 1977). But how does one provide health care to a collection of people? Although there are some who claim such service cannot be done (Kinlein, 1978), we have increasing scientific evidence that supports its feasibility and, in fact, its necessity. It does not mean that nursing must relinquish its service to individuals. On the contrary, one of the distinctive contributions of nursing as a profession is its holistic approach to individual needs. Community health nurses rise to the challenge of adding a unique kind of service, one that has been neglected for too long—service to population groups that include families.

Five guidelines can clarify our understanding of family nursing and enhance practice with families: (1) work with the family collectively, (2) start where the family is, (3) fit nursing intervention to the family's stage of development, (4) recognize the validity of family structural variations, and (5) emphasize family strengths.

WORK WITH THE FAMILY COLLECTIVELY

To practice family nursing, nurses must set aside the usual focus on individuals and remind themselves that several people together have a collective personality, collective interests, and a collective set of needs. Viewing a group of people as one unit becomes less difficult when we examine the way we often think. We often speak, for instance, of an organization as conservative or liberal. We say that a group has taken a stand on abortion or that a business needs to become better organized. In each case, we view the group collectively, as a single entity with attributes and activities in common. So it is with families. A family has its own personality, interests, and needs.

Working with several people at the same time is not as difficult as it may initially seem. We have all experienced being part of a group that was treated as a single unit. A coach admonishes his team, "Let's practice the pivot turn one more time." A teacher says to a group of 12-year-olds, "Now, class, I'd like you to divide into groups of four each and prepare a three-page paper on how we can enjoy winter. This will be due in one week." A mother addresses her family, "This house has got to be cleaned before Grandma gets here." The church school teacher, during final Christmas play rehearsal, begs the cast members to review their lines. In each instance, the group as a whole is addressed. Group action is expected. Evaluation of the outcomes will be based on what the group does collectively.

With families, the approach is very similar. As much as possible, community health nurses want to involve all the members during nurse-client interaction (Miller and Janosik, 1980). This approach reinforces the importance of each individual member's contribution to total family functioning. Nurses want to encourage everyone's participation in the work that the nurse and the family jointly agree to do. Like the coach, the nurse wants to help them work together as a team for their collective benefit.

Consider how you might work with the Stone family collectively. An initial contact by phone call or home visit could be used to determine whether the Stones were interested in family nursing. If not, individual members might want service, and a family focus could be introduced later. If the Stones did want family care, you would ask to meet with the entire family to discuss what the service had to offer and what they would hope to gain from it. You would explain that each person must be involved and committed to the agreed-upon goals; that, like a team of oarsmen, the family would have to pull together to accomplish the purpose of the visits. To help the Stone family improve its health status, you might jointly decide to work first on family communication patterns. A session of brainstorming could uncover many causes of poor communication. More brainstorming might suggest solutions and plans for action . On each visit you would view the Stones as a group. You would expect group responses and actions. Evaluation of outcomes would be based on what the family did collectively.

START WHERE THE FAMILY IS

When working with families, community health nurses begin at their present, not their ideal, level of functioning (Kinlein, 1978). Although you may recognize that the Stones need to develop more facilitative interaction, the family may not wish to, or be ready for, work on its communication patterns. To discover where a family is, community health nurses act in two ways. First, they conduct a family assessment to ascertain the members' needs and level of health. Concurrently, they determine their collective interests, concerns, and priorities.

The Kegler family illustrates this principle. Marcia Kegler brought her baby to the well-child clinic once but failed to keep further appointments. Concerned that the family might be having other difficulties, the community health nurse made a home visit. The mobile home was cluttered and dirty; the baby was crying in his playpen. Marcia seemed uninterested in the nurse's visit. She listened politely but had little to say, only repeating that everything was O.K. and that the baby was doing fine. He was just fussy now because he was teething, she explained. As they talked, Marcia's husband Bob, a delivery van driver, stopped by to pick up a sports magazine to read on his lunch hour. The three of them discussed the problems of inflation and how expensive it was to raise a child. The nurse reminded them that the clinic was free, and that they could at least get good health care without extra cost. They agreed without enthusiasm. After Bob left, the nurse spent the remainder of the visit discussing infant care with Marcia, particularly emphasizing regular checkups and immunizations.

The next visit also focused on the baby, but the nurse had an uncomfortable feeling that this family was not really interested in her help. After consulting her supervisor, the nurse did what she wished she had done in the first place. She asked to talk with Marcia and Bob together and explained frankly why she had first come to their home and what she could offer in the way of counseling, teaching, support, and referral to other community resources. She then asked them what, if anything, they would like. What were their concerns? The Keglers were more than responsive. There followed a listing of financial difficulties so long that sometimes they had felt like giving up. Yet the Keglers believed they would eventually overcome their problems if they just had "someone to lean on," as they put it. Their greatest need at this time was for friends. They were new in the city, and both their families lived some distance away on farms. The neighbors were friendly but not close enough to confide in.

Now the nurse could start where this family was. In addition to providing needed support herself by focusing on the parents instead of the baby, the nurse also introduced them to a young couples' group which met at the community center. She had learned that, although their baby's health should be a concern, the Keglers' present social needs were greater and required her attention first.

FIT NURSING INTERVENTION TO THE FAMILY'S STAGE OF DEVELOPMENT

Although every family engages in the same basic functions, the tasks to accomplish these functions vary with each stage of the family's development. A young family, for instance, will appropriately meet its members' affiliation needs by establishing mutually satisfying relationships and meaningful communication patterns. As the family enters later stages, these bonds change with the release of some members into new families and the loss of others through death. Awareness of the family's developmental stage enables the nurse to assess the appropriateness of the family's level of functioning and to tailor intervention accordingly.

A nurse's work with the Roberts family exemplifies this principle. The Roberts, a couple in their midsixties, had recently moved to a retirement complex. They had received nursing visits following Mrs. Roberts' stroke three years previously but requested service now because Mr. Roberts was feeling "poorly" all the time. He thought that perhaps his diet and lack of activity might be the causes and hoped the nurse would have some helpful suggestions. The couple had eagerly awaited Mr. Roberts' retirement from teaching, planning to be lazy, travel, visit all their children, and do all those things they had never had time to do when they were young. Now neither of them seemed to have any energy or capacity to enjoy their new life. The move from their home of 28 years had been difficult; they were still trying to find space in the tiny apartment for their cherished books and mementos, many of which they had been forced to give away.

The nurse recognized that Mr. and Mrs. Roberts were experiencing a situational crisis (leaving their home of 28 years) and a developmental crisis (entering retirement and the aging stage). Many of the Roberts' expectations for this new life stage were unrealistic; they had not adequately prepared themselves for the adjustments that the loss of their home and retirement would demand. Through discussion, the nurse was able to help the Roberts understand their situation and feelings. They decided on a series of nursing visits focused on adapting to retirement and aging, and they agreed that the Roberts needed to join a support group of persons who were experiencing some of the same difficulties. Such a group was currently meeting in the retirement center; they joined it. Because this nurse was able to help the Roberts through their crisis in a supportive and nonjudgmental manner, she found them receptive later to discussing preparation for the inevitable loss and bereavement that would occur when one of them died. She was suiting her nursing intervention to this family's stage of development.

RECOGNIZE THE VALIDITY OF FAMILY STRUCTURAL VARIATIONS

Many families seen by community health nurses are nontraditional in structure, such as single-parent families and unmarried couples (Hanson, 1986; Loveland-Cherry, 1986). Other families are organized around nontraditional patterns; for example, both parents may have careers or a husband may care for children at home while his wife financially supports the family. There are reasons for these variant structures and organizational patterns. They result from social change—change in employment practices, welfare programs, economic conditions, sex roles, status of women and minorities, birth control, divorce, war, and many other influences. Such variations in family structure and organization lead to revised patterns of family functioning (Smith, 1983). Member roles and tasks often differ dramatically from our expectations, as in a family with a single parent who works full-time while raising children, or a dual-career marriage in which both partners have undifferentiated roles. Community health nurses, many of whom are accustomed to traditional family patterns, may find such variations difficult to understand or accept unless they recognize their validity.

There are two important aspects to consider in this principle. First, what is normal for one family is not necessarily normal for another. Each family is unique in its combination of structure, composition, roles, and behaviors. As long as a family carries out its functions effectively and demonstrates the characteristics of a healthy family, we must agree that its form, no matter how variant, is valid.

Second, families are constantly changing. Marriage transforms two people into a married couple without children. Adding children changes this family's structure. Divorce again alters structure and roles. Remarriage with the addition of children from another family changes the family again. Children grow up and leave the home while the parents, together or singly, are left to adjust to yet another family structure. And so it goes. Throughout the life cycle, a family seldom stays the same for very long. Each of these changes forces a family to adapt to its circumstances. Consider the young woman with a baby whose husband deserts her. She has no choice but to assume a single-parent role. Each change also creates varying degrees of stress and demands considerable adaptive energy on the family's part. Many family changes are predictable; they are part of normal life cycle growth. Some are not. The nurse's responsibility is to help families cope with the changes while remaining nonjudgmental and accepting of the variant forms encountered.

Homosexual unions are difficult for some nurses to deal with. Because homosexual families are not always recognized as a valid family form for religious or other reasons, the nurse may feel uncomfortable relating to them. Yet the nurse's responsibility remains the same. Like any family, homosexual couples need to carry out basic functions and develop characteristics that promote their collective health. The nurse can view these, and all families, as unique groups, each with its own set of needs, whose interests can best be served through unbiased care.

EMPHASIZE FAMILY STRENGTHS

Too often, without meaning to derogate, community health nurses focus their attention on family weaknesses, referring to them as needs or problems. It seems to suit their role as helper to look for things that need help. This negative emphasis can be devastating to a family and demolish any hopes of a truly therapeutic relationship. No one likes to be criticized and people with a lowered self-image (composing a large share of the community health nurse's caseload) like it least of all. Instead, families need their strengths reinforced.

Emphasizing a family's strengths makes that group of people feel better about themselves. It fosters a positive self-image and promotes self-confidence. It energizes the family to cope more effectively with life (Peitze, 1984). This is not to say that nurses should ignore problems. On the contrary, their assessment should explore all aspects of family functioning to determine both strengths and weaknesses. The nurse needs a total picture to achieve adequate perspective in nursing care planning, and to begin work on problems when the family is ready and chooses to. Yet, even as the nurse becomes aware of a family's various behaviors, the emphasis should stay on the positive ones. Emphasizing strengths says, in effect, "Proof that you are important to me is that I see many good things about you."

Family strengths, according to Hill (1971), are "those traits which facilitate the ability of the family to meet the needs of its members and the demands made upon it by systems outside the family unit." Not all traits that appear positive are necessarily strengths, however. Before the nurse selects a trait to emphasize, it is important first to examine it closely and ask whether or not that behavior is actually facilitating family functioning. A strong work orientation may be a strength when balanced with play and relaxation, but a family obsessed by work is experiencing this trait as a weakness. Hott (1977) suggests that the differentiating factor between whether a trait is a strength or a weakness is the amount of free choice, as opposed to compulsive drive, exercised.

Some traits a nurse may consider possible strengths to emphasize are basic family functions, family developmental tasks, and characteristics of family health. For instance, a nurse might wish to commend a family that meets its members' physical, emotional, and spiritual needs; shows respect for various members' points of view; or fosters self-discipline in its children (Peitze, 1984).

We see a vivid illustration of this principle in the family nursing care of the Stevensons. The community health nurse made an initial home visit after referral by an outpatient physician who was concerned about possible child abuse. Alice Stevenson had brought her baby to the emergency room for treatment of a head laceration. He had fallen off the table while she was changing him, she claimed. Bruises on his arms made the physician suspicious, but Alice explained those as caused by his older brother's rough play. The nurse opened the visit by stating she was simply following up on the emergency room treatment and wanted to see how they were progressing. She made no mention of child abuse. She observed the mother and children closely, looking for small things to compliment Alice on while learning all she could about the family's background. Because the nurse appeared approving rather than suspicious or judgmental, Alice agreed to further visits.

During a later session Alice admitted to the nurse that she had dropped the baby on purpose. She could not get him to stop crying, no matter what she did; she just could not endure it any longer. There had been other times when she had physically abused him, too. She had not wanted this baby at all; her husband had gotten her pregnant and then left her shortly before the baby was born. Like many abusive parents, Alice had unrealistic expectations for her children's behavior as well as very inadequate self-esteem (Kempe and Helfer, 1972; Ryan, 1984). Realizing that Alice would be particularly vulnerable to any criticism, the nurse concentrated on her strengths. She complimented her on how well she managed her home and dressed the children, on maintaining her job, and on reading stories to the three-year-old boy. It took many visits before Alice trusted the nurse, but in time they were able to discuss her feelings frankly and work toward improving this family's health. Emphasizing strengths had provided a bridge for the Stevensons into a helping relationship.

Summary

The family as the unit of service has received increasing emphasis in nursing over the years. Today family nursing has an important place in nursing practice, particularly in community health nursing. Its significance results from recognition that the family itself must be a target of service, that family health and individual health strongly influence each other, and that family health affects community health.

Healthy families demonstrate six important characteristics:

1. There is a facilitative process of interaction among family members.
2. They enhance individual member development.

3. Their role relationships are structured effectively.
4. They actively attempt to cope with problems.
5. They have a healthy home environment and life-style.
6. They establish regular links with the broader community.

To assess a family's health systematically, the nurse needs a conceptual framework upon which to base the assessment, a clearly defined set of categories for data collection, and a method for measuring the family's level of functioning. The six characteristics of a healthy family provide one assessment framework that community health nurses can use. In this chapter we described twelve categories for data collection and several methods to facilitate specific assessment of family health.

During assessment, the nurse focuses on the family as a total unit, utilizes goal-directed assessment questions, allows adequate time for data collection, combines quantitative with qualitative data, and exercises professional judgment.

Community health nurses enhance their practice with families by observing five principles:

1. Work with the family collectively.
2. Start where the family is.
3. Fit nursing intervention to the family's stage of development.
4. Recognize the validity of family structural variations.
5. Emphasize family strengths.

Study Questions

1. Construct an ecomap of a family that you know well. Ask a colleague to help you with this task. Make it a simulated interview and alternate role playing the part of the nurse and the client family. Afterward, assess the balance between the family and the resources in its environment.
2. Draw a genogram of your family and ask a colleague to role-play the part of the community health nurse while you play the client. Make your drawing of the genogram as complete as possible. Then analyze your thoughts and feelings (Holman, 1983):

   How did you feel while tracing your family history?
   Did you learn anything new about your family?
   Did any family trends or traits appear?
   Did any uncomfortable or suppressed information come to the surface?
   Do you have any new insights about your family?

3. Assess a family (other than your own) that you know well by completing a family assessment guide. You may use one of the forms in this chapter or a form available to you from some other source. Based on your assessment, determine one nursing intervention that could be used to promote this family's health.

References

Baranowski, T., and P. Nader. (1985). Family health behavior. In D. Turk and R. Kerns (eds.), *Health, illness, and families*. New York: Wiley.

Baranowski, T., P. R. Nader, K. Dunn, and N. A. Vanderpool. (1982). Family self-help: Promoting changes in health behavior. *Journal of Communication* 32(3): 161–72.

Broderick, C. B. (1967). In D. H. Olson (ed.), *Treating relationships*. Lake Mills, Iowa: Graphic.

Chin, S. (1985). Can self-care theory be applied to families? In J. Riehl-Sisca (ed.), *The science and art of self-care*. Norwalk, Conn.: Appleton-Century-Crofts.

Christensen, H. T. (ed.). (1964). *Handbook of marriage and the family*. Chicago: Rand McNally.

Clements, I. W., and F. B. Roberts (eds.). (1983). *Family health: A theoretical approach to nursing care*. New York: Wiley.

Crooks, C. E., et al. (1987). The family's role in health promotion. *Health Values* 11(2): 7–12.

Duffy, M. E. (1988). Health promotion in the family: Current findings and directives for nursing research. *Journal of Advanced Nursing* 13(1): 109–17.

Duvall, E. M., and B. C. Miller. (1985). *Marriage and family development*. 6th ed. New York: Harper & Row.

Edelman, C., and C. L. Mandle (eds.). (1986). *Health promotion thoughout the life span*. St. Louis: C. V. Mosby.

Ford, L. C. (1973). *The development of family nursing*. In D. Hymovich and M. Barnard (eds.), *Family health care*. New York: McGraw-Hill.

Freeman, R. B. and J. Heinrich. (1981). *Community health nursing practice*. Philadelphia: W. B. Saunders.

Friedman, M. M. (1986). *Family nursing theory and assessment*. 2nd ed. New York: Appleton-Century-Crofts.

Hanson, J. (1984). The family. In C. Roy (ed.), *Introduction to nursing: An adaptation model*. 2nd ed. Englewood Cliffs, N.J.: Prentice-Hall.

Hanson, S. M. (1986). Healthy single-parent families. *Family Relations* 35(1): 125–32.

Hartman, A. (1978). Diagrammatic assessment of family relationships. *Social Casework* 59(10): 59–64.

Hill, R. B. (1971). *The strengths of black families*. New York: Emerson Hall.

Hill, R., and D. Hansen. (1960). The identification of conceptual frameworks utilized in family study. *Marriage and Family Living* 22: 299–311.

Holman, A. M. (1983). *Family assessment: Tools for understanding and intervention*. Beverly Hills, Calif.: Sage.

Holmes, T., and R. Rahe. (1967). The social readjustment rating scale. *Journal of Psychosomatic Research* 11: 213–17.

Hott, J. R. (1977). Mobilizing family strengths in health maintenance and coping with illness. In A. Reinhardt and M. Quinn, *Current practice in family-centered community nursing*. St. Louis: C. V. Mosby.

Johnston, R. L. (1987). Approaching family intervention through Rogers' conceptual model. In A. L. Whall (ed.), *Family therapy theory for nursing: Four approaches*. Norwalk, Conn.: Appleton-Century-Crofts.

Kandzari, J. H., J. R. Howard, and M. Rock. (1981). *The well family: A developmental approach to assessment*. Boston: Little, Brown.

Kempe, C. H. and R. E. Helfer (eds.). (1972). *Helping the battered child and his family*. Philadelphia: J. B. Lippincott.

Kinlein, M. L. (1978). Point of view on the front: Nursing and family and community health. *Family and Community Health* 1(1): 57.

Lancaster, J. B., J. Altmann, A. S. Rossi, and L. R. Sherrod. (1987). *Parenting across the life span*. New York: Aldine deGruyter.

Loveland-Cherry, C. J. (1984). Family system patterns of autonomy and cohesiveness: Relationship to family members' health behavior. *Nursing Research* 33(1): 51–52.

Loveland-Cherry, C. J. (1986). Personal health practices in single-parent and two-parent families. *Family Relations* 35(1): 133–39.

McCubbin, H., A. Cauble, and J. Patterson (eds.). (1982). *Family stress coping and social support.* Springfield, Ill.: Charles C. Thomas.

Mendes, H. A. (1979). Single-parent families: A typology of life-styles. *Social Work* 24: 193.

Miller, J. R., and E. H. Janosik. (1980). *Family-focused care.* New York: McGraw-Hill.

Neuman, B. (1983). Family intervention using the Betty Neuman health care model. In I. W. Clements and F. B. Roberts, *Family health: A theoretical approach to nursing care.* New York: Wiley.

Olson, D., H. I. McCubbin, and Associates. (1983). *Families: What makes them work.* Beverly Hills, Calif.: Sage.

Otto, H. A. (1963). Criteria for assessing family strength. *Family Process* 2(2): 329–37.

Otto, H. A. (1973). A framework for assessing family strengths. In A. Reinhardt and M. Quinn (eds.), *Family-centered community nursing: A socio-cultural framework.* St. Louis: C. V. Mosby.

Peitze, C. F.. (1984). Health promotion for the well family. *Nursing Clinics of North America* 19(2): 229–37.

Pesznecker, B., and E. Zahlis. (1986). Establishing mutual help groups for family-member caregivers: A new role for community health nurses. *Public Health Nursing* 3(1): 29–37.

Pratt, L. (1976). *Family structure and effective health behavior: The energized family.* Boston: Houghton Mifflin.

Robischon, P., and J. A. Smith. (1977). Family assessment. In A. Reinhardt and M. Quinn (eds.), *Current practice in family-centered community nursing.* St. Louis: C. V. Mosby.

Ross, M. M., and H. Helmer. (1988). A comparative analysis of Neuman's model using the individual and family as the units of care. *Public Health Nursing* 5(1): 30–36.

Ryan, M. T. (1984). Identifying the sexually abused child. *Pediatric Nursing* 10: 419–21.

Satir, V. (1967). *Conjoint family therapy.* Palo Alto, CA: Science and Behavior Books.

Smith, L. (1983). A conceptual model of families incorporating an adolescent mother and child into the household. *Advances in Nursing Science* 6(1): 45–60.

Stinnett, N. (1981). In search of strong families. In N. Stinnett, B. Chesser, and J. De Frain (eds.), *Building family strengths: Blueprints for action.* Lincoln, Nebr.: University of Nebraska Press.

Stinnett, N., and K. H. Saur. (1977). Relationship characteristics of strong families. *Family Perspective* 11(4): 3–11.

Tanner-Nelson, P., and B. Banonis. (1981). Family consensus and stress identified in Delaware's White House Conference on the family. In N. Stinnett, J. DeFrain, K. King, P. Knaub, and G. Rowe (eds.), *Family strengths* III: Roots of well being (pp. 43–60). Lincoln, Nebr.: University of Nebraska Press.

Turk, D. C., and R. D. Kerns (eds.). (1985). *Health, illness and families: A life span perspective.* New York: Wiley.

Whall, A. L. (1987). *Family therapy theory for nursing: Four approaches.* Norwalk, Conn.: Appleton-Century-Crofts.

Selected Readings

Baranowski, T., and P. Nader. (1985). Family health behavior. In D. Turk and R. Kerns (eds.), *Health, illness, and families.* New York: Wiley.

Baranowski, T., P. R. Nader, K. Dunn, and N. A. Vanderpool. (1982). Family self-help: Promoting changes in health behavior. *Journal of Communication* 32(3): 161–72.

Berg, C. L., and D. Helgeson. (1984). That first home visit. *Journal of Community Health Nursing* 1(3): 207–15.

Chin, S. (1985). Can self-care theory be applied to families? In J. Riehl-Sisca (ed.), *The science and art of self-care*. Norwalk, Conn.: Appleton-Century-Crofts.

Choi, T., L. Josten, and M. L. Christiansen. (1983). Health-specific family coping index for noninstitutional care. *American Journal of Public Health* 73: 1275–77.

Clark, J. (1986). Supporting the family... heading off a breakdown. *Nursing Times* 82(32): 33–34.

Clements, I. W., and F. B. Roberts (eds). (1983). *Family health: A theoretical approach to nursing care*. New York: Wiley.

Crooks, C. E., et al. (1987). The family's role in health promotion. *Health Values* 11(2): 7–12.

Darrill, J., and J. Hyde. (1975). Working with high-risk families: Family advocacy and the parent education program. *Children Today* 4: 23.

Duffy, M. E. (1988). Health promotion in the family: Current findings and directives for nursing research. *Journal of Advanced Nursing* 13(1): 109–17.

Duvall, E. M., and B. C. Miller. (1985). *Marriage and family development*. 6th ed. New York: Harper and Row.

Edelman, C., and C. L. Mandle (eds.). (1986). *Health promotion throughout the life span*. St. Louis: C. V. Mosby.

Friedman, M. M. (1986). *Family nursing theory and assessment*. 2nd ed. New York: Appleton-Century-Crofts.

Gelles, R. J. (1976). Demythologizing child abuse. *Family Coordinator 25*: 135.

Getty, C., and W. Humphreys (eds.). (1981). *Understanding the family: Stress and change in American family life*. Norwalk, Conn.: Appleton-Century-Crofts.

Glasser, P. H., and L. N. Glasser. (1970). *Families in crisis*. New York: Harper and Row.

Hanson, J. (1984). The family. In C. Roy (ed.), *Introduction to nursing: An adaptation model*. 2nd ed. Englewood Cliffs, N.J.: Prentice-Hall.

Hanson, S. M. (1986). Healthy single-parent families. *Family Relations* 35(1): 125–32.

Hill, R. B. (1971). *The strengths of black families*. New York: Emerson Hall.

Holman, A. M. (1983). *Family assessment: Tools for understanding and intervention*. Beverly Hills, Calif.: Sage.

Hymovich, D., and M. Barnard (eds.). (1973). *Family health care*. New York: McGraw-Hill.

Johnston, R. L. (1987). Approaching family intervention through Rogers' conceptual model. In A. L. Whall (ed.), *Family therapy theory for nursing: Four approaches*. Norwalk, Conn.: Appleton-Century-Crofts.

Kandzari, J. H., J. R. Howard, and M. Rock. (1981). *The well family: A developmental approach to assessment*. Boston: Little, Brown.

Kempe, C. H., and R. E. Helfer (eds.). (1972). *Helping the battered child and his family*. Philadelphia: J. B. Lippincott.

Knafl, K. A., and H. K. Grace. (1978). *Families across the life cycle*. Boston: Little, Brown.

Lancaster, J. B., J. Altmann, A. S. Rossi, and L. R. Sherrod. (1987). *Parenting across the life span*. New York: Aldine deGruyter.

Leavitt, M. B. (1982). *Families at risk: Primary prevention in nursing practice*. Boston: Little, Brown.

Lockhart, C. A. (1975). Family assessment of coping ability. In S. E. Archer and R. Fleshman (eds.), *Community health nursing: Patterns and practice* (pp. 333–336). North Scituate, Mass.: Duxbury Press.

Loveland-Cherry, C. J. (1984). Family system patterns of autonomy and cohesiveness: Relationship to family members' health behavior. *Nursing Research* 33(1): 51–52.

Loveland-Cherry, C. J. (1986). Personal health practices in single-parent and two-parent families. *Family Relations* 35(1): 133–39.

Martin, E. P., and J. M. Martin. (1978). *The black extended family.* Chicago: University of Chicago Press.

McCubbin, H. I. (1979). Integrating coping behavior in family stress theory. *Journal of Marriage and the Family* 41: 237–44.

McCubbin, H., A. Cauble, and J. Patterson (eds.). (1982). *Family stress coping and social support.* Springfield, Ill.: Charles C. Thomas.

Mendes, H. A. (1979). Single-parent families: A typology of life-styles. *Social Work* 24: 193–99.

Miller, J. R., and E. H. Janosik. (1980). *Family-focused care.* New York: McGraw-Hill.

Mills, D. (1984). A model for stepfamily development. *Family Relations* 33: 365.

Nelson, M., and G. Nelson. (1982). Problems of equity in the reconstituted family: A social exchange analysis. *Family Relations* 31: 223.

Neuman, B. (1983). Family intervention using the Betty Neuman health care model. In I. W. Clements and F. B. Roberts, *Family health: A theoretical approach to nursing care.* New York: Wiley.

Norton, A. (1980). The influence of divorce on traditional life cycle measures. *Journal of Marriage and Family* 42: 63.

Olson, D., H. I. McCubbin, and Associates. (1981). *Families: What makes them work.* Beverly Hills, Calif.: Sage.

Otto, H. A. (1973). A framework for assessing family strengths. In A. Reinhardt and M. Quinn (eds.), *Family-centered community nursing.* St. Louis: C. V. Mosby.

Papernow, P. (1984). The stepfamily cycle: An experiential model of stepfamily development. *Family Relations* 33: 355.

Peitze, C. F. (1984). Health promotion for the well family. *Nursing Clinics of North America* 19(2): 229–37.

Pender, N. J. (1987). *Health promotion in nursing practice.* 2nd ed. Norwalk, Conn.: Appleton and Lange.

Pesznecker, B., and E. Zahlis. (1986). Establishing mutual help groups for family-member caregivers: A new role for community health nurses. *Public Health Nursing* 3(1): 29–37.

Pratt, L. (1976). *Family structure and effective health behavior: The energized family.* Boston: Houghton Mifflin.

Rhodes, S., and J. Wilson. (1981). *Surviving family life.* New York: G. P. Putnam's Sons.

Robischon, P., and J. A. Smith. (1977). Family assessment. In A. Reinhardt and M. Quinn (eds.), *Current practice in family-centered community nursing.* St. Louis: C. V. Mosby.

Ross, M. M., and H. Helmer. (1988). A comparative analysis of Neuman's model using the individual and family as the units of care. *Public Health Nursing* 5(1): 30–36.

Simons-Morton, B. G., N. M. O'Hara, and D. G. Simons-Morton. (1986). Promoting healthful diet and exercise behaviors in communities, schools, and families. *Family and Community Health* 9(3): 1–13.

Smith, L. (1983). A conceptual model of families incorporating an adolescent mother and child into the household. *Advances in Nursing Science* 6(1): 45–60.

Sobol, E. G., and P. Robischon. (1975). *Family nursing: A study guide.* 2nd ed. St. Louis: C. V. Mosby.

Turk, D. C., and R. D. Kerns (eds.). (1985). *Health, illness and families: A life span perspective.* New York: Wiley.

Weber, T., J. E. McKeever, and S. H. McDaniel. (1985). A beginner's guide to the problem-oriented first family interview. *Family Process* 24: 357.

Whall, A. L. (1987). *Family therapy theory for nursing: Four approaches.* Norwalk, Conn.: Appleton-Century-Crofts.

Wilkie, J. (1981). The trend toward delayed parenthood. *Journal of Marriage and the Family* 43(3): 583.

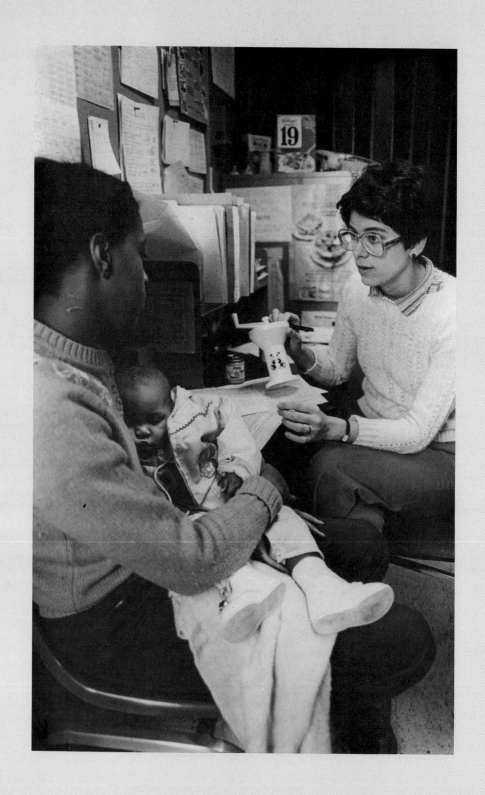

16 Maternal and Infant Health

Michele Hadeka

Working with maternal and infant populations is a primary facet of community health nursing. More than 70 percent of nursing practice in official health agencies involves primary preventive work with mothers and infants, especially adolescent mothers and high-risk infants.

Why should maternal and infant populations require this amount of attention from community health nursing? Despite the existence of advanced technology and availability of excellent perinatal services in our society, certain segments of the maternal and infant populations, particularly those who are economically disadvantaged, remain at high risk. While some women receive excellent prenatal care and benefit from the diagnostic capabilities of advanced technology, other women go without prenatal care and even without enough food to help them produce healthy babies. Each year, 3.7 million women in the United States give birth, and as many as half a million of these women have no medical insurance (Gold, Kenny, and Singh, 1987). Furthermore, many women do not have the financial or emotional resources to sustain minimal health levels for themselves and their infants. Clearly these women and their babies need primary preventive services, but reaching them with well-designed programs presents a considerable challenge for community health nurses. In this chapter, we describe the health status and needs of maternal and infant populations; we discuss how to design, implement, and evaluate maternal and infant health programs; and we outline community resources for maternal and infant health.

HEALTH STATUS AND GOALS FOR PREGNANT WOMEN AND INFANTS

Community health nurses constitute a key group of health care workers involved in both the planning of programs and the actual delivery of services to mothers and babies. A solid understanding of vital statistics and other data regarding maternal-infant populations assists nurses in determining both the appropriateness and the effectiveness of programs and services. Reviewing some of the vital statistics of the past decade provides insight into the problem areas in maternal-infant health.

In 1979, *Healthy People — The Surgeon General's Report on Health Promotion and Disease Prevention* described the changing patterns of disease and death in the United States. The Surgeon General's report identified five major goals aimed at improving the health status of all age groups by the year 1990. Among these goals was the following: "For infants...35 percent lower death rate than the 14.1 deaths per 1000 live births that occurred in 1977. That would mean less than 9 deaths per 1000 live births by 1990." (Public Health Service, 1979). Two subgoals for infants were "to reduce incidence of low-birthweight infants" and "to reduce birth defects" (Public Health Service, 1979).

In 1980, each major goal was further subdivided into specific, achievable objectives and published in *Promoting Health/Preventing Disease: Objectives for the Nation.*

After more than a decade of working toward improving maternal-infant health, the United States has made some progress. However, it is likely that many of the Surgeon General's objectives will not be achieved. The infant mortality rate (deaths for all babies up to 1 year of age) has dropped substantially from the 14.1 per 1000 live births in 1972 to 10.6 per 1000 live births in 1985 (Center for Disease Control, 1988). It is projected that the infant mortality rate will continue to drop to 9.1 per 1000 live births by 1990 (CDC, 1988) but will fall short of the Surgeon General's goal. This infant mortality rate remains higher than those of 17 other nations (Windom, 1987) including France, Japan, and the countries of Scandinavia. It is interesting to note that the Japanese reached the same goal the U.S. is trying to achieve more than a decade ago (Jacobson, 1987). The infant mortality rate among American blacks has decreased from 23.1 per 1000 live births in 1978 (Public Health Reports, 1983) to 18.2 per 1000 live births in 1985 (CDC, 1988) and is projected to continue dropping to 15.9 per 1000 live births by 1990 (CDC, 1988). These projections still fall short of the Surgeon General's target of no more than 12 deaths per 1000 live births.

Two-thirds of infant deaths in this country occur among low-birthweight babies (Figure 16-1). The Surgeon General's objective for decreasing the number of low-birthweight babies stated that by 1990, low-birthweight babies should constitute not more than 5 percent of all live births (Public Health Reports, 1983). We expect that by 1990 the percentage will be 6.7, once again falling short of the Surgeon General's target (CDC, 1988).

There are, however, several objectives that are being met. The neonatal mortality rate (deaths for all infants up to 28 days old) was 9.5 per 1000 live births in 1978 (Public Health Reports, 1983) and is projected to reach a low of 5.7 per 1000 live births by 1990, better than the Surgeon General's targeted 6.5 per 1000 live births (CDC, 1988). A second objective that has been met is for the majority of infants to leave hospitals in car safety carriers (Public

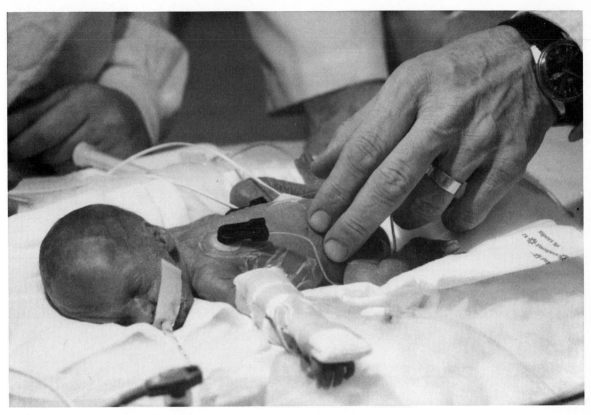

Figure 16-1
Low-birthweight babies need special care and are at high risk for neonatal mortality.

Health Reports, 1983); a 1987 survey indicated that approximately 75 percent of all infants were doing so (CDC, 1988). A third successful objective relates to screening all newborns for metabolic disorders such as PKU and congenital hypothyroidism. Such screening services are now available in all states (CDC, 1988).

FACTORS INFLUENCING THE HEALTH OF PREGNANT WOMEN AND INFANTS

Most pregnant women in the United States are healthy, have normal pregnancies, and produce healthy babies (Burst, 1987). Nevertheless, there are many factors that contribute to the health problems of those mothers and babies who figure in the statistics on infant mortality and low birth weight. Some factors are genetic and largely beyond the individual's control. Some factors are socioeconomic and resistant to change. Other factors are related to lifestyle choices that individual women have made. It is in the realm of lifestyle choices that the work of community health nurses can have the most significant impact. Data related to these factors are provided below.

ALCOHOL USE DURING PREGNANCY

According to recent statistics, one-third of all alcoholics in the United States are women (Mullins and Gazaway, 1985). Approximately 9 percent of pregnant women are heavy drinkers (Abel, 1982), and women classified as heavy drinkers have babies with the highest incidence of fetal alcohol syndrome (Mullins and Gazaway, 1985). Moreover, 40 percent of pregnant women are moderate drinkers, and babies born to these mothers have higher than average incidences of some fetal alcohol characteristics (Mullins and Gazaway, 1985). These include central nervous system deficiencies such as mental retardation, growth deficiencies, abnormal facial characteristics, other system abnormalities such as heart or kidney defects, birthmarks, and abnormalities of the external genitalia.

Alcohol use during pregnancy also increases the risk for abruptio placentae, stillbirth (Marbury et al., 1983), spontaneous abortion, congenital anomalies (Mullins and Gazaway, 1985), prematurity, postmaturity, and infections (Boyd, 1985). Some studies suggest that alcohol use during pregnancy is linked to the incidence of low-birthweight infants (Mills et al., 1984). Beer seems to be the most common alcoholic beverage consumed during pregnancy (Abel, 1982). Eighty-three percent of women reporting alcohol consumption during pregnancy also smoked (Brooten et al., 1987).

CIGARETTE SMOKING DURING PREGNANCY

Approximately 20 percent of pregnant women smoke (Figure 16-2) (Streissguth et al., 1983). Smoking during pregnancy has been associated with stillbirths, spontaneous abortions, higher perinatal mortality, and low birth weights (Nilsen et al., 1984; Feldman, 1985). Infants whose mothers smoke during pregnancy weigh approximately 200 grams less at birth than infants whose mothers did not smoke (Brooten et al., 1987). Perinatal mortality for infants born to women who smoked five or more cigarettes per day is reported to be 44.9 percent higher than that for infants born to women who do not smoke (Rush and Cassano, 1983; Feldman, 1985).

MATERNAL BODY WEIGHT BEFORE AND DURING PREGNANCY

Research has demonstrated a positive correlation between weight gain during pregnancy and normal-birthweight babies (Dimperio and Mahoun, 1985). Weight gains of 25 to 30 pounds during pregnancy are recommended (Neeson and May, 1986). Women of normal weight for their height tend to produce longer babies (Dimperio and Mahoun, 1985). Obese women have a higher incidence of perinatal mortality and medical problems than do women of

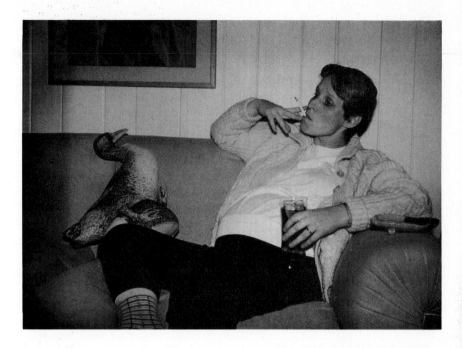

Figure 16-2
Pregnant women who
smoke endanger their
babies' lives as well as
their own.

normal weight (Calandra, Abell and Beischer, 1981), while underweight women have twice as many low-birthweight babies as women whose weight is within normal range (Dimperio and Mahoun, 1985). There is a correlation between poor weight gain in pregnancy and low-birthweight babies (Dimperio and Mahoun, 1985). Low birthweight is associated with higher incidences of growth problems, developmental delays, central nervous system disorders, and mental retardation (Heckler, 1983; Brooten et al., 1987), and two-thirds of infants who die before one year of age weighed less than 5 pounds 7 ounces at birth (Heckler, 1983; Jacobson, 1987). Insufficient caloric intake in pregnant adolescents (who themselves are still growing) is a concern (Brooten et al., 1987).

PREGNANCY DURING ADOLESCENCE

Each year, more than one million American teenagers become pregnant (MacDonald, 1987). There is a strong association between young maternal age and high infant mortality rates (Miller et al., 1986), and infants born to teenagers are at increased risk for neonatal and postneonatal mortality (Friede et al., 1987). Black infants born to adolescents are at higher risk of low birth weight than are white infants (Friede et al., 1987). Infants born to very young adolescents (aged 10 to 15 years) are at very high risk for neonatal mortality (Friede et al., 1987).

PLANNING FOR THE HEALTH OF MATERNAL-INFANT POPULATIONS

Developing quality health care programs and services for specific populations does not happen by chance. Such programs are based upon identified needs and are organized and delivered in a thoughtful, logical fashion. Ideally, they result from coordinated community planning. Effective community planning can save nurses valuable time and resources and can help prevent inappropriate distribution and duplication of services.

THE PLANNING PROCESS

Daly (1986) identifies the specific process of community planning as follows:

1. *Prioritize the problems:* Analyze the relative urgency of problems diagnosed during the assessment phase.
2. *Select nursing responsibilities:* Differentiate those problems that nursing actions can resolve from those that other professionals can best handle.
3. *Identify goals, objectives, and actions:* Identify short-term, intermediate, long-term goals; behavioral objectives oriented to community behavior and derived from the goals; and the specific actions to achieve the objectives.
4. *Develop a nursing plan:* Write the problems, actions, and expected behavior outcomes on a community nursing care plan.

The process of community health planning may be clear, but the work involved may seem somewhat overwhelming. However, it need not be. The nursing process provides a conceptual approach to planning client care and is readily adaptable for planning programs and services for populations of clients. An in-depth discussion of the nursing process applied to population-focused care is provided in Chapter 8 and will not be pursued further here. Instead, we will discuss some specific factors to consider when applying the nursing process to maternal-infant health populations.

COMMON FEATURES OF HEALTH PROGRAMS FOR MATERNAL-INFANT POPULATIONS

It is helpful for the nurse/planner to know that maternal-infant programs across the country share many common features. For example, there are concerted efforts to follow clients closely during the antepartum and postpartum periods. A major focus of community health nurses during this time is teaching. Nurses introduce new information or reinforce existing knowledge of pregnancy, delivery, and postpartum health considerations. Through teaching, nurses assist mothers to adapt to the physiological and emotional changes they are experiencing and help them to anticipate and plan for the impact their infants will have on their daily lives.

While working with a maternal population, community health nurses do comprehensive, ongoing client assessments. In addition to considering their clients' physiological and emotional status, nurses look closely at clients' social support systems, access to medical care, financial status, housing needs, and ability to provide for their babies. If clients need assistance in any or all of these areas, nurses intervene and refer them to other appropriate community resources. Nurses may need to serve as advocates for clients in the referral process. Ideally, once the referral has been made, community health nurses work collaboratively with other professionals to meet clients' needs.

The following outline shows some typical features of maternal-infant health programs.

I.   Antepartum teaching
    a.   Significance of prenatal care
    b.   Self-responsibility
    c.   Physiological changes during pregnancy
    d.   Fetal growth and development
    e.   Nutrition
    f.   Exercise
    g.   Hazards of alcohol consumption and/or smoking
    h.   Breastfeeding
    i.   Stages of labor
    j.   Delivery—process and options available
    k.   Future birth control

II. Introduction to community resources
    a.   Childbirth classes
    b.   Self-help groups
    c.   Women/Infant/Children (WIC) Supplemental Food Program
    d.   Department of Social Welfare
    e.   Planned Parenthood
    f.   School-based clinics
    g.   High-risk clinics

III. Postpartum teaching
    a.   Newborn assessments
    b.   Care of the newborn
    c.   Growth and development of the infant
    d.   Mother/infant bonding
    e.   Postpartum physiological changes in the mother
    f.   Breast/bottle feeding
    g.   Exercise

        h.   Future birth control
        i.   Return to work
        j.   Child care
  IV. Delivery of services
        a.   Clinic visits
        b.   Home visits
        c.   Formal classes
        d.   Self-help groups
        e.   Community education
   V. Coordination with other community resources
        a.   Physicians
        b.   Clinics
        c.   Hospitals
        d.   High schools
        e.   Industries
        f.   WIC
        g.   Department of Social Welfare
  VI. Client advocacy
        a.   Follow-up services
        b.   Efforts to influence legislation and policies
        c.   Testimony on behalf of maternal-infant population

These common features provide a guiding framework for designing maternal and infant services. Each population, however, has specific needs that the community health nurse should assess and incorporate into the program plan. Two important considerations include: (1) specific needs identified through data and client input, and (2) the developmental stage of the population being served.

NEEDS OF SPECIFIC POPULATIONS

To design programs and services for maternal-infant populations, planners need to have a sound understanding of the population they are attempting to serve. Vital statistics assist planners to identify specific problems and pinpoint segments of the population where problems are more likely to occur, yet statistics alone cannot fully characterize the populations they represent. Our society has witnessed numerous ineffective community projects, public works projects (Pressman and Wildavsky, 1984) and health care projects. Such programs often have failed because the targeted populations were assessed incompletely or not involved in the planning process.

Most nurses realize that a predetermined, generalized plan may not meet the needs of any one specific client. To increase effectiveness, the nurse involves the client in designing a plan to meet individual needs. The nurse considers such things as the client's level of education, previous knowledge, life experience, level of motivation, culture, and developmental stage.

The same philosophy of consumer input and attention to clients' specific needs holds true when planning programs for a population. While a broad program to provide services to groups of clients may look and sound logical, such a program will probably need further refining to meet the needs of diverse groups. For example, an agency may develop a generalized program to provide prenatal services to clients. While the program designed may meet the needs of some women, it is very unlikely that one program design will be equally effective with college-educated career women (Figure 16-3), pregnant adolescents, low-income inner-city black women, or women in rural Appalachia. The needs of the women in each of these subpopulations are very different. Women from each of these groups can provide valuable information to planners regarding their culture, characteristics, and specific needs. As with individual clients, input from the targeted population increases the program's chances for success.

Figure 16-3
Pregnant career women share specific needs for prenatal teaching and assistance.

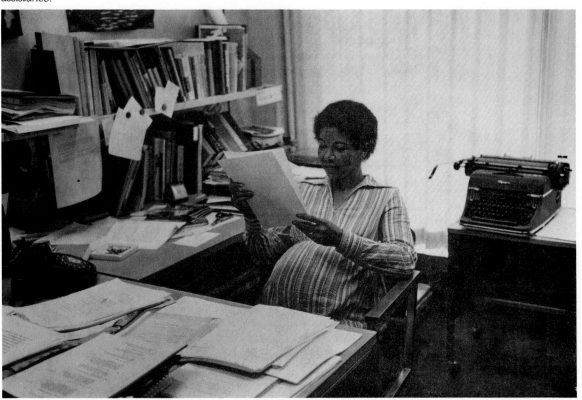

DEVELOPMENTAL STAGE OF THE POPULATION BEING SERVED

As individuals grow and mature, they continually experience physiological changes, personality changes as new psychosocial issues are met (Erikson, 1968), and increasingly sophisticated thought processes (Piaget, 1950). Consequently, a person's most pressing concerns at one stage in life may seem insignificant at the next stage of development.

When planning maternal-infant health programs, it is crucial that the community health nurse consider the developmental stages of the women being served. For example, adolescents are in a stage of intellectual development in which their thinking processes are moving from the concrete to the abstract (Piaget, 1950). Many adolescents can think in the abstract; they can imagine the complexities of life as a single parent and envision the adult role they would be expected to assume. Other adolescents can think only in concrete terms, dealing primarily with the past and present. They have difficulty comprehending the complex psychosocial issues with which they will be faced upon the birth of their infants. Innovative and creative approaches must be used with these adolescents to assist them in better understanding the complex nature of child care. Some maternal-infant health programs and some high schools involve pregnant adolescents (and those judged likely to become pregnant) in child day-care programs. The adolescents participate in the day-to-day care of infants and toddlers and experience the joys of children as well as the intense demands and heavy responsibility involved in providing appropriate child care.

The needs of pregnant women in the developmental stages of young adulthood and middle adulthood differ substantially from those of adolescents and will vary between individuals (Erikson, 1968). A thorough understanding of the developmental tasks and the psychosocial issues confronting each population should be the cornerstone of solid, well-developed programs. Such programs can be adapted to the developmental needs of clients in adolescence, young adulthood, or middle adulthood.

IMPLEMENTATION OF MATERNAL-INFANT HEALTH PROGRAMS

Methods of delivering services to clients often are determined by the financial resources of the agency providing the services. The majority of maternal-infant health programs in the United States receive public funding through local tax dollars and through federal block grants given to each state for allocation by state officials.

Methods of delivering services will vary based upon the population and its specific needs. The geographical distribution of clients and the size of the nursing staff available to deliver the services also play significant roles. For example, in rural areas where clients are scattered over a large area, it may be appropriate to deliver services to the population on a one-to-one basis through nurse-run clinics or home visits.

CLINIC PROGRAMS

In the *clinic setting* each client receives an individualized examination and health teaching. Unfortunately, there are time constraints placed on the nurse and thus the actual time spent in teaching clients is relatively short. Clinics may be effective on Native American reservations where the population is centrally located and in sites where migrant farm workers and their families are temporarily located.

HOME VISITS

Home visits also can provide clients with a one-to-one opportunity for teaching with the community health nurse. There are two major benefits to home visits. First, the client is in the comfortable, familiar surroundings of her own home. Second, the nurse's assessment is enhanced by observations in the home setting of such things as family interactions, values, and priorities. Home visiting to maternal-infant health clients can prove costly for an agency if clients are not at home at scheduled visit times and home visits must be rescheduled.

In metropolitan areas where community health nurses and clients are in close proximity to one another, nurse-run clinics and home visits may still be appropriate mechanisms for the delivery of services. With close proximity, clients can visit the clinic frequently, and nurses can make more home visits with less distance to travel between clients. In addition, metropolitan areas afford community health nurses an opportunity to use a group approach with clients. This may include small, informal group discussions or larger, more formal classes. Whether small or large, groups can provide a vehicle for teaching by the nurse as well as a means for clients to teach and learn from one another. Group discussions can complement clinic and home visits and be ongoing at both neighborhood clinics and WIC clinics.

SELF-HELP GROUPS

The methods presented above for implementation of services are relatively traditional. Nurses also need to use innovative and creative approaches such as *self-help groups,* which are defined as "voluntary small group structures for mutual aid in the accomplishment of a specific purpose. They are usually formed by peers who have come together for mutual assistance in satisfying a common need, overcoming a common handicap or life disrupting problem, and bringing about desired social and/or personal change." (Balgopal,

1986, p. 123). While many groups are formed by peers, establishing self-help groups is also an appropriate role for community health nurses (Pesznecker and Zahlis, 1986).

Self-help groups provide many benefits to participants (Figure 16-4). Within our present health care system, clients often express feelings of insignificance and loss of control. However, in a self-help group environment individuals regain their sense of identity and control. Acceptance of responsibility for health-promoting behaviors is a key concept supported by the majority of self-help groups. Members who lose sight of their self-responsibility are readily confronted by the group. Individuals reach out to help other members and in the process help themselves to become better informed and stronger in their own beliefs.

Self-help groups have been successfully developed for the prenatal population to address common concerns such as prenatal changes, adapting to pregnancy, fetal growth and development, and labor and delivery. For postpartum women, groups have been established for breastfeeding mothers, mothers of infants, mothers of toddlers, and mothers of twins. In each instance, members of healthy populations help one another to remain healthy and prevent potential problems.

While many community health nurses may be unfamiliar with the concept of self-help groups, it is a concept that needs to be integrated into community health nursing practice more consistently. The role of the nurse will vary depending upon the size, interests, and level of sophistication of the group. For example, with a group of well-educated women who are effective prob-

Figure 16-4
Expectant mothers can enjoy and benefit from group activities such as this aerobics class.

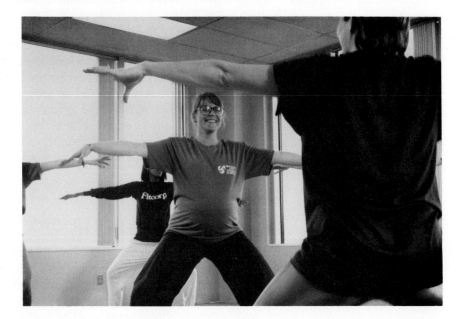

lem-solvers, the nurse may initiate the group and then serve primarily as a resource person. With a group of adolescents, on the other hand, the nurse may need to be present at each meeting to facilitate group process as well as to clarify information shared within the group. In Chapter 9 we describe group work in greater detail.

TEACHING — CONTENT AND METHODOLOGIES

Teaching is an integral part of any maternal-infant program having health promotion as its primary focus. Our discussion of program implementation would be incomplete without a look at teaching methods.

At first glance, content areas for prenatal and postnatal health teaching may appear to be the same for all women. A common mistake is to approach all women of childbearing age with the same content using the same teaching methods. In order for the teaching to be effective, however, the content must vary depending on the needs, characteristics, and developmental stage of each population (Figure 16-5). For example, in the area of nutrition, an appropriate goal for all groups of women may be

> on a daily basis, pregnant women will consume the amount of calories appropriate for their height and weight; those calories will be an appropriate balance of protein, carbohydrates, and fats.

Content presented to well-educated career women may be relatively straightforward in discussing food groups and the appropriate distribution of calories. The content may reinforce information gained in high school, college, or other settings. Nutritional teaching material presented to adolescents may need to include basic nutritional information that the adolescents may not have had the opportunity to receive either through educational programs or life experience. Teaching geared toward adolescents also needs to include discussions based around types of foods that they find appealing. In addition, this younger population needs assistance in planning menus and selecting nutritious and appetizing foods. Nutritional information presented to specific cultural groups such as Hispanic or Asian women needs to go beyond traditional American food patterns to encompass the dietary patterns of the women's native culture.

In addition to tailoring subject matter to fit the client population, community health nurses should select teaching methodologies appropriate to clients. Some groups may respond positively to structured classes; others may prefer a less-formal discussion format. Two community health nurses working in a community-based parent-child center in Middlebury, Vermont, developed a prenatal teaching program for adolescents with a majority of the content taught in small discussion groups at the child care center. These nurses found that the adolescents were very comfortable with this method, learning

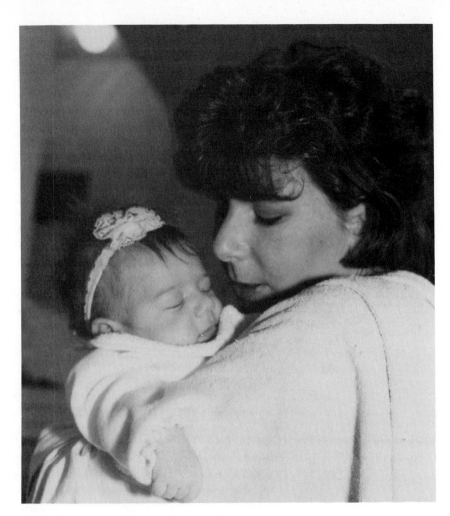

Figure 16-5
This young mother and
infant represent a
population whose learning
needs may include
information about nutrition,
exercise, growth and
development, parenting,
and many other topics. The
nurse tailors teaching to
clients' specific needs and
developmental stages.

not only from the nurses but from one another. These same nurses use the small-group approach to meet in high school settings on a weekly basis with adolescents who are at high risk for pregnancy.

Teaching aids used should be appropriate for each audience. It is important to remember that many of the available teaching aids are in English and depict white, middle-class women and infants. While these will be appropriate for some populations, not all populations will be able to identify with the mothers and babies portrayed. When at all possible, teaching aids should be congruent with the language, race, and culture of the population being served (Wittenberg, 1983).

Teaching and motivating women to promote their own health and the health of their babies is a major challenge, and there is no one "right way" to approach the task. Community health nurses need to be innovative and creative in their approach to teaching. In Chapter 11, we provide further information and resources on teaching in community health nursing.

STAFFING MATERNAL-INFANT HEALTH PROGRAMS

A program may be well designed and appropriate for the population, but if the nursing personnel selected to implement the program are not qualified, the program has little chance for success. The selection of nursing personnel is an area needing much attention. As management recruits nursing staff to work with maternal-infant health populations, we recommend that nurses have the following qualifications:

1. A sound educational background, minimally a baccalaureate degree in nursing
2. A solid understanding of nursing process and ability to use it in working with individuals, families, and groups
3. A knowledge of, and willingness to work with, other community resources
4. Effective communication skills
5. A sincere, nonjudgmental approach to clients

COMMUNITY RESOURCES FOR MATERNAL-INFANT HEALTH

The maternal-infant population has complex needs. It is not unusual for community health nurses to see multiple personal and family problems in this group and, since community health nurses clearly cannot meet all these needs, it is essential that they have a working knowledge of community resources for assistance and referral. Some community resources for maternal and infant health include Planned Parenthood, community childbirth classes, Department of Social Welfare, and the Women, Infants, and Children Special Supplemental Food Program. A clear understanding of the services provided and a positive working relationship between agency personnel will facilitate effective provision of services to this population group.

The Department of Social Welfare assigns each family a trained social worker. After interviewing the family, the social worker determines whether or not the family or individual members of the family meet eligibility criteria for programs administered by the Department of Social Welfare such as the Medicaid program, the Food Stamp program, and the Aid to Families with Dependent Children program. If the social worker establishes family or individual eligibility, she or he starts the process of applying for benefits (Hadeka, 1987).

The Women, Infants, and Children (WIC) Special Supplemental Food Program is a federal program that provides nutritional support to low-income women and children. Established in 1972 as a pilot program, it receives its funding from the Food and Nutrition Service of the U.S. Department of Agriculture. The food provided by the program helps pregnant women to produce healthy, normal-birthweight babies. Food is also provided for the infants through their formative years to facilitate normal growth and development. In the years of the WIC program's existence its funding has increased from 20 million dollars a year in 1974 to over 1.5 billion dollars a year in 1984 (Jacobson, 1987). The WIC program provides supplemental foods and nutrition education to pregnant women up to six months postpartum, nursing mothers up to one year postpartum, and children from birth to age five (Miller, 1984).

Eligibility of the above groups rests on income level, geographical area, and nutritional risk. Determining income eligibility is relatively uncomplicated, as guidelines are clearly defined by each state. Geographical eligibility varies, since many states offer services in all areas while others do not. Clients must live in an area that has been designated to receive funding. Determining nutritional risk is more complex; a nurse or nutritionist interviews individual clients and reviews their previous medical and nutritional history. Factors that put pregnant or postpartum women at risk include the following:

Age (i.e., adolescents or over 40)

Poor obstetrical history, such as previous low-birthweight infants, miscarriages, short periods between pregnancies, and gestational diabetes

Anemia

Poor weight gain (low or high)

Inadequate consumption of food (Jacobson, 1987)

Factors that put infants and children at risk include the following:

Poor growth

Anemia

Obesity

Chronic illnesses

Nutrition-related diseases (Berkenfield and Schwartz, 1980)

Based upon information obtained from clients, the health professional identifies areas of strength and areas for change. The program then offers a supplemental food package to clients for the next six months. The food package contains foods with high-quality protein, iron, calcium, and Vitamins A and C. The specific foods offered tend to be combinations of fruit juice fortified with vitamin C, eggs, milk (lowfat or whole), cheese, fortified cereals, and fortified infant formula (Miller, 1984). Distribution of food packages varies within states. In some states local dairies deliver the food to the home; in other states clients receive vouchers and exchange them for food packages at local grocery stores. The WIC program reevaluates clients at predetermined intervals. It reassesses needs, continues nutrition education, and recertifies food packages if appropriate.

EVALUATION OF MATERNAL-INFANT HEALTH PROGRAMS

Evaluation is a critical aspect of maternal-infant health program planning. Four questions, in particular, should be addressed (Veney and Kaluzny, 1984): (1) Was the program relevant? That is, did it meet the identified needs of this particular maternal-infant population? (2) Did the program meet its goals and objectives? (3) Was the program cost-effective? Did the outcomes justify the resources used? (4) What was the program's long-term impact on the health of this population of mothers and infants?

Community health nurses find the answers to the above questions through a carefully designed, systematic evaluation plan. In Chapter 8 we discuss program evaluation in detail. For our purposes in this chapter we examine three useful methods for obtaining evaluation data.

Vital statistics provide an important data base for evaluating maternal-infant programs. State or national figures can help agency personnel determine whether their own statistics are improving, remaining constant, or worsening. Using vital statistics, nurses can make comparisons between or within population groups. For instance, they might compare the incidence of low-birthweight babies born to their clients with rates reported by similar agencies in other urban areas. One disadvantage of using vital statistics is that the time required to compile this data can make it difficult to have the most current figures.

A second mechanism for evaluation within individual maternal-infant programs is quality assurance. A quality assurance program looks constructively at client services and raises questions such as the following:

How soon after receiving the referral were clients seen?
Was the data base complete?
Was the plan of care appropriate?
Were the established outcomes reasonable and achievable?
Were clients involved in the planning process?
Were appropriate referrals made?
Was there follow-up on the referrals?
Was discharge of the client appropriate?

Quality assurance programs can use various methods to gather this type of information, such as feedback from clients through periodic questionnaires and personal interviews or telephone surveys. Disadvantages of these methods may be the time consumed and the expense for the agency.

A cost-effective mechanism for assessing a program and the client care delivered is through auditing client records. It is not feasible for an agency to review every client record, but random samplings can be done at predetermined times each year. If clearly defined criteria are established, then those conducting the audit can easily review a record and determine, in their professional judgment, whether or not the criteria have been met. Auditing client records can be a positive learning experience, and agency staff should be encouraged to participate in the process. Reading through another nurse's documentation can be a positive reminder of the impact that the community health nurse can have on the effectiveness of services delivered.

Summary

Vital statistics indicate that the status of maternal and infant health in the United States can still be improved when compared with that of other industrialized nations. We are a society that has both the knowledge and the resources to improve the quality of life for mothers and babies.

Factors influencing the health of pregnant women and infants may be genetic, socioeconomic, or related to life-style and individual choices. The latter category is a prime target for community health nursing intervention. Life-style–related factors influencing the health status of pregnant women and infants include alcohol consumption, smoking, and weight gain during pregnancy. Pregnancy during adolescence adds additional risk.

In planning effective maternal-infant programs, community health nurses must consider needs identified by the populations themselves as well as vital statistics. The planning process includes prioritizing problems; selecting nursing responsibilities; identifying goals, objectives, and actions; and developing a nursing plan. Maternal-infant programs across the country have certain features in common, including perinatal follow-up and teaching, client assessment, service delivery, coordination with other community resources, and client advocacy. These common features assist community health nurses in designing maternal and infant programs. Two other planning considerations include specific needs identified through data and client input, and the developmental stage of the population being served.

Creative and innovative methods of implementation such as discussion and self-help groups should be used more widely for teaching and working with maternal-infant populations. Effective implementation of health programs also depends on appropriately qualified staff members. The nature of the maternal-infant population is complex and diverse; thus, appropriate uses of community resources provide an important adjunct to community health nursing services.

To evaluate the effectiveness of maternal-infant health programs, the community health nurse needs to ask the following questions: (1) Was the program relevant? (2) Did it meet identified goals and objectives? (3) Was the program cost-effective? (4) What was the program's long-term impact on the health of the population of mothers and infants? Three methods for obtaining evaluation data are collection of vital statistics, use of quality assurance programs, and use of the auditing process.

Study Questions

1. To support the Surgeon General's "Objectives for the Nation," what specific objectives has your state's health department developed for mothers and infants? How do your state's statistics compare with those of other states on (1) infant death rates (generally and by blacks, whites, hispanics), (2) incidence of low-birthweight infants and (3) incidence of birth defects?
2. Describe three different maternal-infant populations in your county. What are their most pressing health needs? Do any existing services target these populations? How well, in your judgment, are clients' needs being met? Interview a city or county community health nurse as well as other public health professionals to help you find your answers.
3. Select one life-style–related factor that affects pregnant women and infants (such as alcohol, smoking, or nutrition) and design a health program to deal with it. Be sure to include the main factors, discussed in this chapter, for planning a maternal-infant program.

References

Abel, E. (1982). Consumption of alcohol during pregnancy: A review of effects on growth and development of offspring. *Human Biology* 54: 421–53.

Balgopal, P., R. Pallassana, P. Ephross, and T. Vassil. (1986). Self-help groups and professional helpers. *Small Group Behavior* 17(2): 123–27.

Berkenfield, J., and J. Schwartz. (1980). Nutrition intervention in the community: The "WIC" program. *New England Journal of Medicine* 302(10): 579–81.

Boyd, M. D. (1985). Patient motivation during pregnancy. *Maryland Medical Journal* 34(10): 977–81.

Brooten, D., M. A. Peters, M. Glotts, S. E. Goffrey, M. Knapp, S. Cohen, and C. Jordan. (1987). A survey of nutrition, caffeine, cigarette, and alcohol intake in early pregnancy in an urban clinic population. *Journal of Nurse-Midwifery* 32(2): 85–90.

Burst, H. V. (1987). Issues and concerns of healthy pregnant women. *Public Health Reports* July–August Supp.: 57–61.

Calendra, C., D. A. Abell, and N. A. Beischner. (1981). Maternal obesity in pregnancy. *Obstetrics and Gynecology* 57(8): 8–12.

Center for Disease Control. (1988). U. S. falling short on its infant health goals. *The New York Times:* July 10.

Daly, E. B. (1986). Health promotion and the community. In C. Edelman and C. L. Mandle (eds.), *Health Promotion Throughout the Lifespan.* St. Louis, Mo.: Mosby, 234–56.

Dimperio, D. L., and C. S. Mahoun. (1985). Influencing pregnancy through nutrition and dietary changes. *Maryland Medical Journal* 34(10): 997–1002.

Erikson, E. H. (1968). *Identity, youth, and crisis.* New York: W. W. Norton.

Feldman, P. R. (1985). Smoking and healthy pregnancy: Now is the time to quit. *Maryland Medical Journal* 34(10): 982–86.

Gold, R. B., A. M. Kenney, and S. Singh. (1987). Paying for maternity care in the United States. *Family Planning Perspectives* 19(5): 190–206.

Hadeka, M. (1987). Clinical judgment in community health nursing. Boston: Little, Brown.

Heckler, M. (1983). Healthy mothers, healthy babies: A goal we can all help attain. *Public Health Reports* 98(6): 529.

Jacobson, H. N. (1987). Progress on key issues in maternal nutrition. *Public Health Reports* July–August Supp.: 50–52.

MacDonald, D. I. (1987). An approach to the problem of teenage pregnancy. *Public Health Reports* 102(4): 377–85.

Marbury, M. C., S. Linn, R. Monson, S. Schoenbaum, P. G. Stubblefield, and K. Ryan. (1983). *American Journal of Public Health* 73(10): 1165–68.

Miller, C. A., A. Fine, S. Adams-Taylor, and L. B. Schorr. (1986). *Monitoring children's health: Key indicators.* Washington, D.C.: American Public Health Association.

Miller, D. F. (1984). *Dimensions of community health.* Dubuque, Ia.: William C. Brown.

Mills, J., B. Grauband, E. Harley, et al. (1984). Maternal alcohol consumption and birthweight. *Journal of the American Medical Association* 252: 1875–79.

Mullins, C. L., and P. M. Gazaway. (1985). Alcohol and drug use in pregnancy: A case for management. *Maryland Medical Journal* 34(10): 991–96.

Neeson, J., and K. May. (1986). *Comprehensive maternity nursing.* Philadelphia: J. B. Lippincott.

Nilsen, S., N. Sagen, H. Kim, et al. (1984). Smoking, hemoglobin levels, and birth weights in normal pregnancies. *American Journal of Obstetrics and Gynecology.* 148: 752–58.

Pesznecker, B., and E. Zahlis. (1986). Establishing mutual-help groups for family-member caregivers: A new role for community health nurses. *Public Health Nursing* 3: 29.

Piaget, J. (1950). *The psychology of intelligence.* London: Routledge and Kegan Paul, Ltd.

Pressman, J. L., and A. Wildavsky. (1984). *Implementation.* 3rd ed. Berkeley: University of California Press.

Public Health Reports Supplement. (1983). Pregnancy and infant health. *Public Health Reports:* 24–40.

Public Health Service. (1979). *Healthy people: The Surgeon General's report on health promotion and disease prevention* (DHEN Publication No. 79–55071). Washington, D. C.: U. S. Government Printing Office.

Rush, D., and P. Cassano. (1983). Relationship of cigarette smoking and social class to birthweight and perinatal mortality among all births in Britain. *Journal of Epidemiology and Community Health* 37: 249–55.

Streissguth, A. P., B. L. Darby, H. M. Barr, J. R. Smith, and D. C. Mantin. (1983). Comparison of drinking and smoking patterns during pregnancy over a six-month interval. *American Journal of Obstetrics and Gynecology* 145: 716–23.

Veney, J. E., and A. D. Kaluzny. (1984). *Evaluation and decision making for health services programs.* Englewood Cliffs, N.J.: Prentice-Hall.

Windom, R. E. (1987). Seeking answers to the slowing progress in lowering infant mortality. *Public Health Reports* 102(2): 121–22.

Wittenberg, C. K. (1983). Summary of market research for "healthy mothers, healthy babies" campaign. *Public Health Reports* 98(4): 356–59.

Selected Readings

Abel, E. (1982). Consumption of alcohol during pregnancy: A review of effects on growth and development of offspring. *Human Biology* 54: 421–53.

Berkenfield, J., and J. Schwartz. (1980). Nutrition intervention in the community: The "WIC" program. *New England Journal of Medicine* 302(10): 579–81.

Boyd, M. D. (1985). Patient motivation during pregnancy. *Maryland Medical Journal* 34(10): 977–81.

Brooten, D., M. A. Peters, M. Glotts, S. E. Goffrey, M. Knapp, S. Cohen, and C. Jordan. (1987). A survey of nutrition, caffeine, cigarette, and alcohol intake in early pregnancy in an urban clinic population. *Journal of Nurse-Midwifery* 32(2): 85–90.

Burst, H. V. (1987). Issues and concerns of healthy pregnant women. *Public Health Reports* July–August Supp.: 57–61.

Calendra, C., D. Abell, and N. Beishner. (1981). Maternal obesity in pregnancy. *Obstetrics and Gynecology* 57(8): 8–12.

Davis, B., et al. (1988). Implementation and preliminary evaluation of a community-based prenatal health education program. *Family and Community Health* 11(1): 8–16.

Dimperio, D., and C. Mahoun. (1985). Influencing pregnancy through nutrition and dietary changes. *Maryland Medical Journal* 34(10): 997–1002.

Dodds, J. M. (1987). Nutrition and health: An individual responsibility. *Public Health Reports* July–August Supp.: 29–33.

Feldman, P. R. (1985). Smoking and healthy pregnancy: Now is the time to quit. *Maryland Medical Journal* 34(10): 982–86.

Gold, R. B., A. M. Kenney, and S. Singh. (1987). Paying for maternity care in the United States. *Family Planning Perspectives* 19(5): 190–206.

Hadeka, M. (1987). *Clinical judgment in community health nursing.* Boston: Scott, Foresman/Little, Brown.

Heckler, M. (1983). Healthy mothers, healthy babies: A goal we can all help attain. *Public Health Reports* 98(6): 529.

Jacobson, H. N. (1987). Progress on key issues in maternal nutrition. *Public Health Reports* July–August Supp.: 50–52.

MacDonald, D. I. (1987). An approach to the problem of teenage pregnancy. *Public Health Reports* 102(4): 377–85.

McKay, R., and M. Segall. (1983). Methods and models for the aggregate. *Nursing Outlook* 31(6): 328–34.

Mullins, C. L., and P. M. Gazaway. (1985). Alcohol and drug use in pregnancy: A case for management. *Maryland Medical Journal* 34(10): 991–96.

Petze, C. F. (1984). Health promotion for the well family. *Nursing Clinics of North America* 19(2): 229–37.

Public Health Service (1979). *Healthy people: The Surgeon General's report on health promotion and disease prevention* (DHEN Publication No. 79–55071). Washington, D. C.: U. S. Government Printing Office.

Schulze, M. W., et al. (1987). Attitudes of community health nurses toward maternal and child health nursing: Development of an instrument. *Journal of Professional Nursing* 3(6): 347–53.

Tegtmeier, D., and S. Elsea. (1984). Wellness throughout the maternity cycle. *Nursing Clinics of North America* 19(2): 219–27.

von Windeguth, B., M. T. Urbano, J. S. Hayes, and K. Martyn. (1988). Analysis of infant risk factors documented by public health nurses. *Public Health Nursing* 5(3): 165–69.

Windom, R. E. (1987). Seeking answers to the slowing progress in lowering infant mortality. *Public Health Reports* 102(2): 121–22.

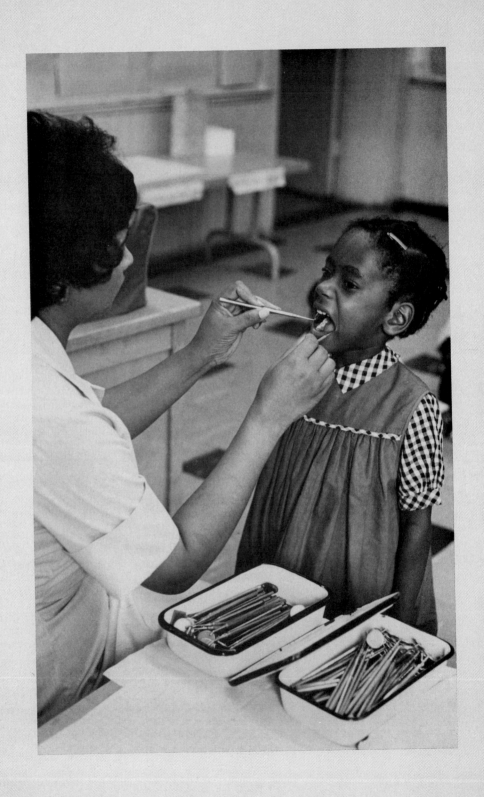

17 Preschool, School-age, and Adolescent Populations

Healthy children are a vital resource to ensure the future well-being of the nation. They are the parents, workers, leaders, and decision makers of tomorrow, and their health and safety depend on today's decisions and actions. Their future lies in our hands.

Children are an important population group of concern to community health nursing. To understand the nurse's role in serving this population, we must first ask some questions. What are the health needs of children as an aggregate? What preschool, school-age, and adolescent populations are at greatest risk of poor health? What health programs are available to serve these groups, and what others are needed? In this chapter we address these questions by summarizing the state of children's health. The subject is treated extensively in many excellent sources; a number are listed at the conclusion of the chapter. The reader is encouraged to explore them for greater depth and breadth of understanding. In this chapter we seek to gain a clearer conception of specific childhood populations at risk and the community health nurse's contribution to those groups.

CHILDREN'S HEALTH NEEDS

The well-being of children has been a subject of great concern in this country for many years. As a nation, we have emphasized its importance through development of numerous laws and services, yet the needs of millions of children continue to go unmet. Consider the following facts about children in the United States (Children's Defense Fund, 1988; Miller et al., 1986):

One in four preschoolers is poor.
One in five children is poor.
One in two of the children born into single-parent families is poor.

493

Minority children are disproportionately poor. (More than 43 percent of all black children and 37.7 percent of all Hispanic children are poor.)

Seven to 20 percent of low-income children suffer from anemia.

Between 1981 and 1986, reported childhood abuse and neglect increased 50 percent (an estimated 1.9 million children).

One in two children has a mother in the labor force, but less than 50 percent of these children have adequate child care.

One in five children is at risk of becoming a teen parent.

One in six children has no health insurance.

One in three children has never been to a dentist.

One in seven children is at risk of dropping out of school.

Families with children comprise nearly one-third of America's homeless population.

Furthermore, the many needs of America's 13 million poor children are only part of the picture. There are millions more children in moderate-income families who are "child care poor, housing poor, health insurance poor, and higher education poor" (Children's Defense Fund, 1988). Added to these are "a growing number of privileged youths (who) suffer from spiritual poverty, afflicted by what John Levy of the Jung Institute labels 'affluenza'" (Children's Defense Fund, 1988). Plagued with boredom, low self-esteem, and lack of motivation, children in wealthy homes are often insulated from challenge and risk and find drugs, alcohol, and sex far too accessible. Many of the same problems exist for children of the urban rich as for those of the urban poor. Clearly there is a need for improvement in our efforts to prepare children adequately for the future.

CHILDHOOD MORTALITY

Specifically, what are children's health needs? The health of children generally has improved a great deal since the early 1900s. Childhood mortality rates have dropped dramatically. We have seen the threat of major child-killing infectious diseases, such as diphtheria, pneumonia, and tuberculosis, significantly reduced. Now, according to the National Center for Health Statistics (1988), injury is the leading cause of death among children over the age of nine months in the United States. Injuries cause approximately 44 percent of all deaths of children from one to four years old, 51 percent of deaths of children from five to nine years old, and 58 percent of deaths of children from 10 to 14 years old (Waller, Baker, and Szocka, 1989). Motor vehicle-related injuries are the most prevalent cause of death for children of all ages except those who are less than one year old, for whom homicide accounts for even more deaths than motor vehicles.

In motor-vehicle-related deaths, infants less than one year old are at greatest risk as passengers, as are children from one to four years old and from 10 to 14 years old. Children five to nine years old are at greatest risk as pedestrians. Use of appropriate restraints in motor vehicles (see Figure 17-1) has proved effective in reducing child deaths and injuries (Avery, 1980). Between 1980 and 1985 the motor vehicle occupant death rate in children declined by 14 percent (Waller, Baker, and Szocka, 1989).

"All other injuries" account for the second leading cause of death in children. Drowning, house fires, and homicide lead the list of threats in this cate-

Figure 17-1
Appropriate use of restraints in motor vehicles can prevent many childhood injuries and deaths.

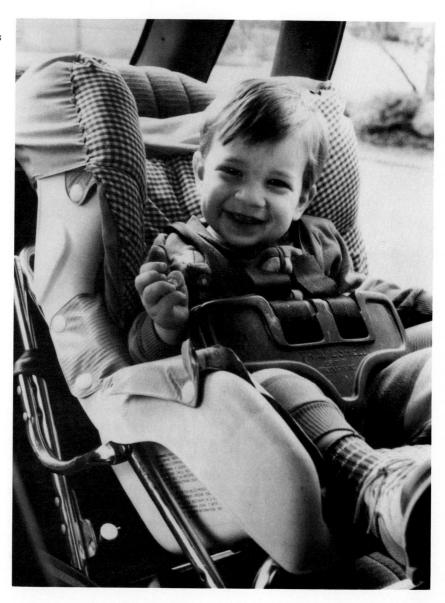

gory. In the "other injuries" category, deaths from drowning are most common, death from house fires account for 11 percent of all childhood deaths, and homicide deaths comprise 9 percent of all childhood injury deaths (National Center for Health Statistics, 1988).

There are noteworthy differences in injury rates across racial groups. House fire and homicide injury rates are three times as high for black children as for white children. Pedestrian deaths are twice as high for blacks as for whites, and the latter have twice as many drownings as blacks between one and four years old. Native Americans have exceptionally high injury death rates in pedestrian non-traffic deaths, poisonings, and motor vehicle occupant categories. Oriental children have higher injury death rates from falls than do children in the other groups (National Center for Health Statistics, 1988).

The loss of children's lives resulting from all injuries combined suggests a staggering number of years of productive life lost to society. Congenital anomalies and homicides are two other major causes of death among children. Homicides have risen at a frightening rate since 1925, showing a sixfold increase for one- to four-year-old children and a twofold increase for the five-to-14 age group. Homicides of children under the age of three most often result from family violence, but homicides involving children over the age of 12 generally involve violence outside the home ("Child Homicide," 1982).

CHILDHOOD MORBIDITY

Although childhood mortality rates have markedly decreased, morbidity rates are high. The most common types of acute conditions are respiratory illnesses (which account for the largest group), infectious and parasitic diseases, injuries, and digestive diseases (U.S. Bureau of Census, 1989). During the preschool and school-age years, children undergo significant physical and emotional changes, increase their contact with other people, and experience many new life events. All these factors serve to increase their vulnerability to injury and disease.

Other child health problems, less easy to detect and measure but often as debilitating, are those of emotional, behavioral, and intellectual development. Emotional disorders are quite prevalent in childhood; it is estimated that 10 percent of school-age children have adjustment difficulties that seriously interfere with academic and social development (Sigman, 1985). Other problems include learning disabilities, behavior disorders, developmental disabilities, speech and vision problems, and neuroses and psychoses. They have been called the "new morbidity" (Public Health Service, 1979). Although these problems are not new, awareness and concern for them has increased as the rates of occurrence for other life-threatening childhood diseases have diminished.

There is no precise etiology for these childhood developmental problems. Usually multiple causes, such as genetic, emotional, environmental, and cultural influences, are involved for children with learning disorders and behavior problems. A deprived environment and poor nutrition have been associated with mental retardation (Public Health Service, 1979). Increased aggressive behavior among children has been attributed to violence on television (Comstock, 1981).

Child abuse and neglect pose serious threats to children's health, both physical and emotional: "Abuse and neglect. . . account not only for many injuries, burns and other seeming accidents in children but also for brain damage, emotional scars, and even deaths. There are also children who are victims of sexual abuse, incest, and rape" (Public Health Service, 1979, p. 37). The problem is difficult to detect and often under-reported (Schetky and Green, 1988). Nationally, the rate of reported child abuse and neglect was 23.6 children per 1000 children in the population (Miller et al., 1986), and this rate is increasing.

Causes of abusive behavior generally derive from family situations where immaturity, stress, poverty, alcoholism, unstable employment, and physical and social isolation may be present, singly or in combination (Schetky and Green, 1988). Abusive adults often were abused themselves as children, carry low self-images into their adult lives, and are unable to cope with the demands of parenting or parent-substitute roles: "Abusing parents are often immature, dependent, unable to handle responsibility. They have low self-esteem, strong beliefs about the value of physical punishment, and misconceptions about children's competence to understand and perform according to their expectations. They frequently make unreasonable demands and, during times of crisis, may direct their anger and frustration at a child. They often are isolated socially and have difficulty seeking help" (Public Health Service, 1979, p. 38).

Families at high risk for child abuse may be those which are chronically troubled or temporarily stressed. Teenage mothers and families with closely spaced children may also be more likely to engage in abusive behavior. Although poverty and lack of education are often linked with child abuse, no socioeconomic level is immune.

A greater incidence of child abuse outside the home is coming to public attention. Physical and emotional maltreatment of children in institutions such as day-care centers, nursery schools, and children's theater should alert the community health nurse to watch for this problem in settings beyond the family home.

HEALTH PROBLEMS OF PRESCHOOL CHILDREN

The preschool population, ages one through four years, has a low mortality rate that is becoming lower every year. Currently it is 0.52 deaths per 1,000 live births, compared with 20 per 1,000 at the beginning of the century (National Center for Health Statistics, 1988). We can credit this dramatic change to the prevention and control of the acute childhood communicable diseases. The major cause of death is injuries (falls, drownings, burns, poisonings) followed by motor vehicle accidents, congenital anomalies, and malignant neoplasms.

As pointed out earlier, however, morbidity rates in this group are exceptionally high. Preschool children experience a high frequency of acute illnesses, the total number of which exceeds that of any other age. These account for a large number of days of restricted activity and disability requiring bed rest. Respiratory illness makes up 67 percent of these acute conditions (U.S. Bureau of Census, 1989). Preschoolers are vulnerable to many types of accidents. Their nutritional and dental health needs are great during this period of rapid growth, and their future mental health as adults will be influenced by how well their emotional needs are met during this phase of their development.

HEALTH PROBLEMS OF SCHOOL-AGE CHILDREN

As with preschool children, the mortality rates of schoolchildren are low and decreasing; they have dropped from 4 per 1,000 in 1900 to 0.32 per 1,000 currently. Again, we can credit this reduction to effective prevention and control of the acute infectious diseases of childhood. In 1900 the leading causes of death among this group were diphtheria, accidents (but not motor vehicle accidents), pneumonia and influenza, tuberculosis, and heart disease. Today motor vehicle accidents lead the list of causes of death for children aged 5 to 14, followed by all other accidents, congenital malformations, and homicide (U.S. Bureau of Census, 1989).

Morbidity in schoolchildren, however, is high. Children of this age group are most often affected by respiratory illness, followed by infectious diseases, injuries, and digestive conditions. Among schoolchildren, the incidence of measles, rubella (German measles), pertussis (whooping cough), and infectious parotitis (mumps) has dropped considerably because of widespread immunization efforts. Yet more cases than should still occur, some with potentially serious complications, such as birth defects from rubella and nerve deafness from mumps. Chicken pox, because no immunization for it is yet widely accepted and used, continues to be a frequent childhood illness.

Behavioral disorders and developmental disabilities are problems of this age group, often because they become exacerbated when the child enters school. The prevalence of these problems is difficult to measure epidemiologically, but one estimate places "clinical maladjustment" rates for schoolchildren at 11 percent (Hanlon and Pickett, 1984).

Handicapped schoolchildren, those with one or more chronic disabilities that limit activities, make up 3.9 percent of the school-age population, and this figure is rising (Newacheck, Budetti, and McManus, 1984). Handicaps include speech (15.2 per 1,000), hearing (14.3 per 1,000), and visual (11.3

per 1,000) defects, and partial or complete paralysis (2 per 1,000) (Hanlon and Pickett, 1984).

Other health problems found in this age group are nutritional problems (primarily overeating and inappropriate food choices) and poor dental health. Obesity often begins in childhood and becomes a risk factor for heart disease, hypertension, and diabetes. Obese children are three times more likely to become obese adults (Jonides, 1982). Schoolchildren's diets, often unreasonably high in sugar and fat, increase the incidence of coronary arteriosclerosis and dental caries in this population group. The average American child between the ages of 5 and 17 has more than four decayed, missing, or filled teeth. The prevalence of dental caries increases with age, with a slightly higher rate among girls than boys (Hanlon and Pickett, 1984).

HEALTH PROBLEMS OF ADOLESCENTS

Adolescents, during the period roughly encompassing the teen years, encounter many complex changes, physically, emotionally, cognitively, and socially. Rapid and major developmental adjustments create a variety of stresses, with concomitant problems, that have an impact on their health.

Mortality and morbidity rates for adolescents are low overall and demonstrate considerable improvement over the early 1900s. However, people in this age group die 2.5 times more often than younger children, and since 1960 the adolescent death rate has been gradually increasing (Public Health Service, 1979).

What are the health problems of adolescents? Violent death and injury head the list of major threats to life and health. For whites (male and female), motor vehicle accidents cause the greatest number of deaths, followed by all other accidents, suicide, and homicide. For nonwhites (male and female), homicides are the leading cause of death, with motor vehicle accidents second and all other accidents third.

The suicide rate for adolescents has more than doubled over recent years. In 1983 there were 205 suicide deaths to U.S. children aged 5 to 14 years. In the same year the number of suicides in youths aged 15 to 24 years was 4,845. Suicide rates are higher in whites than blacks, with adolescent males at greatest risk in this population group, having a death rate nearly three times higher than that of females. Accidents, homicides, and suicides together cause nearly three-fourths of all adolescent deaths (Miller et al., 1986). Responsibility for these has been attributed "to behavior patterns characterized by judgmental errors, aggressiveness, and, in some cases, ambivalence about wanting to live or die. Certainly, greater risk-taking occurs in this period of life" (Public Health Service, 1979, p. 43).

Another set of health problems for adolescents relates to life-style and behavior patterns. They include alcohol and drug abuse, unwanted pregnancies, sexually transmitted diseases (STDs), and poor nutrition.

Alcohol and Drug Abuse

A recent study done by the United States National Institute on Drug Abuse shows that 32 percent of adolescents use alcohol, 12.3 percent use marijuana, and 1.8 percent use cocaine (U.S. Bureau of Census, 1989). Members of this age group tend to consume alcohol less frequently (an average of once monthly) than adults do, but when adolescents do drink they drink large quantities and they experience more frequent episodes of intoxication than adults, thus increasing the chances of violent behavior and motor vehicle accidents. According to one report, 62 percent of tested drivers aged 16 to 19 years had positive blood alcohol levels, compared with 49 percent of drivers 35 years and older (Miller et al., 1986). Cigarette smoking continues to be "the most significant preventable health problem of adolescents" (Hanlon and Pickett, 1984, p. 422). The rates of cigarette smoking are decreasing among males and increasing among females but have been declining overall since 1974. An increasing number of adolescents smoke marijuana and take stimulants—amphetamines—frequently. Illegal use of substances such as cocaine, hallucinogens, and prescription medications tends to be more common with older adolescents and young adults (18 to 25 years of age) than with younger adolescents. Drug abuse among young people was almost unknown before 1950 and rare before 1962. Now, adolescent drug experimentation and use pose serious physical and psychological threats.

Teenage Pregnancies and STDs

Increasing sexual activity among adolescents creates two other significant health problems for this age group. They are teenage pregnancies and sexually transmitted diseases (STDs). The United States leads nearly all developed nations in rates of teenage pregnancy, abortion, and childbearing. Recently in the U.S. 14 percent of all births were to girls in their teens (Miller et al., 1986). Each year 10 percent of all teenage girls become pregnant (two-thirds of these are unmarried), and at least a third terminate their pregnancies. Babies born to teenage mothers are more likely to be premature and underweight (Children's Defense Fund, 1988). Young mothers are at high risk of bearing infants with low birth weight, less because of their biological age (except for preteen mothers whose youth increases their risk) than because of other associated factors, such as smoking and alcohol consumption (Merritt, Laurence, and Naeye, 1980). They are also at risk for a greater number of physical, psychological, and social problems, including disrupted schooling, as a result of pregnancy (President's Commission, 1981). Those who choose to end their pregnancies with abortion encounter other physical and psychosocial complications, including emotionally wrenching ethical dilemmas. STDs, particularly gonorrhea and syphilis, pose another threat to adolescent health and are increasing in this age group despite improved treatment and reporting. Other STDs, notably genital herpes and nonspecific urethritis, have become major public health problems. Combined with gonorrhea and syphilis, they strike approximately 8 million to 12 million young people a year (Public Health Service, 1979). Serious complications can result from these diseases, including sterility in young women who have pelvic inflammatory disease. Acquired Immune Deficiency Syndrome (AIDS) has not been a problem in the past with this age group but poses a serious threat for the future.

Poor Nutrition and Obesity

Poor nutrition and obesity are common among adolescents, whose diets often consist of nonnourishing snacks (Figure 17-2) and unhealthy meals (Langford, 1981). Among adolescent girls, two problems of mounting incidence and gravity are anorexia nervosa and bulimia (Drewnowski et al., 1988). While creating nutritional problems in that they starve their victims, these diseases have emotional etiologies that pose a complex challenge to treatment.

HEALTH SERVICES FOR CHILDREN AND THE NURSE'S ROLE

What is being done to meet children's health needs? In response to the nation's inadequate services for children, the Select Panel for the Promotion of Children's Health, established in 1978, developed health goals for children and expectant mothers in the United States and designed a plan to achieve the goals (Hanlon and Pickett, 1984). The panel, in 1981, found that the current health care system had not kept up with children's changing health needs, with advanced technology, or with epidemiologic research. The panel emphasized a need for more disease and injury prevention through programs addressing environmental concerns. It recommended that health services focus on the relationship between health and behavior, and it urged improved nutrition. Members recommended a reconstitution of the former Children's Bureau into a new Maternal and Child Health Administration, to be housed in the Public Health Service, and the consolidation of maternal–child functions at the state level into a single agency. These recommendations are being carried out in many areas.

A variety of programs now exist that directly or indirectly serve the health needs of children. Community health nurses play a major and vital role in delivering these services. In community health, they fall into three categories approximating the three practice priorities of community health nursing practice: preventive health programs, health protection, and health promotion.

PREVENTIVE HEALTH PROGRAMS FOR CHILDREN

Quality *child care* provides a significant avenue for preventing illness and injury among young children. With 50 percent of all mothers of preschool children in the labor force (Children's Defense Fund, 1988), the demand for

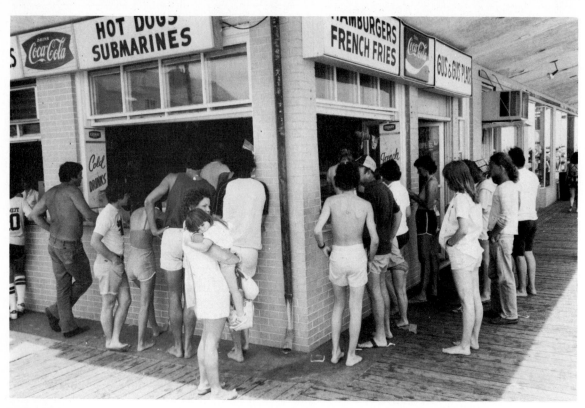

Figure 17-2
Fast foods are popular
with young people whose
frequently poor eating habits
can lead to health problems.

child care has increased by more than 100 percent since 1970 (Children's Defense Fund, 1988). Children in day care tend to contract a significantly higher number of illnesses (19 to 30 percent more) than children cared for at home (Johansen et al., 1988). Many of these disease occurrences can be prevented through improved policies and adherence to those policies regarding sick children (Landis and Earp, 1988). Further preventive measures are needed to ensure cleanliness, good nutrition, proper ventilation, lighting, exercise, and a safe, emotionally secure environment (Aronson and Gilsdorf, 1986; Smith, 1985; Wong, 1986). Many children suffer injuries and even death due to lack of safe child care; one important preventive measure is to ensure lower child-to-caregiver ratios (Children's Defense Fund, 1988). Community health nurses play a vital role in monitoring the quality of child care and educating parents, caregivers, and the public about appropriate preventive actions.

Health departments and private services continue to offer *immunization* against each of the seven major childhood infectious diseases — measles, mumps, polio, rubella, diphtheria, pertussis, and tetanus — which can cause permanent disability and sometimes even death. Although their threat has been substantially reduced, vigilance cannot be relaxed. Low immunization levels in many areas, particularly among the poor, and increased disease rates signal the need for constant surveillance, outreach programs, and educational efforts. Community health nurses are deeply involved in each of these preventive activities. Health departments and schools often work collaboratively to provide immunization services (Table 17-1). A compulsory immunization law, varying in its application from state to state, has enabled public health personnel to carry out these preventive services.

Parental support services, available through many public and private agencies including churches, have long-range effects on children's health. Emotionally healthy parents and stable families offer a healthful environment and support system for growing children. Community health nurses provide teaching and counseling services to parents in their homes and in groups. Discussing parenting concerns and increasing parents' understanding of normal child growth and development allay fears and prevent problems. Through such efforts, family violence and abuse can be averted.

Family planning programs, often stationed strategically near schools and in inner cities, provide birth control information and counseling to young people. Community health nurses, in collaboration with an interdisciplinary team, are usually the primary care providers in these programs. Their major goals are to prevent teenage pregnancy, educate teenagers about reproduction and contraception, and encourage responsible sexual behavior.

Providing *STD services* has been more difficult. Young people affected with one of these diseases are often afraid or embarrassed to seek help. Furthermore, community health professionals receive very little training in this area and may be uncomfortable and judgmental in their approach. Vulnerable groups, particularly minority youths, inner-city residents, and homosex-

Table 17-1
Childhood Immunization Schedule

Age*	Diphtheria Pertussis Tetanus	Polio	Measles	Rubella	Mumps	PRP-D
2 months	x	x				
4 months	x	x				
6 months	x	x(optional)				
15 months**			x	x	x	
18 months***	x	x				x
4-6 years	x	x				
14-16 years****	x					

*It is recommended that immunizations begin in early infancy, but they can be initiated later under direction of a physician.
**Measles, rubella and mumps vaccines may be combined in a single injection and given at about 15 months of age.
***18-month DPT may be given with MMR at 15 months. 18-month OPV may be given with MMR at 15 months.
****A sixth tetanus-diphtheria booster should be given at 14-16 years, then every 10 years.
PRP-D-Haemophilus b diphtheria toxoid conjugate vaccine.
Source: Report of the Committee on Infectious Diseases (1988). American Academy of Pediatrics. Elk Grove Village, Illinois.

uals, are being reached, however. Quality services and nonjudgmental attitudes attract young people who need help, and such help is being offered through STD clinics, family planning clinics, private physicians, schools, and employers. Community health nurses, stationed in most of these settings, are generally the professionals who deal most directly with these clients. Improved public awareness and education, screening of high-risk groups, appropriate antibiotic treatment of infected individuals, and identification and treatment of sexual contacts have served to reduce the threat of STDs.

Treatment and prevention of alcohol and drug abuse is another difficult task. Many social and economic influences promote chemical abuse and dependency, complicating the reversal of these effects (Newcomb et al., 1986). Recommended strategies and areas in which community health nurses working with aggregates can be more involved include the following (Public Health Service, 1979; Perry et al., 1985):

1. Prevention through early and ongoing education
2. Working to make the social climate less accepting of these behaviors
3. Reducing stress factors contributing to chemical abuse
4. Law enforcement

Educational efforts to discourage alcohol and drug use have often been ineffective, some even creating an incentive to experiment with them. Educational strategies that have been most successful have focused on the young person's individual responsibility for daily decisions affecting his or her health (Public Health Service, 1979). Thus, programs such as youth service clubs and community activities that encourage children and adolescents to make wise choices that affect their well-being and promote self-worth can serve as useful preventive measures.

HEALTH PROTECTION PROGRAMS FOR CHILDREN

Accidents and injury control programs serve a critical role in protecting the lives of children. Efforts to prevent motor vehicle accidents, a major killer, include driver education programs, better highway construction (reducing sharp curves and improving signs), improved motor vehicle design and safety features, and continuing research into the causes of various types of crashes. Injury prevention and reduction has been addressed through strategies such as use of safety restraints (particularly specially designed ones for infants and small children), air bags, substituting other modes of travel (air, rail, or bus), lower speed limits, stricter enforcement of and penalties associated with drunk driving laws, safer automobile design, and helmets for motorcyclists.

Falls, the major killer of preschool children and the cause of deaths and injuries for millions of other children each year, occur mostly in the home.

Here the community health nurse plays a major role in observing potential hazards, teaching safety measures, and reinforcing positive practices. Preventive and protective measures may be achieved through simple and inexpensive changes in the home. They include guards on windows and across stairways, safer walking surfaces, elimination of sharp objects or modification of surfaces that a child might fall against, securing of electrical outlets and toxic chemicals, and closer supervision of young children.

Child deaths and injuries from burns result primarily from house fires, but also from electrical burns and scalds. Many local fire departments and public health programs offer safety education in this area, emphasizing the use of heat- and smoke-detecting systems, fire drills, and home evacuation plans; less flammable structural materials, furnishings, and clothing; and careful smoking. Scalds occur in kitchens and bathrooms most often. Adults can protect children by keeping pot handles turned toward the center of the stove and by modifying water temperatures in water heaters.

Safety programs also seek to protect children from the hazards of poisonings, ingestion of prescription and over-the-counter drugs, product-related accidents (unsafe toys, bicycles, skateboards, playground equipment, and furniture), and recreational accidents, including drownings and sport injuries. Safety services assume various forms. Poison control centers in many localities offer information and emergency assistance. Toxic household substances, such as cleaning supplies, must be clearly labeled, and harmful drugs packaged with special seals and safety caps. Product safety is monitored by the Federal Consumer Product Safety Commission. Greater efforts are being made to reduce recreational injuries through improved boating and swimming regulations, water safety measures, team sports safety measures, and better protective equipment and playing fields for sports participants, including football helmets that don't injure other players and obstacle-free zones around playing fields. Generally, the community health nurse can educate families to recognize potentially hazardous situations and encourage efforts to eliminate them (Richardson, 1988).

Programs to reduce environmental hazards begin at the federal level, where the government sets and enforces pollution standards and deals with environmental contamination that poses health risks. At the state and municipal government levels, measures include monitoring air and drinking water safety, providing proper sewage disposal, controlling ionizing radiation, enforcing auto safety and emission standards, and regulating agricultural chemicals and pesticides. Locally, protective measures include educational programs warning against toxic agents in the environment, community surveillance, and enforcement of environmental health standards. At all levels, epidemiologic research probes the causes and seeks answers to provide better protection for the public. Community health nurses need to be alert to environmental hazards and work collaboratively with other members of the public health team to report problems and educate clients. Improved environmental con-

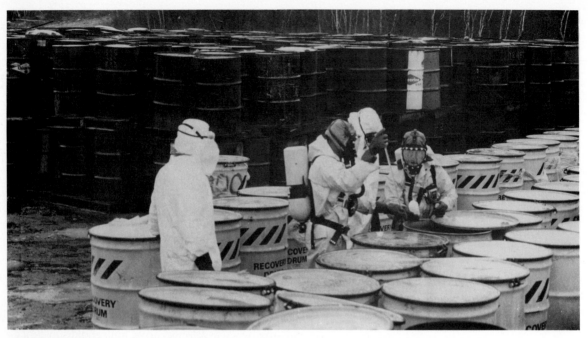

Figure 17-3
Workers wear protective gear during cleanup of illegally dumped chemicals.
Toxic materials in the environment pose serious threats to children's health,
both immediately and in the future.

trol protects today's children against disease and disability and tomorrow's children against birth defects and the long-range hazards of environmental contamination (Figure 17-3).

We have learned in community health that infectious diseases can be controlled and in some cases eliminated. Witness the successful worldwide eradication of smallpox, the dramatic decline in paralytic polio, and the decreasing incidence of the other communicable diseases of childhood. *Control of infectious diseases* comes largely through a two-part effort. One part is wide-scale, persistent immunization programs, discussed earlier. The second part is rigorous monitoring and surveillance of communicable disease incidence. Such surveillance is done continuously in the United States through the efforts of the federal Centers for Disease Control in collaboration with state and local health departments. Surveillance involves four basic activities (Public Health Service, 1979):

1. *Case finding* of disease or exposure to disease, done by community health professionals
2. *Case reporting* to public health officials, by health care providers, schools, and industries

3. *Analysis and interpretation* of communicable disease data to determine implications
4. *Appropriate response* with control measures

Community health nurses do case finding and reporting and assist other health team members in carrying out control measures.

Programs protecting children against infectious diseases encompass efforts such as closing swimming pools with unsafe bacteria counts, conducting immunization campaigns in conjunction with influenza outbreaks, and working with hospital pediatric units to reduce the incidence and threat of iatrogenic disease.

Services to protect children from abuse are much less developed or effective. A variety of factors account for this. Most child abuse occurs in the home; thus, only the most blatant situations become evident to outsiders (Figure 17-4). Community health nurses and physicians who see injured children may find parents' explanations plausible and not suspect or want to believe that foul play might be responsible. Avoidance of legal involvement keeps others from reporting suspected cases. A model law passed in 1963 (Children's Bureau, 1963) required mandatory reporting of suspicious cases of child abuse. In 1966, the American Academy of Pediatrics developed recommendations for an improved reporting, record-keeping, and intervention system that would provide legal immunity to the reporting professional ("Maltreatment of Children," 1966). Currently, all the states have developed adaptations of the model law, professionals and the public are more aware of the problem, and there is an increase in reporting. Nonetheless, it is estimated that only 1 percent of battered-child cases are actually reported (Hanlon and Pickett, 1984). In 1974, the National Center for Child Abuse and Neglect was established as a result of the Child Abuse Prevention and Treatment Act. The center collects and analyzes information on child abuse and neglect, serves as an information clearinghouse, publishes educational materials on the subject, offers technical assistance, and conducts research into the problem. The Surgeon General's report on health promotion and disease prevention suggests a multifaceted approach to dealing with child abuse and neglect. It recommends "parent education, enhancement of community and social support systems, assistance to abusing parents through collaborative efforts of public and private sector, and projects designed to create an integrated health and social service delivery system" (Public Health Service, 1979, p. 38). Education of health care providers as well as parents has been recommended (Johnston, 1988). The effectiveness of local programs depends, in large measure, on the willingness of community health professionals to increase their awareness and work as a team to detect, report, and develop interventions for abusers and abused children (Hanlon and Pickett, 1984). The community health nurse is in a unique position to detect early signs of neglect and abuse, establish rapport with abusing parents, family members, or others, and assist with appropriate interventions and referrals.

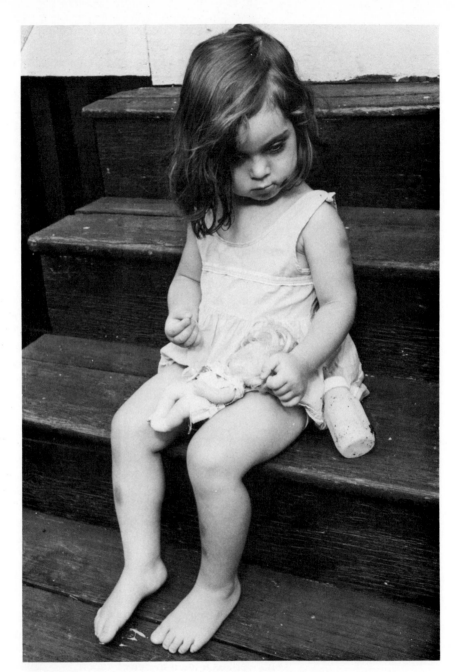

Figure 17-4
The abused child's experiences will strongly influence her future perceptions of the parenting role.

Fluoridation of community water supplies is the most effective, safe, and low-cost means of *protecting children's dental health*. Fluoride makes teeth less susceptible to decay by increasing resistance to the bacteria-produced acid in the mouth. As of 1980, 60 percent of all children in the United States had access to fluoridated water (Hanlon and Pickett, 1984). Fluoride rinses, dietary supplements, and direct applications are other methods used to protect children's teeth, but they have met with less success. Public acceptance of community water fluoridation has been slow, despite 35 years of research demonstrating its unquestioned safety and effectiveness. In addition to regular dental care (Kronmiller and Nirsch, 1985), good nutrition, and proper oral hygiene, community health nurses can safely promote public water fluoridation as an important program for protecting children's dental health.

HEALTH PROMOTION PROGRAMS FOR CHILDREN

Early childhood development programs serve an increasingly important function for the escalating number of children enrolled in day-care centers and preschools. At least half of all children today have mothers who work, and that figure is rising (Children's Defense Fund, 1988). Economic pressures eat into family time together and often diminish the quality of children's physical and psychosocial nourishment. Childhood development programs, such as Head Start, provide physical, emotional, intellectual, and social stimulation during a critical period of children's growth when impressions are being made and patterns formed that will influence what kind of adults these children will be in the future. Comprehensive preschool programs promote good physical health, proper nutrition, a positive self-concept, and cognitive and social skill development. Many such programs exist, but more are needed (Richardson, 1988). The quality of day care and preschool programs varies considerably. Licensing laws can regulate only minimum safety and health standards. In addition, numerous child care operations are too small to require licensing, leaving their quality open to individual discretion. Community health nurses can influence the quality of day care and preschool programs through active educational efforts and through monitoring of health and safety standards.

Nutrition and weight control programs form another important set of health promotion services. Children need to learn sound dietary habits early in life to establish healthy lifelong patterns (Perry et al., 1988). Some preschool and school programs teach, as well as provide, good nutrition and encourage the kinds of eating patterns that prevent obesity. For overweight children and adolescents, there are a number of weight control programs available through schools, health departments, community health centers, health maintenance organizations, and private groups. Adolescents are particularly vulnerable to media and peer pressures for nonnutritive snacks, including diet sodas, based on a desire to be accepted and to look trim. Fad diets can also be harmful if they are not balanced nutritionally. Programs aimed at nutritionally sounder advertising are having a positive effect. Parents and children are becoming more aware of the need to cut down their consumption of saturated fat, salt, sugar, and overprocessed foods in order to feel better and look better. The nurse, through nutrition education and reinforcement of positive practices (Pipes, 1984), plays a significant role in promoting the health of children.

The value of *exercise and physical fitness programs* for young people has been recognized for some time. Organized groups, such as the YMCA, YWCA, Boy and Girl Scouts, and Campfire Girls, have offered sports and character development programs for many years. Good preschool programs provide equipment and opportunities for large-muscle activity as well as fine motor development. Schools, parks, and recreation centers encourage exercise through use of playground equipment and organized sports activities. Despite these opportunities, many young people do not exercise often enough or vigorously enough. Members of minority groups, females, and inner-city residents exercise less than do white, suburban males (Public Health Service, 1979). Even team sports keep players inactive much of the time and are not activities that young people continue in their adult lives. More comprehensive physical education programs that encourage vigorous exercise and self-discipline as lifetime habits would better serve the health needs of this population group. Community health nurses can promote such programs through the schools as well as encourage these activities in their contacts with students of all ages (Figure 17-5).

The demonstrated hazards of cigarette smoking, alcohol, and drug abuse have prompted the development of *substance abuse programs* particularly targeting children and adolescents. Health education efforts involving school nurses have been a major source of influence encouraging students to make responsible decisions about smoking, drinking, and other behaviors affecting their health (Keenan, 1986). Health departments, community health nursing agencies, and private groups such as the American Cancer Society and the National Lung Association also provide educational materials and promote antismoking and drug use prevention campaigns. The more successful programs emphasize how the human body works and how behavior affects it. They also help young people resist social pressures to smoke and take drugs by pointing out that those who do are in the minority and by showing the deleterious effects of these practices. Using students themselves as health educators is a positive use of peer pressure and has proved to be a successful means of influencing attitudes (Public Health Service, 1979). Other groups, such as 4-H clubs, churches, the Catholic Youth Organization, and Scouts, use peer counseling to influence young people to assume responsibility for healthy lifestyles. The community health nurse participates in and supports existing programs in addition to counseling and referring young people who need help.

Stress control programs for children and adolescents do not exist in any great numbers, yet they are needed. Many of the health problems discussed

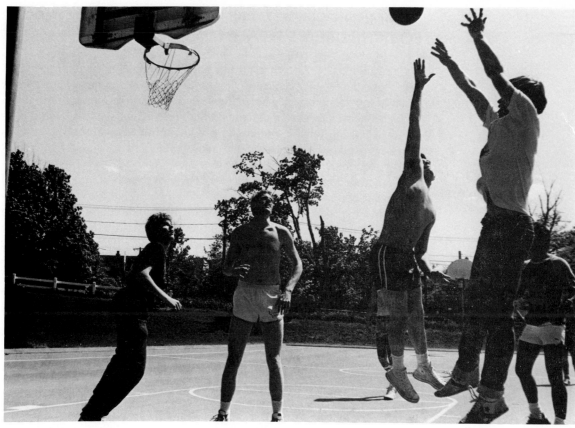

Figure 17-5
Vigorous exercise that promotes fitness and self-discipline is an important
contributor to young people's health. Team sports further enhance the
development of social skills and healthy relationships.

in this chapter relate to the emotional health of young people. Reckless driving, suicide, homicide, unwanted pregnancy, smoking, alcoholism, drug misuse, obesity, anorexia nervosa, and bulimia, as well as other problems — all signal the presence of some kind of stress and coping skills inadequate to handle it. Crisis intervention programs and services that treat a problem after it occurs are helpful and can prevent problems from worsening. More needed, however, for this population group are programs that build coping skills early, including self-help and mutual support activities. Programs offered in a group context, such as those mentioned earlier — 4-H, Scouts, various character-building clubs, and organizations like Outward Bound — have proven most effective. For the nurse, recognition of young people at risk (Child et al., 1980; Killen et al., 1987), counseling, and early referral to sources of help can prevent problems from arising. Reduction of stresses in the family and community environments can further enhance this group's health.

COMMUNITY HEALTH NURSING INTERVENTIONS FOR CHILDREN'S HEALTH

The previous description of programs addressing children's health problems also points out areas of deficiency in services. Community health nurses face the challenge of continually assessing each population group's current health problems as well as determining available and needed services. Some gaps can be filled by nursing interventions. Others must be referred to various members of the community health team with whom the nurse may sometimes collaboratively develop services.

Community health nursing interventions with preschool, school-age, and adolescent populations are those outlined in the basic conceptual model discussed in Chapter 3: education, engineering, and enforcement. We have seen examples of each mentioned in the previous discussion. For instance, the nurse uses educational interventions when teaching proper nutrition, family planning, physical and psychological effects of drug abuse, safety precautions, or weight control. Each of these involves providing information and encouraging client groups to act on that information in a manner that is health-enhancing. Engineering interventions, those strategies in which the nurse uses a greater degree of persuasion or positive manipulation, are evident in conducting voluntary immunization programs, encouraging use of contraceptives, counseling for stress reduction, identifying and treating STD sexual contacts, or encouraging use of safety devices, such as stairway guards. The nurse uses enforcement interventions, those activities employing some form of coercion, when requiring immunizations that are mandated by law, or when reporting illegal drug use, child abuse, or environmental health standards violations, such as rat infestation of a home.

SCHOOL HEALTH

In community health practice, nursing service to a school-age population requires a special mind-set. Nurses must shift from a focus entirely on individual schoolchildren or small groups of children to one that includes aggregates. In order to show how this shift can be made, let us consider what your role as school nurse would involve.

Imagine that you, a community health nurse, recently became school nurse for Keeler Elementary School. You have been working with families and groups in the community for several years, but you have not done school nursing before. Since it is summer and school has not yet started, you take time to get acquainted with the school and the nurse's role.

Mrs. Murray, the principal, is happy to talk with you. She comments that she expects the nurse to keep the children as healthy as possible and be the major consultant on health matters in the school. Because she is very busy with administrative concerns, she prefers that you carve out your own role, although she wants to be kept informed of your plans. She describes the school to you. Built 40 years ago, Keeler has 353 students in grades kindergarten through sixth. With 14 teachers, its pupil-teacher ratio is 25:1. The teachers give some health instruction to their classes. Mr. Jones, a fourth-grade teacher, was a medical corpsman in the army and handles first-aid problems for the school when the nurse is not there. Two PTA mother-volunteers keep the student health records in order. You can ask for more help if you need it. Mrs. Murray gives you material to read that describes school health services generally.

Nursing Services

You learn that school health services incorporate three functions: health services, health education, and improvement of the school environment (Schaller, 1981). Health services include programs such as vision and hearing screening, psychological testing, health examinations, emergency care, and referrals. There are special corrective and training services for speech, hearing, or mental health problems. Student and family counseling are important components; there is a program of communicable disease control. School health services also include health appraisal and services for school personnel.

The health education function of school health services involves planned and incidental teaching of health concepts; classes in health science and healthful living; and use of educational media, library resources, and community facilities. These activities aim to integrate health information with students' daily living experiences, to build positive attitudes toward health, and to establish sound health practices.

The third function of school health services is the promotion of healthful school living. Emphasis on a healthful physical environment includes proper selection, design, organization, operation, and maintenance of the physical plant. Consideration should be shown for areas such as adaptability to student needs; safety; visual, thermal, and acoustic factors; aesthetic values; sanitation; and safety of the school bus system. Healthful school living also emphasizes planning a daily schedule that monitors healthful classroom experiences, extra class activities, school lunches, emotional climate, program of discipline, and teaching methods. It also seeks to promote the physical, mental, and emotional health of school personnel.

The School Health Team

You are impressed with all that can be done in school health and explore the subject further through reading and interviewing school personnel. It quickly becomes apparent that school health, like all health programs in the community, requires a team effort (Butcher et al., 1988). Although the school nurse plays a central role, she collaborates with many other individuals. The school principal influences all phases of the school health program. Mrs. Murray, for example, can promote good school health through actively supporting all the school's health services, setting policies, and tapping community resources. She can reinforce positive efforts, ranging from health teaching to good housekeeping by the custodian, within the school. Because of the principal's influential position, it is absolutely essential that the nurse maintain a positive working relationship with her.

Teachers, whether they are involved in regular instruction, physical education, or special education classes, play a major role in school health. Because they spend so much time with students, their observations, health teaching, and personal health habits have a profound effect on student health and the quality of school health services. Nurse and teachers must collaborate constantly.

Other health team members, such as health educators, health coordinators, psychologists, audiologists, counselors, dentists, dental hygienists, social workers, or health aides, may be present depending on the size and financial resources of the school. All team members, including students, parents, and the custodian, have a specialized role complementary to that of the school nurse. Consultation and referral between team members are crucial to implementing the school health program (Figure 17-6).

The school physician may work full-time, part-time, or be available on a consultation basis. This role focuses largely on advising and consulting in policy and medical-legal matters. The physician often serves as liaison with the community and other health agencies and consults with those who plan and develop school health programs. The physician may also become involved in some student health appraisal and health problem intervention (Schaller, 1981). A good working relationship between the school nurse and school physician is important. The nurse's role, while complementary to and different from the physician's, nonetheless may need clarifying and interpreting to maximize the effectiveness of their collaboration.

Figure 17-6
A school nurse, third from right, meets with a developmental specialist, a psychologist, a speech therapist, two teachers, and a social worker. Their combined knowledge and efforts are essential for promoting a comprehensive school health program.

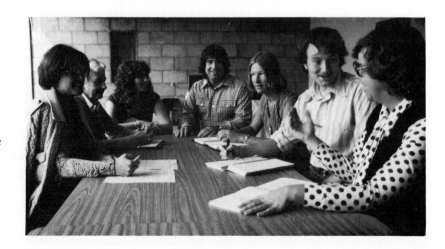

You want to learn more about the school nurse's role. You consult with your nursing supervisor, who explains the difference between specialized school nursing and the generalized school nursing that you will be expected to practice.

SPECIALIZED AND GENERALIZED NURSING ROLES

School nurses operate from one of two administrative bases. In many localities, school nurses are hired through the public school system and maintain a specialized, school-based service. There is growing conviction that such nurses should work under the jurisdiction of the board of health rather than the board of education. With professional instead of educational supervision, better utilization of the nurse and improved quality of health care service would be ensured (American Nurses Association, 1983). An advantage of the specialized school nurse's role is that the nurse can concentrate all her time and effort on the school health program and thus develop specialized skills in school health assessment and intervention. A disadvantage is that school nurses' practice is often limited to the school setting. A specialized role may prevent the school nurse from assessing preschoolers, providing health service to families of schoolchildren, or making broader community assessments and contacts.

School nurse practitioners, nurses with advanced preparation and experience in child care and school health, assume an even more specialized and expanded role — that of identifying and managing many of the health problems of schoolchildren. They have made a significant contribution to the provision of primary health care to schoolchildren (Figure 17-7). They have an important but different function from that of school nurses who are community health nurses.

Generalized school nurses work within the framework of generalized community health nursing, serving private and sometimes public schools as part of their caseloads. The advantage of a generalized school nurse role is the broader community base from which the nurse can operate. This base allows contact with preschoolers and families, strengthened knowledge of the community and its resources, and integration of in-school and out-of-school care (Freeman and Heinrich, 1981). Humes (1975, p. 396) also argues, "A public health nurse working in the schools tends to have more of a working knowledge of the general health needs of the community. With this kind of background information she is better able to view student health problems in a community context." A disadvantage of the generalized role, however, is that the nurse often has less time to meet school health needs.

Whether specialized or generalized, the primary functions of the school nurse are to prevent illness and to promote and maintain the health of the school community. A philosophy of school nursing, adopted in Minnesota, is suggested by your supervisor as a basis for your school nursing practice (Minnesota Nurses Association, 1974, p. 3):

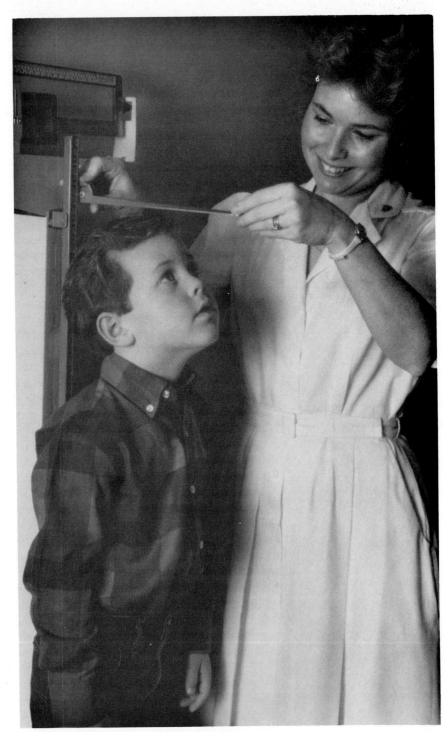

Figure 17-7
Monitoring schoolchildren's growth and development alerts the school nurse to any early signs of potential health problems. This young boy discovers that he is within normal height for his age.

> All children and their families have a right to education which guides them toward self-awareness and self-realization in meeting the needs of complex living. The focus of public health school nursing is the self-motivation of individuals and families to seek and maintain optimum health. The partnership of public health school nursing and education is essential for increasing high level wellness of students, their families, school personnel, and the community.

The community health nurse not only serves individuals, families, and groups within the context of school health, but also the school as an organization and its membership (students and staff) as population groups.

School has started, and the three days a week you spend at Keeler never seem to be enough time to finish all there is to do. You have already looked through student records to determine children with health problems and followed up on your findings. You sent five children home with notes recommending dental work; sent little Norma, a new kindergartner, to the audiologist after testing her hearing; and referred Jimmy Hansen for psychological testing. You found out that Tommy Sandberg had a convulsive disorder but did not take his medication regularly. You visited his family, explained the need for consistent treatment and medical supervision, had him start on a regular treatment program, and gave him his medication during school hours. Many individual children in your school show signs of improved health as a result of your efforts. Several families of children in the school are now part of your regular caseload. The group you started with sixth-graders on how to become good baby-sitters is going well. Yet there are so many children you have not assessed. Moreover, what about the teachers' needs? You know that you are not really providing service to the whole school community. You realize that you must shift your focus.

NURSING GOALS

Previously your primary goal as a school nurse had been to assess and promote the health of the preschool and school-age child. Changing your focus means you now adopt a broader set of goals for school nursing that involve the school organization and population levels. You want to include the individual, family, and group levels. Basing your goals on those outlined by the Minnesota Nurses Association (1974), you aim to do the following:

1. Assess the health and developmental status of the preschool and school-age child
2. Promote and maintain optimal health of students, families, and school personnel
3. Implement an appropriate plan for the education and care of each exceptional and each handicapped child

At these levels, you concentrate on selected individuals, selected families, or special groups needing nursing or other professional intervention. For example, you may seek to identify children with speech and language delays (Goldberg, 1984). Many of these clients will be referred to other community resources for assistance. You plan to get to know personally each member of the school family and staff, including the secretary and the custodian, in order to cultivate their good will, sharpen their observation skills regarding the students, and assess their own health needs. A faculty or staff member who is not well physically or emotionally may significantly influence the health of the school community.

Organizational Level

At the organizational level, you aim to fulfill the following responsibilities (Minnesota Nurses Association, 1974):

1. Establish and revise school and district health policies, administration, and philosophy pertaining to school health services.
2. Develop and maintain a system of emergency care.
3. Provide for school safety and a healthful school environment.
4. Facilitate comprehensive community health care planning and resources development to include the health needs of the preschool and school-age populations and their families.

This level requires more attention than you have given to it in the past. True, you have worked out a system with Mr. Jones to handle basic first aid for injuries and have updated physician orders to cover emergencies. Now you make certain everyone understands what to do and where to go in the event of an emergency such as a tornado. Some school safety issues have been addressed, but now you need to examine the overall safety of the building and check with administration about safety of the school buses. You look into the effectiveness of fire drills and alternate routes for emptying the building. You oversee the handling of dangerous materials in the science laboratories.

The school environment needs more careful assessment. You start checking the nutritional value of the school lunches and the ventilation of classrooms. You begin to analyze seating arrangements in each classroom while observing students, and you consult with teachers about your observations. The dingy halls of the old building soon take on a more cheerful appearance through the work of your volunteer paint crew from the PTA.

As an organization, Keeler Elementary School is functioning fairly well, you decide. The pupil-teacher ratio is slightly high by some standards, but a class of 25 students is generally considered a manageable load. To provide students with more individual attention, you suggest adding more teacher aides. Faculty on the whole get along well with each other and with Mrs. Murray. There is open communication and positive feedback. Working conditions are pleasant, and faculty requests are answered in a reasonable amount of time. There is also adequate space, equipment, personnel assistance, and support for your school health program.

To influence school health policy and resource planning, you volunteer to serve on a district committee that meets once a month. Meeting other professionals concerned about school health broadens your understanding of school and community needs and also gives you ideas on intervention strategies and ways to tap community resources.

Population Group Level

At the population group level, you aim to achieve the following goals (Minnesota Nurses Association, 1974):

1. Assess the collective needs of preschool and school-age children and school personnel.
2. Identify existing and potential health problems in the school population (and in the larger community affecting it), determine those at greatest risk, develop a plan, and intervene to minimize or prevent problems.
3. Promote and maintain optimal health of the student body and the school personnel population.
4. Prevent and control communicable disease in the student population (in order to protect the well-being of students and the community).
5. Evaluate and upgrade the contribution of the school nurse role toward promoting the health of the school community.

During a conference with your community health nursing supervisor, you review the new goals and make plans for conducting a broader assessment of the school population's health. Journal articles and discussion with other school nurses give you additional ideas. For example, one school nurse, instead of performing a routine physical examination on every child, developed a systematic method of classroom assessment. She evaluated an entire class of 25 to 30 children at one time through regular observation of their behavior and developmental status and through close consultation with teachers that alerted them about special student behaviors to observe (Withrow, 1979). You decide to try this method in combination with further data gathering on selected children through screening, interviews, and family visits. The yearly vision and hearing screening, which you are required to give students, offers another opportunity to observe them closely for signs of child abuse, malnutrition, or other physical or emotional problems that might be prevalent among this population group.

You assess preschool-age children who will be starting kindergarten next year by holding a Saturday afternoon preschool fair. Invitations are sent out to all the families in the community with four-year-old children. PTA volunteers help you organize games and refreshments and conduct school tours. Registered nurse volunteers from the community assist you in cursory physical exams that include vision and hearing screening. You notify parents immediately if children need follow-up care.

While conducting this preschool assessment, you keep in mind that you want a profile of this population of four-year-olds, not just each individual child's health picture. You look for recurring problems that are common to the group, such as skin rashes, orthopedic defects, headaches, eating or respiratory difficulties, and signs of communicable diseases. Such population screening has sometimes uncovered widespread community health problems. For instance, recognition of common symptoms among people residing near Love Canal in New York led to a discovery that the canal was contaminated with poisonous industrial wastes. In 1980, a community in Memphis, Tennessee, whose incidence of miscarriages, cancer, and infant deaths had markedly increased, discovered that nearby chemicals buried many years previously were the cause. Identifying common problems among the preschool or school-age populations, including problems specific to each age group such as adolescents (Keenan, 1986), enables you to take corrective action on a broader scale and thus to help many children at once as well as to take preventive action.

You begin to collect data on the needs of the school personnel population by observing and talking informally with faculty and staff. You discover that some of the teachers seem on the verge of burning out. They do not enjoy their teaching, feel tired most of the time, take piles of work home with them every night, do not sleep well, and often feel irritable toward the children. With school administration's approval, you plan a workshop to prevent teacher burnout. Expert consultants help the teachers learn to recognize symptoms and avoid burnout. During the workshop the teachers develop specific plans to help them cope with their present situations and design strategies for alleviating future stress.

The three sets of goals for school nursing have helped you refocus your thinking and expand your service to include not only individual, family, and group levels of nursing intervention but school organization and school population group levels as well.

Summary

Children are an important population group. Community health nurses need to understand children's health problems and how they can be addressed.

Mortality rates for children have decreased dramatically since the early 1900s. Causes of death have also changed. Infectious diseases used to be the leading threat to the lives of children; now accidents are the leading cause of death for children over one year of age. Morbidity rates among children, in contrast to their mortality rates, remain high. Children are still vulnerable to many illnesses, injuries, and emotional problems.

For preschoolers, the major threat to life and health is accidents (falls, drownings, burns, and poisonings). Other health concerns include acute illnesses, particularly respiratory illness, and nutritional, dental, and emotional needs. Motor vehicle accidents are the leading cause of death for school-age children. Further health problems for this group include respiratory illnesses, injuries, infectious diseases, digestive conditions, emotional and behavioral problems, handicaps, and nutritional problems. Mortality rates for adolescents are twice as high as those for younger children. Violent deaths and injuries are the leading threats to life and health in this population group. Accidents (motor vehicle and other), homicides, and suicides are the three major causes of death. Other health problems include alcohol and drug abuse, unwanted pregnancies, STDs, and poor nutrition.

Health services for children span three categories: preventive, health protecting, and health promoting. The community health nurse plays a vital role in each. Preventive services include quality child care, immunization programs, parental support services, family planning programs, services for those with STDs, and alcohol and drug abuse prevention programs. Health protection services include accident and injury control, programs to reduce environmental hazards, control of infectious diseases, services to protect children from child abuse, and fluoridation of community water supplies to protect children's dental health. Health promotion services include programs in early childhood development; nutrition and weight control; exercise and physical fitness; smoking, alcohol, and drug abuse education; and stress control.

Community health nurses use three basic interventions while serving children's health needs. With educational interventions, such as nutrition teaching, nurses provide information and encourage clients to act responsibly on behalf of their own health. With engineering interventions, such as encouraging use of contraceptives, nurses employ persuasive tactics to move clients toward more positive health behaviors. With enforcement interventions, such as reporting and intervening in child abuse, nurses practice some form of coercion to protect children from threats to their health.

Nursing of the school-age population involves providing health services and health education and ensuring a healthful school environment. School nurses may be generalized or specialized, but overall they seek to improve the health of schoolchildren as an aggregate.

Study Questions

1. What is the major cause of death among school-age children? What community-wide interventions could be initiated to prevent these deaths? Select one intervention and describe how you and a group of community health professionals might develop this preventive measure.
2. Describe one health promotion program you, as a community health nurse, could initiate and carry out to improve the health of children in a day-care center.
3. How can environmental health protection programs affect the future health of infants? Why is control of environmental hazards important for

A Prayer/Pledge of Responsibility for Children*

We pray [accept responsibility] for children
    who put chocolate fingers everywhere,
    who like to be tickled,
    who stomp in puddles and ruin their new pants,
    who sneak popsicles before supper,
    who erase holes in math workbooks,
    who can never find their shoes.
And we pray [accept responsibility] for those
    who stare at photographers from behind barbed wire,
    who can't bound down the street in a new pair of sneakers,
    who never "counted potatoes,"
    who are born in places we wouldn't be caught dead,
    who never go to the circus,
    who live in an X-rated world.
We pray [accept responsibility] for children
    who bring us sticky kisses and fistfuls of dandelions,
    who sleep with the dog and bury goldfish,
    who hug us in a hurry and forget their lunch money,
    who cover themselves with Band-aids and sing off key,
    who squeeze toothpaste all over the sink,
    who slurp their soup.
And we pray [accept responsibility] for those
    who never get dessert,
    who have no safe blanket to drag behind them,
    who watch their parents watch them die,
    who can't find any bread to steal,
    who don't have any rooms to clean up,
    whose pictures aren't on anybody's dresser,
    whose monsters are real.
We pray [accept responsibility] for children
    who spend all their allowance before Tuesday,
    who throw tantrums in the grocery store and pick at their food,
    who like ghost stories,
    who shove dirty clothes under the bed, and never rinse out the tub,
    who get visits from the tooth fairy,
    who don't like to be kissed in front of the carpool,
    who squirm in church or temple and scream in the phone,
    whose tears we sometimes laugh at and whose smiles can make us cry.
And we pray [accept responsibility] for those
    whose nightmares come in the daytime,
    who will eat anything,
    who have never seen a dentist,
    who aren't spoiled by anybody,
    who go to bed hungry and cry themselves to sleep,
    who live and move, but have no being.
We pray [accept responsibility] for children who want to be carried and
    for those who must,
    for those we never give up on and for those
    who don't get a second chance.
For those we smother... and for those who will grab the hand of anybody kind
enough to offer it.

                                       —Ina J. Hughs

*"Accept responsibility" is CDF's addition.

children of any age? List three things a nurse can do to protect children from environmental hazards.

4. A 14-year-old girl from a middle-class family and a 14-year-old girl from a poor family both come to the family planning clinic where you work. The girls have similar symptoms that possibly indicate gonorrhea. Would your assessment and interventions be the same or different for the two girls? What are your values and attitudes toward people with diseases that are sexually transmitted? Does social class, race, age, or sex make any difference in how you feel about them? What is one action the community health nurse can take to prevent such diseases in this population group?

References

American Academy of Pediatrics. (1988). *Report of the Committee on Infectious Diseases.* Elk Grove Village, Ill.: Author.

American Nurses Association. (1983). *Standards of school nursing practice.* Kansas City, Mo.: Author.

Aronson, S., and J. R. Gilsdorf. (1986). Preventive management of infectious diseases in day-care. *Pediatrics in Review* 7: 259–62.

Avery, J. (1980). The safety of children in cars. *Practitioner* 224: 816–21.

Butcher, A. H., et al. (1988). Heart smart: A school health program meeting the 1990 Objectives for the Nation. *Health Education Quarterly* 15(1): 17–34.

Child, A., C. M. Murphy, and M. C. Rhyne. (1980). Depression in children: Reasons and risks. *Pediatric Nursing* 6: 9–15.

Child homicide—United States. (1982). *Morbidity and Mortality Weekly Report* 31: 292–94.

Children's Bureau. U.S. Department of Health, Education and Welfare. (1963). The abused child—Principles and suggested language for legislation on reporting of the abused child. Washington, D.C.: U.S. Government Printing Office.

Children's Defense Fund. (1988). *What every American should be asking political leaders in 1988.* Washington, D.C.: Author.

Comstock, G. (1981). Influence of mass media on child health and behavior. *Health Education Quarterly* 8(1): 32.

Drewnowski, A., S. Hopkins, and R. Kessler. (1988). The prevalence of bulimia nervosa in the U.S. college student population. *American Journal of Public Health* 78(10): 1322–25.

Freeman, R., and J. Heinrich. (1981). *Community health nursing practice.* 2nd ed. Philadelphia: W. B. Saunders.

Goldberg, R. (1984). Identifying speech and language delays in children. *Pediatric Nursing* 10: 252–59.

Hanlon, J. J., and G. E. Pickett. (1984). *Public health: administration and practice.* 8th ed. St. Louis: Times Mirror/Mosby.

Humes, C. W., Jr. (1975). Who should administer school nursing services? *American Journal of Public Health* 65: 394.

Johansen, A., A. Leibowitz, and L. Waite. (1988). Child care and children's illness. *American Journal of Public Health* 78(9): 1175–77.

Johnston, C. (1988). Last chance for change?...Education and training relating to child abuse. *Nursing Times* 84(7): 30–31.

Jonides, L. (1982). Childhood obesity: A treatment approach for private practice. *Pediatric Nursing* 8: 320–22.

Keenan, R. (1986). School-based adolescent health care programs. *Pediatric Nursing* 12: 365–69.

Killen, J., et al. (1987). Depressive symptoms and substance use among adolescent binge eaters and purgers: A defined population study. *American Journal of Public Health* 77(12): 1539–41.

Kronmiller, J. E., and R. F. Nirsch. (1985). Preventive dentistry for children. *Pediatric Nursing* 11: 446–49.

Landis, S. E., and J. L. Earp. (1988). Day care center illness: Policy and practice in North Carolina. *American Journal of Public Health* 78(3): 311–13.

Langford, R. (1981). Teenagers and obesity. *American Journal of Nursing* 81: 556–59.

Maltreatment of children: Recommendations of Committee on the Infant and Pre-school Child of the American Academy of Pediatrics. (1966). *Pediatrics* 37: 377.

Merritt, T., R. Laurence, and R. Naeye. (1980). The infants of adolescent mothers. *Pediatric Annals* 9(3): 32.

Miller, C. A., A. Fine, S. Adams-Taylor, and L. Schorr. (1986). *Monitoring children's health: Key indicators.* Washington, D.C.: American Public Health Association.

Minnesota Nurses Association, Special Committee, School Nurse Branch. (1974). *Goals of school nursing: An interpretive tool.* St. Paul, Minn.: Minnesota Nurses Association.

National Center for Health Statistics. (1988). *Vital statistics of the United States, 1986, Volumes I and II, Mortality, Parts A and B.* Washington, D.C.: U.S. Government Printing Office.

Newacheck, P., P. Budetti, and P. McManus. (1984). Trends in childhood disability. *American Journal of Public Health* 74: 232–36.

Newcomb, M., E. Maddahian, and P. Bentler. (1986). Risk factors for drug use among adolescents: Concurrent and longitudinal analyses. *American Journal of Public Health* 76(5): 525–31.

Perry, C. L., et al. (1985). The concept of health promotion and the prevention of adolescent drug abuse. *Health Education Quarterly* 12(2): 169–84.

Perry, C. L., et al. (1988). Parent involvement with children's health promotion: The Minnesota Home Team. *American Journal of Public Health* 78(9): 1156–60.

Pipes, P. L. (1984). *Nutrition in infancy and childhood.* 3rd ed. St. Louis: C. V. Mosby.

President's Commission for a National Agenda for the Eighties. (1981). Helping families — to help themselves. *International Journal of Family Therapy* 3(3): 208–33.

Public Health Service. (1979). *Healthy people: The Surgeon General's report on health promotion and disease prevention* (DHEW Publication No. 79-55071). Washington, D.C.: U.S. Government Printing Office.

Richardson, S. F. (1988). Child health promotion practices. *Journal of Pediatric Health Care* 2(2): 73–78.

Schaller, W. (1981). *The school health program.* 5th ed. Philadelphia: W. B. Saunders.

Schetky, D., and A. Green. (1988). *Child sexual abuse.* New York: Brunner/Mazel.

Sigman, M. (1985). *Children with emotional disorders and developmental disabilities.* Orlando, Fla.: Grune and Stratton.

Smith, D. P. (1985). Common day care diseases: Patterns and prevention. *Pediatric Nursing* 12: 175–78.

United States Bureau of Census. (1989). *Statistical abstract of the U.S.,* 109th edition. Washington, D.C.: U.S. Department of Commerce.

Waller, A., S. Baker, and A. Szocka. (1989). Childhood injury deaths: National analysis and geographic variations. *American Journal of Public Health* 79(3): 310–15.

Withrow, C. (1979). The school nurse takes a look at her charges. *Nursing '79,* 1: 48–51.

Wong, D. L. (1986). Helping parents select day care. *Pediatric Nursing* 12: 181–87.

Selected Readings

American Nurses Association. (1983). *Standards of school nursing practice.* Kansas City, Mo.: Author.

American Public Health Association. (1980). Health of school-age children (Resolution No. 7905). *American Journal of Public Health* 70: 304–5.

Avery, J. (1980). The safety of children in cars. *Practitioner* 224: 816–21.

Blum, R. (ed.). (1982). *The clinical practice of adolescent medicine.* New York: Academic Press.

Boyd, J. H., and E. K. Moscicki. (1986). Firearms and youth suicide. *American Journal of Public Health* 76(10): 1240–42.

Boyle, M., E. Koff, and L. Guidas. (1981). Assessment and management of anorexia nervosa. *Maternal Child Nursing Journal* 6: 412–18.

Budetti, P., J. Butler, and P. McManus. (1982). Federal health program reforms: Implications for child health care. *Milbank Memorial Fund Quarterly,* 60(1): 155.

Butcher, A. H., et al. (1988). Heart smart: A school health program meeting the 1990 Objectives for the Nation. *Health Education Quarterly* 15(1): 17–34.

Cadman, D., et al. (1987). Evaluation of public health preschool child developmental screening: The process and outcomes of a community program. *American Journal of Public Health* 77(1): 45–51.

Children's Defense Fund. (1979). *America's children and their families: Basic facts.* Washington, D.C.: Author.

Committee on School Health. (1981). School health: A guide for health professionals. Evanston, Ill.: American Academy of Pediatrics.

Comstock, G. (1981). Influence of mass media on child health and behavior. *Health Education Quarterly* 8(1): 32.

Cushner, I. (1981). Maternal behavior and perinatal risks: Alcohol, smoking, and drugs. *Annual Review of Public Health* 2: 201.

Daniel, W. (1977). *Adolescents in health and disease.* St. Louis: C. V. Mosby.

Daniel, W. (1981). Overview of adolescent health problems. *Southern Medical Journal* 74: 569.

Dibble, J. (1981). ABC for teens: Parent education after the baby comes. *Pediatric Nursing* 7: 21–25.

Doyle, K., and C. Cassell. (1981). Teenage sexuality: The early adolescent years. *Obstetrics and Gynecology Annual* 10: 423.

Drewnowski, A., S. Hopkins, and R. Kessler. (1988). The prevalence of bulimia nervosa in the U.S. college student population. *American Journal of Public Health* 78(10): 1322–25.

Freeman, R., and J. Heinrich. (1981). *Community health nursing practice* 2nd ed. Philadelphia: W. B. Saunders.

Goldberg, R. (1984). Identifying speech and language delays in children. *Pediatric Nursing* 10: 252–59.

Green, L., and D. Iverson. (1982). School health education. *Annual Review of Public Health* 3: 321.

Hanlon, J. J. and G. E. Pickett. (1984). *Public health: Administration and practice.* 8th ed. St. Louis: Times Mirror/Mosby.

Holt, S., and T. Robinson. (1979). The school nurse's family assessment tool. *American Journal of Nursing* 79: 950.

Johansen, A., A. Leibowitz, and L. Waite. (1988). Child care and children's illness. *American Journal of Public Health* 78(9): 1175–77.

Johnston, C. (1988). Last chance for change? . . . Education and training relating to child abuse. *Nursing Times* 84(7): 30–31.

Jonides, L. (1982). Childhood obesity: A treatment approach for private practice. *Pediatric Nursing* 8: 320–22.

Keenan, R. (1986). School-based adolescent health care programs. *Pediatric Nursing* 12: 365–69.

Keller, O. L. (1986). Bulimia: Primary care approach and intervention. *Nurse Practitioner* 11: 42–51.

Kronmiller, J., and R. F. Nirsch. (1985). Preventive dentistry for children. *Pediatric Nursing* 11: 446–49.

Langford, R. (1981). Teenagers and obesity. *American Journal of Nursing 81*: 556–59.

Levey, L., M. MacDowell, and S. Levey. (1986). Health care of poverty and non-poverty children in Iowa. *American Journal of Public Health* 76(8): 1000–1003.

Long, G., C. Whitman, M. Johansson, C. Williams, and R. Tuthill. (1975). Evaluation of a school health program directed to children with history of high absence — A focus for nursing intervention. *American Journal of Public Health* 65: 388–93.

Lyons, J. F., et al. (1987). Research generated nursing diagnoses for healthy school-age children. *Issues in Comprehensive Pediatric Nursing* 10(3): 149–59.

McAlister, A. (1981). Social and environmental influences on health behavior. *Health Education Quarterly* 8(1): 25.

Merritt, T., R. Laurence, and R. Naeye. (1980). The infants of adolescent mothers. *Pediatric Annals* 9(3): 32.

Miller, C. A., A. Fine, S. Adams-Taylor, and L Schorr. (1986). *Monitoring children's health: Key indicators.* Washington, D.C.: American Public Health Association.

Newacheck, P., P. Budetti, and P. McManus. (1984). Trends in childhood disability. *American Journal of Public Health* 74: 232–36.

Newcomb, M., E. Maddahian, and P. Bentler. (1986). Risk factors for drug use among adolescents: Concurrent and longitudinal analyses. *American Journal of Public Health* 76(5): 525–31.

O'Brien, M., M. Manley, and M. Heagarty. (1975). Expanding the public health nurse's role in child care. *Nursing Outlook* 23: 369–73.

Perry, C. L., et al. (1985). The concept of health promotion and the prevention of adolescent drug abuse. *Health Education Quarterly* 12(2): 169–84.

Perry, C. L., et al. (1988). Primary prevention of cardiovascular disease: Community-wide strategies for youth. *Journal of Consulting Clinical Psychology* 56(3): 358–64.

Pipes, P. L. (1984). *Nutrition in Infancy and Childhood.* 3rd ed. St. Louis: C. V. Mosby.

Porter, P. (1981). Realistic outcomes of school health service programs. *Health Education Quarterly* 8(1): 81.

President's Commission for a National Agenda for the Eighties. (1981). Helping families — to help themselves. *International Journal of Family Therapy* 3(3): 208–33.

Public Health Service. (1979). *Healthy people: The Surgeon General's report on health promotion and disease prevention* (DHEW Publication No. 79-55071). Washington, D.C.: U.S. Government Printing Office.

Rice, M., and P. Kibee. (1983). Review: Identifying the adolescent substance abuser, *Maternal Child Nursing Journal* 8: 139–42.

Richardson, S. F. (1988). Child health promotion practices. *Journal of Pediatric Health Care* 2(2): 73–78.

Ryan, M. T. (1984). Identifying the sexually abused child. *Pediatric Nursing* 10: 419–21.

Sapala, S., and G. Strokosch. (1981). Adolescent sexuality: Use of a questionnaire for health teaching and counseling. *Pediatric Nursing* 7: 33–35.

Schaller, W. (1981). *The school health program.* 5th ed. Philadelphia: W. B. Saunders.

Schetky, D., and A. Green. (1988). *Child sexual abuse.* New York: Brunner/Mazel.

Schlechter, F. (1981). An experiment in group adolescent weight loss guidance. *Journal of School Health* 51(2): 123–24.

School-age day care: Developing a responsive curriculum. (1980, January). *Child Care Information Exchange,* pp. 17–20.

Sigman, M. (1985). *Children with emotional disorders and developmental disabilities.* Orlando, Fla.: Grune and Stratton.

Silver, G. (1981). Redefining school health services: Comprehensive child health care as the framework. *Journal of School Health* 51(3): 157–62.

Sloan, R. S., and B. D. Porter. (1984). Preventing sexual abuse of children: A model school education program . . . the community health nurse in elementary education. *Journal of Community Health Nursing* 1(3): 181–88.

Smith, D. P. (1985). Common day care diseases: Patterns and prevention. *Pediatric Nursing* 12: 175–78.

Tackett, J., and M. Hunsberger (eds.). (1981). *Family-centered care of children and adolescents.* Philadelphia: W. B. Saunders.

Tauxe, R., K. Johnson, J. Boase, S. Helgerson, and P. Blake. (1986). Control of day care shigellosis: A trial of convalescent day care in isolation. *American Journal of Public Health* 76(6): 627–30.

Tyrell, S. (1981). Accidents will happen. *Health and Social Science Journal* 9: 263–65.

Waller, A., S. Baker, and A. Szocka. (1989). Childhood injury deaths: National analysis and geographic variations. *American Journal of Public Health* 79(3): 310–15.

Weiss, B., and B. Duncan. (1986). Bicycle helmet use by children: Knowledge and behavior of physicians. *American Journal of Public Health* 76(8): 1022–23.

Wintemute, G., J. Kraus, S. Teret, and M. Wright. (1987). Drowning in childhood and adolescence: A population-based study. *American Journal of Public Health* 77(7): 830–32.

Withrow, C. (1979). The school nurse takes a look at her charges. *Nursing '79,* 1: 48–51.

Wold, S. (1980). *School nursing: A framework for practice.* St. Louis: C. V. Mosby.

Wong, D. L. (1986). Helping parents select day care. *Pediatric Nursing* 12: 181–87.

Zabin, L., and S. Clark. (1981). Why they delay: A study of teenage family planning clinic patients. *Family Planning Perspective* 13(5): 205.

Zapka, J. G., et al. (1985). College health services: Setting for community, organizational, and individual change. *Family and Community Health* 8(1): 18–34.

Zuckerman, D., A. Colby, N. Ware, and J. Lazerson. (1986). The prevalence of bulimia among college students. *American Journal of Public Health* 76(9): 1135–37.

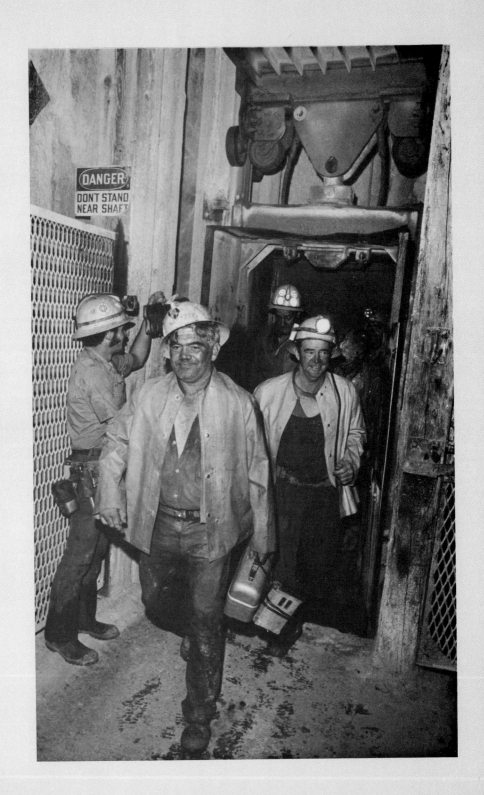

18 Health of the Working Population

Elaine Richard

Barbara W. Spradley

One of the largest population groups of concern to community health is the working population. In the United States it is made up of 120 million people, 40 percent of whom are women (U.S. Bureau of Census, 1989). This aggregate is composed of generally well adults whose health and safety at work, until a few decades ago, were viewed as their own responsibility. In recent years we have come to recognize that safety and health in the workplace have a major influence on the public's health and that employers and others must share in the responsibility for workers' safety and health on the job. Potential or actual injuries and illnesses associated with the workplace are the focus of the field known as occupational health.

In this chapter we examine selected aspects of occupational health. First we define the working population and look at the impact of the work environment on this group's health. Then we review and summarize historical perspectives and legislation affecting the health of the working population. Finally, we describe the health needs of workers, ways to meet those needs, and the community health nurse's contribution to the health of the working population.

DEFINING THE WORKING POPULATION

What is the working population? When we think of workers we generally think of people who are gainfully employed, and we visualize the most obvious types: an executive in a three-piece suit carrying a briefcase, a professional person in uniform, or a jeans-clad worker with a lunch pail. In actuality there are almost infinitely varied types of workers and jobs encompassing nearly every conceivable activity. Most workers are paid monetarily for what they do. Others, such as housewives and volunteers, also work but are not identified in the labor (worker) statistics. Yet all these workers have health needs that should be addressed by community health practitioners.

The working population, composed of all people who work, includes most of the country's well adults. At the federal level it is appropriate to consider the total working population as a single group whose need for safe and healthful working conditions can be enhanced through public education and enabling legislation. We shall discuss these efforts in a later section. For assessment of needs and provision of health services, however, the community health nurse must view this aggregate in terms of smaller groups or subpopulations. That is, the nurse must assess the health safety needs and worksite hazards of a specific group of workers, whether they are assembly-line workers in a plant, bank tellers, farmers, or operators of video display terminals, and then design health interventions and mechanisms for service provision appropriate to that working group. Let us look more closely at the work environment and factors in it that affect worker health.

THE WORK ENVIRONMENT

The healthy adult working population, although scattered throughout the nation in a myriad of urban and rural settings, still shares characteristics of its work environment in common. We shall examine five environmental factors common to every work setting and discuss their potential impact on the health of workers. These factors can be grouped into five categories: (1) physical, (2) chemical, (3) biological, (4) ergonomical, and (5) psychosocial.

Physical factors are structural elements of the workplace that influence worker health and productivity. Various features on the job form an assemblage of parts that defines the physical work environment. These include such factors as work space, temperature, lighting, noise, vibration, color, radiation, pressure, and soundness of building and equipment construction. The quality of such elements can make an impact on worker health (Office of Technology Assessment, 1985). Excessive noise, for example, may disrupt concentration; interfere with on-the-job communication, job performance, and safety; and, over a period of time, cause hearing loss (Levy and Wegman, 1988). Extremes of temperature are another problem. Field laborers, road construction crews, or persons working around furnaces may experience heat extremes that, if compounded by excessive physical exertion, can cause heatstroke. Excessive levels of electromagnetic and ionizing radiation found in certain manufacturing operations or hospitals also may create serious deleterious effects (Clever, 1981). Pressure extremes, experienced by deep-sea divers or by persons working at high altitudes or in tunneling operations, may cause improper gas exchange and tissue damage affecting ears, sinuses, and teeth (Levy and Wegman, 1988). Many physical factors can threaten safety, such as lack of protection from acetylene torch sparks, sharp or falling objects, or weak scaffolding. Despite awareness of these hazards, occupational injury rates continue to rise (Robinson, 1988).

Chemical factors are the chemical agents present in the work environment that may threaten worker health and safety. Numerous chemicals are found in the raw materials, production processes, and day-to-day operations of industries and businesses such as dry cleaners, painters, food companies, photographers, automobile manufacturers, plastics factories, farms, pharmaceutical companies, and hospitals. In recent years, chemical agents have become an increasing menace to the health of the working population (Public Health Service, 1979). The giant petroleum industry followed by the modern chemical industry have introduced new chemicals at the alarming rate of several hundred basically untested new compounds a year, subjecting workers to unknown hazards (Last, 1987). Chemicals are present in many forms. Frequently chemicals are associated with gases; however, they are also present in the form of solvents, mists, vapors, dusts, and solids. Depending on their form and structure, chemicals enter the human body through the lungs, gastrointestinal tract, and skin. Therefore, an understanding of the toxicology of chemicals is essential for identifying (1) the amount of chemical exposure that produces toxicity, (2) the routes through which chemicals enter the body, and (3) the appropriate personal protection for workers (Williams and Burson, 1985). For example, lead enters the body through the gastrointestinal tract and the lungs. Workers exposed to toxic levels must maintain good hand-washing practices, avoid eating on the job to prevent the ingestion of this chemical, and at the same time employ appropriate respiratory protection to prevent inhaling this agent.

Many toxic chemicals such as insecticides are taken for granted in daily use and their toxicity frequently ignored. Careless handling and needless exposure can lead to serious burns, poisoning, asphyxia, tissue damage, or even cancer. For example, a significant number of workers applying hot coal tar to wood block floors developed malignant neoplasms (Silverstein et al., 1985). Some inert, nontoxic industrial materials, such as resins and polymers, may decompose and form toxic byproducts when heated. Workers need to be warned and protected from all potential hazards associated with the materials they must use on the job (Sax, 1986). With proper handling and protection, many toxic conditions can be prevented. Ideally, all toxic substances would be eliminated through substitution of nontoxic agents, when such chemicals exist.

Biological factors are the organisms and potential contaminants found in the work environment. These include bacteria, viruses, rickettsias, molds, fungi, parasites of various types, insects, animals, and even toxic plants that may be present. Potential hazards, such as infectious or parasitic diseases, may derive from exposure to contaminated water or to insects. Other vehicles include improper waste or sewage disposal, unsanitary work environments (Arbab and Weidner, 1986), improper food handling, and unsanitary personal practices.

Workers in every setting have their own unique set of potential biological hazards (Levy and Wegman, 1988). Agricultural workers, for instance, are subject to a condition called "farmer's lung" that comes from inhaling fungi-contaminated grain dust. Staphylococcal and other infectious agents threaten hospital workers. Brucellosis (undulant fever) and Q fever from infected cattle are a threat to slaughterhouse workers. Outdoor workers, such as builders, forest rangers, or environmental specialists, face the hazards of insect and animal attack as well as contact with toxic plants, such as poison oak and ivy.

Ergonomical factors also affect workers' well-being. These are all the interactions between the worker, the demands of the job, the work setting, and the overall environment. Ergonomics is sometimes called human factors engineering. It has become a field of study in occupational health and is defined as "an applied science concerned with the design of facilities, equipment, tools, and tasks that are compatible with the anatomical, physiological, biochemical, perceptual, and behavioral characteristics of humans" (Levy and Wegman, 1988, p. 112). In short, ergonomics deals with people interacting with their work environments.

For our purposes in describing the elements of the work environment, ergonomical factors are the customs, laws, design, and expectations of the work itself. They include all the physiological and psychological demands (and potential stressors) that the job makes on the worker. The design of necessary tools, work space, physical positions workers must assume and motions they must make to do the job, standards and habits associated with carrying out the work — all these have an impact on workers' health. (Figure 18-1). Health problems can arise from improper lifting habits, inadequate or unsafe tools, poor lighting (Jacobsen et al., 1987), or unrealistic job demands; from a work design that promotes interruptions, provides inadequate space, and offers only poor ventilation; or from any other stress-producing working conditions. For example, Mexican field laborers in some southwestern states as recently as 1984 were required to use short-handled hoes to speed production and maximize crop yield. Hours of stooping over plants in this doubled-up position, however, caused serious skeletal and internal injuries, some of which were permanent. In another situation, workers on variable shifts (as opposed to fixed schedules) exhibited higher rates of heavy drinking, job stress, and emotional problems (Gordon et al., 1986).

Psychosocial factors include all the responses and behaviors that workers exhibit on the job based on the attitudes and values learned from their cultural backgrounds, life experiences, and worksite norms. They are the workers' responses to the work and the work milieu. Some people may appear (and feel) fatigued, tense, bored, angry, depressed, or agitated. Others may

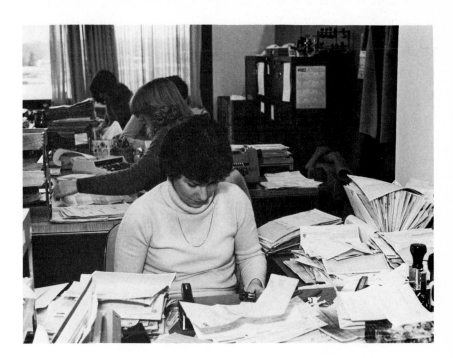

Figure 18-1
Ergonomical factors can create stressful working conditions that affect employees' health. Several studies have demonstrated that secretaries are among the most highly stressed workers.

be enthusiastic and energized. Similar work conditions can evoke different responses from people. Repetitive work may be boring for some people, but for others it offers an opportunity for reflection. Certain types of work can be challenging for some, but not challenging enough for others. Worksite norms about such things as smoking cessation have influenced worker behavior (Sorensen et al., 1986).

The nature of the work itself evokes worker responses as much as the work conditions do. Work that is time pressured or that conflicts with personal values may create tremendous stress for employees (Gough et al., 1988). Ethical dilemmas, such as being asked to promote a product whose sales will benefit the company (and preserve the employee's job) but whose use may be injurious to the public, can tear people up emotionally. Peer pressure can create another set of stressors, as is evident in personal conflict experienced by many workers during a strike. Yet another psychosocial factor that can make the work situation hazardous to employee health involves unrealistic personal expectations on the part of workers for what they can and hope to accomplish on the job. Unattainable aspirations can lead to chronic stress and fatigue and eventual burnout (Veninga and Spradley, 1981).

Depending on the work setting, the presence of these five factors will vary in intensity and potential for threat to worker health. They present a core of critical data for occupational health assessment and planning. Table 18-1 summarizes these five environmental factors.

Table 18-1
Factors Influencing Health and Productivity in the Work Environment

Variable	Physical	Chemical	Biological	Ergonomical	Psychosocial
Definition	Structural elements of workplace	Chemical agents present in work environment	Biological organisms and potential contaminants in work environment	Customs, rules, design, and expectations of the work itself	Workers' values, attitudes, and responses
Selected Types	Radiation Noise Vibration Light Temperature Space Color Pressure Construction	Mists Vapors Gases Solids Liquids Dusts Solvents	Viruses Insects Molds Fungi Bacteria Animals Plants Parasites Rickettsias	Design of work space Design of job Work habits Required motions Design of tools Work standards Work flow	Emotional: Boredom Anger Depression Behavioral: Fatigue Tension Cultural: Values Norms
Illustrative Potential Hazards	Excessive noise Electromagnetic radiation Excessive ionizing radiation Temperature extremes Excessive vibration Pressure extremes Unsafe objects or structures	Excessive airborne concentrations Topical irritants Toxic absorption through skin Toxic ingestion	Contaminated water or food Improper waste or sewage disposal Unsanitary work environment Improper food handling Insect or animal attack Unsanitary personal practices	Improper lifting Poor motions or positions Improper tools Inadequate space to do work Interruptions Unrealistic work expectations Repetitive motion	Boring work Unchallenging work Time pressure Conflicts with worker values Group dissatisfaction Unrealistic personal expectations Peer pressure

HEALTH AND THE WORKPLACE: HISTORICAL PERSPECTIVES

The work setting clearly presents many hazards to workers' health; nonetheless, conditions in the work setting have improved considerably from previous years. Modern occupational health is an outgrowth of the nineteenth-century Industrial Revolution in England. Deplorable work conditions and exploitation of workers created a growing public concern and spawned the development of many protective laws. This influence was felt in the United States, whose early agricultural character in the 1800s was rapidly being replaced by industrialization. By 1900 the United States supplied more than one-third of the world's annual demand for iron and steel (Lee, 1978). As industrial growth escalated, immigrants poured into the United States, forming a large portion of the labor force. Workers, both adults and children, commonly worked 12- to 14-hour shifts, seven days a week, under unspeakable conditions of grime, dust, physical hazards, smoke, and noxious fumes. People accepted work-related illnesses and injuries as necessary risks and expected to live shorter lives, into the forties and fifties, death being common in the thirties for workers in some trades (Lee, 1978).

The connection between work conditions and health was ignored. Employers attributed employees' poor health and early deaths to the workers' own personal habits on the job or their home living conditions. Physicians, uneducated in the relationship between work and health, blamed industrial-related diseases, such as silicosis, lead poisoning, and tuberculosis, on other causes. But the evidence was there. In the early 1900s the Public Health Service conducted one of the first scientific studies in occupational hazards by investigating dust conditions in mining, cement manufacturing, and stone cutting. Other studies followed. Lead poisoning was as high as 22 percent among a group of pottery workers studied. A 1914 study of garment workers showed a high incidence of tuberculosis related to poor ventilation, overcrowding, and unsanitary work conditions. Other investigations revealed phosphorous poisoning among workers in the match industry (1912), radium poisoning in the watch industry (1920s), and mercury poisoning in the felt hat industry (1930s) (Lee, 1978). The public was awakening to the effect of work conditions on people's health.

With development of the labor movement came the demand for healthful and safe working conditions. Workers' compensation laws provided for occupational injury and disease coverage, and other efforts were made to protect workers against the health hazards of the workplace. The health of American workers is better today than it has ever been, but health hazards still exist and new ones continue to develop as technology and environmental influences change. Occupational health faces the challenge of continued protection and promotion of worker health and improvement of the work environment.

SIGNIFICANT LEGISLATION AFFECTING THE HEALTH AND SAFETY OF WORKERS

The preceding historical summary clearly emphasizes the need for public awareness and understanding before changes could occur to improve the health of the working population. Such understanding has resulted from knowledge based on experience and research.

The earliest systematic study of occupational disease was recorded in 1700 by Bernardino Ramazzini, now known as the "father of occupational medicine" (Lee, 1978). This Italian physician had the foresight, when attempting a diagnosis, to ask what occupation the patient was engaged in. Despite his influence, interest in and information concerning worker health evolved slowly. A few classic studies, some of which are mentioned in the previous section, influenced the gradual development of protective legislation. Further influence came from disastrous events in the workplace. One notable event was the Triangle Waist factory fire in New York City in 1911 in which 154 workers, mostly young women, died. Fire escapes ended in midair and the factory doors were locked. This tragic event resulted in the first serious safety laws to protect working people (Morris, 1976). Today a growing body of legislation exists to protect the health and safety of workers. Current laws that employers must implement include the following.

The Workmen's Compensation Act of 1911 was enacted in several states initially and finally in all states by 1948. This law requires employers to carry employee insurance that provides compensation for wages lost and costs of medical and rehabilitative care associated with work-related diseases and injuries. Application of the law varies from state to state. A trend across all states, however, is to emphasize early intervention and rehabilitation.

Second Injury Funds, established under most state workers' compensation laws, encourage employers to hire the handicapped. Employees who acquire a "second injury" (for example, loss of a limb or an eye, or a worsened chronic condition) from their work are covered. When the second injury results in permanent, total disability, the employer is then liable only for the amount of disability directly attributable to the worker's employment while the funds cover the difference to which the employee is entitled. Again, coverage varies with each state. The Department of Labor enforces the provision of these funds.

The Federal Coal Mine Health and Safety Act of 1967 is a unique law in that it is the only federal program that deals with a specific occupational disease. The act originally provided for the establishment of health standards in coal mines and medical examinations for actively employed underground coal miners. Through the Social Security Administration, it also provided black lung (pneumoconiosis) benefits. Specifically, it required all exposed workers to have radiographic examinations and provided federal funds to compensate mine victims and survivors of deceased miners. The subsequent Federal Mine Safety and Health Amendments Act of 1977 retains most of the original provisions.

The Occupational Safety and Health Act of 1970 has had tremendous significance for the working population. Generally it seeks to provide workers with protection against personal injury and illness resulting from hazardous working conditions. More specifically, its purpose and functions are "to assure safe and healthful working conditions for working men and women by authorizing enforcement of the standards developed under the Act; by assisting and encouraging the States in their efforts to assure safe and healthful working conditions; by providing for research, information, education, and training in the field of occupational safety and health and for other purposes" (Lee, 1978, p. 80).

The act created two federal agencies. The Occupational Safety and Health Administration (OSHA), housed in the Department of Labor, became its regulatory branch. Its research branch became the responsibility of the National Institute for Occupational Safety and Health (NIOSH), based in the Public Health Service (under the Department of Health and Human Services). Specifically, OSHA responsibilities include the following (Levy and Wegman, 1988):

Develop and update mandatory occupational safety and health standards

Monitor and enforce regulations and standards

Require employers to keep accurate records on work-related injuries, illnesses, and hazardous exposures

Maintain an occupational safety and health statistics collection and analysis system (collaborating with NIOSH)

Supervise employer and worker education and training to identify and prevent unsafe or unhealthy working conditions (collaborating with NIOSH)

Provide grants to states to assist in compliance with the Act

NIOSH responsibilities include the following (Hanlon and Pickett, 1984; NIOSH, 1986):

Research on occupational safety and health problems

Hazard evaluation

Toxicity determinations

Work force development and training

Industry-wide studies of chronic or low-level exposures to hazardous substances

Research on psychological, motivational, and behavioral factors as they relate to occupational safety and health

Training of occupational safety and health professionals

The Privacy Act of 1974 ensures that only necessary information be collected on individuals by federal agencies. Furthermore, this information, such as medical history, education, or financial and employment history, must be maintained so that the individual's privacy is protected (Lee, 1978).

The Toxic Substances Control Act of 1976 serves to ensure that chemical substances do not present an "unreasonable risk of injury to health or the environment" (Lee, 1978, p. 83). The act requires that certain chemical substances and mixtures be tested and their use restricted. It is also concerned with the manufacture, processing, commercial distribution, and disposal of such substances. The Environmental Protection Agency enforces the Act.

Worker Right-to-Know Legislation, passed federally in 1986 as the Hazard Communication Act, ensures that workers are adequately informed regarding hazards in their places of work. A growing sentiment in the nation says that workers should know what risks they face on the job.

HEALTH NEEDS OF THE ADULT POPULATION

The working population, as mentioned previously, is made up of adults whose health determines the productivity and well-being of our communities and our nation. For all American adults, aged 25 to 64, the major causes of death are cancer, heart disease, accidents, stroke, and suicide. Table 18-2 shows the leading causes of death for this population group.

Chronic diseases pose the most significant threat to the health of American adults (U.S. Bureau of the Census, 1989). Cancer, formerly second, has moved into first place as the leading cause of death among American adults. Environmental and work-related factors play a major role in the increase in cancer for this population. Lung, large intestine, and breast cancers cause the most fatalities among this age group. An increasing number of these are occupational and smoking-related malignancies whose direct etiology often remains unclear since there may have been repeated and prolonged exposure to several carcinogenic agents over many years.

Major preventable risk factors contributing to cancer are smoking, alcohol consumption, diet, radiation, sunlight, occupational exposure, water and air pollution, and heredity (Public Health Service, 1979). For the working population, occupational exposure presents an increasing set of health hazards as new chemicals and other potential cancer-causing materials are produced and used every year. In addition, known carcinogenic agents such as asbestos and vinyl chloride continue to threaten the health of workers who, without adequate protection, develop malignancies not commonly found in the general population. Mesothelioma, a lung cancer related to asbestos expo-

Table 18-2
Leading Causes of Death and Numbers of Deaths (in Thousands) for American Adults Aged 25 to 64 Years

Cause of Death	Total	Male	Female
Cancer	157.2	83.2	74.0
Heart Disease	143.4	102.0	41.4
Accidents	41.9	31.9	10.0
Cerebrovascular problems	19.8	10.5	9.3
Suicide	19.2	14.6	4.6
Liver disease and cirrhosis	16.2	11.0	5.2
Chronic obstructive pulmonary diseases	13.4	7.8	5.6
Diabetes	9.8	5.0	4.8
Pneumonia and flu	7.6	5.0	2.6

Source: U.S. Bureau of the Census. (1989). *Statistical Abstract of the United States, 1989.* 109th ed. Washington, D.C.: U.S. Government Printing Office.

sure, has even been documented among people whose only known exposure was to the contaminants carried home on the shoes and clothes of the worker (Lee, 1978). It has been estimated that up to 20 percent of total cancer deaths may be due to occupational hazards (Public Health Service, 1979) (Figure 18-2). More than one-fourth of all deaths among adults aged 25 to 64 are due to cardiovascular diseases, primarily coronary artery (heart) disease and stroke. Heart disease has been the leading cause of death for men above age 40. Women, on the other hand, prior to menopause have only one-third the heart disease rate of men. After menopause the incidence in women increases. By age 70 it is nearly the same, and by age 85 the rates are equal (National Center for Health Statistics, 1988).

Figure 18-2
Some workers must deal with known carcinogenic agents on the job.
Adequate protection is essential for their health and safety.

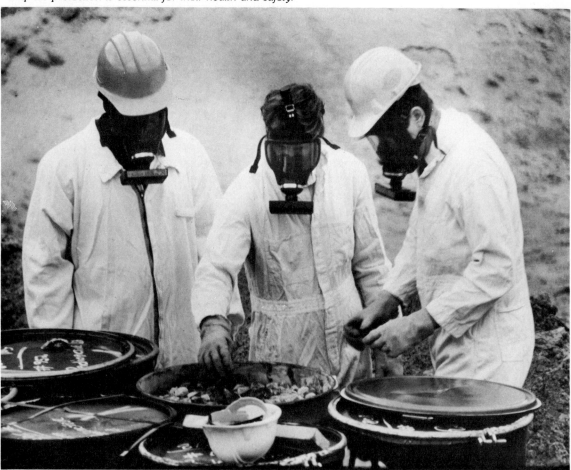

In addition to its impact on mortality rates, heart disease has a tremendous impact on worker health. It is the largest contributor to permanent disability claims for workers under 65 and accounts for more days of hospitalization than any other single disorder. It is the principal cause of limited activity for some 5 to 6 million Americans under age 65 (U.S. Bureau of the Census, 1989).

Strokes, too, in addition to being a significant cause of death (7 percent of the total mortality rate), leave many American adults disabled with paralysis, speech problems, and memory loss. Furthermore, "nearly 10 percent of nursing home admissions in people under 65 are because of strokes" (Public Health Service, 1979, p. 56). Blacks between the ages of 25 and 64 are more than twice (2.5 times) as susceptible to strokes as whites, largely because of the high prevalence and incidence of hypertension among black Americans.

Risk factors associated with coronary heart disease can be separated into three main categories: personal, hereditary, and environmental. Personal risk factors include sex, age, race, high cholesterol (specifically low-density lipo-proteins to cholesterol ratio), high blood pressure, and cigarette smoking. The most preventable of these include cholesterol, high blood pressure, and cigarette smoking. Heredity is a risk factor category which cannot be changed by the individual. Our understanding of environmental risk factors, especially as they relate to occupational exposures, is quite limited at this point (Levy and Wegman, 1988). The likelihood of heart disease or stroke occurring multiplies with the increasing number of risk factors present.

Three other problems posing major threats to the health of American adults, and thus to the working population, are accidents, alcohol abuse, and mental illness. Each has taken a tremendous toll in lives lost and health and productivity diminished. The Surgeon General's report on health promotion and disease prevention states a compelling case for the preventability of these problems (Public Health Service, 1979).

WORK-RELATED HEALTH PROBLEMS

What are the health problems of the working population specifically? American workers are exposed to numerous safety and health hazards in the work environment, which we examined earlier in this chapter. Their impact on worker health has led to identification (Baker et al., 1988) of the ten leading work-related health problems:

1. Occupational lung disease
2. Musculoskeletal injuries
3. Occupational cancer
4. Severe occupational traumatic injuries
5. Cardiovascular diseases
6. Reproductive problems

7. Neurotoxic illness
8. Noise-induced hearing loss
9. Dermatological problems
10. Psychological disorders

It is estimated that 20 million work-related injuries and 390,000 new work-related illnesses occur in the United States each year. However, the actual number of injuries and illnesses reported each year is much lower. It is also estimated that there may be 100,000 or more work-related deaths in the United States each year (Levy and Wegman, 1988). While the incidence of some of these diseases will diminish through preventive efforts, epidemiologic research will continue to shed new light on the nature, causes, and linkages of occupational diseases, contributing to a likely increase in their reporting (Hanlon and Pickett, 1984).

Collection of occupational disease data has been difficult since the lag time is so great between exposure and onset of the disease and actual clinical evidence. Silicosis, for example, takes 15 years to develop. Some cases of mesothelioma have not become evident until 25 years after the worker was last exposed to asbestos (Hanlon and Pickett, 1984). The lag time for solid tumors is at least 10 to 20 years and possibly as long as 50 years (Levy and Wegman, 1988). Lung disease in workers occurs gradually over time. Most often exposures do not result in acute symptoms, and once the symptoms do occur, little can be done. It is for this reason that respiratory disease prevention is so important. Many workers who have moved on to other jobs or retired are only now discovering disease that may be connected to previous employment. Documenting this connection poses problems. Nonetheless, more sophisticated epidemiologic methods and an improved data base are enabling public health and industrial researchers to demonstrate linkages and make more accurate predictions. They have estimated, for instance, that of the 6,000 current and previous uranium workers, approximately 600 to 1,100 will die of lung cancer in about 20 years because of radiation exposure (Key et al., 1977). More than 12 percent of active coal miners have radiographic evidence of pneumoconiosis, or "black lung" (Baker et al., 1988), and workers exposed to heavy metals, such as lead, mercury, and arsenic, will likely develop related diseases. Researchers have also demonstrated the relationship between cotton mill dust and byssinosis, a lung disease formerly thought not to exist in the United States. Epidemiologists are studying the connections between skin diseases and materials used on the job, a problem of considerable magnitude since dermatological problems are among the most common of occupational diseases. It is estimated that seven million industrial workers have exposure to noise levels that cause impaired hearing (Hanlon and Pickett, 1984). As the knowledge base regarding occupational illnesses increases, nurses will be better equipped to design more effective protective and preventive measures.

A final set of health problems affecting workers encompasses all the ergonomic and psychological stresses that workers experience on the job or bring to the job from their personal lives. With our increasing technology and changing work environments, new concerns over such things as "tight building syndrome," or problems associated with working indoors, have surfaced (Whorton et al., 1987). There is also an increasing amount of research being devoted to the study of "visual display terminal exposure," or visual problems associated with computer use (Centers for Disease Control, 1988). There is some evidence that up to 30 percent of absenteeism is due to emotional disturbances (Hanlon and Pickett, 1984). Pressures at work to be more productive, or a physically stressful work environment (for example, excessive noise, heat, or vibration) can send a worker home to take out his or her frustrations through such outlets as domestic violence or alcohol abuse. Problems at home, like financial or interpersonal difficulties, can, on the other hand, affect the worker's performance on the job. Either source of stress creates a vicious cycle perpetuating and escalating the problems in both settings with the potential for unsafe practice at work and harm to self or family at home. Clearly workers' mental health influences their safety, their productivity, and their levels of health.

OCCUPATIONAL SAFETY AND HEALTH PROGRAMS

What efforts are being made to address the above problems and to promote the health of the working population? Of primary concern to occupational health and safety professionals are the factors in the work environment that have an impact on workers' health and safety. Clearly the business of occupational health is the prevention of work-related hazards, the protection of workers from known health risks, and the promotion of fitness and productivity among workers.

Occupational health programs, generally speaking, have grown tremendously since World War II. Many manufacturing plants, service organizations such as the Kansas Farm Bureau, and commercial establishments, including department stores, have instituted some kind of health program for employees. Many programs still concentrate on providing emergency care, but others are beginning to recognize the importance of prevention and health promotion. For example, Sperry Univac of St. Paul, Minnesota, has held an Employee Health Promotion Day, and Ball Electronics keeps employees fit with exercise breaks. The Resource Trust Company of Minneapolis, Minnesota, pays the initial fee and half the weekly dues of any employee who attends Weight Watchers. As an added incentive, the firm reimburses the other half of the costs to employees when they meet their weight objectives (*Wellness Gazette*, 1980).

Because the nature of work, as well as the number and type of workers employed, varies in different businesses, the potential hazards and the need and type of on-site health programs varies. For example, construction and mine workers are a high-risk group for certain types of injuries and illnesses. These workers require an aggressive surveillance program that focuses on prevention and personal protection. On the other hand, professionals, such as lawyers and accountants, who in general do not encounter physical safety and health hazards on the job but may experience psychological stresses, would benefit more from a health promotion program that includes emphasis on stress management and physical fitness.

In order to determine the priorities for intervention and the appropriate health goals and objectives for an aggregate of workers, it is essential that an environmental and workers' assessment be conducted. Knowledge of workers' job classifications, materials handling, and exposures will provide clues to potential hazardous substances and working conditions. This information, together with data on the characteristics of the aggregate in terms of age, sex, race, and existing health conditions, should be compiled. In addition, one should examine workers' compensation claims and occupational safety and health reports to identify subpopulations at risk for occupational illness and injury (Wegman and Froines, 1985; Sundin et al., 1986; Froines et al., 1986).

The two professionals who generally provide on-site services are the occupational health nurse (OHN) and the safety specialist. Other members of the interdisciplinary team may include an industrial hygienist, ergonomist, toxicologist, and occupational health physician. However, these specialists are generally employed only by large corporations or provide only selected part-time services on a contractual basis. Therefore, the occupational health nurse position in a large company or the community health nurse serving smaller companies provides the cornerstone to occupational health (Babbitz, 1984).

Because the working population is primarily composed of healthy adults, the goal of occupational health is to provide a healthy and safe work environment and to promote personal health behaviors of workers in an attempt to maintain a healthy, productive work force. Thus, occupational health programs encompass the entire spectrum of the health continuum involving the practice components of disease prevention, health protection, and health promotion (White, 1982). In Table 18-3 we list these practice priorities.

The practice priority of prevention holds primary importance in occupational health because work-related injuries and illnesses are frequently not reversible. Limb loss or mesothelioma from asbestos exposure are conditions for which there are no cures. Interventions, therefore, are aimed at eliminating the hazards by such methods as redesigning the equipment to provide safety guards and to substitute materials that are effective but less toxic. The Surgeon General's report points out, "Once these occupational hazards are defined, they can be controlled. Safer materials may be substituted; manufacturing processes may be changed to prevent release of offending agents; hazardous material can be isolated in enclosures; exhaust methods and other engineering techniques may be used to control the source; special clothing and other protective devices may be used (Figure 18-3); and efforts can be

Table 18-3
Practice Priorities in Occupational Health

Goal and Function	Prevention	Protection	Promotion
Goal	Elimination of hazardous substance or condition	Avoidance of injury or illness of high-risk workers	Attainment of an optimal level of personal health
Function	Job analysis Preplacement exams Hazard communication Materials handling and training Industrial hygiene sampling Health surveillance Safety measures on equipment Safer work procedures Walk-through evaluations	Personal safety measures: Hard hats Ear muffs or plugs Safety glasses Respirators Foot protection Skin barrier creams Legislation and regulation: OSHA standards Employees right-to-know laws	Wellness: Physical fitness Smoking cessation Nutritional awareness Stress management Screening: Health risk appraisal Cancer detection Diabetes and hypertension screening Health policy formulation: Smoking Alcohol Cafeteria meal planning

made to educate and motivate workers and managers to comply with safety procedures" (Public Health Service, 1979, p. 8).

The practice priority of protection becomes essential when hazardous exposures cannot be eliminated. Construction workers, for example, wear hard hats and steel-toed safety shoes to protect themselves from falling objects. Protection of workers is frequently achieved through legislation and regulation. The Occupational Safety and Health Act of 1970, discussed previously, provided the impetus for worker protection. More recently, employee right-to-know legislation has been passed in several states, focusing on training of employees who are working with potentially hazardous agents. The enforcement of such regulations will continue to be the key intervention for ensuring that workers are adequately protected on their jobs (Cheremisinoff, 1984).

Occupational safety programs available in many industries include plant surveillance, safety violation reporting, and worker safety education. Genetic screening, present in a few settings, identifies workers with sensitivity to specific hazards; however, it is a controversial program, criticized by labor and civil rights groups as an invasion of privacy. It may be more appropriate to protect all workers from those hazards (Hanlon and Pickett, 1984).

The practice priority of health promotion has appropriately received much attention and activity in the workplace over the past decade (Bruhn et al., 1987; Christenson et al., 1988; Fuchs et al., 1985). The workplace is an ideal setting in which to conduct health promotion efforts for two important reasons: (1) the vast majority of the healthy population may be reached at the work-

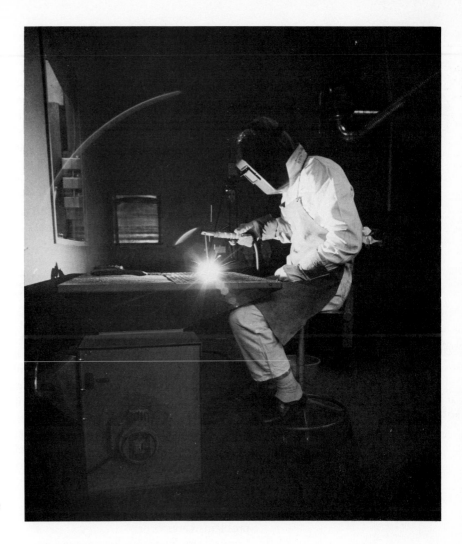

Figure 18-3
A welder wears protection
against ultraviolet light.

site, and (2) employers have viewed wellness programs as legitimate, worthwhile employee benefits to promote and support (Warner, 1987).

Of significance for community health is the fact that health promotion activities in the workplace can involve long-term interventions that will allow for a variety of educational and motivational strategies to be employed as well as a systematic plan for ongoing monitoring and evaluation of programs. The work environment itself can serve as a model healthy community. The adoption of positive health policies on such issues as smoking (Fielding, 1986), cafeteria meal planning, alcohol, and seat belt use will establish health norms for company personnel. Many of these positive health behaviors could also have an impact on employees' homes and families.

Typical health promotion programs include exercise, weight loss, smoking cessation, and nutrition education. There is growing evidence that wellness efforts are effective. Some research indicates that, as a result of wellness promotion, employees have shown increased self-esteem, improved job performance and job satisfaction, decreased absenteeism, and less use of company health services (Azarow and Cardy, 1981; Christenson et al., 1988; Warner, 1987; McGill, 1979). Health promotion programs in the workplace have the potential for providing a significant contribution to adult health as well as to research and development in this new arena of wellness. Cost and production incentives increasingly cause greater receptivity among employers to methods that enhance employee wellness (Warner, 1987). More research is needed to demonstrate the correlation between healthy employees and increased productivity on the job. Health promotion will continue to be a vital area of emphasis for the working community.

NONOCCUPATIONAL HEALTH SERVICES

Although employers are not required to provide treatment of nonoccupational (not incurred as a result of being on the job) injuries and illnesses, many companies do provide such services. One reason is that the location in which some health problems, such as muscle strain, influenza, and minor rashes, are acquired cannot easily be determined, thus making it simpler to provide service regardless of source. The on-site treatment of minor acute injury and illness as well as employee counseling is dependent on the philosophy of the company, the employment of an OHN, and the company's prior experience with offering these services as an employee benefit.

From the nurse's perspective, the advantages of offering nonoccupational health services are the following:

1. The OHN develops rapport with employees and can detect health problems early.
2. Loss of employee productive time is minimized when treatment is given on-site.
3. The OHN, through triage, can decide which cases require medical attention and which can be managed by the nurse (Figure 18-4).
4. The OHN can provide needed on-going personal health education and counseling in the context of a more holistic view of the worker.
5. On-site chronic disease management, such as hypertension monitoring, increases compliance, thereby saving costs of physician visits and complications associated with noncompliance with treatment.
6. The OHN provides employees with personal contact—a valued commodity in our high-technology work environments.

A concern expressed by a number of OHNs is that too much time can be spent in nonoccupational illness management to the neglect of a more ag-

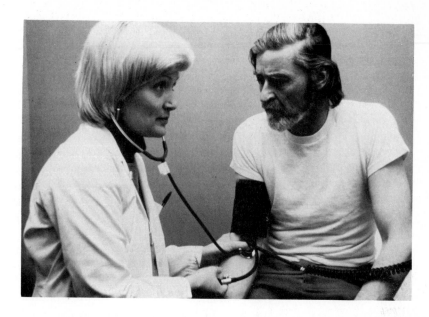

Figure 18-4
Early detection of warning signs that might lead to coronary artery disease or other illness is an important part of the occupational health nurse's preventive program.

gressive occupational health surveillance program. As OHNs learn more concerning the environmental factors that threaten the health of this population group, they will likely spend less time with illness management and move more aggressively into primary prevention, protection, and health promotion efforts (American Association of Occupational Health Nurses, 1984).

OCCUPATIONAL HEALTH: NURSING'S CONTRIBUTION AND CHALLENGE

Community health nurses have a long history of involvement in occupational health. In 1895, the Vermont Marble Company hired the first industrial nurse in the United States to care for its employees and their families. It was an unusual demonstration of interest in employee welfare at that time. The nursing service, consisting almost entirely of home visiting and care of the sick, was free to employees and their families. Gradually this nursing role changed. By World War II there was a striking increase in employment of industrial public health nurses who practiced illness prevention and health education among employees at work. In addition to emergency care and nursing of ill employees, the activities of many industrial nurses involved safety education, hygiene, nutrition, and improvement of working conditions. Yet a significantly high number of industrial injuries and sick employees kept many nurses too busy to do anything but illness care. They might see as many as 75 or more patients a day in the plant dispensary, where they provided first aid and medications (Kalisch and Kalisch, 1978). More recently, as we have seen, employee health programs have improved as socioeconomic and political pressures have created improved safety and health standards for the work environment. These changes have caused the role of the nurse to expand and change also.

As we examine occupational health and the role of the occupational health nurse, we must remind ourselves that traditional nursing practice with individuals and groups of employees is very different from aggregate nursing. We must again broaden our perspective to include the health needs of working population groups.

In 1979, Arthur D. Little, Inc. conducted a study of occupational health nursing. The findings revealed that occupational health nursing services contributed positively to employee health and morale. The study also concluded that on-site services were cost-effective because they reduced (1) lost work time, (2) insurance premiums, and (3) medical costs (Little, 1980).

The nurse's role in occupational health, as previously mentioned, has traditionally focused on illness and injury care. This has been the direct result of the knowledge and skills obtained in basic nursing education. During the last decade a number of nursing education programs (primarily on the graduate level) have developed a specialty focus in occupational health. In addition, many continuing education programs provide OHNs with updated information and skill training for identifying and assistance in managing the physical, chemical, biological, ergonomical, and psychosocial factors in the work environment that contribute to the health and safety of workers. As a result, the OHN's role is not universal; it is dependent on the type and philosophy of the company, type and number of workers, the health professionals involved, exposures and potential hazards in the work environment, and the knowledge and skills of the nurse.

Nurses who select the field of occupational health and safety will encounter significant differences from employment in the acute care setting (Bey et al., 1988). In order to make the adjustment, the nurse should be aware of the factors that make practice in occupational health unique (American Association of Occupational Health Nurses, 1988; Babbitz, 1984; Cox, 1985).

The *setting,* unlike hospitals or ambulatory care centers, is in a non-healthcare institution where production or service (not health care) is the goal of the organization. The OHN participates in the organization's goals through activities that will contribute to a productive work force.

The *position* of the OHN, in the organization is as staff (versus being a line employee). Although the nurse is generally responsible for the management of the occupational health unit, the OHN serves in the capacity of health consultant to line management personnel. Therefore, the power to effect change is not in any position of authority but in the OHN's expertise.

The *location* of the OHN contributes to isolationism. It is estimated that more than 65 percent of OHNs are the only health professionals in the industrial setting (Jacobson and Richard, 1982). This lack of on-site supervision and direction requires OHNs to be comfortable, competent, and independent decision makers. Because of their isolation, OHNs need to network with other nurses and professional organizations in the community for peer support and setting of appropriate occupational health standards (Jacobson and Richard, 1982).

The *client* served in occupational health is a well population with whom long-term contact is possible. For this reason, OHNs know their clients well and have opportunities to work with them through various stages of personal as well as health-service-related incidents. Exposure to this continuum of health care challenges OHNs to utilize all the community health nursing model interventions — education, engineering, and enforcement — described in Chapter 3.

Finally, the *practice focus* is aggregate oriented; the nurse serves a worker population group. Environmental factors significantly influence the health and safety of workers. Therefore, OHNs need to constantly monitor the work environment and assess the health needs of the entire worker population in order to identify populations at risk, such as men in hazardous lines of work (Ossler, 1986) or older workers (Poore, 1986), and develop prevention, promotion, and protection programs. Nurses with community health experience, an aggregate focus, and strong managerial skills are in the best position to meet the needs of this population.

COMMUNITY-BASED OCCUPATIONAL HEALTH

Agencies external to business and industry also provide occupational health nursing services. Historically, public health nurses of visiting nurse associations made home visits to sick employees and their families. In subsequent years, public health agencies provided part-time nursing services to small companies. These services included supervising the work environment, conducting health examinations, keeping records, teaching health, health counseling, providing first aid, giving immunizations, and referring workers to community resources. More recently, community health nursing services have offered health screening and health promotion programs (American Association of Occupational Health Nurses, 1988). Furthermore, OHN consultants based in state departments of health provide consultation and continuing education programs to nurses employed in occupational health settings.

Hospital-based occupational health programs, large medical-industrial health clinics, and insurance companies also provide occupational health nursing services. These services may be in the form of direct care (rehabilitation of an injured worker) or indirect care (consultation on implementing regulations regarding record keeping or compiling health data statistics).

A continuing unmet public health need is the health of workers in smaller companies (approximately 100 or fewer employees). These companies have more hazards because equipment and controls are often inadequate. They seldom, if ever, have a health professional on site, nor has the community provided health services that would meet their needs. Attempts have been made by some communities, but no sustained efforts exist. Community health nurses are in a position to accept this challenge and develop a system that will ensure ongoing service to this high-risk population.

Community health nurses continue to have a significant role in occupational health, both directly and indirectly. Let us consider how you as an OHN might practice nursing with the working community.

EMPLOYEE HEALTH CASE STUDY

You have just been hired, let us imagine, as a full-time OHN for Allied Electronics, a firm that manufactures and sells electronic components and equipment. Allied's 450 employees are scattered through its sprawling five-acre plant located on the edge of the city. At present, Allied's health program consists of several components. The health service, run by the nurse, provides emergency care for employees who are injured or become ill on the job. An on-call physician has left standing orders for the nurse to use in emergencies and sick care. Regular checking for real or potential hazards in the work environment is done through the safety division by the plant safety engineer. Allied pays for a large percentage of employee health care through its health benefits program; this is precisely why Allied has hired you. Health insurance premiums per employee have skyrocketed, and managers are looking for alternative solutions to lower health provision costs. They would like you to develop a new approach to employee health.

NURSING GOALS

A broad goal for occupational health is to promote and maintain the highest level of physical, social, and emotional health of all workers (Hanlon and Pickett, 1984; American Association of Occupational Health Nurses, 1988). In actual practice, this goal is only beginning to be realized in selected instances. Nevertheless, it is a worthy and, more important, an essential objective in the realization of an energized and productive working community.

We can address this goal more specifically through the following five working goals that guide occupational health nursing practice. These goals summarize a comprehensive listing of occupational health nursing competencies developed by M. J. Keller (1971) and combine them with the AAOHN job descriptions for OHNs (1984).

1. Assess the health needs of employees and intervene to promote and maintain their highest possible level of wellness.
2. Monitor and study factors in the work environment that pose real or potential hazards to employee health, and take action to minimize their impact or prevent their occurrence.
3. Provide early diagnosis and prompt treatment for injury or illness on the job.

4. Provide programs for employees with disease or disability aimed at restoring and maintaining their maximum level of functioning.
5. Maintain accurate records of employee illness and injury to provide an on-going data base for research and program planning.

THE OCCUPATIONAL HEALTH TEAM

Even as you consider these goals, you realize that you will not be pursuing them alone. Like most community health efforts, your work will require collaboration with others. Company management and administrative personnel will be important partners with you in this venture. As Keller (1979, p. 414) points out, "The philosophy and vision of these administrative persons can make or break the contribution of the nurse and the development of her full potential." Collaboration may take time but will be worth the investment. Your goal is to gain the respect and trust of management and establish open communication lines in order that you may influence company policies regarding the nature and scope of its health program.

The company physician is another important health team member with whom the nurse collaborates. Whether working full-time, part-time, or on-call, the physician has a strong influence on the company's health policies and programs. Development of a positive working relationship with the physician gives the nurse a powerful supporter of proposals and program efforts.

Based in health service, usually a part of personnel services, the nurse works closely with other professional, technical, and clerical personnel, particularly those from the safety, engineering, and industrial hygiene departments. Any comprehensive assessment of employee health and safety problems, as well as any health promotion program, requires cooperation and assistance from many individuals working in various departments within the organization.

Finally, the occupational health team is not complete without the workers themselves (Babbitz, 1984). You will want to encourage employees to identify problems and needs. They can also contribute to decision making regarding health programs. Their cooperation in implementing and evaluating programs is essential for an effective health protection and promotion effort.

As the only nurse at Allied, you will particularly need skills in effective communication, leadership, change management, and assertiveness. These tools will be crucial to effectively interpreting your role and promoting your ideas. Your goal is to establish positive working relationships with the other team members, on whom your success depends.

NURSING SERVICES

Nurses involved in occupational health have a unique opportunity to help shape the health profile of the working population. The degree of that influence depends on how the nurse defines her role. Also, the nurse must be able to overcome the many obstacles incurred in the occupational setting, including restrictive company policy, misunderstanding of the nurse's role, and lack of time for innovative program development. The nurse's role in occupational health, therefore, still varies considerably. It ranges from only providing emergency care for injuries or illness on the job to establishing comprehensive policies and programs covering health promotion, accident and disease prevention, and innovative care for disease and disability (Cox, 1985).

Meeting Employee Needs

Occupational health nursing applies the philosophy and skills of nursing and community health to protecting and promoting the health of people in the context of their employment (Brown, 1981; Jacobson and Richard, 1982; Babbitz, 1984). In other words, the OHN relies on in-depth nursing preparation as well as a strong community health background to provide the tools and perspectives necessary for meeting the challenges of occupational health. Many nurses in occupational health acquire additional physical assessment and management skills as well.

Specifically, some of your typical nursing activities in the new job will include history taking, partial physical examinations, ordering of tests, and emergency care. You will refer many employees for further treatment and follow-up care. Keeping health records will be an expected part of your job, but it can be largely delegated to clerical help. You will participate in conducting health education and health counseling sessions for groups as well as for individual employees. Health assessment, screening, and monitoring are also important aspects of your role.

In order to keep a proper perspective on your goals and also to begin developing a more innovative approach to meeting the employees' health needs (the reason you were hired), you do some strategic planning. You review your five main goals, develop specific objectives for each one, and schedule times when the activities to meet those objectives will be done.

Meeting most of the individual and group needs of employees can be accomplished by scheduling health service hours, classes, and counseling sessions. You plan time to visit departments, observe, and interview selected personnel as part of your health assessment process.

You know there is a relationship between the health of the employees (a population group) and the health of Allied Electronics (an organization). Consequently, you keep a running log of observations on how the company functions and what its effects are on the employees. For example, you notice that some departments seem to place greater stress on their workers than other departments. Among these workers there is a higher incidence of hypertension, headaches, gastrointestinal disturbances, and other somatic complaints. You collect data on the working conditions in those departments. Is there high production pressure? Are there any opportunities to relieve stress on the job? Do workers receive any positive feedback about their work? Could the symptoms be caused or aggravated by some environmental factor such as chemical gases, or noise? (See Figure 18-5.)

Assessment Strategies

To assess the health needs of the total employee population and selected smaller population groups within the company, you use several approaches. You first enlist the assistance of the company computer services, compile the results of individual health histories and physical examinations, and analyze the findings. A picture emerges of dominant health problems among the employees and of the workers at greatest risk for other problems.

It appears that hypertension, overweight, excessive smoking, and inadequate exercise are the major problems common to Allied's employee population. You can attack these problems on several fronts. You start a regular program of blood pressure monitoring. The employee health education program can be upgraded with new videotapes and literature to make workers more health concious and show them how to improve their health. Specifically, they learn how to lose weight, manage stress, stop smoking, and maintain an exercise program. More important than information, however, is motivation. You convince management that company inducements, such as Resource Trust Company's payment for Weight Watchers costs, are important in stimulating employee participation. You tell them about the Speedcall Corporation of Hayward, California, which pays its workers a seven-dollar weekly bonus if they do not smoke on the job. After two years on this program, 20 of 24 smokers had quit smoking on the job (*Minnesota Council on Health News-*

Figure 18-5
The work environment can contribute to or detract from employees' health. Effects of hazards, noise, and toxic chemicals are examples of the nurse's concerns for the workers in this auto assembly plant.

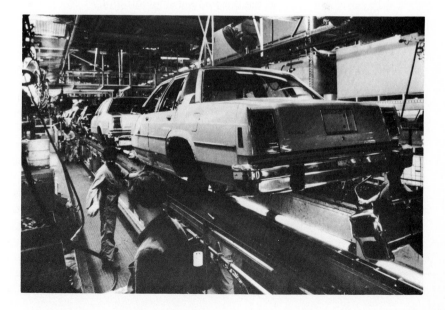

letter, 1979, January). Ball Electronics gives workers time for exercise breaks (*Wellness Gazette,* 1980, January). A number of Milwaukee, Wisconsin, companies, some of them splitting the cost between employer and employee, have enrolled employees in the Milwaukee YMCA fitness programs. Allied's management agrees to give time for exercise breaks, a weekly bonus to employees who stop smoking on the job, and a quarterly bonus to those whose blood pressure readings are within normal limits.

Another approach that you use to assess the health needs of the employee population is to conduct an environmental survey of health hazards. Using data from the safety division's regular spot checking, you collaborate with the division on systematic observations of working conditions and interviews of workers. In addition, you post suggestion boxes and gain management's approval to give any employee half a day off with pay for suggesting a safety or health improvement that is implemented into the health program. You gain further ideas from other companies' measures. For example, Scherer Brothers Lumber Company in Minneapolis has removed cigarette machines and stocked other vending machines with nutritionally beneficial foods, such as granola bars, yogurt, and fruit drinks. The company provides fresh fruit instead of sweet rolls to its employees without charge. It has reduced its noise levels, provided a health maintenance organization medical insurance option to encourage illness prevention, and initiated a committee of employees to plan wellness activities (*Minnesota Council on Health Newsletter,* 1979, October).

To assess employee population health further, you participate in a committee composed of the company physician and other personnel to analyze accidents, injuries, and illnesses. The findings reveal a high percentage of injuries and absenteeism. One possible solution is to offer incentive pay similar to the programs instituted by other companies. Parsons Pine Products, Inc., an Ashland, Oregon, manufacturing plant, had a high rate of accidents and absenteeism. Management offered incentive pay to encourage employee wellness. For each month that workers were not absent or late they received eight hours of extra pay. In addition, if they had no injury accidents during the quarter, they received two more hours of pay per month. As a result, absenteeism was reduced by 30 percent, accident rates dropped from 86 percent above average to almost zero, and the company's medical insurance costs dropped (*Minnesota Council on Health Newsletter,* 1978, September). Scherer Brothers also uses "wellness pay." For each month that employees are not absent from work because of illness, they receive two hours of extra pay (*Minnesota Council on Health Newsletter,* 1979, October).

Another problem uncovered in your analysis is a rising incidence of back injuries among Allied's production workers. You learn that Ball Electronics has a similar problem, and you consider its approach. Ball has instituted a voluntary exercise program. Once or twice a day, assembly line workers engage in five-minute limbering and strengthening exercises near their work stations. They are also invited to use the company exercise room, attend optional exercise classes offered at break times (lasting five extra minutes for employees on company time) and after work, and join the company running club. The program resulted in improved productive efficiency and job satisfaction but had not been in effect long enough to measure direct impact on back injuries (*Minnesota Council on Health Newsletter,* 1979, October). In the meantime you offer literature on backache prevention and present two classes, one at noon and the other at the beginning of the afternoon shift, on ways to strengthen back muscles and prevent injuries.

Each set of data gathered through the various assessment approaches gives you material to guide your planning and development of health programs. An important dimension in this process is accurate record keeping. Exact figures on incidence and prevalence of health problems in the company give you ammunition to justify your programs and data with which to compare the result when you evaluate program outcomes.

Occupational health nursing demands a great deal from the nurse. Individual needs in the workplace will always compete for the nurse's time and attention with aggregate needs, often to the detriment of the latter. To maintain a proper focus on aggregate needs requires discipline and commitment, commitment based on a different mind-set and the realization that health and productivity of workers is interrelated with the health of the community. The factors that contribute to the health of workers, namely the workplace and the community-at-large, are a responsibility of all who serve as community health nurses.

Summary

The working population, composed of well adults, makes up the majority of the American people. The profile of this aggregate is changing from an industrialized labor force to a greater proportion of white-collar workers and professionals.

Five types of environmental factors, common to all work settings, can influence worker health or safety. Physical, or structural, elements include such things as temperature and noise extremes. Chemical factors are the potentially hazardous chemical agents present. Biological organisms, such as viruses, bacteria, and fungi, may contaminate the work environment and cause disease. Ergonomical factors include the customs, design, and expectations of the job that influence the way people interact with their work environment. Psychosocial factors are the workers' feelings and behavior in response to the job. Assessment of all these is critical in determining appropriate occupational health interventions.

Worker health has only recently become a target for health intervention. Historically, workers have suffered unhealthy, dangerous working conditions and contracted debilitating, often fatal, diseases and injuries directly attributable to their employment. The labor movement and workmen's compensation laws turned the tide in favor of workers' rights in the early 1900s.

Several important laws affecting worker health and safety have been passed since 1911. Two of the more significant of these are the Occupational Safety and Health Act of 1970 and the Hazard Communication Act of 1986.

Chronic diseases are the prime threat to the health of the adult working population. Cancer ranks highest in mortality rates, heart disease second, and accidents third. Leading work-related health problems include occupational lung disease, injuries, and occupational cancers.

Programs designed to serve the health needs of the working population vary with occupational site and assessment of needs unique to that setting. Occupational health services encompass the three public health practice priorities — prevention, protection, and health promotion. Preventive programs seek to eliminate potential hazards to worker health and safety. Protective services shield workers from remaining hazards. Health promotion, or wellness, programs seek to maintain and improve the personal health of workers. Health services for workers may also cover nonoccupational illness.

OHNs practice in settings where the production of goods and services is the goal of the organization. The OHN's role requires management skills and expertise in environmental and adult health. OHNs generally work independently and serve population groups on a long-term basis. Community health nurses based in other agencies may also serve occupational health clients, often on a contractual basis with the company.

Occupational health nursing applies the philosophy and skills of nursing and community health to protecting and promoting the health of people in the context of their employment. The nurse must view the client population as a whole, work with other company professionals to assess worker health needs and the needs associated with the work environment, and then design, implement, and evaluate health services.

Study Questions

1. The hospital work environment poses many potential threats to its employees' health. Select a unit in the hospital with which you are familiar, and identify one health hazard for each of the five factors described in this chapter.
2. What is one method of control (protection or prevention) that you would suggest for each of the five factors identified above?
3. If you were asked to offer a weight control program for a local industry of 100 employees, what steps would you consider taking to develop such a program?

References

American Association of Occupational Health Nurses. (1984). *Job descriptions for occupational health nurses.* Atlanta: Author.

American Association of Occupational Health Nurses. (1988). The year 2000: Health objectives for the nation. *American Association of Occupational Health Nurses' Journal* 36(6): 285–88.

Arbab, D., and L. Weidner. (1986). Infectious diseases and field water supply and sanitation among migrant farm workers. *American Journal of Public Health* 76(6): 694–95.

Azarow, J., and W. Cardy. (1981, November). Health on the job: Change the worker or change the workplace. Paper presented at the Annual Meeting of the American Public Health Association, Los Angeles.

Babbitz, M. A. (1984). The practice of occupational health nursing in the United States. *Occupational Health Nursing* 31(6): 23–25.

Baker, E., J. Melius, and J. Millar. (1988). Surveillance of occupational illness and injury in the U.S.: Current perspectives and future directions. *Journal of Public Health Policy* (Summer): 198–221.

Bey, J. M., et al. (1988). How management and nurses perceive occupational health nursing. *American Association of Occupational Health Nurses' Journal* 36(2): 61–69.

Brown, M. L. (1981). *Occupational health nursing: Principles and practice.* New York: Springer.

Bruhn, J. G., et al. (1987). Promoting healthy behavior in the workplace. *Health Values* 11(5): 39–48.

Centers for Disease Control. (1988). NIOSH recommendations for occupational safety and health standards. *Mortality and Morbidity Weekly Report* 37(S-7): 1–29.

Cheremisinoff, P. N. (1984). *Management of hazardous occupational environments.* Lancaster, Pa.: Technomic Publishing.

Christenson, G., et al. (1988). Highlights from the National Survey of Worksite Health Promotion Activities. *Health Values* 12(2): 29–33.

Clever, L. H. (1981). Health hazards of hospital personnel. *Western Journal of Medicine* 135: 162–65.

Cox, A. R. (1985). Profile of the occupational health nurse. *Occupational Health Nursing* 33(12): 591–93.

Fielding, J. E. (1986). Banning worksite smoking. *American Journal of Public Health* 76(8): 957–59.

Froines, J., C. Dellenbaugh, and D. Wegman. (1986). Occupational health surveillance: A means to identify work-related risks. *American Journal of Public Health* 76(9): 1089–96.

Fuchs, J. A., et al. (1985). The evolving concept of worksetting health promotion. *Health Values* 9(4): 3–6.

Gordon, N., P. Cleary, C. Parker, and C. Czeisler. (1986). The prevalence and health impact of shiftwork. *American Journal of Public Health* 76(10): 1225–28.

Gough, P., et al. (1988). Combating the pressure . . . occupational stress. *Nursing Times* 84(2): 43–45.

Hanlon, J., and G. Pickett. (1984). *Public health: Administration and practice.* 8th ed. St. Louis: Times Mirror/Mosby.

Jacobsen, F., T. Wehr, D. Sack, S. James, and N. Rosenthal. (1987). Seasonal affective disorder: A review of the syndrome and its public health implications. *American Journal of Public Health* 77(1): 57–60.

Jacobson, R., and E. Richard. (1982). Occupational health nursing: A public health perspective. In B. Spradley (ed.), *Readings in community health nursing.* 2nd ed. Boston: Little, Brown.

Kalisch, P., and B. Kalisch. (1978). *The advance of American nursing.* Boston: Little, Brown.

Keller, M. (1979). Health needs and nursing care of the labor force. In M. J. Fromer (ed.), *Community health care and the nursing process.* St. Louis: C. V. Mosby.

Keller, M. J., in association with W. T. May. (1971). *Occupational health content in baccalaureate nursing education.* Cincinnati, Ohio: National Institute of Occupational Safety and Health.

Key, M., A. Henschel, J. Butler, R. Ligo, and I. Tabershaw, (eds.). (1977). *Occupational diseases: A guide to their recognition* (rev. ed.) (DHEW [NIOSH] Pub. No. 77-181). Washington, D.C.: U.S. Government Printing Office.

Last, J. (1987). *Public health and human ecology.* East Norwalk, Conn.: Appleton and Lange.

Lee, J. (1978). *The new nurse in industry: A guide for the newly employed occupational health nurse* (DHEW [NIOSH] Pub. No. 78-143). Cincinnati, Ohio: U.S. Government Printing Office.

Levy, B. S., and D. H. Wegman. (1988). *Occupational health: Recognizing and preventing work-related disease.* 2nd ed. Boston: Little, Brown.

Little, A. D. (1980). *Costs and benefits of occupational health nursing.* (DHEW [NIOSH] Pub. No. 80-140). Cincinnati, Ohio: U.S. Government Printing Office.

McGill, A. M. (ed.). (1979). *Proceedings of the National Conference on Health Promotion Programs in Occupational Settings.* DHHS, Office of the Assistant Secretary for Health. Washington, D.C.: U.S. Government Printing Office.

Minnesota Council on Health Newsletter. (1978, September). Minneapolis, Minn.: Minnesota Council on Health.

Minnesota Council on Health Newsletter. (1979, January). Minneapolis, Minn.: Minnesota Council on Health.

Minnesota Council on Health Newsletter. (1979, October). Minneapolis, Minn.: Minnesota Council on Health.

Morris, R. B. (ed.). (1976). *The United States Department of Labor bicentennial history of the American worker.* Washington, D.C.: U.S. Government Printing Office.

National Center for Health Statistics. (1988). *Vital Statistics of the United States, 1986, Volume II, Mortality, Part A.* DHHS Pub. No. (PHS)88-1122. Public Health Service, Washington, D.C.: U.S. Government Printing Office.

National Institute for Occupational Safety and Health. (1986). *NIOSH recommendations for occupational safety and health standards.* Atlanta: Center for Disease Control, DHHS.

Office of Technology Assessment, U.S. Congress (1985). *Preventing illness and injury in the workplace* (a), Publication No. OTA-H-256. Washington, D.C.: U.S. Government Printing Office.

Olishifski, J. B. (ed.). (1979). *Fundamentals of industrial hygiene.* 2nd ed. Chicago: National Safety Council.

Ossler, C. C. (1986). Men's work environments and health risks. *Nursing Clinics of North America* 21(1): 25–36.

Poore, M. (1986). Older workers. *Journal of Occupational Safety and Health* 55(8): 12–15.

Public Health Service. (1979). *Healthy people: The Surgeon General's report on health promotion and disease prevention* (DHEW Publication No. 79-55071). Washington, D.C.: U.S. Government Printing Office.

Robinson, J. C. (1988). The rising long-term trend in occupational injury rates. *American Journal of Public Health* 78(3): 276–81.

Sax, N. I. (1986). *Dangerous properties of industrial materials.* 5th ed. New York: D. VanNostrand.

Silverstein, M., et al. (1985). Mortality among workers exposed to coal tar pitch volatiles and welding emissions: An exercise in epidemiologic triage. *American Journal of Public Health* 75(11): 1283–87.

Sorensen, G., T. Pechacek, and U. Pallonene. (1986). Occupational and worksite norms and attitudes about smoking cessation. *American Journal of Public Health* 76(5): 544–49.

Sundin, D. S., D. H. Pedersen, and T. M. Frazier. (1986). Occupational hazard and health surveillance. *American Journal of Public Health* 716(9): 1083–84.

U.S. Bureau of the Census. (1989). *Statistical abstract of the United States, 1989.* 109th ed. Washington, D.C.: U.S. Government Printing Office.

Veninga, R., and J. Spradley. (1981). *The work-stress connection.* Boston: Little, Brown.

Warner, K. E. (1987). Selling health promotion to corporate America: Uses and abuses of the economic argument. *Health Education Quarterly* 14(1): 39–55.

Wegman, D. H., and J. R. Froines. (1985). Surveillance needs for occupational health. *American Journal of Public Health* 75(11): 1259–61.

Wellness Gazette. (1980, January). Minneapolis, Minn.: Minnesota Council on Health.

White, M. S. (1982). Construct for public health nursing. *Nursing Outlook 30:* 527–530.

Whorton, M., S. Larson, N. Gordon, and R. Morgan. (1987). Investigation and workup of tight building syndrome. *Journal of Occupational Medicine* 29(2): 142–47.

Williams, P. L., and J. L. Burson (eds.). (1985). *Industrial toxicology: Safety and health implications in the workplace.* New York: VanNostrand Reinhold.

Selected Readings

American Association of Occupational Health Nurses. (1984). *Job descriptions for occupational health nurses.* Atlanta: Author.

American Association of Occupational Health Nurses. (1988). The year 2000: Health objectives for the nation. *American Association of Occupational Health Nurses' Journal* 36(6): 285–88.

American Public Health Association. (1975). *Chart book: Health and work in America.* Washington, D.C.: U.S. Government Printing Office.

Arbab, D., and L. Weidner. (1986). Infectious diseases and field water supply and sanitation among migrant farm workers. *American Journal of Public Health* 76(6): 694–95.

Babbitz, M. A. (1984). The practice of occupational health nursing in the United States. *Occupational Health Nursing* 31(6): 23–25.

Baker, E., J. Melius, and J. Millar. (1988). Surveillance of occupational illness and injury in the U.S: Current perspectives and future directions. *Journal of Public Health Policy* (Summer): 198–221.

Bey, J. M., et al. (1988). How management and nurses perceive occupational health nursing. *American Association of Occupational Health Nurses' Journal* 36(2): 61–69.

Bezold, C., R. J. Carlson, and J. Peck. (1986). *The future of work and health.* Dover, Mass.: Auburn Publishing.

Brown, M. L. (1981). *Occupational health nursing: Principles and practice.* New York: Springer.

Bruhn, J. G., et al. (1987). Promoting healthy behavior in the workplace. *Health Values* 11(5): 39–48.

Bulow-Hube, S., et al. (1987). The innovation-decision model and workplace health promotion programs. *Health Education Research* 2(1): 15–25.

Centers for Disease Control. (1988). NIOSH recommendations for occupational safety and health standards. *Mortality and Morbidity Weekly Report* 37(S-7): 1–29.

Cheremisinoff, P. N. (1984). *Management of hazardous occupational environments.* Lancaster, Pa: Technomic Publishing.

Christenson, G., et al. (1988). Highlights from the National Survey of Worksite Health Promotion Activities. *Health Values* 12(2): 29–33.

Clever, L. H. (1981). Health hazards of hospital personnel. *Western Journal of Medicine* 135: 162–65.

Cox, A. R. (1985). Profile of the occupational health nurse. *Occupational Health Nursing* 33(12): 591–93.

Dobson, E. A. (1987). Good health for women. *Health Visitor* 60(11): 363.

Fielding, J., and L. Breslow. (1983). Health promotion programs sponsored by California employers. *American Journal of Public Health* 73(5): 538–42.

Fielding, J. E. (1986). Banning worksite smoking. *American Journal of Public Health* 76(8): 957–59.

Froines, J., C. Dellenbaugh, and D. Wegman. (1986). Occupational health surveillance: A means to identify work-related risks. *American Journal of Public Health* 76(9): 1089–96.

Fuchs, J. A., et al. (1985). The evolving concept of worksetting health promotion. *Health Values* 9(4): 3–6.

Girdano, D. A. (1986). *Occupational health promotion: A practical guide to program development*. New York: Macmillan.

Goodman, A., S. Freidman, S. Beatrice, and S. Bart. (1987). Rubella in the workplace: The need for employee immunization. *American Journal of Public Health* 77(6): 725–26.

Gough, P., et al. (1988). Combatting the pressure . . . occupational stress. *Nursing Times* 84(2): 43–45.

Hanlon, J., and G. Pickett. (1984). *Public health: Administration and practice*. 8th ed. St. Louis: Times Mirror/Mosby.

Jacobson, R., and E. Richard. (1982). Occupational health nursing: A public health perspective. In B. Spradley (ed.), *Readings in community health nursing*. 2nd ed. Boston: Little, Brown.

Keller, M. (1983). Health needs and nursing care of the labor force. In M. J. Fromer, *Community health care and the nursing process*. 2nd ed. St. Louis: C. V. Mosby.

Last, J. (1987). *Public health and human ecology*. East Norwalk, Conn.: Appleton and Lange.

Lee, J. (1978). The new nurse in industry: A guide for the newly employed occupational health nurse. (DHEW [NIOSH] Publication No. 78-143). Cincinnati, Ohio: U.S. Government Printing Office.

Lee, J. S. (1983). Environmental evaluation of the workplace. *Family and Community Health* 6(2): 16–23.

Levy, B. S., and D. H. Wegman. (1988). *Occupational health: Recognizing and preventing work-related disease*. 2nd ed. Boston: Little, Brown.

Levy, S. R. (1986). Worksite health promotion. *Family and Community Health* 9(3): 1–13.

Little, A. D. (1980). Costs and benefits of occupational health nursing. (DHEW [NIOSH] Publication No. 80-140). Cincinnati, Ohio: U.S. Government Printing Office.

Mattson, M. T., et al. (1988). Worksite health promotion: Some important questions. *Health Values* 12(1): 23–28.

Morris, R. B. (ed.). (1976). *The United States Department of Labor bicentennial history of the American worker*. Washington, D.C.: U.S. Government Printing Office.

National Center for Health Statistics. (1988). *Vital Statistics of the United States, 1986, Volume II, Mortality, Part A*. DHHS Pub. No. (PHS)88-1122. Public Health Service, Washington, D.C.: U.S. Government Printing Office.

National Institute for Occupational Safety and Health. (1983). *Program plan by program areas for FY 1983*. (DHHS Publication No. 83-102). Washington, D.C.: U.S. Government Printing Office.

Office of Technology Assessment, U.S. Congress. (1985). *Preventing illness and injury in the workplace* (a). Publication No. OTA-H-256. Washington, D.C.: U.S. Government Printing Office.

Office of Technology Assessment, U.S. Congress. (1985). *Reproductive hazards in the workplace* (b). Publication No. 052-003-01001-1. Washington, D.C.: U.S. Government Printing Office.

Olishifski, J. B. (ed.). (1979). Fundamentals of industrial hygiene. 2nd ed. Chicago: National Safety Council.

Ossler, C. C. (1986). Men's work environments and health risks. *Nursing Clinics of North America* 21(1): 25–36.

Poore, M. (1986). Older workers. *Journal of Occupational Safety and Health* 55(8): 12–15.

Public Health Service. (1979). *Healthy people: The Surgeon General's report on health promotion and disease prevention* (DHEW Publication No. 79-55071). Washington, D.C.: U.S. Government Printing Office.

Richter, E., and Kretzmer, D. (1980). Prevention through pre-review in occupational health and safety. *American Journal of Public Health* 70(2): 157–59.

Robinson, J. C. (1988). The rising long-term trend in occupational injury rates. *American Journal of Public Health* 78(3): 276–81.

Rutstein, D., et al. (1983). Sentinel health events (occupational): A basis for physician recognition and public health surveillance. *American Journal of Public Health* 73(9): 1054–62.

Sax, N. I. (1986). *Dangerous properties of industrial materials*. 5th ed. New York: D. VanNostrand.

Seligman, P., W. Halperin, R. Mullan, and T. Frazier. (1986). Occupational lead poisoning in Ohio: Surveillance using worker's compensation data. *American Journal of Public Health* 76(11): 1299–1302.

Sundin, D. S., D. H. Pedersen, and T. M. Frazier. (1986). Occupational hazard and health surveillance. *American Journal of Public Health* 716(9): 1083–84.

U.S. Bureau of the Census. (1989). *Statistical abstract of the United States, 1989*. 109th ed. Washington, D.C.: U.S. Government Printing Office.

Veninga, K. A. (1983). How to establish a nutrition education program. *Occupational Health Nursing* 31(12): 34–38.

Veninga, R., and J. P. Spradley. (1981). The work–stress connection. Boston: Little, Brown.

Warner, K. E. (1987). Selling health promotion to corporate America: Uses and abuses of the economic argument. *Health Education Quarterly* 14(1): 39–55.

Wegman, D. H., and J. R. Froines. (1985). Surveillance needs for occupational health. *American Journal of Public Health* 75(11): 1259–61.

Whorton, M., S. Larson, N. Gordon, and R. Morgan. (1987). Investigation and workup of tight building syndrome. *Journal of Occupational Medicine* 29(2): 142–47.

Williams, P. L., and J. L. Burson (eds.). (1985). *Industrial toxicology: Safety and health implications in the workplace*. New York: VanNostrand Reinhold.

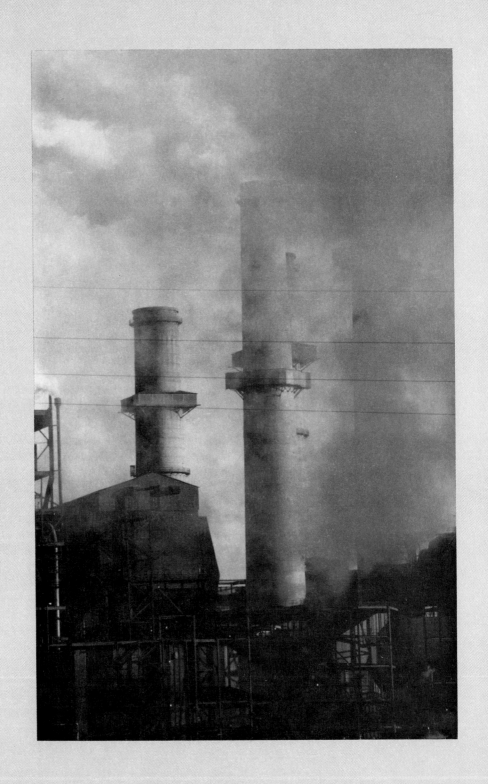

19 Environmental Health

Laura Spradley Harris
Barbara Walton Spradley

Environmental conditions strongly influence people's health status, so the study of environmental health has tremendous meaning for community health nurses. Broadly defined, environmental health encompasses all those elements of the environment that influence people's health and well-being, such as the conditions of workplaces, homes, communities, or cities. It also includes the many forces—chemical, physical, and psychological—that are present in the environment and affect human health.

Different environments pose different health problems and benefits (Figure 19-1). Consider the effects of acid rain, soil erosion, and insect invasions on the inhabitants of a rural community, as opposed to the effects of industrial toxic wastes and airport noise on those living in an urban setting. The health effects of a hot, dry climate are different from those of an arctic area, and the environmental conditions of an industrialized nation are dramatically different from those of a third-world country.

The concept of environmental health encompasses many topics. Some areas of community health nursing that involve environmental health, such as occupational health, home health care, and epidemiology, are covered in more detail in other chapters. In this chapter we address these areas broadly and focus specifically on other environmental considerations affecting public health, including historical perspectives and discussions of toxic agents in the environment, chemical hazards, air pollution, radiation, environmentally related accidents, safety, psychological hazards related to the environment, and governmental and private-sector roles in controlling environmental health. Throughout the chapter, we discuss implications for the community health nurse, and we conclude with a set of assessment and intervention guidelines for community health nursing practice.

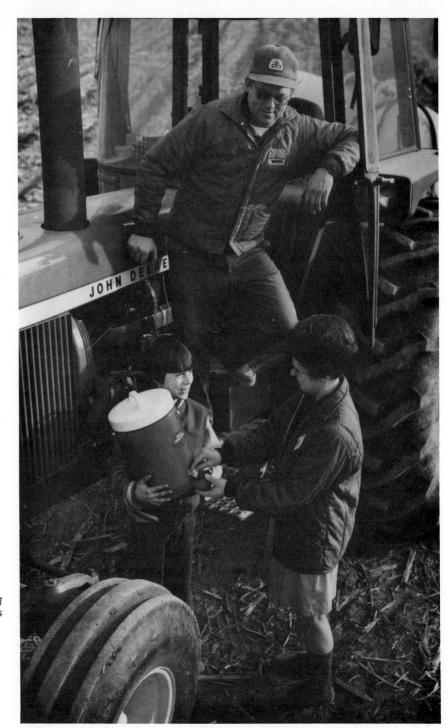

Figure 19-1
Every environmental setting
offers unique advantages as
well as unique problems.
Here a farm family enjoys
work and refreshment
together, yet the dangers
posed by use of heavy
farm equipment and
pesticides present safety
and health threats.

ENVIRONMENTAL HEALTH CONSIDERATIONS

Determining environmental health means more than looking for illness or disease-causing agents; it also means assessing the quality of the environment. Do the conditions of both the man-made and the natural environment combine to provide a health-enhancing milieu? One needs to ask not only whether people's surroundings have clean air and are free from hazardous substances, but whether they are clean and aesthetically pleasing. Is the environment not only physically comfortable but also sufficiently stimulating?

PREVENTIVE MEASURES

The study of environmental health has become increasingly complex as people's influence on the environment has increased. With the unprecedented advances in science and technology that have taken place in the past few decades, our ability to affect the environment has expanded and the implications are not fully comprehended. New forms of energy and new synthetic chemical substances appear each year with such rapidity that we cannot anticipate all the potential side effects on our environment and in turn on our health. For each advance and "improvement" the toll we must pay is frequently not known. Therefore, scientists must use foresight as they design innovations, government officials must play watchdog, and those concerned with human and environmental health must monitor new developments and intervene when appropriate. Health practitioners need to determine causal links between people and their environment with an eye to improving the health and well-being of both. Community health nurses should be aware of environmental health factors when treating either communities or individuals as clients. Nurses should be alert to potential problems in the environment, whether they are physical hazards, such as lack of stair railings, or psychological factors, such as the stress of poverty or overcrowded living conditions. Not only do community health nurses need to be able to identify possible causal agents of health problems, they must also be aware enough to help prevent environmentally related illness, and know who to contact if an environmental health hazard is detected.

HOLISTIC/ECOLOGICAL PERSPECTIVE

When considering environmental health, it is important to keep in mind the total relationship between people and their environment. One cannot isolate a single causal factor in many cases, since there may be many causal relationships. Furthermore, the development of a cure for one evil may create another.

We need a holistic, or ecological, viewpoint. The concept of environmental health is often reduced to a focus on specific health hazards, or factors in an environment that pose a health threat to the people living there, but "for those charged with the protection and enhancement of the environment, a broad concept of human–environment relationships is of critical importance" (Hanlon and Pickett, 1984, p. 319).

By taking an ecological approach in studying environmental health, the community health nurse can examine how environmental conditions affect humans and their health and also how humans affect their environments. Hanlon and Pickett describe this ecological perspective as "a recognition of the fact that we can affect our environment and our environment can affect us and that preventive and promotive measures may be applied to all aspects of our environment as well as to ourselves" (Hanlon and Pickett, 1984, p. 362). An ecological perspective takes into account the interconnectedness of all living organisms and their physical environment. It recognizes that any manipulation of one element or organism may have hazardous effects on the rest of the environment, upsetting the balance of the ecosystem. No one factor, whether organism or substance, can be viewed in isolation from the rest of its environment. For example, several years ago the spraying of pesticides on a watermelon crop on the west coast of the United States resulted in a serious outbreak of anticholinesterase intoxication. The food-borne pesticide caused 264 reported cases in Oregon, Washington, and California. After eating aldicarb-contaminated watermelons, people experienced nausea, vomiting, abdominal pain, diarrhea, blurred vision, dysarthria, and other neurological signs (Green et al., 1987). We must keep in mind that our actions affect other living organisms. We share this planet with millions of other living creatures, so we must consider the ecological balance and anticipate the far-reaching consequences of our actions before introducing environmental change.

VIEW OF THE CLIENT

In studying environmental health it is important for us to consider our clients not only as individuals and communities but as a species. Providing the necessities for a healthy human environment and the survival of the human species, we must take into account not only present generations but future ones as well. We must consider food and fuel limitations of the natural environment, attend to conservation by balancing present and future needs, and prevent the consequences of environmental abuse. This last point broadens the focus even more. Not only should we determine how current practices and toxins are hurting humans, but also discover what threats they pose to the biosphere and thus to future generations. For example, carbon monoxide gas given off by factories and automobiles is toxic and can be lethal. Not only does it cause dizziness, headaches, and lung diseases in humans who inhale it, but it is also found to reduce the protective ozone layer, thus increasing ultraviolet irradiation and posing a serious ecological threat for the future.

HISTORICAL PERSPECTIVES

Environmental influences on people's health span all of human history. People's interactions with their environment and the conditions of that environment have shaped their mental, emotional, and physical health since the beginning of time. From ancient tribal practices of burial of excreta to modern-day sewage treatment, humans have been concerned with how the environment would provide for their needs and affect their well-being.

In an effort to promote human health, people have taken steps to control, alter, and adapt to their environment. Demonstrations of this concern go back to Biblical times, when the Israelites observed strict rules governing food preparation, practiced sanitation, and quarantined people with infectious diseases, such as leprosy.

As populations became more settled and urbanized, many different environmental health concerns developed. Community actions to deal with these developments have been recorded as far back as 2500 B.C. Archeologists have discovered ancient cities of northern India and the Middle Kingdom of Egypt that used sophisticated water and waste disposal systems. Early Roman civilizations built aqueducts, or drainage systems, for supplying fresh water, and they developed management operations for overseeing water and sewage systems (McGrew, 1985).

A major environmental issue in the medieval world was the spread of infectious diseases brought about by the growth of cities, increased trade, and wars. "Plague, spread by rodents, appears in the writings of Dionysius in the third century" (Blumenthal, 1985). The most severe infectious diseases were outbreaks of leprosy and bubonic plague during the thirteenth and fourteenth centuries (McGrew, 1985). As leprosy spread and peaked in Europe in the early thirteenth century, people recognized a connection between the environment and the spread of disease. They instituted epidemic control by isolating people with signs of the disease and checking newcomers to the community. Thus, long before science had discovered the true cause of these diseases, people were instinctively changing or avoiding harmful environmental circumstances in an effort to promote health (Purdom, 1980). Simple city ordinances restricted locals from washing their clothes or tanners from cleaning their skins in rivers that supplied drinkng water. A law passed in London in 1309 governed the disposal of wastes into the Thames river. Similarly, people passed rules governing the sale of old or spoiled meat to local residents, and "in Basel, leftover fish were displayed at a special inferior food stall and sold only to strangers" (McGrew, 1985). This early concern for sanitary conditions became a major focus in public health, reaching its peak between 1840 and 1880.

The social hygiene movement called for societal transformation to create a truly healthful environment (McGrew, 1985). During the mid- to late-1800s, Florence Nightingale in England and Dr. Ignace Semmelweiss in Vienna were early pioneers in the promotion of clean hospital and surgical conditions to prevent illness. Oliver Wendell Holmes made the connection between exposure to sepsis and childbed fever in Boston in 1843. John Snow first documented environmental spread of disease in 1850 when he linked the spread of cholera in London with contaminated drinking water (Blumenthal, 1985). The work of Pasteur and Koch demonstrated the role of bacteria in disease. All of these, in addition to greater use of the microscope, shed further light on the relationship of the environment to health.

Awareness of environmental impact on health was first documented in "Report on an Inquiry into the Sanitary Conditions of the Labouring Population of Great Britain" by Edwin Chadwick in 1842. This document addressed the necessity for a healthy environment. About the same time, a similar report in the United States called "Report of the Sanitary Commission of Massachussetts," by Lemuel Shattuck, provided original insights into environmental health issues including smoke prevention, pest control, sanitation programs, and food regulations. These documents marked the first organized concern for public health and environmental health controls (Hanlon and Pickett, 1984).

Since that time, the focus has gradually shifted from sanitation to the problems generated by advances in technology, chemical production, and pollution. We are only beginning to understand the complex and far-reaching threats these pose to the public's health. In the next section we will look at specific environmental factors that affect public health today.

TOXIC AGENTS IN THE ENVIRONMENT

Many of the earliest major environmental hazards affecting public health have been eliminated through improved technology and scientific advances. At the same time, technology has created new and more complex hazards. For example, more effective methods of hygiene and sterilization have reduced the spread of disease, but the chemicals introduced to accomplish these goals pose other unintended and unknown health hazards. Increased urbanization has also had major effects on the environment and on people's health. Because community health nurses may be called on to assess environmental health hazards, they need a general knowledge of how environmental factors affect people's health. In this section we explore the role of toxic agents in the environment, especially those carried through water, food, vectors, and wastes.

WATER CONTAMINANTS

Water is such an essential element to human survival that the available quantity and quality of water within a community becomes a prime environmental health issue. In the Middle Ages disease epidemics spread as people drank water contaminated by human waste; this is still a problem in developing countries today. Water has many uses other than consumption by humans. It serves as a means of transportation. It cleans and cools the body or other objects. It is the basis for many forms of recreation and sports such as swimming and boating, and it provides a vehicle for disposing of human and industrial wastes and controlling fires. Apart from serving human needs, water also serves as a medium for sustaining other living organisms, a home to plant and animal life, and as a means of carrying and distributing necessary nutrients in the environment. Although our main environmental health concern deals with the consumption of water by humans, it is important, taking an ecological perspective, to keep in mind water's other uses and users.

How does one assess whether the purity of drinking water is affecting the health of a population? First, one should be familiar with possible contaminants. Although this is a broad subject, we can summarize the basics here.

Drinking water comes from two main sources: surface water, such as lakes and streams, and underground sources, such as wells and springs. In general, underground sources are thought to be less subject to contamination than are surface sources, which are open to runoff from agricultural pesticides or industrial wastes. But groundwater, too, may become affected with the seepage of toxins through the soil, such as hazardous wastes that are buried near the source.

In most industrialized nations an adequate amount of water has not been a serious issue. Areas with limited water supplies have devised facilities to store water during high flow periods so that it would be available to satisfy the year-round needs of a given community. Adequate water supply to meet agricultural demands still has not been achieved, however. The 1988 drought in the Midwest gives testimony to this fact.

The major concern with regard to water is its purity. Water can be contaminated and made unsafe for drinking in many different ways. It may be infected with parasites, such as giardia lamblia, which can cause giardiasia, a gastrointestinal disease that results in diarrhea and malabsorption of nutrients. A recent study showed an association between the risk of giardiasis and unfiltered surface water systems (Kent et al., 1988). Giardia enter a water supply by contamination from human or wild animal feces that carry the parasite. Beavers in the north Cascade mountains often contaminate water (Blumenthal, 1985) and make it essential for humans using the area for recreation to treat the water with iodine before drinking it. Water may also be contaminated with bacteria such as vibrio cholerae, resulting in cholera, or with viruses leading to hepatitis-A (Blumenthal, 1985).

Toxic substances introduced by humans are another source of water pollution. Streams that run near farmland may be contaminated by pesticides from the runoff that then find their way into communities' drinking water downstream. Other industrial pollutants may enter drinking water through oil spills, careless dumping, or buried hazardous wastes that seep into underground water sources. Such wastes not only harm the quality of the water but can affect the quality of local fish and shellfish, making them unfit for consumption. Mercury poisoning from contaminated seafood on the Atlantic coast is a case in point. By 1988 one third of the nation's shellfish beds had been closed because of pollution. Finally, pollutants may affect other organisms in the water which, in turn, affects the water quality. These organisms may play a role in the purification of water, and removing them may upset the ecological balance (Purdom, 1980). Another potential problem is thermal pollution; some organisms in water are affected by a rise in water temperature due to power plants or other industries dissipating excess heat into lakes and streams.

In response to the various potential water pollutants, most cities and local communities with public or semipublic water systems in operation have set up water testing and treatment purification centers to ensure safe drinking water. Unfortunately, testing for bacteria and toxins often does not occur until after illness has been reported. Another major problem arises in rural areas where most water supplies are private and thus not assured of systematic testing and treatment. Testing water for coliforms as indicator organisms has proven useful (Purdom, 1980), and water frequently is treated with chlorine to disinfect it. Caution must be exercised with purification methods, however; it was recently discovered that carcinogens are produced from the reaction of chlorine with humic acids found in treated waters (Purdom, 1980).

A final health issue related to water involves its use for recreational purposes such as public swimming. Lakes, oceans, rivers, and even whirlpools often carry infectious agents and result in a number of health problems including swimmers' itch and diarrheal diseases (WHO, 1986; Blumenthal, 1985). Many outbreaks have been caused by polluted water systems serving campgrounds, parks, and other public areas (DeWailly et al., 1986).

Most of the responsibility for maintaining water quality rests with state and local governments. The federal government took a needed step in 1974 by passing the Safe Drinking Water Act, which gave the Environmental Protection Agency (EPA) authority to establish water standards and to ensure that these standards were upheld. The federal government also provided funds to assist state and local governments in this effort.

On an international scale, because of enormous health problems in developing nations due to unclean water, the World Health Organization (WHO) declared that the 1980s would be the International Clean Water Decade. WHO established a goal to have safe drinking water for all by the year 1990 (Blumenthal, 1985; Last, 1987). Efforts to address water purity at the international level continue to assume high priority.

What role can community health nurses play in the effort to keep water safe? As nurses make visits in a community, they can help by examining household or city drinking water. Is there a strange odor or discoloration? Are particles or sediment visible in the water? Being aware of drinking water quality and possible contaminants in a given county alerts the nurse to consider possible causal relationships if a problem exists. Asking clients to observe and report changes in water quality further assists the nurse in the monitoring process. When such changes occur, the proper authorities, such as health department officials, should be notified and water samples tested. Community health nurses can also be alert to increased incidence of illnesses that might be water related. For example, if several children exhibit similar symptoms, the nurse might inquire as to whether all have been swimming in the same pool or drinking from the same water fountain. While water quality monitoring is ultimately the responsibility of environmental health authorities, it behooves the nurse, as a contributing member of the health team, to observe and report any information that would further the goal of safe and healthy water for the community.

UNSAFE FOOD

The significance of infectious agents carried through food is often underestimated. "Although their true incidence is unknown, food-borne infections and poisonings are outnumbered only by the common cold as causes of short-term illness. Estimates vary considerably, but one million cases or more are thought to occur annually in the United States" (Hanlon and Pickett, 1984). The relationship of food to the health of an individual or a community can be examined from many diverse angles. From famine and starvation to malnutrition, food-related health hazards are found not only in less developed countries but also in the United States. These topics, as well as those dealing with individual nutritional needs such as specific deficiencies or allergies, are usually left to the clinician or dietician. We will describe how our supply of food, particularly the quality of that food, is affected by the environment, and we will look at health hazards associated with food.

The community health nurse needs to ask, "How does the environment influence the safety of food for human consumption?" Three types of hazardous foods must be considered when examining food as a possible health problem: inherently harmful foods, contaminated foods, and foods with toxic additives. The first type, which includes poisonous foods such as certain types of mushrooms, does not pose a serious threat to most people. The general public can identify and avoid harmful plants and substances, so that cases of poisonings are rare (Green and Anderson, 1986).

Contaminated foods pose a more serious health problem. Food may be infected with harmful bacteria such as Salmonella, staphylococcus aureus, or clostridium botulinum, causing outbreaks of Salmonella poisoning or botulism. Blumenthal reports that "33 percent of poultry, 15 percent of pork, and up to 10 percent of beef products are contaminated with Salmonella" (1985, p. 33) because of inadequate processing and shipping methods. Cooking destroys the organism, but problems may be caused by undercooking foods, such as rare roast beef, or handling raw meats. Viral food transmission is rare. Parasitic transmission generally takes the form of trichinosis, caused by ingesting trichinella spiralis in undercooked pork. Various types of worm infestations have created serious health problems, particularly in third world countries. Different types of chemical food contamination result from improper food handling or processing. Examples include dirty machines used in food processing factories, pesticides and herbicides used by farmers to grow their crops, and mercury in fish that live in polluted water (Figure 19-2) (WHO, 1986).

A third health hazard from food comes from the intentional introduction of additives to food products. Because present-day consumers demand convenience foods and time-saving devices, and businesses want to produce food items with long shelf lives, enhanced flavor, and lasting, vibrant colors, many foreign chemicals and synthetic products have been added to foods. As consumers shift toward healthier eating they do not know and are only starting to question the effects these additives may have over time. For example, red dye #2 once was added to improve the color of certain food products but has since been proven carcinogenic. Preservatives and chemical flavorings such as saccharine have also proven hazardous in large doses; it is still questionable what small doses may do with prolonged use. Recently, questions have been raised about potential long-range effects of NutraSweet,

Figure 19-2
Industrial pollutants in lakes and oceans affect the safety of fish and shellfish for human consumption.

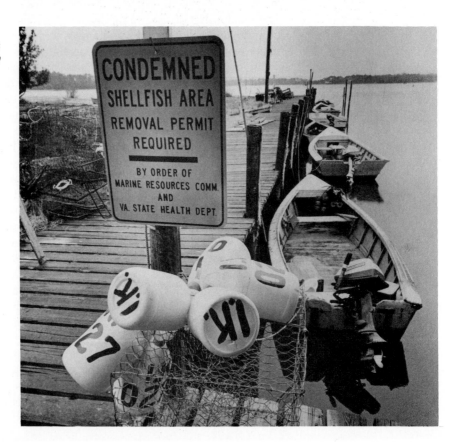

a sugar substitute. Furthermore, such natural flavor enhancers as salt and processed sugars appear in excessive quantities in some canned and packaged foods and are linked to unhealthy dietary consequences such as hypertension or obesity. In small doses none of these additives may be harmful, but when additives are consumed in combination over prolonged periods of time, they may create serious health consequences.

It is the legal responsibility of food producers, processors, and manufacturers to guarantee the quality and safety of food products. However, conflicting motives, such as concern over loss of profit, often lead to careless or inadequate monitoring (Green and Anderson, 1986). Governmental regulatory agencies exist on the local, state, and federal level to set standards and control the quality of food sold to the public. Such public health authorities as the Food and Drug Administration and the Departments of Agriculture and Health are all necessary to help ensure the purity of commercial food products. Included in their jurisdiction is the supervision of the food service industry. Licensing requirements, sanitation standards, and inspections serve as control measures.

Governmental agencies cannot cover all the bases, however. Inadequate inspection of the quality of commercial fish sold for eating, for example, has led to numerous outbreaks of hepatitis and other illnesses. With the wide variety of possible contaminants and potential dangers, consumers' best protection is to supervise their own food quality. Community health nurses can have a significant impact through health education. Most bacterial and viral foodborne diseases can be prevented if people know and practice simple food handling techniques. Nurses can teach the basics of keeping perishable products sufficiently refrigerated, discarding foods that may be old or spoiled, cooking foods thoroughly, and bringing water to a full boil to be certain of eliminating microbes. Nurses can emphasize washing and cleaning produce and equipment used in food processing, including the preparer's own hands. Finally, nurses can educate people to watch for signs of contamination, such as an indented can that may signal the presence of living bacteria using the oxygen within the container and contaminating its contents. Nurses can also raise public awareness regarding the conditions of supermarkets, restaurants, and other food handlers and help to promote community standards and policies for safer eating.

VECTORS

All human communities are affected by the insects and rodents living in their environment. Not only are these creatures a nuisance in people's homes, but they may do economic damage and create serious health hazards as well. On the least dangerous level they serve as annoying pests that may cause irritation, such as mosquito or fly bites, and discomfort, such as infestations of bedbugs or lice. They can also pose a direct threat through such things as attacks by rats or squirrels. They can consume and, in turn, contaminate our food. But by far the most serious health hazard that they impose is through their role as vectors.

A *vector* is defined as "a nonhuman carrier of disease organisms that can transmit these organisms directly to humans" (Blumenthal, 1985). The most common vectors are mosquitos, flies, ticks, roaches, fleas, rats, mice, and ground squirrels. All of these agents can serve as reservoirs for germs that they then transmit through physical contact with humans or by contaminating human foodstuffs or water. Table 19-1 summarizes some of the diseases spread

Table 19-1
Some Insect Vectors and Diseases Transmitted by Them

Vector	Disease	Pathogen
Mosquitoes		
Anopheles sp.	Malaria	*Plasmodium sp.* (protozoa)
Culex sp.	Filiariasis	*Wucheraria bancrofti* and *malayi* (nematodes)
Culex sp.	Encephalitis	arbovirus
Aedes aegypti	Yellow fever	arbovirus
Aedes aegypti	Dengue	arbovirus
Biting Flies		
Deerfly	Filariasis	*Loa loa* (nematode)
Black fly	River blindness	*Onchocerca volvulus* (nematode)
Tsetse fly	Sleeping sickness	*Trypanosoma gambiense* and *rhodesiense* (protozoa)
Sand fly	Kala-azar	*Leishmania donovani*
	Tropical ulcer	*Leishmania tropica*
	Cutaneous leishmaniasis	*Leishmania mexicana*
	Espundia	*Leishmania braziliense* (protozoa)
	Phlebotomus fever	arbovirus
Other Insects		
Gnats	Filariasis	*Mansonella ozzardi* (nematode)
Rat flea	Plague	*Yersinia pestis* (bacteria)
	Murine typhus	*Rickettsia mooseri*
Body louse	Epidemic typhus	*Rickettsia prowazekii*
	Trench fever	*Rickettsia quintana*
Tick	Rocky Mountain spotted fever	*Rickettsia rickettsia*
Tick	Colorado tick fever	arbovirus
Mite	Rickettsialpox	*Rickettsia akari*

Source: D. Blumenthal (1985), *Introduction to Environmental Health.* New York: Springer, p. 35.

by vectors. Cases of vector-spread diseases range from the fourteenth-century bubonic plague epidemic spread by rat fleas, which killed a quarter of the European population, to the continuing problem of mosquito-spread malaria in nonindustrialized nations.

Vector surveys, research, and control are usually left to local and state health departments. These agencies have also implemented community awareness and pest control programs. The community health nurse can contribute through awareness of the presence and possible health threat of rodents and insects. By remaining alert to the presence of vectors in homes, schools, and communities, nurses can take measures to educate affected persons and notify proper authorities when corrective action is needed.

Once vectors have been found, health workers can attempt to control them through many methods. Approaches used in the past include trapping rodents, poisoning, spraying with pesticides, and eliminating areas where vectors breed, as by draining or filling marshes to control mosquito populations. It is essential in planning any approach to consider the possible health hazards to humans or other living organisms and the effect the method will have on the ecosystem — how it may upset the ecological balance. "The most fundamental and effective approach is to improve sanitary conditions and practices to the extent that conditions no longer exist that encourage the multiplication of insects and rodents" (WHO, 1986, p. 110). Community health nurses can assist this effort by surveying homes for exposed rubbish, watching for openings in structures where rodents might enter, and helping people take measures to secure their homes from the entrance and infestation of rodents and insects.

WASTES

In the United States more than five pounds of refuse or solid waste is produced per person per day. According to the Office of Solid Waste Management, that number is expected to increase to more than six pounds per person per day in the next decade (Purdom, 1980). (See Figure 19-3.) With the vast amounts of waste produced in the form of human excreta, household garbage, and agricultural and industrial by-products, including hazardous chemical and radioactive substances, it is no wonder that waste management has become an important and pressing topic in recent decades. New technology has effectively addressed some of the problems but there is still much need for improvement. These wastes pose a wide range of public health concerns. Therefore, it is imperative that health officials, including nurses, become aware of the possible health hazards that these wastes present to individuals and to communities.

One of the oldest environmental health hazards comes from improper disposal of human excreta. Although industrialized nations successfully address the problem, it continues to be a widespread problem in third-world nations and in rural, poverty-stricken communities. Human wastes, particularly feces,

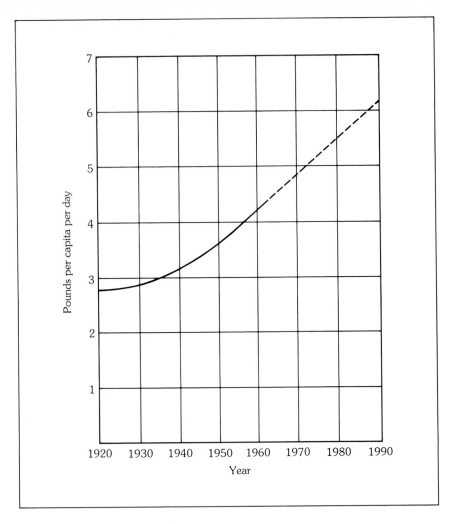

Figure 19-3
United States trend in per capita refuse production.

provide a perfect environment in which bacteria and disease-causing parasites can live and reproduce. Therefore, contamination through drinking water, food grown in contaminated soil, and even direct contact with the soil can cause infections. For example, hookworm, a problem in the U.S. in the early part of this century, usually entered the body through the skin of bare feet (Blumenthal, 1985). In most modernized urban areas the public sewage system handles waste. Most communities handle the dangers inherent in raw sewage through treatment and disposal into a body of water. Some communities, including Tokyo, with its population of more than 12 million inhabitants, use collection trucks and tanks (Green and Anderson, 1986). In most instances in the United States, state health departments oversee proper waste treatment and disposal. In rural areas where individuals usually have private cesspools or septic tanks, the supervision of proper waste handling is difficult and not as consistent. Health workers in rural settings should be alert to the potential dangers posed by inconsistent monitoring.

Societies have developed various ways to dispose of their garbage, none of which provide a perfect solution (Hanlon, 1984). Dumping and burning are the most common disposal methods. Dumping is problematic because garbage dumps provide perfect conditions for the breeding of rats, flies, and other vectors. Dumps also are eyesores that take up valuable land resources. Burning, although it reduces the volume of garbage, produces noxious odors and pollutes the air. Sanitary landfills keep refuse out of sight by burying it, but this method can cause problems by contaminating the groundwater and surrounding soil, thereby posing a threat to organisms living on top of the landfill. Love Canal (Figure 19-4) was a frightening example of a community whose health was jeopardized because its homes were built on top of an old landfill where chemical waste had been buried (Blumenthal, 1985). New technology is being considered and tried in some communities to handle solid waste.

A grave concern of the modern world focuses on how to dispose of toxic chemical and radioactive wastes produced by industry. The threat is serious since we are not certain how all these wastes affect us, or whether our present methods of disposal are foolproof. Furthermore, many of these wastes escape containment or accidentally leak into water systems and into the soil to contaminate drinking water and food. The current method of disposal is storage, but storage containers may not always be leakproof, and interference with dump sites or storage facilities may expose the environment to these toxic substances. Many examples of chemical contamination exist in communities such as Elizabeth, N.J., Times Beach, Mich., Love Canal, N.Y., and Minamata, Japan (Blumenthal, 1985). We also face the continuing problem of securing disposal sites for the increasing volume of hazardous wastes. Communities seek the advantages of new technology but do not wish to bury the resulting wastes in their backyards. In many instances legislators and public officials have faced serious conflict in their efforts to locate acceptable toxic waste dump sites.

The industrialized world creates a constant demand for new and better goods, services, and means of production. Industry and technology have accommodated this desire by developing more sophisticated means of energy production, labor-saving devices, and practical as well as novel products. A major problem has emerged out of this concentration on mass production: how to handle the vast amount of waste created from discardable goods, by-products of production, and the "throw-away" ethic. Not only does mass production take an enormous toll on our natural resources, but the quantity and nature of the resulting wastes also pose serious health hazards. Improper disposal of domestic products such as some household cleaners causes health dangers (Tuthill et al., 1987). It is imperative that we learn not only to dispose of these wastes safely — to protect humans, the environment, and future generations — but that we also look seriously at other options. More emphasis could be placed on transforming waste into usable products, increasing

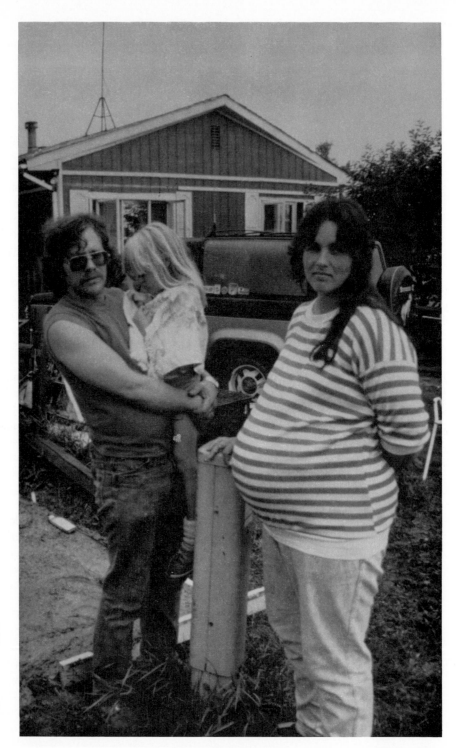

Figure 19-4
Environmental
contamination from
industrial waste poses
serious threats to the
long-term health of
community residents. The
Freiermuth family, shown
here outside their Forest
Glen mobile home (near
Niagara Falls, N.Y.), had to
move from the Love Canal
area in 1980 because of
toxic wastes. Several years
later the family had to
move again because
hazardous substances were
found in the soil near their
new home.

the amount and kinds of recycling done, and reducing the amount of refuse produced in the first place. Community health nurses can encourage these actions by educating the public and lobbying for enabling legislation.

CHEMICALS

The list of chemicals, both natural and synthetic, in the environment and the threats they pose to human and environmental health is overwhelming. "Approximately 55,000 chemicals are in use in the United States; of these, 1000 to 1500 constitute the greatest part of hazardous exposures, but only about 450 have established threshold limit values and adequate toxicity testing. Several hundred new chemicals come into use each year, basically untested" (Last, 1987, p. 146). We have touched on many of these chemicals in our discussions of air, water, soil, and food contaminants, and most specifically in our discussion of hazardous wastes. It is not within the scope of this chapter to explore in detail all the specific chemical substances present in the environment and their potential effects on humans. We will, however, present a general overview of the different categories of environmental chemicals, where they are found, the dangers they impose, and community health nurses' role in forestalling or detecting those dangers.

Inorganic Chemicals

This first category of chemical pollutants includes those that do not contain carbon, are not derived from living matter, and are usually of mineral composition. Substances such as zinc, cadmium, lead, iron, calcium, sodium, potassium, magnesium, and copper often play an important role in human physiology, but they are poisonous if a person is exposed to large quantities.

Lead, whether in organic or inorganic form, is a toxic agent frequently found in occupational or industrial settings. Workers must be careful to avoid inhaling lead fumes and exposing their families to lead dust on their clothing. Lead is also used in paint, leaded gasoline, and batteries. Lead poisoning usually produces symptoms of cerebral or central nervous system disorders. It is especially dangerous in children, whose high metabolic activity makes them more susceptible (Last, 1987). Community health nurses need to check with clients for possible exposure, and examine client homes for lead-based paint, now restricted in residential use. In particular, nurses can warn parents to keep their young children from eating old paint chips from windowsills, walls, or furniture painted with lead-based paint.

Mercury, in both organic and inorganic form, is also highly toxic. It is used in many scientific instruments, electronic equipment, crop fungicides, and the processing of dental fillings. Inorganic mercury can be changed through bacterial action in industrial processes to more toxic organic compounds, as in the bleach used for paper manufacturing. Toxic mercurials then escape into the environment and contaminate the food chain. In Minanata Bay, Japan, for example, many persons were crippled with nervous system disorders caused by eating mercury-contaminated seafood.

Other harmful metals include aluminum, which recently has been associated with certain mental disorders and has been found in high levels in the brain tissue of patients with Alzheimer's disease (Last, 1987). Chromium, nickel, and arsenic are among other toxic compounds. (See Table 19-2).

Organic Chemicals

This second category of chemical contaminants includes those containing carbon. Many of these chemicals are by-products of the petroleum industry, including many alcohols, ethers, hydrocarbons such as benzene, medicines, and plastics. Ingestion or exposure may cause cancer, liver and kidney disease, birth defects, and many other health problems. Pesticides for household and crop use, particularly DDT (Dichlorodiphenyl Trichloroethane), have created major health hazards (Blumenthal, 1985). DDT, a very dangerous chemical used for pest control, was banned in 1972 because of environmental and health concerns. However, it is still present in the environment and continues to be used illicitly, posing a danger to farmers and migrant farmworkers in particular.

Dusts

Dusts can contain numerous types of chemical irritants and poisons. Many hazardous dusts are associated with the workplace; for example, coal miners have developed black lung disease from inhaling coal dust, and a respiratory disease called silicosis is caused by exposure to silica dust (common in mining, sandblasting, and tunnel work). Asbestos fibers, which are found in insulation and fireproofing materials, textiles, and many other products, have been associated with lung cancer. Exposed individuals who smoke are at 30 times greater risk of developing lung cancer than those who do not smoke (Green and Anderson, 1986).

Gases and Fumes

A long list of gaseous pollutants, including sulfur oxide and nitrogen oxides produced by industrial emissions, pose additional problems for community health. Not only do such gases cause respiratory disease, asphyxiation, or toxicity in humans, but they harm the environment as well. Some, for example, are associated with acid rain. We will discuss this problem in a later section.

Another gas that has been a topic of concern in recent years is radon. This colorless, odorless radioactive gas is formed by uranium breakdown in soil and rock. Radon enters buildings through cracks in basement walls or through

Table 19-2
Occupational Carcinogens

Carcinogen	Cancer Site	Examples of Exposed Occupations
4-Aminodiphenyl Auramine B-napthylamine Magenta Benzidine	Bladder	Dye manufacturing; rubber manufacturing
Arsenic	Skin; lung; liver	Metal smelting; arsenic pesticide production; metal alloy workers
Asbestos	Lung; mesothelium; gastrointestinal tract	Asbestos miners; insulators; shipyard workers
Benzene	Leukemia (blood-forming organs)	Petrochemical workers; chemists
Bischloromethyl ether (BCME)	Lung	Organic chemical synthesizers
Cadmium	Prostate	Cadmium alloy workers; welders
Chromium/Chromates	Lung; nasal sinuses	Chromate producers; metal workers
Coke oven emissions	Lung; kidney	Coke oven workers
Foundry emissions	Lung	Foundry workers
Leather dust	Nasal cavity; nasal sinuses; bladder	Shoe manufacturing
Nickel	Lung; nasal passages	Nickel smelting; metal workers
Radiation (x-rays)	Leukemia (blood-forming organs; skin; breast; thyroid; bone	Radiologists; industrial radiographers; atomic energy workers
Radon gas	Lung	Uranium and feldspar miners
Soots, tars, and oil (aromatic hydrocarbons)	Skin; lung; bladder; scrotum	Roofers; chimney sweepers; petroleum workers; shale oil workers
Ultraviolet light	Skin	Outdoor workers
Vinyl chloride	Liver; brain; lung	Polyvinyl chloride synthesizers; rubber workers
Welding fumes	Lung	Welders
Wood dust	Nasal passages	Hardwood workers; furniture makers

Source: D. Blumenthal (1985), *Introduction to Environmental Health*. New York: Springer.

sewer openings. Furnaces and exhaust fans can help pull radon into a house, although the highest levels tend to be found in basements where the gas enters. Home testing for radon was recommended by the EPA and the U.S. Public Health Service in 1988, (Weinstein et al., 1988) although safe levels had not been established by the EPA at that time. Sealing cracks in basement walls and covering dirt floors can substantially reduce radon levels.

Other gases, including chlorine, ozone, sulfur dioxide, and carbon monoxide, are all harmful to individual health as well as to the broader environment and the ecosystem. We will discuss the health effects of these gases in the section on air pollution.

Exposure to chemicals can have far-reaching effects on humans. People may come in contact with them in their homes through building materials, cleaning products, or airborne dust. Another source is the workplace, where many different compounds are created and used each day. Toxic substances also may be transferred home from the workplace. In the greater community, pollutants in the air and food chain create further hazards. Toxic chemicals can cause illness when they are inhaled, come into contact with the skin (as in industrial accidents where chemicals are spilled), or ingested (as when a child drinks from a liquid cleaning solvent bottle). The federal government and local health agencies do their best to set standards of exposure and to monitor chemical use and production, but the job is enormous and often difficult to accomplish.

Chemical exposure is an area where community health nurses can play a vital role in prevention and correction. It is difficult to monitor all the possible contacts a person or community may be experiencing with toxic chemicals, but such monitoring is necessary in order to estimate health risks and establish correlations. By being aware of the possible chemical hazards in an individual's personal environment, a community health nurse can help not only the individual but also the larger community of people who might be in danger. Multiple exposures in small doses from many different sources may add up. Are clients' homes well ventilated? Are wood-burning stoves polluting the air with sulfur oxide? Does home insulation contain asbestos? Are all household chemical agents stored in a childproof place? Monitoring difficulties arise from the vast number of chemicals people may be exposed to, the cumulative exposures to a certain chemical people may experience over time, and the fact that disease symptoms may not appear until years after exposure, when the toxic chemical may no longer be in the immediate environment. All these make finding a specific environmental cause for a given disease or symptom frustrating and sometimes impossible.

AIR POLLUTION

Air pollution is now recognized as one of the most hazardous sources of chemical contamination (Figure 19-5). It is especially prevalent in highly industrialized and urbanized areas where concentrations of people, motor vehicles, and industry produce large volumes of gaseous pollutants. "More than 200 million tons of toxic material are released into the air above the United States each year, about one ton per person" (Hanlon and Pickett, 1984,

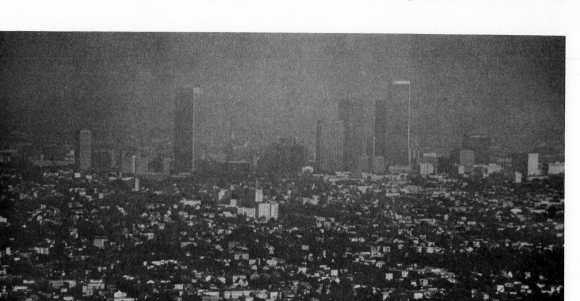

Figure 19-5
Afternoon smog shrouds
downtown Los Angeles.

p. 330). These airborne pollutants have adverse effects on many areas of human life. Blumenthal (1985) cites six:

Property
Aesthetics
The economy
Human health
Vegetation and agricultural output
Weather

The last three have the most far-reaching consequences.

Most air pollution results from industrial and automotive emissions. Pollutants include lead, ozone, carbon monoxide, sulfur dioxide, hydrocarbons, nitrogen oxides, and particulates such as dust and ash. (These were mentioned in the section on chemical contaminants.) The list of diseases and symptoms of ill health associated with air pollutants is lengthy, ranging from minor nose and throat irritations, respiratory infections, and bronchial asthma, to emphysema, cardiovascular disease, lung cancer, and genetic mutations (see Figure 19-6).

As with other toxic chemicals, it is often difficult to establish a cause-effect relationship between air pollution and illness. A relatively short, high level of exposure is normally easier to identify. There have been a number of poignant

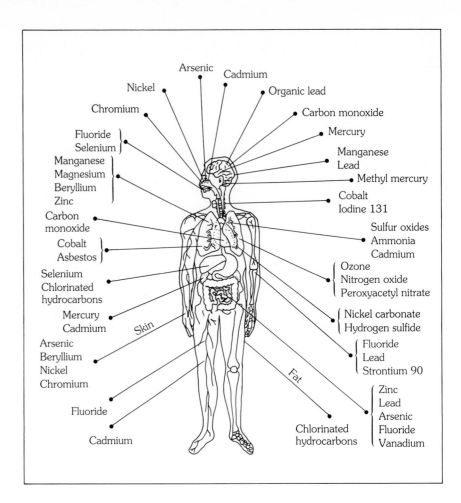

Figure 19-6
*Body system targets of
major air pollutants.*

examples. One occurred in London in 1952, when weather conditions trapped smoke and fog over the city for nearly a week. Four thousand more people died than was normal, with a sharp increase in deaths from respiratory diseases. A second incident occurred in Bhopal, India, in 1984. A chemical plant leaked methyl isocyanate into the atmosphere, taking approximately two thousand lives (Green and Anderson, 1986). Although these disasters and others like them are dramatic and frightening, the effects of long-term exposure to low levels of pollution are perhaps even more threatening. They are definitely more difficult to record, to measure, to understand, to define, to correlate, and to control. We may never understand their total effects.

Certain geographical areas are more susceptible to the ill effects of air pollution because of their weather conditions or physical terrain. The episode in London, which was an extreme but not isolated incident, occurred when a lack of wind combined with low temperatures to create a temperature inversion — a phenomenon in which air that normally rises is trapped under a layer of warm air, allowing air contaminants to build up to intolerable levels. Los Angeles, another city troubled by air pollution, is surrounded by mountains that prevent winds from clearing away smoke and fumes. A further condition occurs in urban areas where city buildings create a "heat island effect." Warm air traps pollution in the atmosphere around the city (Blumenthal, 1985). Thus, in examining the effects of air pollution, it is necessary to take into account meteorological and topographical characteristics of an area.

Although much air pollution results from some type of human activity, naturally occurring dusts and ash can also pose problems. Elements in the environment, such as pollen from plants and flowers, ash from volcanic eruptions, or airborne microorganisms, can have ill effects on health.

The health hazards of air pollution include wide-ranging ecological effects. The emission of hazardous chemicals into the earth's atmosphere has a serious effect on our environment. Air pollutants, such as sulfur dioxide from power plant emissions or nitrogen oxides from motor vehicle exhaust, combine with water vapor to produce sulfuric and nitric acid, known as "acid rain," in many parts of the northern United States (Last, 1987). Although acid rain does not seem to pose any direct danger to humans, it kills small forms of life and endangers the forest and fresh water ecologies. An increased accumulation of carbon dioxide in the atmosphere from fuel combustion is altering the climate. Scientists believe that this carbon dioxide buildup traps infrared heat near the earth's surface and raises the earth's temperatures (Lemonick, 1987). Known as the "greenhouse effect," this too could have catastrophic consequences (Last, 1987) for the world's food supply and living conditions. Once again the community health nurse can have an influence through community education and lobbying for appropriate legislation.

Government regulation in the realm of air quality has been relatively slow. In 1963 the federal government finally passed a series of Clean Air Acts. These set standards for air quality and industrial emissions, and delegated funds to assist in pollution control programs. Although progress has been made, further public health efforts are needed to help identify pollution sources and related health hazards. Table 19-3 summarizes seven major air pollutants and their health effects.

One area in which community health nurses can promote health is in detecting indoor pollutants. People are exposed to numerous impurities in the air in their homes and workplaces. Many household products and building materials emit vapors that can cause problems. Cigarette and cigar smoke are common indoor pollutants that can have ill effects on nonsmokers as well as smokers. Carbon monoxide poisoning may result from stove emissions or car exhaust accumulating in a garage. Radon gas trapped in basements or tightly insulated homes is also a concern. Nurses can assist with prevention or elimination of these health hazards by ensuring a well-ventilated indoor environment and looking for possible sources of pollution.

Table 19-3
National Air Pollutant Emissions, by Pollutant and Source, 1980 (million metric tons per year)

Source	Particulates	Sulfur Oxides	Nitrogen Oxides	Hydro-carbons	Carbon Monoxide
Transportation	1.4	0.9	9.1	7.8	69.1
Highway vehicles	1.1	0.4	6.6	6.4	61.9
Aircraft	0.1	0.0	0.1	0.2	1.0
Railroads	0.1	0.1	0.7	0.2	0.3
Vessels	0.0	0.3	0.2	0.5	1.5
Other off-highway vehicles	0.1	0.1	1.5	0.5	4.4
Stationary source fuel					
Combustion	1.4	19.0	10.6	0.2	2.1
Electric utilities	0.8	15.9	6.7	0.0	0.3
Industrial	0.3	2.3	3.3	0.1	0.6
Commercial-institutional	0.1	0.6	0.3	0.0	0.1
Residential	0.2	0.2	0.3	0.1	1.1
Industrial processes	3.7	3.8	0.7	10.8	5.8
Solid waste disposal	0.4	0.0	0.1	0.6	2.2
Incineration	0.2	0.0	0.0	0.3	1.2
Open burning	0.2	0.0	0.1	0.3	1.0
Miscellaneous	0.9	0.0	0.2	2.4	6.2
Forest fires	0.8	0.0	0.2	0.7	5.5
Other burning	0.1	0.0	0.0	0.1	0.7
Miscellaneous organic solvents	0.0	0.0	0.0	1.6	0.0
TOTAL	7.8	23.7	20.7	21.8	85.4

Source: Council on Environmental Quality. *Environmental Quality 1981.* Washington, D.C.: U.S. Government Printing Office, 1982.

RADIATION

Radiation can be found in many areas of our environment. It occurs naturally as background radiation from the sun, soil, and minerals. In its manmade form, it has numerous uses in science and industry for lasers, various types of testing, and production. It is found in many home electronic devices, such as television sets and microwave ovens. Radiation is present in countless areas of the medical field, including X rays and radioisotopes used in diagnosis and treatment. Health concerns over radiation exposure have perhaps been most dramatized with the potential exposure from nuclear energy plants and nuclear weapons.

Regardless of its source, radiation is dangerous to human health. The extent of danger depends on the dose and type of radiation. For example, casualties among miners can be attributed to their prolonged and intense exposure to radioactive minerals such as uranium. Prolonged exposure may cause skin ulcers, damage to cells, cancer, premature aging, kidney dysfunction, and genetic disorders in the children of those whose cells have been damaged.

A major area of concern centers on the problems associated with nuclear energy and nuclear weapons. The production of radioactive wastes, the threat of accidental exposure from unsafe reactors, and possible fallout from weapons testing create real fears that have been confirmed by such incidents as Three Mile Island and Chernobyl. In the latter two settings accidents allowed radioactive ions to escape into the atmosphere. "Such accidents, however, are not very common. Further, the normal operation of nuclear power plants exposes the population to considerably less radiation than other man-made sources, such as medical radiation, or natural radiation" (WHO, 1986, p. 18).

Because of intense public concern, steps have been taken to protect people against exposure to radiation. The medical and dental fields have developed simple safety procedures, such as having patients wear lead aprons during X rays and technicians stand behind metal walls (Figure 19-7). Federal legislation and many other efforts address setting standards and researching the biological effects of radiation. The United States Public Health Service holds responsibility for monitoring nuclear plants and other possible sources of radiation to protect the public. "One of the most difficult problems that confronts the public health worker is the maintenance of an appropriate balance between the benefits that may result from the use of radioactive materials and radiation-generating equipment and the risks that might possibly be entailed" (Hanlon and Pickett, 1984, p. 378). The community health nurse can encourage compliance with government standards, keep the public informed of safety measures, and promote research efforts.

Figure 19-7
Protective bibs or aprons are now routinely used in dentists' and doctors' offices to avoid unnecessary radiation exposure.

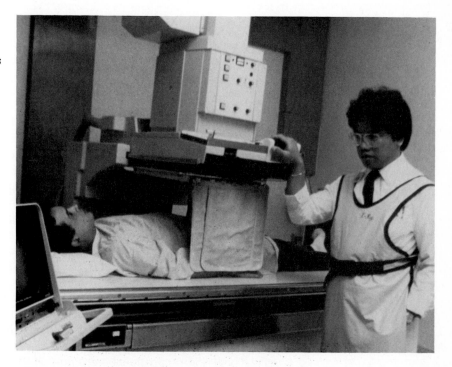

ACCIDENTS AND NATURAL DISASTERS

Another environmental characteristic that must be considered in assessing health risks is a community's level of safety. How likely is it that accidents will occur? This is a very important question when one considers that the leading cause of death in people between the ages of 1 and 44 years is unintentional injuries (Green and Anderson, 1985). Injury victims take up more hospital beds than any other type of patient—20 million beds in the U.S. per day (Hanlon and Pickett, 1984). Considering these facts, any steps that public health workers can take to prevent accidents or limit their impact may greatly improve the overall health of a community.

Green and Anderson (1986) list five sources of injuries that can be prevented and six target area settings in which to concentrate preventive measures.

Injury Sources	*Environments*
Falls	Home
Burns	Occupational
Poisonings	School
Vehicle crashes	Highway
Drownings	Farm
	Recreational

Simple steps can be taken to prevent many accidents and make people's environments safer. One approach to creating a safer environment is to modify products to make them safer and reduce their potential harm (Green and Anderson, 1986). Seat belts and airbags have helped to lessen the injury potential of automobiles (Latimer and Lave, 1987; Williams and Lund, 1986). Because companies are held strictly liable for the safety of their products, they have invested considerable resources into researching and designing safe goods. Childproof caps on medication bottles are an example. Industry also has a duty to warn consumers if a product is inherently dangerous, as when toys have sharp edges or parts small enough to be ingested. Bright orange frowning faces on bottles that contain harmful substances have helped to warn consumers and reduce the number of poisonings. Children learn to avoid poisonous plants and other potential hazards through school and community education efforts. Organizations such as the Consumer Protection Agency, and consumer advocates like Ralph Nader continue to watchdog environmental safety.

Community safety organizations, government agencies, and public health officials all play their parts in assessing community safety and taking measures to prevent accidents. Federal legislation to enforce speed limits has helped to reduce the number of automobile accidents, and supervision of recreational and occupational areas has led to discovery of health hazards and promoted the development of safety programs. State-established boating safety regulations, or the assigning of extra lifeguards to patrol a lake with a record of previous drownings, are measures that help to reduce the number of recreational accidents. Community surveys of intersections where multiple traffic accidents have occurred have led to installation of traffic signals and a reduction of accidents.

One area in which community health nurses can promote safety is the home environment. Locks can be put on cupboards where toxic materials are kept. Railings can be installed on stairways and in bathrooms used by the elderly. Gates can be used at the tops of stairways to prevent small children from falling. Non-skid decals can be used in bathtubs to prevent slipping. Generally, the nurse's role in health education will promote safe behaviors and prevent injury.

Safety education offers one of the most vital preventive measures. When people are made aware of possible dangers and unsafe areas within an environment, they can avoid injuring themselves. Local community programs to educate people on the dangers of driving while intoxicated or to instruct them on the proper handling of home machinery such as chainsaws can also help to reduce accident potential. In the event that an accident does occur, educating the public about appropriate actions to take can help to reduce the potential impact of the accident. First-aid and CPR classes are very beneficial. Education as a preventive measure applies particularly in the case of natural disasters. Although we cannot prevent a tornado or earthquake, we can be prepared in the event that one does occur. By running fire drills in schools and workplaces, or informing people of the location of safe and unsafe places to take shelter during an electrical storm or hurricane, we can help to forestall or minimize tragic events.

PSYCHOLOGICAL HAZARDS

Our discussion of environmental health would not be complete if we were to overlook the psychological hazards that people must face in their environments. Environment plays a significant role in the mental health of a community. The psychological variables that affect individuals often lead to physiological illnesses. Such elements as noise, overcrowding, traffic, lack of privacy, unavailability of work, and boredom can be detrimental to peoples' well-being.

Noise is often cited as a major environmental health problem. Extremely loud noises, such as pneumatic drills or loud rock music, can cause temporary or permanent hearing loss. Other noises, perhaps from machinery at the workplace or residential exposure to airport traffic, can lead to headaches, sleep disruption, lowered body resistance to disease, ulcers, and aggravation of existing physical disorders (Hanlon and Pickett, 1984). The effects vary in severity depending on the intensity and duration of the noises and the disposition of the individuals concerned.

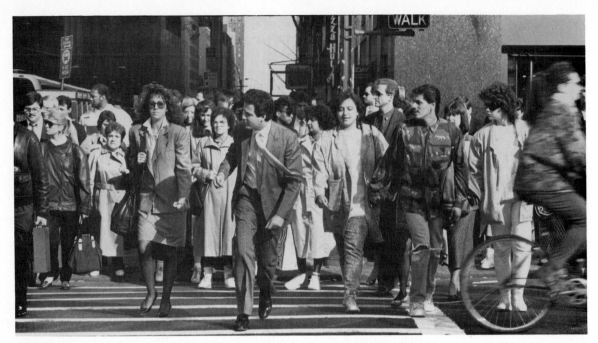

Figure 19-8
Crowds and congestion add to the environmental stressors affecting the
health of city dwellers.

Another psychological hazard is urban crowding (Figure 19-8). Early studies on crowding done by J. B. Calhoun demonstrated gross effects on behavior. When healthy, naturally clean laboratory mice were forced to live in overcrowded conditions, they broke down in almost all aspects of normal behavior (Hanlon and Pickett, 1984). Gross insanitation led to aggressive behavior, strong mice attacking the weak, symptoms of regression and mental disturbance, mating decline, homosexual activity, and neglect or cannibalization of weaker offspring. Although this is an extreme example, it perhaps gives us some insight into the conditions of our urban areas and the psychological stress that urban conditions may create.

The daily psychological stresses of the modern world are innumerable. Excessive stimulation comes from rapid societal changes created by new technology, an accelerated pace of living, increased work production demands, and other causes. All can create potential health hazards. It is necessary for community health nurses to be aware of these stressors, to recognize the potential they have for affecting both psychological and physiological health, and to encourage stress reduction wherever possible. Some specific ways that community health nurses can promote a psychologically healthy environment include active lobbying for reasonable airport traffic patterns, neighborhood crime prevention, reduction of workplace stressors, and development of educational and support programs to reduce life-style stressors.

HUMAN CONTROL OVER ENVIRONMENTAL HEALTH

Maintaining a healthy environment and balanced ecology, and promoting the health of humans living in it, remain challenges. Past efforts to accomplish these goals have been only partially successful. However, increased public awareness and concern for future generations has exerted tremendous pressure to create new and more effective measures. In this final section we consider some of the efforts, both public and private, being made to foster a healthier environment.

GOVERNMENTAL SECTOR

In the United States, all levels of government have worked diligently to assess, prevent, and correct environmental health hazards. In previous sections, we mentioned many activities and organizations on the local, state, and federal levels that deal with environmental health issues. Local governments assume responsibility for proper waste disposal, pure water supply, and efficient sanitary and safety conditions within the community. State governments, represented by different agencies, handle broader issues that deal with the creation of state regulations, policies, and supervision of local health efforts (Hanlon and Pickett, 1984). The federal government is charged with establishing and enforcing health standards and regulations.

The major environmental health efforts of the federal government have come primarily in the last two decades. During this time public concern for people's health in relation to the environment, as well as concern for the environment itself, has stimulated increased government actions. During this time the Environmental Protection Agency (EPA) was established. Created in 1970, this agency was given extensive authority over all environmental concerns and protection of the public health. Other related agencies were also established, including the Food and Drug Administration (FDA), the Occupational Safety and Health Administration (OSHA), and the Product Safety Commission. Because there are so many different organizations and levels of government involved in environmental health issues, responsibilities and areas of concern overlap tremendously. Confusion and disorganization result when people do not know who has authority in any one particular area or who should be contacted to handle a problem when it arises. Public health agents, including nurses, can help to work through the red tape and "complexities of the interagency-intergovernmental relationships" (Hanlon and Pickett, 1984, p. 389).

An important international agency, the World Health Organization, has helped to identify and address world health problems, including issues of environmental concern. Since many modern technological discoveries cause far-reaching health hazards that affect the environment and the health of the entire world population, this organization and others like it may play increasingly important roles in the future (WHO, 1986).

PRIVATE SECTOR

The role of the private sector in environmental health remains unclear. Legislation such as the Products Liability Law has made private business more conscious of health and safety issues. The private sector is usually labeled as the enemy of the environment, concerned only with profit and its own survival. Private business and industry have often been accused of having total disregard for the health of the environment and its effect on human health. This image is changing slowly. Many companies, confronted by concerned environmentalists or consumer protection groups, have been forced to change their practices. Boycotts of products, listings of environmentally conscientious firms, and general public outrage have put a stop to many harmful practices. A number of companies have been concerned for some time with the environmental impact of their business operations; they have sought not only reduction of health hazards but ways to promote environmental and public health. Timber companies, for example, have actively engaged in reforestation projects. Private business has been a major contributor to many nonprofit environmentally concerned projects and agencies, such as the Sierra Club. Furthermore, the benefits that private business brings to an area may outweigh the disadvantages. This raises a question that is difficult to answer. Is it acceptable to allow a new industry to develop in an economically depressed area in order to create jobs when that industry is stripping the area of its natural resources or polluting the environment and endangering the health of residents? The community health nurse, through health education and committee or board involvement, can enhance private-sector awareness of these issues.

ROLE OF THE COMMUNITY HEALTH NURSE IN ENVIRONMENTAL HEALTH

In each of the preceding sections we have discussed actions and given examples of ways that the community health nurse can help to promote a healthy environment. We summarize these in four main guidelines.

1. *Be aware and informed* about possible environmental health threats. The nurse has a responsibility to keep abreast of current environmental issues and know the proper authorities to whom problems should be reported.
2. *Assess clients' environments* and detect health hazards. Careful observation and an environmental checklist can assist in this assessment.

3. *Implement programs to prevent health threats* to clients and the environment. This can be done by direct intervention, especially through client education.
4. *Take action to correct situations* in which health hazards exist. Nurses can use direct intervention or notify proper authorities when corrective measures are beyond their sphere.

Summary

Environmental health is a discipline encompassing all the elements of the environment that influence the health and well-being of its inhabitants. Public health workers, including community health nurses, need to monitor and determine causal links between people and their environment with a concern as to how they may promote the health and well-being of both.

A holistic or ecological perspective of environmental health is important for understanding human–environmental relationships. It provides the context for dealing with current environmental health issues and preventing or minimizing future problems.

Infectious agents in the environment may be carried through water, food, vectors, and wastes. Chemical hazards can cause illness in humans, and air pollution and radiation pose additional threats to human and environmental health. Accidents and safety issues associated with the environment create yet another set of challenges for health professionals. Finally, communities face psychological hazards related to environmental conditions such as overcrowding or noise.

Both government and the private sector play roles in the regulation, monitoring, and prevention of environmental health issues. The community health nurse is an important member of the team of health professionals monitoring the reciprocal relationship between the environment and client health. Nurses can do their share by practicing four important guidelines:

1. Be informed about environmental health threats.
2. Assess clients' environments for health hazards.
3. Prevent environmental health threats.
4. Correct situations in which environmental health hazards exist.

Study Questions

1. If you make a home visit and notice particles in the client's drinking water, what steps should you take to (1) determine whether there is a health threat, and (2) take corrective action?
2. You notice that five babies born in the past year from the same rural community all have cancer. What actions would be appropriate for you to take to determine whether there is an environmental relationship?

3. Design a list of items to include in a checklist for assessing clients' environmental health.

References

Blumenthal, D. (1985). *Introduction to environmental health*. New York: Springer.

Dewailly, E., C. Poirier, and F. Meyer. (1986). Health hazards associated with windsurfing on polluted water. *American Journal of Public Health* 76(6): 690–91.

Green, L. W., and C. L. Anderson. (1986). *Community health*. St. Louis: Times Mirror/Mosby.

Green, M., et al. (1987). An outbreak of watermelon-borne pesticide toxicity. *American Journal of Public Health* 77: 1431–34.

Hanlon, J., and G. Pickett. (1984). *Public health: administration and practice*. St. Louis: Times Mirror/Mosby.

Kent, G., J. Greenspan, J. Herndon, L. Mofenson, J. Harris, T. Eng, and H. Waskin. (1988). Epidemic giardiasis caused by a contaminated public water supply. *American Journal of Public Health* 78: 139–43.

Last, J. M. (1987). *Public health and human ecology*. East Norwalk: Appleton and Lange.

Latimer, E., and L. Lave. (1987). Initial effects of the New York State Auto Safety Belt Law. *American Journal of Public Health* 77: 183–86.

Lemonick, M. D. (1987). The heat is on: Chemical wastes spread into the air threaten the earth's climate. *Time* (Oct. 19): 53–67.

McGrew, R. (1985). *Encyclopedia of medical history*. New York: McGraw-Hill.

Purdom, P. W. (1980). *Environmental health*. New York: Academic Press.

Tuthill, R., E. Stanekill, C. Willis, and G. Moore. (1987). Degree of public support for household hazardous waste control alternatives. *American Journal of Public Health* 77: 304–6.

Weinstein, N., M. Klotz, and P. Sandman. (1988). Optimistic biases in public perceptions of the risk from radon. *American Journal of Public Health* 78(7): 796–800.

Williams, A., and A. Lund. (1986). Seat belt use laws and occupant crash protection in the United States. *American Journal of Public Health* 76(12): 1438–42.

World Health Organization. (1983). *Health impact of different energy sources: A challenge for the end of the century*. Copenhagen: WHO Regional Publications, European Series, No. 16: 19–22.

World Health Organization. (1986). *Health and the environment*. Vienna: WHO Regional Publications, European Series, No. 19: 12–16.

Selected Readings

American Public Health Association. (1988). Labor calls new OSHA rule on formaldehyde insufficiently protective of workers. *The Nation's Health* 18(1): 1, 6.

Bale, T. (1987). A brush with justice: The New Jersey radium dial painters in the courts. *Health/PAC Bulletin* 17(5):18–21.

Blumenthal, D. (1985). *Introduction to environmental health*. New York: Springer.

Cohen, S. (1981). Sound effects on behavior. *Psychology Today* 15: 38–46.

Dewailly, E., C. Poirier, and F. Meyer. (1986). Health hazards associated with windsurfing on polluted water. *American Journal of Public Health* 76(6): 690–91.

Draggan, S., J. Cohrssen, J. and R. Morrison (eds.). (1987). *Environmental impacts on human health: The agenda for long-term research and development*. New York: Praeger Publishers.

Fetter, S., and K. Tsipis. (1981). Catastrophic releases of radioactivity. *Scientific American* 4:41–47.

Geller, E. S. (1986). Prevention of environmental problems. In B. Edelstein and L. Michelson (eds.), *Handbook of prevention*. New York: Plenum Press.

Goldsmith, J. R. (ed.). (1986). *Environmental epidemiology: Epidemiological investigation of community environmental health problems*. Boca Raton, Fla.: CRC Press.

Green, L. W., and C. L. Anderson. (1986). *Community health*. St. Louis: Times Mirror/Mosby.

Hanlon, J., and G. Pickett. (1984). *Public health: Administration and practice*. St. Louis: Times Mirror/Mosby.

Lancaster, J. (1980). *Community mental health nursing: An ecological perspective*. St. Louis: C. V. Mosby.

Last, J. M. (1987). *Public health and human ecology*. East Norwalk, Conn.: Appleton & Lange.

Latimer, E., and L. Lave. (1987). Initial effects of the New York State Auto Safety Belt Law. *American Journal of Public Health* 77(2): 183–86.

Lemonick, M. D. (1987). The heat is on: Chemical wastes spread into the air threaten the earth's climate. *Time* (Oct. 19): 53–67.

Nelson, K. W. (1981). Government regulations—Environmental and occupational health. *American Industrial Hygiene Journal* 42: 633–36.

Proceedings of the Conference on Pesticides, Groundwater, and Health. (1987). Pesticides: Balancing risks and benefits. *Health and Environment Digest* 1(1): 1–5.

Purdom, P. W. (1980). *Environmental health*. New York: Academic Press.

Tuthill, R., E. Stanekill, C. Willis, and G. Moore. (1987). Degree of public support for household hazardous waste control alternatives. *American Journal of Public Health* 77: 304–6.

Weinstein, N., M. Klotz, and P. Sandman. (1988). Optimistic biases in public perceptions of the risk from radon. *American Journal of Public Health* 78(7): 796–800.

Williams, A., and A. Lund. (1986). Seat belt use laws and occupant crash protection in the United States. *American Journal of Public Health* 76(12): 1438–42.

World Health Organization. (1983). *Health impact of different energy sources: A challenge for the end of the century*. Copenhagen: WHO Regional Publications, European Series, No. 16: 19–22.

World Health Organization. (1986). *Health and the environment*. Vienna: WHO Regional Publications, European Series, No. 19: 12–16.

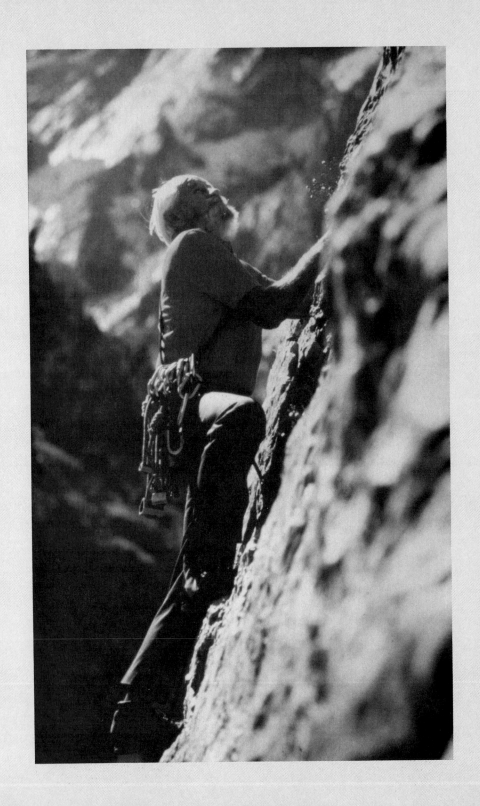

20 Health of the Elderly

The elderly constitute a large and growing population group in our country. They make up a group whose health needs we do not fully understand, and we have yet to offer the full complement of services they require and deserve.

For community health nursing, this population group poses a special challenge. The increasing number of elderly people in the community multiplies the need for health-promoting and preventive services to maximize their ability to remain independent and contributing citizens. This group's greater longevity, replete with all the problems brought on by diminishing functional capacity and increasing chronic disease and disability, brings another dimension of concern. Significant economic, environmental, and social changes create a demand for greater protective and preventive services for older adults in addition to requiring adjustments in health care provision patterns. The challenge is clear. Nursing must study the needs of this group and respond with appropriate, effective interventions.

Our focus in this chapter is on population-based nursing for the elderly. There are four fundamental requirements for effective nursing of any population:

1. Know the characteristics of the population.
2. Set aside stereotypes based on misconceptions about the population.
3. Know the health needs of the population as a basis for nursing intervention.
4. View the population from an aggregate, public health perspective that emphasizes health protection, health promotion, and disease prevention.

In this chapter we first examine the characteristics of the aging population and look at some misconceptions about the elderly. Next, we explore the health needs of older adults. Finally, we discuss population-based health services and nursing interventions applied to the health of the aging population.

CHARACTERISTICS OF THE ELDERLY POPULATION

Never before has the population of elderly people been so large. Moreover, it is increasing in size. Nearly 30 million people in the United States, or 12.2 percent of the country's population, are over 65 years of age (U.S. Bureau of Census, 1989), and by 2050 that number is expected to double to more than 67 million (Andreopoulos and Hogness, 1989). Women outnumber men in the older population because they live an average of 8 years longer. In fact, "women outlive men every place in the world where women no longer perform backbreaking physical labor and where adequate sanitation and a reduced maternal mortality are present" (Butler and Lewis, 1982, p. 6). In the United States, there are 5.6 million more women than men, a proportion of approximately 106 women for every 100 men (U.S. Bureau of Census, 1989).

People are living longer. In 1900 the average life expectancy in the United States was 47 years, and only 4 percent of the population was over 65 years of age. Now, as a result of improved health care, a reduction in infant mortality, and new medical discoveries, the average life expectancy has increased to 74.9 years (71.5 for men, 78.3 for women). For those who reach age 65, the life expectancy becomes even higher by an average of 15 or more additional years; men can expect to live an average of 14.7 additional years, and women an average of 18.6 additional years. The average life expectancies (as of 1987) for blacks (69.7 years), Hispanics (mid-50s), and American Indians (47 years), however, are considerably lower (Andreopoulos and Hogness, 1989).

Within the elderly population, the number of people living into "older" old age has increased. Forty-one percent of elderly people in the United States are over 75 years of age, more than 1 million are 85 or more years of age, and more than 110,000 claim to be over 100 years of age. Until 2030 the 85-years-and-over age group is projected to be the most rapidly growing segment of the entire U.S. population (Andreopoulos and Hogness, 1989). As the number of "older" elderly increases, so too does the size of the group needing assistance with activities of daily living. Dressing, eating, toileting, and bathing become more and more difficult for the over-85 group whose dependency and activity limitations predictably grow with age. Public health observers predict that "with more and more people living through their seventh and eighth decades of life, the size of the potentially dependent population may increase even more dramatically" (Hanlon and Pickett, 1984, p. 434). In the past, women in this age group have been more dependent than men. By the time they reach 85 and over, these women are also likely to outnumber older men two to one, adding to the potential care needs of this population group.

Other facts about the elderly are also useful for community health nurses to know. Most elderly men (81.5 percent of those 65 to 74 years old and

70 percent of those 75 and older) are married and thus have some companionship. Two-thirds of elderly women (40 percent of those 65 to 74 years old and 67 percent of those 75 and older) are widows. Most senior citizens live in the central part of the cities (about 60 percent), and the remainder in rural areas (5 percent on farms, 35 percent in small towns). Some speculate that in 15 or 20 years this demographic picture will change, and more elderly will be living in the suburbs. One-eighth of older Americans are poor, many of them living in profound poverty, unable to afford clothing, recreation, transportation, or other assets that younger people consider necessary for mental health, social status, avoidance of isolation, and personal growth. Among the elderly poor, 33.9 percent of black elderly and 27.4 percent of Hispanic elderly live below the poverty level (U.S. Bureau of Census, 1989).

MISCONCEPTIONS ABOUT THE ELDERLY

All of us have had personal experiences with the elderly. We have watched an older person cross the street; we have observed elderly relatives and neighbors; we have seen older people shopping in the supermarket. During professional training, nurses encounter many sick elderly people. These past experiences with individuals often become the data upon which we base our assumptions about this population. When we generalize our knowledge about a few older persons to the entire aging population, we are stereotyping. Many people, including health professionals, have misconceptions about the elderly. These misconceptions often arise from negative personal experiences. Practitioner bias can interfere with effective practice and prevent the kind of service aging persons need or deserve. Let's take a look at some of the more common misconceptions (Butler and Lewis, 1982; Kee, 1984; Older Women's League, 1987).

It is not true that most old people are dependent. On the contrary, 95 percent of the elderly live in the community, outside formal institutions. Approximately 70 percent live in families and 25 percent live alone or with nonrelatives. Of those living alone or with nonrelatives, some live in boarding homes or personal care homes where assistance is provided in the activities of daily living. The majority of the elderly are vigorous and functioning independently. Of the total elderly population, 45 percent (49.1 percent for males, 43.9 percent for females) have some limitations in activity (Figure 20-1), usually caused by physical handicaps such as arthritis, heart conditions, or vision or hearing loss. Only 5 percent live in formal institutions such as nursing homes, long-term care facilities, supervised living facilities, and mental institutions. And not all of these are permanent residents. Many are recovering from illnesses and will go back to the community.

It is not true that chronological age determines "oldness." One 75-year-old woman is actively involved in community organizations, drives her own car,

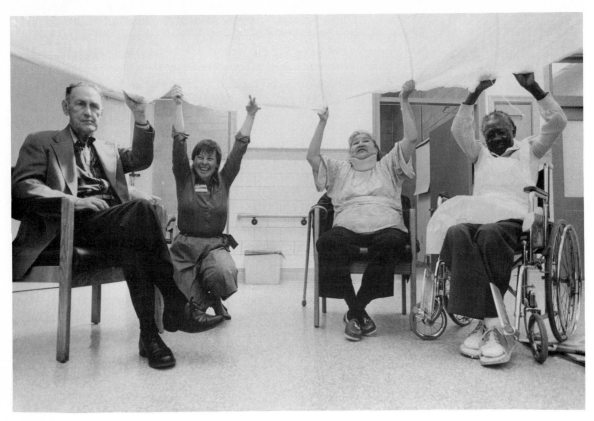

Figure 20-1
Healthy elderly people remain active despite physical limitations. Here a nurse
in an adult day care center uses a parachute to conduct range-of-motion
exercises with frail elderly and disabled clients.

and plays golf. She still has some dark hair and has few wrinkles. Another 75-year-old woman is stooped, wrinkled, slow, and confined to her room. Most old people are quite distinct from one another, and they age at widely disparate rates (Kee, 1984). Physical, social, and mental health parameters, life experiences, and genetic traits all combine to make aging an individualized process.

It is not true that most old people are senile. Senility, while not a legitimate medical diagnosis, is widely cited by health professionals and laymen alike to denote deteriorating mental faculties associated with old age. Such stereotypical labeling often provides an easy escape for practitioners impatient with an older person's complaints. It interferes with proper diagnosis and treatment. Senility, or dementia, may in actuality have its etiology from some treatable source (Public Health Service, 1979, p. 75):

Among the many causes of apparent senility which can be treated to reverse the condition are drug interactions, depression, metabolic disorders (thyroid, kidney, liver, and pituitary malfunction, as well as hypercalcemia and Cushing's Syndrome), chronic subdural hematoma, certain tumors, alcohol toxicities, chemical intoxications (arsenic and mercury), nutritional deficiencies, sensory deprivation due to social isolation or failing sight or hearing, chronic infections, hypoxia or hypercapnia associated with chronic lung disease, and anemia.

Certainly arteriosclerosis and senile brain disease may cause mental disorders among the elderly. But many so-called senile cases, compounded by anxiety, loss, grief, or psychosomatic problems, are treatable and sometimes preventable (Kee, 1984).

It is not true that all old people are content and serene. The tranquil picture of Grandma sitting in her rocker with her hands folded in her lap is misleading. It is true that many older people have learned to accept rather than fight the hardships and vicissitudes of life. Yet, for most people, old age brings increasing problems — physical, emotional, social, and financial — to harass and worry them. Depression, sometimes confused with dementia because the symptoms of disorientation, failing memory, and eccentric behavior are similar, is a frequent problem among the elderly.

It is not true that old people cannot be productive or active. More than 3 million Americans over 65 years of age work full- or part-time, and many others, not counted in labor statistics, work but do not report their earnings because of Social Security restrictions. Healthy old people do not disengage; rather, they are active and involved (Figure 20-2). Kee (1984) emphasizes that activity instead of disengagement produces the best psychological climate for the elderly.

It is not true that most older people have diminished intellectual capacity. Studies show that intelligence, learning ability, and other intellectual skills do not decline with age (Butler and Lewis, 1982). Intelligence is more directly affected by health; poor health and approaching death cause a drop in intellectual functioning (Jarvik, Eisdorfer, and Blum, 1975). Speed of reaction tends to decrease with age, but basic intelligence does not. In fact, some abilities, such as judgment, accuracy, and general knowledge, may increase with age. Most older people are largely capable of making their own decisions; they want and need the freedom to make choices and to be as independent as their limitations will allow (Kee, 1984).

Misconceptions about their intelligence often lead to the treatment of older people as children. Practitioners who infantilize their approaches to and programs for the elderly may create self-fulfilling prophecies: old age may indeed resemble a second childhood if the elderly are stripped of their rights and dignity.

It is not true that all old people are resistant to change. In a study of nursing home residents, Carp (1966) concluded that rigidity is not intrinsic to aging but rather tends to result from difficult social or physical situations. When

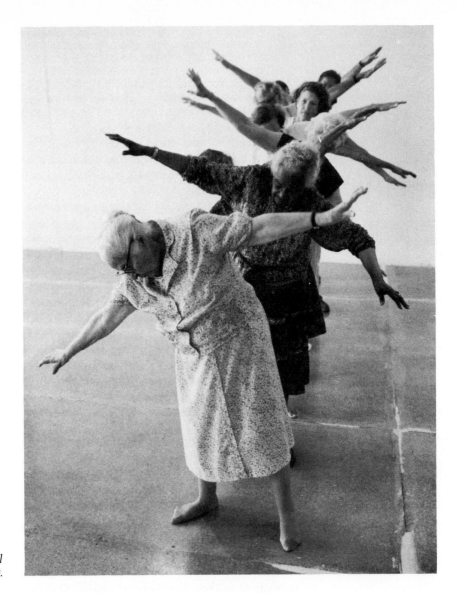

Figure 20-2
These senior citizens in Washington, D.C., have turned to modern dance as a form of creative expression. Their active involvement in a meaningful activity signals healthy aging.

these pressures are lifted, the rigidity disappears. The elderly have spent a lifetime adapting to change, with varying measures of success (Gooding et al., 1986). The ability to change does not depend on age but rather on personality traits acquired throughout life (Butler and Lewis, 1982). An older person's apparent resistance to change may be a factor of her established personality. Then again, her conservatism may be caused by socioeconomic pressures. Financial concern, for example, may cause an older property owner to vote against a school levy that would increase her taxes.

CHARACTERISTICS OF THE HEALTHY ELDERLY

To counter our misconceptions about the elderly, we need to ask, "What does it mean to age successfully?" Healthy old age has been a topic of growing interest among gerontologists. The Andrus Gerontology Center at the University of Southern California and others have been conducting research in this area for many years. No one knows conclusively all the variables that influence healthy old age, but we do know that a lifetime of healthy habits and circumstances, a strong social support system, and a positive emotional outlook all have a major influence on the resources people bring to their later years. Most of us recognize a healthy older person when we meet one. Let us meet such a person.

Case Example

> Minerva Blackstone, affectionately called Minnie by her friends, is a lively 87-year-old woman who enjoys life. Every day, except in bad weather, she walks the half mile to the house of her granddaughter, Karen, for a visit. There she works on the quilt, stretched on a frame, that she is making for Karen. Twice a week Minnie takes the city bus to the senior citizens' center to join her friends in an exercise class. Although her eyesight has failed somewhat, Minnie enjoys reading in the evening and crocheting while she watches T.V. Mysteries and comedies are her favorite kinds of stories. She is not content, however, unless she has kept up on the latest political developments. She always has opinions on current events and expresses them with vigorous shakes of her curly white hair at her monthly group meeting on women and politics. She has a good appetite and generally sleeps well. Minor arthritis does not hamper her activities, nor does the hypertension that she controls by taking her medication with conscientious regularity. Minnie is enjoying healthy, successful old age.

What is healthy old age? As we said earlier, the vast majority (95 percent) of the elderly, like Minnie Blackstone, are living outside institutions and maintaining relative independence, even those with chronic diseases and other disabilities. They are able to function. The ability to function is a key indicator of health and wellness and is an important factor in understanding healthy aging. Good health in the elderly means maintaining the maximum degree of physical, mental, and social vigor of which one is capable. It means being able to adapt, to continue to handle stress, and to be active and involved. In short, healthy aging means being able to function with, and despite, disabilities, with no more than ordinary help from others (Public Health Service, 1979; Speake, 1987).

Wellness among the elderly population varies considerably. It is influenced by many factors such as personality traits, life experiences, current physical health, and current societal supports. Some elderly people, like Minnie Blackstone, demonstrate maximum adaptability, resourcefulness, optimism, and activity. Others, often those from whom we tend to draw our stereotypes, have disengaged and present a picture of dependence and resignation. Most of the elderly population is somewhere in between these two extremes. Although the level of wellness varies among the elderly, that level can be raised. The challenge in community health nursing is to maximize the wellness potential of the elderly. Nurses must analyze and capitalize on the elderly's strengths, not focus only on their problems; the goal is to enable older people to thrive, not merely survive (Boyle et al., 1988; Kiehn, 1987).

HEALTH NEEDS OF THE ELDERLY

Effective nursing with any population requires familiarity with that group's health problems and needs. Aging in and of itself is not a health problem. Rather, aging is a normal, irreversible physiological process. Its pace, however, can sometimes be delayed, researchers are discovering (Rosenfeld, 1976), and many of the problems associated with aging can be prevented (Hanlon and Pickett, 1984). The aging process is subtle, gradual, and lifelong. One can see remarkable differences between individuals' rates of aging; even in a single individual, various systems of the body age at different rates (Kee, 1984). Thus, chronological age cannot serve as an indicator of health needs; "nevertheless, the proportion of people with health problems increases with age and, as a group, the elderly are more likely than younger persons to suffer from multiple, chronic, and often disabling conditions" (Public Health Service, 1979, p. 71).

The leading causes of death among the population aged 65 and over are heart disease, cancer, and stroke, followed by pneumonia, chronic obstructive pulmonary diseases, and diabetes mellitus (National Center for Health Statistics, 1988). Deaths in the group aged 65 to 74 years have declined, but the sharpest rise occurs for those over age 85. While most of the elderly population is healthy, 80 percent have at least one chronic condition, causing nearly half of the elderly population to experience some kind of activity limitations (Mundinger, 1983). A small proportion are dependent and disabled, requiring more extensive care.

The most frequent health problems experienced by older people in the community are arthritis, reduced vision, hearing losses, heart conditions, and hypertension. In those over 65, two in five persons have high blood pressure. "Hypertension increases with age, is twice as prevalent among blacks as whites, and generally affects men more than women. But older black women have the highest rates of hypertension of any group" (Older Women's League, 1987). Acute illness, such as influenza and pneumonia, or injuries, such as burns and those from falls, occur less frequently and can often be prevented (Gooding et al., 1986).

A significant health problem for the elderly arises from adverse drug effects. Older people's bodies handle drugs differently from the bodies of younger people on whom most clinical trials take place. Thus, overprescription of medications or complicated drug regimens for many older persons lead to unexpected and dangerous drug interactions. The elderly need education about the drugs they take and their possible effects. They also need proper supervision of their overall medication intake.

Depression, too, is a difficult problem for older adults. Loss of a spouse, loss of friends, economic problems, physical disease and disability, loneliness, or drug side effects can make an elderly person feel that life holds no meaning. Social and emotional withdrawal often occurs, as does suicide.

In addition to these problems, elderly people have specific health needs. At all stages of life, people have the same basic needs. We know that the elderly, like any age group, have physiological, safety, love and belonging, esteem, and self-actualization needs. Their physical, emotional, and social needs are complex and interrelated (Kee, 1984). As community health nurses assess the health of the elderly population, however, some needs in particular demand extra attention.

Among these is the need for *good nutrition*. People who have maintained sound dietary habits throughout life need change little in old age. Many have not established such habits but may wish to. One study of an elderly population group revealed their desire for help with weight control, cooking, and shopping for good nutrition (Archer, Kelly, and Bisch, 1984). Older people need to maintain their optimal weight by eating a generally low-fat, moderate-carbohydrate, and high-protein diet. They should avoid habitual use of laxatives, adding instead more fiber and bulk to their diet. Loss of teeth will cause some to need foods that are easier to chew. Eating should be a pleasurable experience, preferably taking place in the company of other people.

Older people continue to need *exercise* (Figure 20-3). Aging does not and should not involve passivity; instead, physical activity and movement contribute to quality of intellectual and physical performance in old age. Exercise, such as a daily walk, can keep muscles in good tone, enhance circulation, and promote mental health. Exercise may occur in connection with such activities as homemaking chores, gardening, hobbies, or recreation and sports. Often such physical outlets are done in the company of other people, meeting social and emotional needs as well.

Economic security is another major need for older adults. Worry over finances is often one of the most debilitating factors in old age. Fearing the potential costs of major illness and not wanting to be a burden on family or friends, many older people will conserve their limited financial resources by eating cheaply, using health resources sparingly, and spending little on themselves: "Too often, the fear—let alone the reality—of financial straits prevents elderly people from leading the full and active lives of which they are capable" (Public Health Service, 1979, p.77). Putting older people in touch with appropriate community resources can do much to relieve this source of stress.

Older people need *independence*. As much as possible, the elderly need to make their own decisions and manage their own lives. Even those with activity limitations because of disability can still exercise decision-making

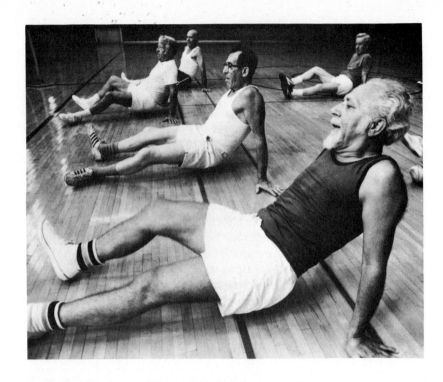

Figure 20-3
Community health nurses must learn the needs of each population group, such as elderly persons' need for physical fitness. Here, senior citizens exercise in a community center's gymnasium.

options about many, if not most, aspects of their daily living. The need for autonomy—to be able to assert ourselves as separate individuals—is great for all of us. With life's restrictions ever increasing for the elderly person, this need is all the greater (Eliopoulus, 1984). Independence helps to meet another need, that of self-respect and dignity. The elderly need to have their ideas and suggestions heard and acted upon and to be addressed by their preferred names in a respectful tone of voice. Respect for the old is not a strong value in our culture, but it is one that needs to be cultivated. Older people represent a rich resource of wisdom, experience, and patience that we are generally wasting in our country.

Older people need *companionship and social interaction*, particularly when they live alone. The company of other people as well as the companionship of a household pet offers avenues for expression and response and adds meaning to life. Many studies of mortality patterns demonstrate that older adults living together have a greater survival rate and retain their independence longer than those who live alone (Hanlon and Pickett, 1984). The problem is of greatest significance for women, who outnumber men considerably in the later years and who live alone more frequently.

Meaningful activity is another need of the elderly. It too adds purpose to life. Some kind of active role in community life is essential for mental health, satisfaction, and self-esteem. It can range from involvement in hobbies, such as gardening or crafts, to volunteer work or even full-time employment (Fig-

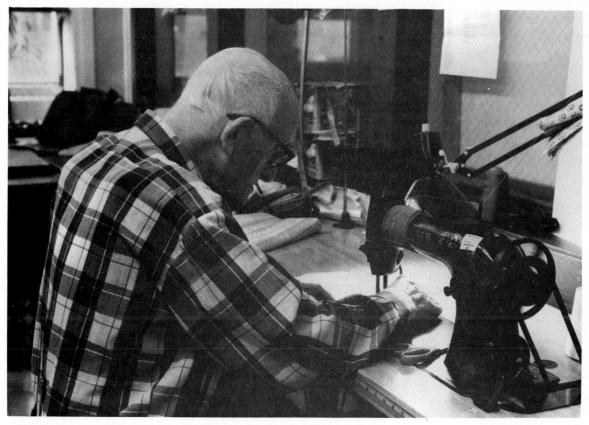

Figure 20-4
Elderly people, like other adults, benefit from satisfying activities. This man
continues to perform work that is valued by himself and others.

ure 20-4). One current example is the federally supported Foster Grandparents and Senior Companions program that engages the help of more than 18,000 seniors. These older adults work 20 hours a week offering companionship and guidance to 63,500 handicapped children across the country. Another program, the Foundation for Grandparenting in New York, plans to use grandparent volunteers to work with schoolchildren on a long-term relationship basis ("America's forgotten resource: Grandparents," 1984, p. 77).

A final need of the elderly, and one that is receiving increasing attention, is that of a *dignified death*. Quality of life has become an important issue, and as Kübler-Ross (1975) describes it, death is the final stage of growth, deserving that same measure of quality. A dignified death — as free as possible from pain, humiliation, discomfort, or financial concerns — can be the end product of a high-quality aging process. For most elderly persons this means having a choice, whenever possible, about where and under what circumstances death will occur. Freedom from financial worries, knowledge that their affairs and family members are taken care of, opportunity for spiritual counseling, and peaceful surroundings, preferably at home with the support of loved ones, are all important quality considerations.

COMMUNITY HEALTH PERSPECTIVE

Another requirement for nursing of the elderly as a population group is to view them from a broad, community health perspective. In general, we can divide nursing service to the elderly into two approaches. One approach emphasizes the science of geriatrics; the other, the science of gerontology. Although these fields overlap, they tend to differ in at least one significant way. Geriatrics is the study of diseases of old age, while gerontology studies the broader phenomena of aging iself (Butler and Lewis, 1982). Geriatric nursing in the past has been oriented primarily toward care of the sick aged. Gerontological nursing, a broader practice, concentrates on preventing illness and promoting the health and maximum functioning of older adults (Elio-poulus, 1984). While both are important dimensions of nursing practice, a community health perspective emphasizes the gerontological approach.

Community health nurses work with many elderly people. In one instance, the nurse may promote and maintain the health of a vigorous 80-year-old man who lives alone in his home. As another example, the nurse may give postsurgical care at home to a 69-year-old woman, teach her husband how to care for her, and help them contact needed community resources for shopping, meals, housekeeping, and transportation services. Perhaps the focus is on teaching nutrition and a healthful life-style to a family, including the 73-year-old grandmother who lives with them. Yet again, the nurse may lead a support group for senior citizens who have recently lost their spouses through death. Mortality after bereavement is high (Kaprio et al., 1987) and can be prevented through nursing intervention.

A large portion of the community health nurse's work with the elderly is at the individual, family, and group levels. However, a community health perspective also leads to concern for and work with large aggregates of the elderly. There are many population groups composed of elderly persons. All the seniors attending an adult day-care center, belonging to a retirement community, living in a nursing home, or using Meals on Wheels are some examples. Others include residents of a senior citizens' high-rise apartment building, retired business and professional women, elderly residents in a community at risk for glaucoma, the elderly poor, and skid-row alcoholics.

Having a community perspective means that the nurse sees the "forest," not just the "trees." Problems in individual segments of a population group can negatively affect the rest of the group. Witness the spread of influenza when people are unprotected. Conversely, health-promoting and disease-preventing measures aimed at an entire population group enhance the health of the individuals involved (Hanlon and Pickett, 1984). For example, a positive life-style emphasis in a retirement community or a comprehensive nutrition and meal-planning program in a senior day-care center can have far-reaching health benefits for the older adults who make up each of those populations. A community health "forest thinker" keeps the big picture in mind and designs interventions for the public good.

HEALTH SERVICES FOR THE ELDERLY POPULATION

How well are we meeting the needs of our older adults? To answer this question, we must first raise other questions. Do health programs for the elderly encompass the full range of needed services? Are they close enough that they can be reached easily when needed? Do they encourage elderly clients to function independently? Do they treat senior citizens with respect and preserve their dignity? Do they recognize older adults' need for companionship, economic security, and social status? When appropriate, do they promote meaningful activities instead of overworked games like bingo and shuffleboard? Games can be useful diversions but must be balanced with opportunities for creative outlets, continued learning, and community service.

Several criteria emerge from this list of questions that describe an effective community health service delivery system for the elderly. Four, in particular, deserve our attention.

Criteria for Effective Service

Comprehensiveness. An effective community health service delivery system for the elderly should be comprehensive. Many communities provide some programs, such as limited health screening or selected activities, but do not offer a full range of services that would more adequately meet the needs of their senior citizens. Gaps and duplication in programs most often result from poor or nonexistent community-wide planning. Furthermore, such planning should be based on thorough assessment of elderly people's needs in that community. A comprehensive set of services should provide the following (Burns, 1984; Ford, 1987; Jameison and Martinson, 1983):

Health care services (prevention, early diagnosis and treatment, rehabilitation)

Health education (including preparation for retirement)

Recreation and activity programs (See Figure 20-5.)

Adult day-care programs

Specialized transportation services

In-home services

Adequate financial support

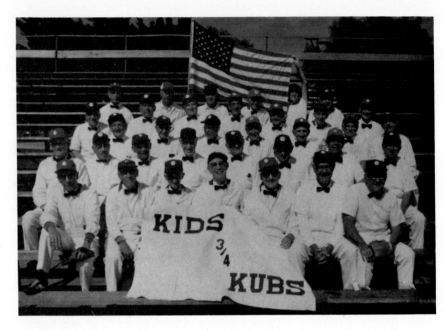

Figure 20-5
Senior citizens are a group whose needs must also be viewed from an aggregate perspective if community health services are to be effective. Recreational activities, such as this baseball team (whose members range in age from 75 to 92) are part of the many programs needed in a comprehensive system serving the elderly population.

Coordination. A second criterion for a community service delivery system for the elderly is coordination (Burns, 1984). Often older persons go from one agency to the next. After visiting one place for food stamps, they may go to another for answers to Medicaid questions, another for congregate dining, and still another for health screening. Such a potpourri of services reflects a system organized for the convenience of providers rather than consumers. It encourages nonuse or misuse. Instead, there should be coordinated, community-wide assessment and planning. Communities must consider alternatives such as multiservice agencies that can meet many needs in one location. As a surgeon general's report indicates, "Many elderly people . . . need a range of services—dietary guidance, eye care, foot care, dental care, and social assistance, as well as routine medical care. And these are best provided at one center" (Public Health Service, 1979, p. 76).

A coordinated information and referral system provides another needed link. Most communities need a better information network. A directory of all resources and services for the elderly with the name and telephone number of a contact person for each listing is available in some communities and should be developed in those without one. A simplified information and referral system—a system that includes one number to call to find out what resources and services are available and how to get them—is particularly helpful to older people.

Accessibility. A third criterion is accessibility. Too often, services for the elderly are not conveniently located or are prohibitive in cost. Some communities are considering multiservice community centers to bring programs and services for the elderly closer to home. More convenient and perhaps specialized transportation services and more in-home services, such as Meals on Wheels, may further solve accessibility problems for many older adults. Federal, state, and private funding sources can be tapped to ease the burden on the economically pressured elderly population.

Quality. Finally, an effective community service system for older people promotes quality programs. By that is meant services that truly address the needs and concerns of a community's senior citizens. Evaluation of the quality of a community's services for the elderly is closely tied to their assessed needs. What are this specific population group's needs in terms of nutrition, exercise, economic security, independence, social interaction, meaningful activities, and preparation for death? Planning for quality community services depends on having adequate, accurate, and current data. Periodic needs assessment is a necessity to ensure updated information and to promote quality services. Unfortunately, in most communities this is not done at all, or is done without any regularity or thoroughness. Many agencies in a given community are involved in delivering services for the elderly. Collaboration and surveys of seniors, perhaps spearheaded by community health nurses as was done in northern California (Archer, Kelly, and Bisch, 1984), can provide vital information for planning needed programs.

Institutional Care

While only 5 percent of the elderly population live in formal institutions, such organizations remain the most visible type of health service for older adults. Of these, nursing homes make up the largest portion. More than 1.5 million elderly persons live in nursing homes, and despite government attempts to protect these individuals and contain costs through admission and care standards, costs have increased along with questions about quality of care.

There is widespread fear and despair associated with nursing homes. Too many older people and their families have been exploited by an industry that frequently puts profit ahead of meeting this group's needs. The book *Tender Loving Greed* (Mendelson, 1974) graphically describes the problem. Even in institutions where the quality of care is acceptable, costs are so high that family resources are soon depleted. Although Medicaid and other government sources pay a large share of nursing home costs, patients and families pay more than half (51%) (Waldo, 1986). Life savings that older parents had hoped to leave for their children may be quickly consumed, forcing them into indigence and dependence on public funds. Dread of nursing homes arises, too, from dehumanizing institutional regulations such as segregation of sexes, strict social policies, and overuse of tranquilizers, and from demeaning or even abusive conditions that promote institutional control rather than the clients' well-being.

Institutions housing the dependent elderly involve several levels of nursing care. Those involving the highest level are called skilled nursing facilities. Less costly are intermediate-care facilities that still provide health care but decrease the amount and type of care given. Medicare generally only pays for skilled nursing facilities services. Medicaid pays for care in skilled as well as intermediate-care facilities. Personal-care homes offer basic social supports, such as bathing and grooming, without medical services. Payment may come from private funds, Title XX (Social Security Act) funds, old age assistance, or aid to the disabled. Boarding homes house elderly persons needing meal service and light housekeeping but who can manage their own personal care. Government funds are not available to support these institutions. Congregate care and group homes are an alternative for specific elderly populations, such as alcoholics or developmentally disabled, and are often subsidized by concerned community organizations.

An alternative to nursing home care is foster home care for the frail elderly. A study of one such program showed that it was less costly than nursing home care and improved clients' health status (Oktay and Volland, 1987).

Deinstitutionalization

"Deinstitutionalizing" people, or promoting their living outside institutions, has received considerable emphasis recently. The trend started several decades ago when it became evident that tuberculosis patients improved more readily and cost of care was less if they were treated on an outpatient basis. Care of the mentally ill began to be deinstitutionalized in the 1950s for the same reasons, and treatment of the developmentally disabled followed suit. For the elderly population we now see an increasing emphasis on avoiding needless institutionalization and maintaining functional independence.

The trend toward deinstitutionalized care for the elderly stems from several incentives. The potential for cost savings appears to be much greater if dependent older people can be discharged from institutions and maintained at home. We know that many nursing home residents are there needlessly (Hanlon and Pickett, 1984) and could manage outside the institution if given adequate assistance. Deinstitutionalization encourages functional independence as well as emotional well-being.

On the other hand, deinstitutionalization is not the panacea that many believe it to be. Although some studies have demonstrated cost savings (Oktay and Volland, 1987), others have shown that community-based systems are more expensive (Toff, 1981). We do not yet have complete data for comparisons. Research has not yet fully assessed the costs to the community for health and social services incurred in maintaining deinstitutionalized dependent people. Nor have most studies been able to determine the change in functional level of people being deinstitutionalized (Hanlon and Pickett, 1984). Furthermore, services for the dependent elderly in the community are often fragmented, inadequate, and inaccessible, with little or no maintenance of standards or quality control. Institutions, despite their problems, are at least regulated and must be accountable for their clients' safety and care.

There is a solution. The dependent elderly need someone in the community to assess their particular needs, assemble and coordinate the appropriate resources and services, and serve as their advocate. It is a role most appropriately filled by the community health nurse. This case management approach tailors services to fit the needs of clients and enables them to function longer outside of institutions (Hanlon and Pickett, 1984; Grau, 1984).

Various techniques are available to assess the needs of older adults. A comprehensive one, the Older Americans Resources and Services Information System (OARS), developed by Duke University, established baseline data on clients' well-being, available economic and social resources, physical and mental health status, and clients' capacity for self-care (Eliopoulus, 1984; Pfeiffer, 1978; Fillenbaum and Smyer, 1981). Clients' capacity for self-care is assessed by means of the Capacity for Self-Care Index, which ascertains clients' ability to go outdoors, climb stairs, move about their homes, bathe, dress, and cut toenails (Shanas, 1980). Other techniques, like the Ability to Perform Work-Related Activities survey (Kovar and LaCroix, 1987), determine an elderly person's physical, psychological, and social needs. A frequently overlooked area for assessment is elderly clients' spiritual needs. Religious dedication and spiritual concern often increase in later years. Limited ability or lack of transportation may prevent older people from attending religious services or engaging in spiritually enhancing activities. Self-health ratings, including clients' reporting on their spiritual needs, is another useful assessment technique.

The case management concept has been practiced by community health nurses for many years with a primary focus on the health needs of their clients. Social workers use case management to address their clients' problems in the area of social needs, including financial problems. Some health maintenance organizations provide a coordinated system of services for their enrolled clients. Unfortunately, many elderly people in the community have no such advocate; a more comprehensive, community-wide system is needed in many localities to serve the total elderly population (Jameison and Martinson, 1983). Such a system could be based on establishment of an agency specifically designed to serve as case manager, or "agent," to assess clients' needs and assemble existing agencies and services to meet those needs (Kodner and Feldman, 1981).

Other alternatives to institutionalization include home services and partial day-care services. Home care provides services such as skilled nursing care, physical or speech therapy, homemaker services, and dietetic counseling. Day-care services include shelter, social activities, nutrition, nursing care, and physical and speech therapy. Both alternatives are useful for families unable to care for an elderly member during work or school hours.

Services for the Well Elderly

Services for the other 95 percent of the elderly population should have as their primary goals the avoidance of needless institutionalization and the maintenance of functional independence. Needs assessment, using techniques such as OARS or the activities survey mentioned in the previous section, forms the basis for determining appropriate services. Although most of the well elderly can assess their own health status, many are reluctant to seek needed help. Thus, *outreach programs* serve an important function in many communities. They locate elderly persons in need of health or social assistance and refer them to appropriate resources.

Geriatric screening is another important program for early detection and treatment of health problems among older adults. Conditions to watch for include hypertension, glaucoma, hearing disorders, cancers, diabetes, anemias, depression, and nutritional deficiencies (Itzin, 1987). At the same time, assessment of elderly clients' socialization, housing, and economic needs, with proper referrals, can prevent further problems from developing that would influence their health status.

Health maintenance programs may be offered through a single agency, such as a health maintenance organization, or coordinated by a case management agency with referrals to other providers. These programs should cover a wide range of health services needed by the elderly, such as those given below (Public Health Service, 1979; Burns, 1984):

Dietary guidance and food services such as Meals on Wheels or group meal services

Dental care

Podiatry

Vision tests and eyeglasses

Hearing tests and hearing aid assistance

Exercise and fitness programs

Speech or physical therapy

Home health services, including skilled nursing and home health aide services

Routine medical care

Medical supplies or equipment

Health education

Medication supervision

Social assistance services may well be offered in conjunction with health maintenance programs since the two are so interrelated. The elderly have many needs in this area. They include the following:

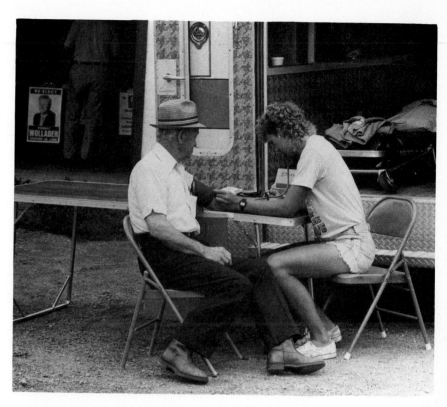

Figure 20-6
Having his blood pressure taken, part of geriatric screening, can lead to early detection of health problems for this older man.

Financial aid and counseling

Safe and affordable housing

Transportation services

Home maintenance assistance (housekeeping, chores, repairs)

Recreational and educational programs

Religious ministries

Community centers for social opportunities

Communication services (phones, access to health professionals)

Legal aid and counseling

Volunteer and employment opportunities

Library services, including talking books and large-print publications

Escort and protective services

Friendly visiting and companions

Senior citizens' discounts (food, drugs, transportation, recreation)

Respite care is a service receiving increasing attention and is aimed primarily at caregivers' needs (Andreopoulos and Hogness, 1989). Many elderly persons at home are cared for by a spouse or other family member. The demands of such care can be exhausting unless the caregiver can get some relief, or respite—thus the name of this service. Respite care may be available through an agency that provides volunteers to relieve caregivers, giving them time away on a regular basis or permitting a periodic vacation. Some hospitals and nursing homes provide extra rooms to give temporary institutional housing for the elderly while caregivers take a break. Elderly clients may also need a change from the constant interaction with their caregivers.

Hospice care may be offered through an institution such as a hospital, or it may be a program providing services that enable dying persons to stay at home (Andreopoulos and Hogness, 1989). Its purpose is to make the dying process as dignified, free from discomfort, and emotionally, spiritually, and socially supportive as possible. Some community health nursing agencies offer hospice programs staffed by their nurses. For the elderly, it is a service that has been well received, meets important needs, and is growing in use.

IMPLICATIONS FOR COMMUNITY HEALTH NURSING

Community health nurses can make a significant contribution to the health of the elderly population. Because these nurses are in the community and already have contact with many older adults, they are in a prime position to begin needs assessment and planning for the health of this group. Though many of the services named above are not within the scope of nursing's practice, the case management role can and often should be a critical aspect of the nurse's contribution to this population (Grau, 1984).

The health care scene in terms of services available for the elderly is changing dramatically. The numbers and types of home care services, for example, are mushrooming. Many entrepreneurs, recognizing the potential of this growing market, are offering goods and services targeted for older adults. Nursing must keep abreast of these changes—aware of new developments, new programs, new regulations, new social and economic forces (like prospective payment) and their potential impact on the provision of health services. Even more important, community health nurses will need to be proactive, designing interventions that maximize nursing's resources and provide the greatest benefit to elderly clients. For example, community health nurses could develop a case management program for older adults as a community-wide assessment, information, and referral service. Such a program might contract with existing agencies to serve as a clearinghouse for the elderly and channel clients to appropriate services. Financing of such a program might be based on tax dollars (if a public agency), grants, or some innovative fee-for-service reimbursement system.

Many of the elderly population's health problems can be prevented and their health promoted (Gooding, 1986; Kiehn, 1987). Change to a healthier life-style is one of the most important preventive measures the nurse can emphasize. Examples include stopping smoking, eating regular and well-balanced meals, exercising regularly, keeping weight within 15 pounds of normal for body build, consuming little or no alcohol, getting proper rest, and maintaining a healthy emotional outlook. Educating the elderly about their health conditions and use of their medications is another important way to prevent problems. Influenza and pneumonia can be prevented through regular health maintenance and immunizations. Other problems associated with environmental conditions and the aging process, such as arthritis, diabetes, and some cancers, can be diagnosed and treated early, thereby minimizing their effect on functional independence.

With an elderly population that is increasing in size and age, community health nurses face a serious challenge in addressing its needs. At the same time nursing can be on the forefront of developing innovative health services for this group, rising to meet the opportunity and the challenge.

Summary

The elderly population is increasing in size and age. Accompanying these changes are this group's escalating health needs and concomitant requirements for new and improved services. Community health nursing has an opportunity to accept the challenge, study the needs of older adults, and develop effective, population-based nursing interventions. Population-based nursing requires four emphases: (1) know the characteristics of the population, (2) avoid misconceptions about them, (3) know the group's health needs, and (4) maintain an aggregate perspective.

The number of adults aged 65 and over is growing. Their percentage of the total population is increasing. Women still live longer than men, and more women are alone in their later years. Given these facts, the potential for a growing number of dependent elderly is great.

Misconceptions or practitioner bias about older adults can interfere with effective community health nursing practice. Contrary to some beliefs, most (95 percent) of the elderly live outside institutions and are relatively independent. Chronological age does not determine "oldness." Senility is not a problem for most older people, but depression and worry often are. Many elderly people are active in the community, most maintain their intellectual ability, and many adapt well to change.

Healthy aging involves the ability to function as independently as possible. It means maintaining the maximum degree of physical, mental, and social vigor of which one is capable. It includes the ability to adapt, to handle stress and change, to be meaningfully active and involved.

The health needs of the elderly center around chronic, often progressive, and disabling conditions. Leading causes of death are heart disease, cancer, and stroke. The most frequent health problems are arthritis, vision and hearing losses, heart conditions, and hypertension. Acute illnesses common to the elderly, primarily influenza and pneumonia, are preventable. Other health problems of older adults include drug reactions and depression.

To promote and maintain health and prevent illness, elderly people need good nutrition, exercise, economic security, independence, companionship and social interaction, and meaningful activity. They also deserve, when possible, a dignified and peaceful death.

An aggregate, community health perspective means that the nurse sees and seeks to serve the entire population of older adults, not just individuals. This is enhanced by examining what services are available and needed, and analyzing their effectiveness when used. Effective community health services for the elderly should be comprehensive, coordinated, accessible, of high quality, and targeted to the specific needs of the older population.

Institutions house 5 percent of the elderly. Most of these are nursing homes where elderly residents receive skilled nursing care. Intermediate-care facilities, personal-care homes, and boarding homes offer decreasing amounts and levels of care.

A trend toward deinstitutionalization is creating many more alternatives for older adults to maintain functional independence at home. It has the potential for being more cost-effective but poses new problems with evaluating quality and coordinating services. A solution can be application of the case management concept, which offers a centralized system for assessing the elderly population's needs and matching those needs with appropriate services.

Services needed by the well elderly include outreach programs, geriatric screening, health maintenance programs that cover a wide range of health services, social assistance services, respite care, and hospice care.

Community health nurses can promote and preserve the health of the elderly by practicing from a perspective of population-based nursing, by developing more effective services such as comprehensive case management, and by promoting healthy life-styles and activities among older adults.

Study Questions

1. Picture in your mind an elderly person whom you know well or know a great deal about. Make a list of characteristics that describe that person. How many of these characteristics fit your picture of most senior citizens? What are your biases about the elderly?
2. If you were Minnie Blackstone's community health nurse, what interventions would you consider using to maintain and promote her health? Why?
3. As part of your regular community health nursing workload, you visit a senior day-care center one afternoon a week. You take the blood pressures of several people who are on hypertensive medications and do some nutritional counseling. The center accommodates 60 senior clients, and you would like to serve the health needs of the entire ag-

gregate. What are some potential health needs of this group? What actions might you consider taking at an aggregate level?

4. Assume you have been asked by your local health department to determine the needs of the elderly population in your community. How would you begin conducting such a needs assessment? What data might you want to collect? How would you find out what services are already being offered and whether or not they are adequate?

References

America's forgotten resource: Grandparents (1984, April 30). *U.S. News & World Report,* pp. 76–77.

Andreopoulos, S., and J. Hogness. (1989). *Health care for an aging society.* New York: Churchill Livingstone, Inc.

Archer, S. E., C. D. Kelly, and S. A. Bisch. (1984). Senior life-style survey. In S. E. Archer, C. D. Kelly, and S. A. Bisch (eds.), *Implementing change in communities: A collaborative process.* St. Louis: C. V. Mosby.

Boyle, J. S., et al. (1988). Toward healthy aging: A theory for community health nursing... in an Appalachian community. *Public Health Nursing* 5(1): 45–51.

Burns, G. B. (1984). Coordinated community health services for the elderly... liaison public health nurse acts as a resource. *Canadian Journal of Public Health* 75(6): 458–62.

Butler, R. N., and M. I. Lewis. (1982). *Aging and mental health: Positive psychosocial approaches.* 3rd ed. St. Louis: C. V. Mosby.

Carp, R. M. (1966). *A future for the aged: Victoria Plaza and its residents.* Austin: University of Texas Press.

Eliopoulus, C. (1984). A self-care model for gerontological nursing. *Geriatric Nursing* 5(8): 366–69.

Fillenbaum, G. G., and M. A. Smyer. (1981). The development, validity, and reliability of the OARS multidimensional functional assessment questionnaire. *Journal of Gerontology* 36(4): 428.

Ford, A. B. (1987). Looking after the old folks. *American Journal of Public Health* 77(12): 1499–1500.

Gooding, H., et al. (1986). The value of preventive care service for the elderly. *Health Visitor* 59(10): 305–6.

Grau, L. (1984). Case management and the nurse... long-term community care to the elderly. *Geriatric Nursing* 5(8): 372–75.

Hanlon, J. J., and G. E. Pickett. (1984). *Public Health: Administration and practice* 8th ed. St. Louis: Times Mirror/Mosby.

Itzin, C. (1987). Screening elderly people. *Nursing Times* 83(48): 47–50.

Jameison, M., and I. Martinson. (1983). Block nursing: Neighbors caring for neighbors. *Nursing Outlook* 31(5): 270–73.

Jarvik, L. F., C. Eisdorfer, and J. E. Blum. (eds.). (1975). *Intellectual functioning in adults.* New York: Springer/Verlag.

Kaprio, J., M. Koskenvuo, H. Rita. (1987). Mortality after bereavement: A prospective study of 95,647 widowed persons. *American Journal of Public Health* 77(3): 283–87.

Kee, C. C. (1984). A case for health promotion with the elderly. *Nursing Clinics of North America* 19(2): 251–62.

Kiehn, M. (1987). A brighter future for the elderly. *Health Visitor* 60(10): 340–42.

Kodner, D. L., and E. S. Feldman. (1981). The service coordination/delivery dichotomy: A critical issue to address in reforming the long-term care system. Paper presented at annual meeting of the American Public Health Association, Los Angeles.

Kovar, M. G., and A. Z. LaCroix. (1987). Aging in the eighties, ability to perform work-related activities, data from the supplement on aging to the National Health Interview Survey: United States, 1984. *National Center for Health Statistics Advance Data* Number 136 (May 8), DHHS Pub. No. (PHS)87–1250. Hyattsville, Maryland: Public Health Service.

Kübler-Ross, E. (1975). *Death: The final stage of growth.* Englewood Cliffs, N.J.: Prentice-Hall.

Mendelson, M. A. (1974). *Tender loving greed.* New York: Knopf.

Mundinger, M. (1983). *Home care controversy: Too little, too late, too costly.* Rockville, Md.: Aspen.

National Center for Health Statistics. (1988). Vital statistics of the United States, 1986, Volume II, Mortality, Part A. DHHS Pub. No. (PHS)88-1122. Public Health Service. Washington, D.C.: U.S. Government Printing Office.

Oktay, J. S., and P. J. Volland. (1987). Foster home care for the frail elderly as an alternative to nursing home care: An experimental evaluation. *American Journal of Public Health* 77(12): 1505–10.

Older Women's League. (1987). The picture of health for midlife and older women in America. *Older Women's League Mother's Day Report 1987.* Washington, D.C.: OWL.

Pfeiffer, E. (ed.). (1978). *Multidimensional functional assessment: The OARS methodology.* 2nd ed. Durham, N.C.: Duke University Center for Study of Aging and Human Development.

Public Health Service. (1979). *Healthy people: The Surgeon General's report on health promotion and disease prevention* (DHEW Publication No. 79-55071). Washington, D.C.: U.S. Government Printing Office.

Rosenfeld, A. (1976). *Prolongevity.* New York: Avon Books.

Shanas, E. (1980). Self-assessment of physical function: White and black elderly in the United States. In S. Haynes and M. Feinleib (eds.), *Epidemiology of aging* (NIH Pub. No. 80-969). Washington, D.C.: U.S. Department of Health and Human Services.

Speake, D. L. (1987). Health promotion activity in the well elderly. *Health Values* 11(6): 25–30.

Toff, G. E. (1981). *Alternatives to institutional care for the elderly: An analysis of state initiatives.* Washington, D.C.: Intergovernmental Health Policy Project.

U.S. Bureau of Census. (1989). *Statistical Abstracts of the United States, 1989,* 109th ed. Washington, D.C.: U.S. Government Printing Office.

Waldo, D. (1986). National health expenditures, 1985. *Health Care Financing Review* 8(Fall): 1–21.

Selected Readings

Andreopoulos, S., and J. Hogness. (1989). *Health care for an aging society.* New York: Churchill Livingstone, Inc.

Archer, S. E., C. D. Kelly, and S. A. Bisch. (1984). Senior life-style survey. In S. E. Archer, C. D. Kelly, and S. A. Bisch (eds.), *Implementing change in communities: A collaborative process.* St. Louis: C. V. Mosby.

Archer, S. E., C. D. Kelly, and S. A. Bisch. (1984). Senior resources survey. In S. E. Archer, C. D. Kelly, and S. A. Bisch, *Implementing change in communities: A collaborative process.* St. Louis: C. V. Mosby.

Birenbaum, A., M. Aronson, and S. Seiffer. (1979). Training medical students to appreciate the special problems of the elderly. *The Gerontologist* 19: 575–79.

Boyle, J. S., et al. (1988). Toward healthy aging: A theory for community health nursing... in an Appalachian community. *Public Health Nursing* 5(1): 45–51.

Branch, L., S. Katz, K. Kneipmann, and J. Papsidero. (1984). A prospective study of functional status among community elders. *American Journal of Public Health* 74: 266–68.

Burns, G. B. (1984). Coordinated community health services for the elderly... liaison public health nurse acts as a resource. *Canadian Journal of Public Health* 75(6): 458–62.

Burnside, I. M. (ed.). (1976). *Nursing and the aged.* New York: McGraw-Hill.

Butler, R. N., and M. I. Lewis. (1977). *Aging and mental health: Positive psychosocial approaches.* 2nd ed. St. Louis: C. V. Mosby.

Clemons, B. (1982). Teaching longevity. *Friendly Exchange* 3(1): 21.

Cohen, C., and J. Sokolvsky. (1980). Social engagement versus isolation: The case of the aged in SRO hotels. *The Gerontologist* 20: 36–43.

Collins, R. (1982). Toward a theory of gerontological nursing. *Nursing and Health Care* 3: 550–56.

Crawford, G. (1987). Support networks and health-related change in the elderly: Theory-based nursing strategies. *Family and Community Health* 10(2): 39–48.

deTornyay, R. (1980). Public health nursing: The nurse's role in community-based practice. *Annual Review of Public Health* 1: 83.

Eisdorfer, E., and F. Wilke. (1976). Research in aging. In A. Hoffman (ed.), *Daily needs and interests of older people.* Springfield, Ill.: Charles C. Thomas.

Ekerdt, D., L. Baden, R. Bossé, and E. Dibbs. The effect of retirement on physical health. *American Journal of Public Health* 73: 779–83.

Eliopoulus, C. (1984). A self-care model for gerontological nursing. *Geriatric Nursing* 5(8): 366–69.

Fahey, C. (1981). Some political, economic, and social considerations. In R. Morris (ed.), *Allocating health resources for the aged and disabled.* Lexington, Mass.: D. C. Heath.

Ford, A. B. (1987). Looking after the old folks. *American Journal of Public Health* 77(12): 1499–1500.

Fowles, D. (1978). *Some prospects for the future elderly population: Statistical reports on older Americans.* Washington, D.C.: U.S. Department of Health, Education and Welfare, Office of Human Development, National Clearinghouse on Aging.

Fries, J., and L. Crapo. (1981). *Vitality and aging: Implications of the rectangular curve.* San Francisco: W. H. Freeman.

Gooding, H., et al. (1986). The value of preventive care service for the elderly. *Health Visitor* 59(10): 305–6.

Grau, L. (1984). Case management and the nurse... long-term community care to the elderly. *Geriatric Nursing* 5(8): 372–75.

Hanlon, J. J. and G. E. Pickett. (1984). *Public health: Administration and Practice.* 8th ed. St. Louis: Times Mirror/Mosby.

Hayter, J. (1983). Modifying the environment to help older persons. *Nursing and Health Care* 84(5): 265–69.

Hickey, R., and R. Douglass. (1981). Mistreatment of the elderly in the domestic setting: An exploratory study. *American Journal of Public Health* 71: 500.

Itzin, C. (1987). Screening elderly people. *Nursing Times* 83(48): 47–50.

Jameison, M., and I. Martinson. (1983). Block nursing: Neighbors caring for neighbors. *Nursing Outlook* 31(5): 270–73.

Kane, R. A., and R. L. Kane. (1981). *Assessing the elderly.* Lexington, Mass.: Lexington Books.

Kane, R. L., and R. A. Kane. (1980). Long-term care: Can our society meet the needs of its elderly? *Annual Review of Public Health* 1: 227.

Kaprio, J., M. Koskenvuo, H. Rita. (1987). Mortality after bereavement: A prospective study of 95,647 widowed persons. *American Journal of Public Health* 77(3): 283–87.

Kee, C. C. (1984). A case for health promotion with the elderly. *Nursing Clinics of North America* 19(2): 251–62.

Kiehn, M. (1987). A brighter future for the elderly. *Health Visitor* 60(10): 340–42.

Kovar, M. G., and A. Z. LaCroix. (1987). Aging in the eighties, ability to perform work-related activities, data from the supplement on aging to the National Health Interview Survey: United States, 1984. *National Center for Health Statistics Advance Data* Number 136 (May 8), DHHS Pub. No. (PHS) 87-1250. Hyattsville, Md.: Public Health Service.

Managan, D., J. Wood, C. Heinichen, M. Hoffman, G. Hess, and D. Gillings. (1974). Older adults: A community survey of health needs. *Nursing Research* 23: 426.

McDaniel, S. A. (1988). Challenges to health promotion among older working women. *Canadian Journal of Public Health* 79(1): Centre Appl. Health Research: S29–32.

Muller, C. (1982). Health status and survival needs of the elderly. *American Journal of Public Health* 72: 789–90.

Oktay, J. S., and P. J. Volland. (1987). Foster home care for the frail elderly as an alternative to nursing home care: An experimental evaluation. *American Journal of Public Health* 77(12): 1505–10.

Older Women's League. (1987). The picture of health for midlife and older women in America. *Older Women's League Mother's Day Report 1987.* Washington, D.C.: OWL.

Olson, I. (1982). Attitudes of nursing students toward aging and the aged. *Gerontology and Geriatrics Education* 2: 233–36.

Pfeiffer, E. (ed.) (1978). Multidimensional functional assessment: The OARS Methodology. 2nd ed. Durham, N.C.: Duke University Center for Study of Aging and Human Development.

Satariano, W. A., S. H. Belle, and G. M. Swanson. (1986). The severity of breast cancer at diagnosis: A comparison of age and extent of disease in black and white women. *American Journal of Public Health* 76(7): 779–82.

Schrock, N. (1980). *Holistic assessment of the healthy aged.* New York: Wiley.

Shanas, E. (1980). Self-assessment of physical function: White and black elderly in the United States. In S. Haynes and M. Feinleib (eds.), *Epidemiology of aging* (NIH Pub. No. 80-969). Washington, D.C.: U.S. Department of Health and Human Services.

Seigel, J. (1980). Recent and prospective demographic trends of the elderly population and some implications for health care. In S. Haynes and M. Feinlein (eds.), *Epidemiology of aging* (NIH Pub. No. 80-969). Washington, D.C.: U.S. Department of Health and Human Services.

Speake, D. L. (1987). Health promotion activity in the well elderly. *Health Values* 11(6): 25–30.

Stefl, B. (1976). Prevention measures and safety factors for the aged. In I. M. Burnside (ed.), *Nursing and the aged.* New York: McGraw-Hill.

Stone, V. (1977). Nursing of older people. In E. Busse and E. Pfeiffer (eds.), *Behavior and adaptation in late life.* 2nd ed. Boston: Little, Brown.

Training materials guide: Community care for the aging. (1981). Washington, D.C.: The Washington School of Psychiatry, Special Projects Division.

U.S. Department of Health, Education and Welfare, Public Health Service. (1969). *Working with older people: A guide to practice* (Vol.1). Arlington, Va.: Author, Division of Health Care Services.

Waldo, D. (1986). National health expenditures, 1985. *Health Care Financing Review* 8(Fall): 1–21.

Winnick, S., et al. (1985). A new role for community nurses in geriatric care. *Canadian Nurse* 81(6): 50–51.

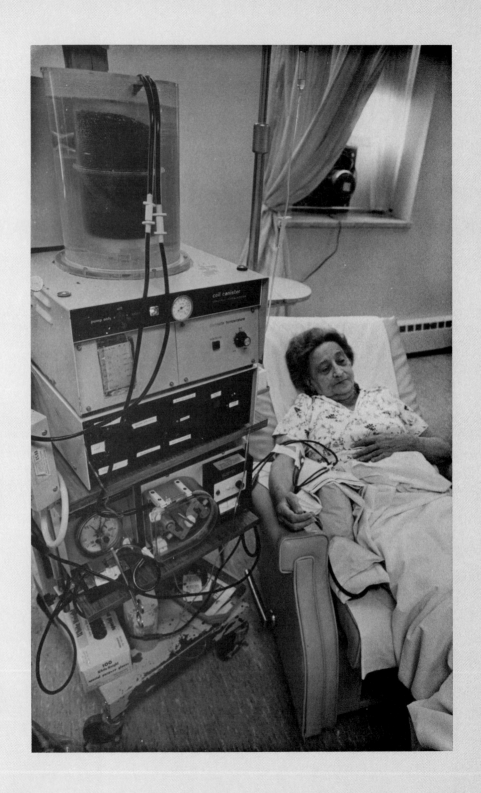

21 Health of the Home Care Population

Barbara W. Spradley
Beverly Dorsey

There are people of all ages who need health services at home. Handicapped children, postsurgical patients, diabetics, quadriplegics, cancer patients, disabled elderly—all are part of a population group needing home health care. Often this group is referred to as the homebound population. It is true that many people are, in fact, confined to their homes. Others can leave home with assistance but also need home services, although they are not technically homebound. An additional group of well people have traditionally utilized home health services. Among them are new mothers and babies receiving postpartum follow-up and infant care, families receiving mental health counseling or parental guidance, and elderly people receiving assistance with medication supervision or nutritional counseling. Both homebound and well clients represent long-standing targets for community health nursing service in the home.

The picture in home health care is changing, however. New home care provision structures are emerging, along with dramatic shifts in financing and provider roles (Phillips et al., 1988; Brown, 1987). These changes are having a profound and continuing impact on community health nursing practice (Burbach et al., 1988; Daubert, 1987). In addition, the population needing home services is growing dramatically for several reasons. The number of dependent elderly is increasing, with a corresponding rise in the incidence of chronic illnesses. Earlier hospital discharges, driven by cost-containment pressures, cause an escalating number of people of all ages to require care in the community. Public awareness and demand for home services as an alternative to institutional care, broader third-party payment coverage for home care, and greater physician acceptance of this phenomenon further enlarges the size of the group utilizing home health care. Finally, more acutely ill clients of all ages, who previously would have remained hospitalized or institutionalized, can be maintained outside the hospital or other institution because of sophisticated technological advances (Lutz, 1987) that allow such complex procedures as intravenous chemotherapy to be provided routinely at home.

In this chapter we examine the nature of home health services — how they have evolved and what they are today. We explore the needs of the subpopulations utilizing home health care, the services available to meet those needs, and community health nursing's role in home health care.

WHAT IS HOME HEALTH CARE?

Home health care, broadly defined, refers to all the services and products provided to clients in their homes to maintain, restore, or promote their physical, mental, and emotional health. Its purpose is to maximize clients' level of independence and minimize the effects of existing disabilities through noninstitutional, supportive services (Lundberg, 1984; Stewart, 1979). In other words, a primary aim of care in the home is to prevent institutionalization (Mundinger, 1983).

The generally accepted definition of home health care has been stated by Warhola (1980):

> Home health care is that component of a continuum of comprehensive care whereby health, social and support services are provided to individuals and families in their places of residence and in the community for the purpose of promoting, maintaining or restoring health, or of maximizing the level of independence, while minimizing the effects of disability and illness, including terminal illness. Services appropriate to the needs of the individual and family are planned, coordinated, and made available by providers organized for the delivery of home care through the use of employed staff, contractual arrangements, or a combination of the two patterns.

Because the population utilizing home health care is so varied in age and needs, home health care covers a broad range of services: nursing; medical and dental care; pharmaceutical services; social services counseling; physical therapy; speech therapy; occupational therapy; laboratory testing; nutrition advice; homemaker or home health aide services; medical equipment and supplies provision; chore services; and transportation (Warhola, 1980). These services consist of two basic types: professional and support.

Home health care aims to accomplish the following (*Home Care Guidelines,* 1981; Davis, 1987):

1. Support families and individuals to avoid premature or inappropriate admission to an institutional care setting
2. Provide respite for families and responsible caretakers from continuous care and supervision of elderly and physically impaired persons, and assist caretakers in providing appropriate services
3. Maintain or restore elderly and physically impaired persons to optimal functional potential, and retard physical and emotional deterioration

4. Provide for support and follow-up services to persons residing in their own or a family member's home
5. Facilitate appropriate release of elderly and physically impaired persons from acute and long-term care facilities to family care or to other community-based programs
6. Provide home-based services to the terminally ill and their families in cooperation with other community-based health and social services

These goals are not easily accomplished without an effective, coordinated home care system (Hughes, 1987). Recent changes are forcing community health nurses and other providers to reexamine how this can be done. Home health care today has changed dramatically from its beginnings. Let us examine those changes and the forces shaping home health practice today.

HISTORICAL VIEW OF HOME HEALTH SERVICES

Early home health services in the United States were organized and administered by laypersons in the late 1800s. They provided nursing care and taught cleanliness and home care techniques to the ill and their families. In 1877, the Women's Branch of the New York City Mission was the first group to employ a graduate nurse to deliver home care (Spiegel, 1983). Since that time nurses have played a primary role in home care.

The Visiting Nurse Service of New York City, established in 1893 by Lillian Wald, was the first U.S.-organized home nursing service. Through Lillian Wald's influence, the Metropolitan Life Insurance Company began a home nursing service for its New York City policyholders in 1909 that later became a model for other insurance companies in the 1920s. This included full coverage for home services (Mundinger, 1983). The first government health department offering visiting nurse care was the Los Angeles Health Department, established in 1898 (Spiegel, 1983).

Home care continued to be a part of nursing practice as the nursing profession developed. Twenty visiting nurse agencies serving the urban poor were operating by 1900, and in 1912 the Red Cross initiated a visiting nurse service for rural communities. Service was provided to the sick, to well babies, and to schoolchildren. County health departments, too, were soon providing home nursing care in rural areas, with service delivery enhanced by the development of automobiles.

Physicians were actively involved in home care before World War II. The war, however, created a physician shortage, and for the sake of efficiency, patients came to physicians. The cost-effectiveness of this pattern prompted its continuance, leaving a gap in home care that was filled by a growing number of visiting nurse associations.

The first hospital-based home care program was founded in 1947 by Dr. E. M. Bluestone at Montefiore Hospital in New York City. This program was prompted by the fact that many people with chronic illnesses were hospitalized for excessive periods of time. A team approach was utilized for posthospital acute care and was the beginning of the concept of convalescent care in the home. The program was also unique in that services were not limited to the poor or the elderly. The first paraprofessional home services—homemakers—were instituted then also. By 1958, this program had added therapy, nutrition, and X-ray and laboratory services to the initial team of physicians, nurses, and social workers. Housekeeping and chore services were provided indirectly through community resources (MacNamara, 1982).

The passage of Medicare and Medicaid legislation in 1965 drastically changed the home care delivery system. Before Medicare was created, most home care was provided by voluntary visiting nurse associations (VNAs). The majority of home care clients were elderly persons, suffering from various chronic conditions, whose greatest need was for nursing care complemented by some health aide and homemaker services. According to Mundinger (1983, p. 39), "A typical visit included bathing the patient, reviewing self-care (nutrition, elimination), and attending to such tasks as vitamin or insulin injections or dressings for chronic ulcers." Payment came either from welfare or from personal payment based on a sliding fee scale subsidized by charity.

With the advent of Medicare, not only did the payment source change but client eligibility, the provision of home care and the purpose of that care changed as well. For more than 70 years before Medicare, ever since Lillian Wald's establishment of the first visiting nurse service, nurses had successfully provided home care on their own to the sick, the disabled, and children. Prior to federal payment, "it was not seen as necessary or even appropriate for physicians to direct home care" (Mundinger, 1983, p. 40). The need for some kind of gatekeeper to ensure provision of services to those who truly needed them as well as political pressures from medical groups concerned about Medicare's impact on medical practice led the federal government to appoint physicians to direct the traditionally nonmedical home services. Home care became more narrowly defined as a substitute for costly, extended hospitalization, and it changed to a medical-based model of practice (Mundinger, 1983). Eligibility for Medicare reimbursement of home care costs was based on patients' acute care conditions; they must be homebound, in need of skilled care (medically directed service given by a nurse or other professional), and under the treatment of a physician. Furthermore, the referring physician must plan, review, and certify as necessary the care to be given.

The medical model radically changed what had been historically the mission of home health care. Previously home services sought to provide nursing care, assistance, and support. Community health problems, after Medicare's advent, were viewed as medical problems whose solution was disease eradication. Home care became medical care. This view overlooked the need for preventive and health-promoting services and discounted the clear need of homebound clients for support services. Physicians and policymakers did not seem to be truly aware of the range of health needs clients had in the home

(Neiman et al., 1986). Somehow there was an assumption that if people could go home from the hospital they could manage meals, laundry, shopping, cleaning, and psychosocial support without supplemental assistance. Home services during these years still included health promotion, health teaching, and holistic family care. Medicare and Medicaid, however, did not cover these services; instead, public health agencies through their nurses provided the services without charge.

The passage of Medicare also influenced the structure of home care services. For the first time, home care agencies, in order to be certified for Medicare reimbursement, were required to provide one other service in addition to nursing. This service could be physical therapy, occupational therapy, speech therapy, social services, or home health aide services. About 250 of the existing 1163 agencies qualified for Medicare participation in 1966. The total number of home care agencies declined after the implementation of Medicare, many smaller voluntary organizations going out of business because they could not develop the service scope and complexity required. This led to the growth of public home health agencies, proprietary agencies, and hospital-based agencies. During the first decade after passage of Medicare, those that met the standards increased by 71 percent to about 430. The most growth was in hospital-based agencies.

From a historical perspective, the escalation in home health care would seem to suggest that we are back where we started. New Mexico Democratic Senator Jeff Bingaman commented in testimony at budget committee hearings in 1984: "Health care in America has come full circle. Health care originated in the home and moved to the hospital with the advent of technology and improved diagnostic and treatment methodologies. Now a new emphasis is being placed on the home to control costs," ("Legislative Roundup," 1984, p. 5). Although home care is back in the spotlight, its mission, services, financing, and providers have all changed. Let us examine some of those changes.

HOME HEALTH SERVICES

What groups utilize home health services and how can we be certain that programs address their needs? The first part of the question is more readily answered than the second.

THE HOME CARE POPULATION

The largest subpopulation in the United States using home care is the elderly. According to "Research news..." (1984), the National Center for Health Statistics reported that, in 1979, "4.9 million adults living in communities needed the help of another person in carrying out everyday activities." The report went on to say that "4.1 million adults needed or received the help of another person for shopping, household chores, preparing meals, or handling money." Of the total number reported, 2.9 million were 65 years or over, and the need for assistance rose sharply with age. In the 65 to 74 age group, less than one in ten needed help, but of those 85 years and over, four in ten needed help. Bakken (1983) adds that these elderly could avoid institutionalization if they received support for their personal care (Figure 21-1).

According to another national study, an estimated 5.8 million persons make up the noninstitutionalized long-term care population. This figure includes persons of all ages and diagnoses who "due to a long-lasting condition, require or receive human help in personal care, mobility, household activities or home delivered health care services" ("Research news...," 1984, p. 13).

Figure 21-1
The care and support of family members play a critical role in enabling the homebound population to avoid institutionalization.

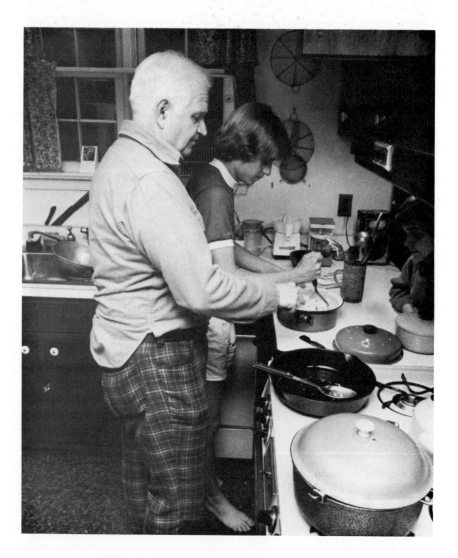

This study, too, showed that dependency increases with age, dramatically so after age 75. Among older adults, those most likely to be dependent were nonwhite females. White males were slightly more dependent than white females under age 75, but after 75, white males were the least likely to be dependent for personal care ("Research news...," 1984, p. 13). Two other studies, describing Medicare patients receiving home health care, showed that two-thirds of all home care patients are women, and approximately one-third of all home care patients live alone (*Home Health,* 1979). We can conclude from the above reports that approximately 4.9 million adults and 1.1 million children need some type of home health services.

Besides the elderly and long-term care populations, another group needing home care is made up of discharged acute care patients. Although exact figures on the size of this group are not available, we know that it is increasing rapidly. Rising hospital costs and prospective payment incentives, in conjunction with dramatic technological advances that make it possible for complicated procedures to be administered in the home, contribute to an enlarging population receiving home care (Griffith, 1987; Lutz, 1987). Many of these are elderly persons who have been hospitalized with an episode of acute illness or disability and need convalescent home care. Others include babies and children with disabilities or individuals sent home with monitors, medications, IVs, and various therapies. (See Figure 21-2.) An increasing number of AIDS clients need home care. Some, such as children, women, and drug users, have additional special needs (Bohland et al., 1986; Young et al., 1988).

Another subpopulation receiving home services is what one health planner calls the "wellness home care market" (Louden, 1983, p. 109). These people do not need medical care but have concerns about their health and well-being and are receptive to health promotion and illness prevention strategies. They use services such as diagnostic testing and screening (for example, blood pressure monitoring); educational counseling (for example, nutrition information); support for daily living, including home maintenance and housekeeping; and illness prevention (for example, information about exercise and stress management). People of all ages make up this group, and it includes a good portion of the elderly population, many of whom are well elderly persons whose functional dependency has increased to the point that they need support for activities of daily living.

NEEDS OF HOME HEALTH SERVICE RECIPIENTS

The majority of home health service recipients are elderly. Their home health needs fall into six categories described by Mundinger (1983, pp. 171–75):

1. *Chronic illness and disability care.* The most common diagnoses of elderly home care clients are cancer, diabetes, and cardiovascular disease. Each is chronic, degenerative, and disabling. Each can lead to

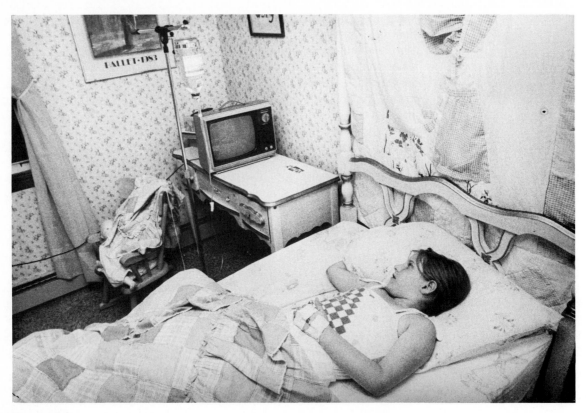

Figure 21-2
Intravenous therapy and other treatments now can be routinely administered
in the home, serving the needs of a home care population that spans all ages.

progressive pathology and deterioration with increased possibility of complications and growing dependency care needs. The large majority (80 percent) of older adults over age 65 live with at least one chronic illness, and many with a mixture of several acute and chronic illnesses and disabilities. (Fedder, Abrams, and Lamy, 1984). Many clients, for example, have arthritis and hypertension in addition to cancer or diabetes. The complexity of their conditions leads to a greater variety of home care service needs.

2. *Social networks.* Meaningful contact with other people is a basic human need, and the elderly homebound, many of whom live alone, especially need this. Social supports are a vital component of home care. Research demonstrates that when social supports are present, clients live longer and are happier (Weissert, 1980) — a reflection on the quality of life for home care clients that should consume more of home care providers' attention (Hughes, 1987).

3. *Sheltered or congregate housing.* As more families are scattered geographically and unable to care for their elderly members and as more older persons live longer, group living for the mostly independent elderly fills an important need. Minor supervision or assistance with activities of daily living are available in sheltered or congregate housing. Residents can assist one another with tasks, meals may be taken in the company of other people, if desired (Figure 21-3), and a nurse is often available or on call. This family-type housing enables older people to maintain their independence for a longer period of time.

4. *Personal services.* We have already seen that a large number of elderly persons need assistance with personal care. This includes preparing meals, doing laundry, shopping, bathing, housecleaning, and being transported to community care centers, such as the physician's office, dentist's office, or hairdresser's salon. Many elderly people

Figure 21-3
Congregate dining in a home-like atmosphere enables these elderly friends to enjoy a meal together and strengthen their social networks.

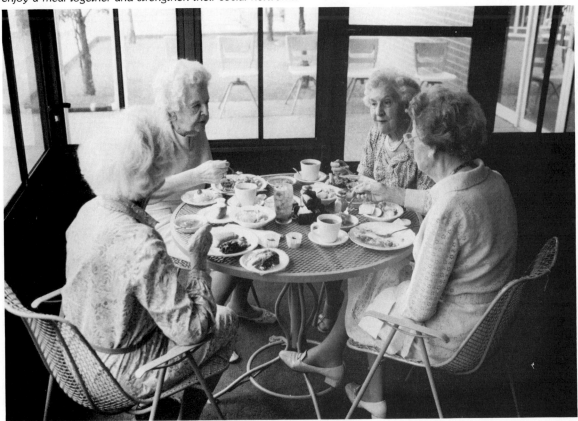

in institutions would be living at home if their personal care needs could be met there (Gary, 1979; Kane and Kane, 1978; Martinson et al., 1985). Sometimes these needs are met voluntarily by family members, a spouse, or friends. Without these resources, elderly people are forced to use up their own funds before becoming eligible for public monies, but by then they may have lost the home in which to live independently: "Requiring the independent and economically stable elderly to become dependent if they are to receive assistance is a financially foolish and socially questionable policy" (Mundinger, 1983, p. 173).

5. *Payment for drugs, eyeglasses, preventive podiatry, and dentistry.* All of these represent ongoing needs of elderly persons whose limited resources frequently prevent them from being met. Mundinger (1983) points out that the increasing number of accidents among the elderly (causing a greater number of referrals for home care than illness in her study population) may well be due to lack of proper glasses, medications, or other necessary care. Poor vision, inadequate medication for hypertension or arthritis, improper foot care, or dental disease can cause accidents or illness leading to institutionalization.

6. *Day care.* Many elderly persons living at home are cared for by family members whose schedules require them to be away during the day. Day care for the elderly frees family members for work or recreation and gives elderly persons a social outlet as well. It may be the deciding factor in living at home versus institutionalization.

All home health service recipients, including the elderly, have needs, varying with their ages and the demands of their health conditions. Both long-term and acute care conditions require assistance that can be divided into two categories: one is services and the other is supplies and equipment (Louden, 1983). The professional services of nurses, physicians, aides, and physical, respiratory, speech, and occupational therapists, meeting the home-bound's first category of needs, are a major component of home health care. An interdisciplinary team is necessary to meet the many and complex needs of this population whose major needs, more than medically related care, are in areas of health teaching, psychological and social support, and prevention or reduction of disability (Mundinger, 1983). Social support personnel (such as social workers, ministers, or family members) and nutritional services (such as Meals on Wheels and congregate dining) fill other vital areas of need. Important additional services may include data and claims processing, equipment service, and home telemetry.

The second category of need is for supplies and equipment. An increasing number of new products are available to maintain ill or disabled people at home (Carter, 1987). They include oxygen and respiratory devices; durable medical equipment, such as wheelchairs, lifts, and walkers; rehabilitation equipment, such as an exercise "horse" or hand grips; nursing care supplies, such as dressings, decubiti cushions, or catheters; drug therapy supplies, such as disposable syringes and intravenous therapy supplies, oxygen concentrator, or needleless insulin injector; nutritional supplies (including oral and total parenteral nutrition); and home kidney dialysis equipment and supplies.

"Wellness" home services recipients have a different set of needs. Their concerns focus on health-promoting and illness-preventing activities. Services used by this group have already been discussed. They include diagnostic screening, educational counseling and information, daily living support services, and illness prevention services (such as exercise guidance and weight and stress control). This group uses certain supplies and equipment such as products for self-diagnosis and screening and for self-treatment, vitamin and nutritional supplements, exercise equipment, products that assist in the activities of daily living, and communications and security devices (Louden, 1983).

DESIGNING RELEVANT HOME HEALTH SERVICES

Assessment of home health clients' needs is essential for appropriate program development. A growing body of research data is shedding light on this area, and nurses should review this information (Martin, 1988). Further research and community needs assessment should be conducted to make sure home care services are appropriately focused. Mundinger (1983), for example, has demonstrated that home health care, when efficiently organized with good backup services, is a highly cost-effective way of caring for the elderly. She also demonstrated that many critically needed services, such as home safety assessment, extensive family medications review, care adapted to the home setting, and coordination of care with medical and other community resources, were nonreimbursable (Mundinger, 1983). This is one of many studies pointing out deficiencies in the reimbursement system for home health services (Cowart, 1985).

The U.S. Department of Health and Human Services has published a quantitative formula for analyzing community need for home care services that is helpful in program development (Warhola, 1980). It enables the home service planner to estimate the number of potential home care users in a given service area by examining the elderly population, the acute care discharged patients, and those inappropriately placed in skilled or intermediate care nursing facilities.

Planning for effective home health services must take into account the fact that the majority of clients have chronic conditions compounded by periodic acute episodes. A diversified service system is necessary to meet this range of needs. Figure 21-4 lists the four major components necessary to provide a full range of home care services. The VNA of Dallas has developed a system of services that provides a useful alternative model (Holt, 1984). It includes three service divisions — home health care, hospice care, and long-term care. Each division offers a variety of specialty services. For example, home health

Day Care
Home Health Care
  nursing   social work
  medical   nutrition
  homemaker/home health aide   pharmaceutical services
  homemaker services   other services:
  attendant services   inhalation therapy
  physical therapy   renal therapy
  occupational therapy   mental health
  speech pathology   lab & diagnostic
                                               supplies/equipment

Hospice

Respite

Other Service Components
  call-in assurance   home delivered meals
  chore services   housekeeping services
  congregate meals   night care
  family subsidies   sheltered housing
  financial & legal counseling/services   special transportation/escort services
  friendly visitor

Figure 21-4
*Components of a local
home health care system.*

care includes nursing services, extended (24-hour) services, patient education, medical social services, homemaker and home health aides, nutritional consultation, durable medical equipment, and rehabilitative services such as physical therapy. Hospice services include care, support, and mobilization of resources for clients in the final stage of life and for their families (McCabe et al., 1987; Paradis et al., 1987). Hospice benefits cover such things as continuous care, respite care, and bereavement counseling. Long-term care includes meals delivered to the home, family care, and primary home care (personal care, housekeeping, meal preparation, and other home chores). A major contributing factor in the success of this VNA is its community-based planning and partnership with community care contract providers and appropriate state agencies and legislators. All were "committed to finding alternatives to institutionalization" (Holt, 1984, p. 53). This home service agency packaged a diversified set of services that met a much broader range of home care clients' needs than "the traditional medically-oriented, single-purpose skilled services offered by home care agencies under Medicare" (Holt, 1984, p. 53).

Ideally, home health services are centrally coordinated by health professionals and operated by means of a case management system based on assessed clients' needs (Mundinger, 1984; Newton, 1986; Warhola, 1980). A case manager may or may not provide direct care and serves as "broker" to see that clients receive needed home care and supportive services (National Association for Home Care, 1984). Providing continuity of care between institutions, such as the hospital, nursing home, or long-term care facility, and the home is one emphasis of this case management approach, as is assignment of appropriate services and resources.

CURRENT STATUS OF HOME HEALTH SERVICES

Home health services are on the cutting edge of change in health care provision. Spurred on by multiple forces (Carter, 1987; Louden, 1983; Moxley, 1984; Mundinger, 1983; Spiegel, 1983), home care is growing rapidly. One major force is cost-containment pressures by government and third-party payers and employers who appreciate home care's lower costs. More research is needed to substantiate these claims, however, and some challenge their validity (Blazer, 1988; Harris et al., 1987b; Weinstein, 1987). Another force for change is the expanding aging population that has increasing dependency needs. In addition, hospitals and nursing homes will eventually be unable to handle the load created by the rise in the number of elderly people needing medical attention. Fewer family caregivers are available since more women work outside the home (Callahan, 1988). Consumers have increased health awareness and concern. Patients are demanding greater satisfaction and quality of life, and care in the home responds to these desires. A final force of growing significance in home health care is the impact of medical and computer technology. Advanced equipment design, electronics, and communication systems have the potential for enabling the ill and disabled to live near-normal lives outside institutions with home services as the sustaining intermediary.

As the demand for home health care increases, so too do the number and variety of agencies providing services. No longer is home care the sole province of public health nursing agencies and VNAs. Palley and Oktay (1983) state that in 1981, according to a Health Care Financing Administration report, there were 3136 home health agencies certified by Medicare in the United States. Of these, 1231 were govenmental, 544 were private and nonprofit, 436 were hospital-based nonprofit programs, 515 were run by VNAs, and 297 were proprietary agencies. By 1989 there were approximately 11000 home care providers, 6000 of which were certified by Medicare. In addition, there were 5000 homemaker–home health aide agencies and 1200 hospices. Nearly half of the hospices were based in home health agencies (Brown, 1984; Paradis, 1987; National Association for Home Care, 1989).

Today one of the fastest growing types of home health care agencies is the hospital-based agency (Lerman, 1987). The number of not-for-profit hospitals offering home care services increased by 67 percent between 1976 and 1982 (Louden, 1983). Escalating costs and a declining census are forcing many hospitals to explore alternative revenue sources; expansion into home care is viewed as a logical extension of hospital services (Lundberg, 1984). One argument is that continuity of care can be maintained for patients. Another is that hospital staff are better trained to handle the demands of highly technological and skilled care now required in many home care situations. We will see many more hospitals developing home care programs in the near future.

Proprietary, for-profit agencies form the other fastest growing group moving into home care. The percentage of home health agencies owned privately grew from 54.6 percent in 1966 to 73.7 percent in 1984 (Phillips et al., 1987), and the proprietary companies have managed to create a business where they supply the majority of home care personnel throughout the nation (Spiegel, 1983). Pharmaceutical companies, insurance companies, temporary staffing agencies, nursing homes, and many others have entered the competitive and mushrooming field of home care. Even some durable medical equipment and supply companies have expanded into providing skilled nursing and other comprehensive services in the home. Companies such as Abbott Laboratories of Chicago, American Hospital Supply Corporation of Evanston, Illinois, Baxter Travenol Laboratories, Inc., of Deerfield, Illinois, and Johnson & Johnson of New Brunswick, New Jersey, are offering home care services along with their home care product businesses (Louden, 1983).

Home care services in the past were generally provided by not-for-profit agencies while the for-profit sector sold home care equipment and supplies. These patterns are changing. The traditional equipment and supply companies see an opportunity for financial profit in offering services, and the not-for-profit providers find the supply and device market, which offers even higher profit margins, financially attractive (Louden, 1983). Hospitals are important customers of supply companies. To avoid direct competition, many supply companies are attempting joint ventures with hospitals.

Products and services that are frequently used in the home care market include incontinence products, self-diagnostic or treatment products, and supplies or services for home parenteral nutrition, intravenous therapy, chemotherapy, kidney dialysis, and respiratory therapy.

Total parenteral nutrition (TPN) is one of the fastest growing high-tech procedures being performed in the home. Home TPN was introduced about ten years ago as a technique to facilitate hospital discharge of those patients whose primary reason for hospitalization was parenteral nutrition support. Nearly 3000 patients in the United States have been involved in such home care programs since their introduction (Ament, 1983). TPN is a method of intravenous feeding used to sustain people who have intestinal obstructions, malabsorption syndromes or other digestive disorders, or anorexia nervosa, and occasionally for those who during the postoperative period following gastrointestinal surgery need feeding. At first patients needed to be connected to intravenous equipment for 24 hours a day, but technological advances in the early 1970s permitted more rapid infusion of the nutritional solutions so that clients can now be free from tubes and solution bags for more than 16 hours a day. It is estimated that between 0.3 percent and 5.5 percent of all patients hospitalized in the United States are receiving TPN. In 1982, 2200 clients received TPN intravenous feedings in their homes, compared with 1200 in 1980, and this number is expected to double in the near future (News Briefs, 1982).

Home administration of many complex high-technology procedures is proving to be cost-effective. One study showed a reduction in costs for TPN from $200 per day to $65 per day (Ament, 1983). Others demonstrated significant reductions in the cost of home intravenous antibiotic administration (News Briefs, 1982; *Hospital Peer Review,* 1983). A home intravenous cancer chemotherapy program in Houston estimated a cost savings of more than half a million dollars in one year (*Hospital Peer Review,* 1983).

Numerous problems have yet to be resolved in providing home care services. While cost savings have been clearly demonstrated in studies of home care, studies have not addressed all the questions that need answering. For example, care of a severely disabled person in the home may appear less costly than in a nursing home, but what is it costing the family or the community (Harris, 1987b)? It may be prohibitive in terms of the drain on physical and emotional as well as financial resources (Figure 21-5). In some instances nursing home care may be less costly than maintaining people at home. Utilization of home care benefits under Medicare and Medicaid is increasingly subject to fraud and abuse (Mundinger, 1983). Costs to the federal government of subsidizing home health care are increasing at a shocking rate (31 percent annually for Medicare from 1972 to 1982 and 23 percent annually for Medicaid from 1977 to 1982) (*Home Health Journal,* 1983). Some studies show that home health services are simply add-ons. There is little evidence that these services have contributed to decreased hospital stays or have substituted for extended institutionalization (Hammond, 1979). Health and Human Services Secretary Margaret Heckler commented in 1983, "The issue is not whether the per-visit cost of home care is lower than the per-diem cost of inpatient care, but the degree to which home care substitutes for more expensive institution care. Overall costs may well increase unless expanded home care is targeted to individuals who would otherwise require institutional care" (*Home Health Journal,* 1983).

A further problem in home care is the quality issue. With so many proprietary agencies entering the field, many uncertified by Medicare and not subject to any standards of care, the potential for reduced quality of services is great. There is an increasing emphasis in the field on assuring quality home care services (Bayer, 1986; Hughes, 1987; Lalonde, 1988), including recognition of homebound clients' rights (see Figure 21-6). Closely tied to quality is the problem of fragmented and overlapping services, emphasizing the need for coordination and case management.

COMMUNITY HEALTH NURSING AND HOME CARE

The changing picture in home health services has significantly affected community health nursing (Daubert, 1987). Formerly the sole providers of home health care, community health nursing agencies now find hospitals, once

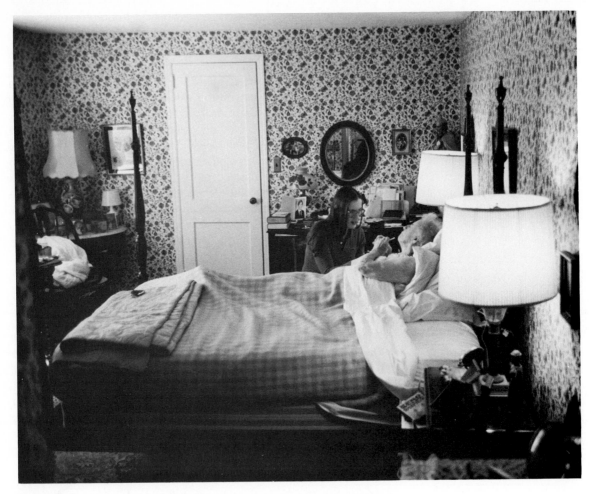

Figure 21-5
*Although care at home has many benefits for homebound clients, the demands
on caregivers' physical, emotional, and financial resources can be heavy.*

their primary referral sources, serving those clients themselves. Medicare and
other reimbursements for home care used to generate a sizable portion of community health nursing agencies' budgets. With decreased referrals those revenues are diminishing. Furthermore, home care providers, whether operating
for profit or not, will often refer clients to public agencies when Medicare
benefits or third-party coverage has run out, requiring taxes or charity to sub-
sidize the care.

The changing financial structure of home health services poses a dilemma
for community health nursing agencies faced with a conflict in values between
the competition model and basic public health values (Phillips et al., 1987).
Although hospitals and other technologically skilled home care providers can
offer important and necessary services to clients at home, their personnel are

Home Care Bill of Rights

Clients have the RIGHT TO:

—Receive written information about rights, including what to do if those rights are violated;

—Receive services according to a suitable and up-to-date plan and subject to accepted medical or nursing standards, and take an active part in creating and changing the plan and evaluating services;

—Be informed about the services being provided or suggested, about other available choices, and about the consequences of these choices, including the consequences of refusing services;

—Refuse services or treatment;

—Know, in advance, any limits to the services available from a provider, whether the services are covered by health insurance, medical assistance, or other health programs, and the provider's grounds for a termination of services;

—Know what the charges are for services, no matter who will be paying the bill;

—Know that there may be other services available in the community, including other home care services and providers, and know where to go for information about these services;

—Choose freely among available providers and be able to change providers after services have begun, within the limits of health insurance, medical assistance, or other health programs;

—Have personal, financial, and medical information kept private;

—Have access to records and written information in accordance with the Minnesota Data Practices Act;

—Be served by properly trained and competent people;

—Be treated with courtesy and respect;

—Receive reasonable notice of changes in services or charges;

—Receive a coordinated transfer when there will be a change in the provider of services;

—Know how to contact an individual associated with the provider who is responsible for handling problems and the name and address of the state or county agency to contact for additional information or assistance;

—Assert these rights without retaliation.

Figure 21-6
An increasing number of home care agencies provide written statements of clients' rights similar to the one shown here. Clients are given information about whom to call if they have questions or comments. (Adapted from the University of Minnesota Home Health Care Services and Ramsey County Public Health Nursing Services Statements of Home Care Bill of Rights, 1987.)

not usually oriented to giving holistic, family-focused, preventive, and health-promoting care so essential for the health of this client population, nor are most home care providers able to offer this broader range of services because of their added expense.

The solution appears to lie in new forms of public-private partnerships. Some innovative programs are already proving successful, such as the VNA of Dallas (Holt, 1984) cited earlier in this chapter. This agency's partnership with public agencies and diversified services offered along a continuum of care place it in a favorable position for government reimbursement. Some agencies are forming coalitions to work collaboratively for referrals and case management. Minnesota has a preadmission screening program that assesses persons before they enter nursing homes to determine their ability to remain in the community. This comprehensive screening, done in part by community health nurses, provides revenue for the agency and is a potential source of new referrals for home care.

Community health nurses face new challenges and new roles in home care (Humphrey, 1988). The home care client population still has the same basic needs, but the changing health care delivery structure requires that nurses develop creative new ways of meeting them (Daubert, 1987). One role that community health nurses are particularly suited for is case management (Mundinger, 1984). Coordination of needed services and resources and provision of continuity of care are critical elements of an effective home health program.

Community health nurses are demonstrating the value of assessment of client health status using functional level as a predictor of need rather than gauging need only by diagnostic category (Bedrosian, 1988). Both the VNS of Omaha, Nebraska, and the Ramsey County Nursing Service of St. Paul, Minnesota, have been using a function code system for determining client health status and ability to manage the activities of daily living. Providers and legislators have been debating for some time about the appropriateness of applying a classification system like Medicare's diagnosis-related group categories to community health clients (Phillips et al., 1989). Research in home care client assessment is an area for greater community health nursing involvement.

A final consideration for nursing is the development and application of outcome measures for determining the effectiveness of home care (Buck, 1988; Lalonde, 1988). Outcome standards in home care are available (Harris, et al., 1987a; Lalonde, 1987; Day, 1987; Rinke, 1988); community health nurses, through the use of such measures, can contribute significantly to the health of the home care population.

Summary

A large group of people of all ages make up the population receiving home health services. Home health care, broadly defined, refers to all the services provided to clients at home that maintain, restore, or promote their health. Historically these services have been provided primarily by public health nurses who combined illness care in the home with comprehensive family care and health promotion. The passage of Medicare and Medicaid legislation drastically changed the home care system in terms of payment source, client eligibility, provision of home care, and the purpose of the care. Physicians were appointed gatekeepers of the system, and home care became medical care. Traditional preventive and health-promoting services continued as separate programs delivered by community health nurses.

The major target subpopulations for home health services are the elderly, the disabled (those needing noninstitutionalized long-term care), discharged acute care patients, and those interested in wellness and self-care. Needs of the elderly home care population include chronic illness or disability care; social networks; sheltered or congregate housing; personal services; payment for drugs, glasses, preventive podiatry and dentistry; and day care. All home care recipients need a variety of services from a multidisciplinary group of professionals and support personnel. They also use a variety of equipment and supplies.

A relevant system for home health services requires a proper needs assessment, and providers should plan diversified services to accommodate the complex and wide-ranging needs of this population. A full range of services includes day, home health, hospice, and respite care. Case management is a critical factor for coordinating continuity of care.

Many forces are influencing the current and future status of home health services. Among them are cost-containment pressures, an increasing elderly population, demands for consumer satisfaction, and advanced technology. In addition to the traditional VNAs and public health nursing agencies, a variety of other agencies offers home health services. The fastest growing of these are the hospital-based and the proprietary for-profit home care programs. As the home care market expands, so does the competition for providing services and products.

Many problems exist in the home care field, including misuse of home care funding, not enough research to demonstrate its cost-effectiveness, and the difficulty of providing quality service to those who need it most.

Community health nursing faces a critical time of challenge and opportunity. Competing home health agencies are greatly influencing the number and type of clients that community health nurses normally serve. Changing financial structures and costs require that community health nursing develop new partnerships and innovative service delivery patterns. A critical service they can provide is using case management in addition to conducting more research and developing more effective ways to measure home care client needs, health status, and outcomes of care.

Study Questions

1. Assume you have been assigned to provide home care to a 75-year-old woman with arthritis, hypertension, and chronic leukemia who

lives alone. What are some general areas of information you will need to gather before beginning to plan her care? Contrast what her care will involve now with what it might have been forty years ago.

2. As part of your community health nursing agency planning team, you are concerned about developing a comprehensive home health services system. What elements should you consider including in it? How would you determine the exact programs to include?

3. From the home care client population's point of view, quality of care is probably the most important criterion for home health services today. What are the needs of the elderly homebound and what actions might you take to ensure that these needs are met? Design a hypothetical home care program for an agency's elderly population.

References

Ament, M. (1983). The economic growth of the total parenteral nutrition. *Nutrition and the M.D.* 9(6): 11.

Bakken, K. L. (1983). Integrated health care: The whole person in community. *Nursing Economics* 1(2): 178–80.

Bayer, R. (1986). Ethics in home care and quality assurance. *Caring* 5(1): 50, 52–53, 55–56.

Bedrosian, C. A. (1988). *Home health nursing: Nursing diagnoses and care plans.* East Norwalk, Conn.: Appleton and Lange.

Blazer, D. (1988). Home health care: House calls revisited. *American Journal of Public Health* 78(3): 238–39.

Bohland, M. G., et al. (1986). AIDS: The implications for home care. *Maternal/Child Nursing* 11(6): 404–11.

Brown, K. (1984). Speakers stress home health agency diversification. *Home Care/ Rehabilitation Product News* (Jan./Feb.): 10.

Brown, R. E. (1987). Home health care—Are the rules changing? *Health Industry Today* (July): 27–32.

Buck, J. N. (1988). Measuring the success of home health care. *Home Health Care Nurse* 6(3): 17–19, 22–23.

Burbach, C. A., et al. (1988). Community and home health nursing: Keeping the concepts clear. *Nursing and Health Care* 9(2): 96–100.

Callahan, D. (1988). Families as caregivers: The limits of morality. *Archives of Physical Medicine and Rehabilitation* 69(5): 323–28.

Carter, K. (1987). Home health agencies and durable medical equipment dealers expanded despite reimbursement woes. *Modern Healthcare* (June) 5: 156–60.

Cowart, M. E. (1985). Policy issues: Financial reimbursement for home care. *Family and Community Health* 8(2): 1–10.

Daubert, E. (1987). Strategic planning in home care. *American Journal of Nursing* (Sept.): 1161–63.

Davis, E. J. (1987). Home care—What's needed? *Public Health Nursing* 4(2): 82–83.

Day, S. R. (1987). *Outcome measures: Research.* Washington, D.C.: National League for Nursing Publication No. 21-2194: 109–27.

Fedder, D., M. K. Abrams, and P. Lamy. (1984). The pharmacist in home health care: Part I—Drugs and the elderly. *Caring* 3(5): 28–31.

Gary, L. R. (1979). *Home health care regulation: Issues and opportunities.* New York: Hunter College.

Griffith, E. (1987). The changing face of home health care. *Public Health Nursing* 4(1): 1.

Hammond, J. (1979). Home health care cost effectiveness: An overview of the literature. *Public Health Reports* 94(4): 305–11.

Harris, M. D., et al. (1987a). *Outcome measures in home care.* Washington, D.C.: National League for Nursing Publication No. 21-2194: 187–204.

Harris, M. D., et al. (1987b). Tracking the cost of home care. *American Journal of Nursing* 87(11): 1500–1502.

Holt, S. W. (1984). Continuity of care in the home: Building a diversified service system that works. *Caring* 3(5): 49–56.

Home care guidelines. (1981). Minnesota Community Health Services, Office of Community Development, Minneapolis, Minn.: Minnesota Department of Health.

Home health and other in-home services. (1979). Department of Health, Education and Welfare. Report to Congress. Washington, D.C.: U.S. Government Printing Office.

Home Health Journal. (1983). Jacksonville, Fla: Home Care Management Consulting, Inc. (Nov.) 4(11): 9–11.

Hospital Peer Review. (1983, April, June; 1984, January). Atlanta: American Health Consultants, Inc. 8(4), 8(6), 9(1).

Hughes, F. (1987). Quality assurance in home care services. *Nursing Management* 18(12): 33–36.

Humphrey, C. J. (1988). The home as a setting for care: Clarifying the boundaries of practice. *Nursing Clinics of North America* 23(2): 305–14.

Kane, R., and R. Kane. (1978). Care of the aged—An old problem in search of new solutions. *Science* 200: 913–18.

Lalonde, B. (1987). The general symptom distress scale: A home care outcome measure. *Quality Review Bulletin* (July): 243–50.

Lalonde, B. (1988). Assuring the quality of home care via the assessment of client outcomes. *Caring* 7(1): 20–24.

Legislative roundup: Durenberger sees home care prospective payment near. (1984). *Caring* 3(5): 5–6.

Lerman, D. (ed.) (1987). *Home Care: Positioning the hospital for the future.* New York: American Hospital Publishing, Inc.

Louden, T. L. (1983). Opportunities—and competition—in home healthcare are on the rise. *Modern Healthcare* 13(12): 109–12.

Lundberg, C. J. (1984). Home health care: A logical extension of hospital services. *Topics in Health Care Financing* 10(3): 22–32.

Lutz, S. (1987). Technology fueling growth in pediatric home care programs. *Modern Healthcare* (July) 31: 60–63.

MacNamara, E. (1982). Home care: Hospitals rediscover comprehensive home care. *Hospitals* 16(21): 60–66.

Martin, K. (1988). Research in home care. *Nursing Clinics of North America* 23(2): 373–85.

Martinson, I. M., M. K. Jameison, B. O'Grady, and M. Sime. (1985). The block nurse program. *Journal of Community Health Nursing* 2(1): 21–29.

McCabe, P., et al. (1987). Home care trends for the terminally ill: Challenges and responsibilities. *Caring* 6(11): 4–6.

Moxley, J. H., III. (1984). New opportunities for out-of-hospital health services. *New England Journal of Medicine* 310(3): 193–97.

Mundinger, M. (1983). *Home care controversy: Too little, too late, too costly.* Rockville, Md.: Aspen Systems.

Mundinger, M. (1984). Community-based care: Who will be the case managers? *Nursing Outlook* 32(6): 294–95.

National Association for Home Care. (1984). *Position paper on legislative and regulatory issues: A blueprint for action.* Washington, D.C.: Author.

National Association for Home Care. (1989). *1990 National home care directory.* Washington, D.C.: Author.

Neiman, E., et al. (1986). Bridging the gap: Hospital to home in a changing health care environment. *Emphasis on Nursing* 2(1): 12–17.

News Briefs. (1982). Home health care may help hospitals live with 7.9% caps. *Modern Health Care* 12(12): 9.

Newton, G. A. (1986). Sharing responsibility for home care of the indigent. *Journal of Nursing Administration* 16(5): 25–27.

Palley, H. A., and J. S. Oktay. (1983). In-home and other supportive community-based services for the chronically limited elderly: Problems, prospects, and proposals. *Home Health Care Services Quarterly* 4(2): 3–9.

Paradis, L., et al. (1987). Home health agencies and hospices — stronger together or alone? *Nursing and Health Care* 8(3): 166–72.

Phillips, E. K., et al. (1987). Home health care: Who's there? *American Journal of Public Health* 77(6): 733–74.

Phillips, E. K., et al. (1988). Public home health: Settling in after DRGs. *Nursing Economics* 6(1): 31–35.

Phillips, E. K., et al. (1989). DRG ripple and the shifting burden of care to home health. *Nursing and Health Care* 10(6): 325–27.

Research news: Studies on elderly show need for home care. (1984). *Caring* 3(5): 11–13.

Rinke, L. T. (1988). *Outcome standards in home health: State of the art.* Washington, D.C.: National League for Nursing Publication No. 21-2204: 1–63.

Speigel, A. D. (1983). *Home health care: Home birthing to hospice care.* Owings Mills, Md.: National Health Publishing.

Stewart, I. E. (1979). *Home health care.* St. Louis: C. V. Mosby.

Warhola, C. (1980). *Planning for home health services — A resource handbook* (DHHS Pub. No. [HRA] 80-14017). Washington, D.C.: U.S. Government Printing Office.

Weinstein, S. M. (1987). Home care forum: Cost viewpoints. NITA 10(6): 401–9.

Weissert, N. (1980). Effects and costs of day care and homemaker services for the chronically ill elderly. Bethesda, Md.: National Center for Health Services Research.

Young, S., et al. (1988). Ambulatory AIDS care for those with special needs — children, women, and drug users. *Journal of Ambulatory Care Management* 11(2): 67–80.

Selected Readings

Bakken, K. L. (1983). Integrated health care: The whole person in community. *Nursing Economics* 1(2): 178–80.

Ballard, S., and R. McNamara. (1983). Quantifying nursing needs in home health care. *Nursing Research* 32: 236–41.

Bayer, R. (1986). Ethics in home care and quality assurance. *Caring* 5(1): 50, 52–53, 55–56.

Bedrosian, C. A. (1988). *Home health nursing: Nursing diagnoses and care plans.* East Norwalk, Conn.: Appleton and Lange.

Belair, P. S. (1986). Home health nursing: A rediscovered concept. *Imprint* 33(1): 19–20.

Berkman, L., and S. Syme. (1979). Social networks, host resistance, and mortality. *American Journal of Epidemiology* 110(5): 583–89.

Bohland, M. G., et al. (1986). AIDS: The implications for home care. *Maternal/Child Nursing* 11(6): 404–11.

Boyle, T. E. (1987). Home care contracting with HMOs and Preferred Provider Organizations. *Caring* 6(1): 23–25.

Brook, R., and K. Lohr. (1981). Quality of care assessment: Its role in the 80s. *American Journal of Public Health* 81: 681–82.

Brown, K. (1984). Speakers stress home health agency diversification. *Home Care/Rehabilitation Product News* (Jan./Feb.): 10.

Buck, J. N. (1988). Measuring the success of home health care. *Home Health Care Nurse* 6(3): 17–19, 22–23.

Burbach, C. A., et al. (1988). Community and home health nursing: Keeping the concepts clear. *Nursing and Health Care* 9(2): 96–100.

Callahan, D. (1988). Families as caregivers: The limits of morality. *Archives of Physical Medicine and Rehabilitation* 69(5): 323–28.

Callahan, J. (1980). Responsibilities of families for their severely disabled elders. *Health Care Financing Review* 4: 29–48.

Cetron, M. (1985). The public opinion of home care: A survey report executive summary. *Caring* 4(10): 12–15.

Cowart, M. E. (1985). Policy issues: Financial reimbursement for home care. *Family and Community Health* 8(2): 1–10.

Cruse, J., et al. (1987). Screening the elderly: A neglected aspect of health visiting. *Geriatric Nursing Home Care* 7(10): 13–17.

Daubert, E. (1987). Strategic planning in home care. *American Journal of Nursing* (Sept.): 1161–63.

Davis, E. J. (1987). Home care — What's needed? *Public Health Nursing* 4(2): 82–83.

DeCrosta, T. (1984). Home health care: It's red hot and right now. *Nursing Life* 2: 54–60.

Donlan, T. G. (1983). No place like home. *Barron's* (March 21): 6, 7, 32.

Ebner, M. E. (1987). Home care economics: Challenges and opportunities for future nursing practitioners. *Deans' Notes* (March) 8(4): 1–2.

Feldman, J., et al. (1988). *Patients and purse strings: The productivity, effectiveness, and efficiency of home care programs for the elderly.* Vol. 2. New York: National League for Nursing Publication No. 201-2191: 367–87.

Fine, D. R. (1986). The home as the workplace: Prejudice and inequity in home health care. *Caring* 5(4): 12–19.

Fish, C. W. (1984). *Administrators' handbook for community health and home care services.* New York: National League for Nursing Publication No. 21-1943: 1–423.

Frietag, E. M. (1988). Marketing in home health care: A practical approach. *Nursing Clinics of North America* 23(2): 415–29.

Gary, L. R. (1979). *Home health care regulation: Issues and opportunities.* New York: Hunter College.

Griffith, E. (1987). The changing face of home health care. *Public Health Nursing* 4(1): 1.

Hamilton, C. L, and B. J. Neubauer. (1989). Hospice nursing: Serving ambivalent clients. *Nursing and Health Care* 10(6): 320–22.

Hammond, J. (1979). Home health care cost effectiveness: An overview of the literature. *Public Health Reports* 94(4): 305–11,

Harrington, C. (1988). Quality, access, and costs: Public policy and home health care. *Nursing Outlook* 36(4): 164–66.

Harris, M. E., et al. (1987a). Outcome measures in home care. New York: National League for Nursing Publication No. 21-2194: 187–204.

Hartshorn, N. R. (1985). The use of volunteers in a home health agency. *Home Healthcare Nurse* 3(6): 26–28.

Harvey, S. (1987). The key to survival: Productivity incentives for home health. *Caring* 6(7): 34–37.

Hildebrandt, E. D. (1983). Respite care in the home. *American Journal of Nursing* (Oct.): 1428–31.

Holt, S. W. (1984). Continuity of care in the home: Building a diversified service system that works. *Caring* 3(5): 49–56.

Home health and other in-home services. (1979). Department of Health, Education and Welfare. Report to Congress. Washington, D.C.: U.S. Government Printing Office.

Home health care: Its utilization, costs and reimbursement. (1977). New York: Health Services Agency of New York City.

Home health: The need for a national policy to better provide for the elderly. (1977). Department of Health, Education and Welfare. Report to Congress. Washington, D.C.: U.S. Government Printing Office.

Hughes, F. (1987). Quality assurance in home care services. *Nursing Management* 18(12): 33–36.

Humphrey, C. J. (1988). The home as a setting for care: Clarifying the boundaries of practice. *Nursing Clinics of North America* 23(2): 305–14.

Inui, T., K. Stevenson, D. Plorde, and I. Murphy. (1980). Needs assessment for hospital-based home care services. *Research in Nursing and Health* 3(3): 101–6.

Kane, R., and R. Kane. (1978). Care of the aged—An old problem in search of new solutions. *Science* 200: 913–18.

Kuntz, E. F. (1983). Hospitals move into home care by striking partnership deals. *Modern Healthcare* 13(12): 116–18.

Lalonde, B. (1988). Assuring the quality of home care via the assessment of client outcomes. *Caring* 7(1): 20–24.

Lerman, D. (ed.) (1987). *Home care: Positioning the hospital for the future.* New York: American Hospital Publishing, Inc.

Louden, T. L. (1983). Opportunities—and competition—in home healthcare are on the rise. *Modern Healthcare* 13(12): 109–12.

Louden, T. L. (1987). The evolution of the home healthcare industry: Developing new levels of business sophistication. *Health Industry Today* (July): 17–24.

Lundberg, C. J. (1984). Home health care: A logical extension of hospital services. *Topics in Health Care Financing* 10(3): 22–32.

Lutz, S. (1987). Technology fueling growth in pediatric home care programs. *Modern Healthcare* (July) 31: 60–63.

MacNamara, E. (1982). Home care: Hospitals rediscover comprehensive home care. *Hospitals* 16(21): 60–66.

Magilvy, J., N. Brown, and J. Dydyn. (1988). The experience of home health care: Perspectives of older adults. *Public Health Nursing* 5(3): 140–45.

Maraldo, P. J. (1989). Home health care should be the heart of a nursing-sponsored national health plan. *Nursing and Health Care* 10(6): 300–304.

Martin, K. (1988). Research in home care. *Nursing Clinics of North America* 23(2): 373–85.

Martinson, I. M., M. K. Jameison, B. O'Grady, and M. Sime. (1985). The block nurse program. *Journal of Community Health Nursing* 2(1): 21–29.

McCabe, P., et al. (1987). Home care trends for the terminally ill: Challenges and responsibilities. *Caring* 6(11): 4–6.

Moxley, J. H., III. (1984). New opportunities for out-of-hospital health services. *New England Journal of Medicine* 310(3): 193–97.

Moyer, N. (1986). Public policy, politics, and home health care. *Home Healthcare Nurse* 4(5): 7–10, 12.

Mundinger, M. (1983). *Home care controversy: Too little, too late, too costly.* Rockville, Md.: Aspen Systems.

Mundinger, M. (1984). Community-based care: Who will be the case managers? *Nursing Outlook* 32(6): 294–95.

National Association for Home Care. (1984). *Position paper on legislative and regulatory issues: A blueprint for action.* Washington, D.C.: Author.

Neiman, E., et al. (1986). Bridging the gap: Hospital to home in a changing health care environment. *Emphasis on Nursing* 2(1): 12–17.

Newton, G. A. (1986). Sharing responsibility for home care of the indigent. *Journal of Nursing Administration* 16(5): 25–27.

Paradis, L., et al. (1987). Home health agencies and hospices — stronger together or alone? *Nursing and Health Care* 8(3): 166–72.

Pasquale, D. K. (1987). A basis for prospective payment for home care. *Image Journal of Nursing Scholarship* 19(4): 186–91.

Pegels, C. (1980). *Health care and the elderly.* Rockville Md.: Aspen Systems.

Phillips, E. K., et al. (1988). Public home health: Settling in after DRGs. *Nursing Economics* 6(1): 31–35.

Phillips, E. K., et al. (1989). DRG ripple and the shifting burden of care to home health. *Nursing and Health Care* 10(6): 325–27.

Powell, D. J. (1984). Nurses — "High touch" entrepreneurs. *Nursing Economics* 2(1): 33–36.

Public Health Nursing Section. (1982). *Assessment of health risks in the home environment: A manual designed to assist public health nurses perform an environmental assessment.* Minneapolis, Minn. Department of Health.

Ramage, N. B. (1985). In-home health services: A policy perspective. *Family and Community Health* 8(2): 11–21.

Rinke, L. T. (1988). *Outcome standards in home health: State of the art.* New York: National League for Nursing Publication No. 21-2204: 1–63.

Robinson, J. (1987). Care in the community: Support for informal carers of chronically ill and disabled people. *International Disability Studies* 9(2): 78–80.

Snow, D., and L. Kleinman. (1987). The impact of crime on home care services *American Journal of Public Health* 77(2): 209–10.

Somers, A. (1978). The high cost of health care for the elderly: Diagnosis, prognosis, and some questions for therapy. *Journal of Health Policy, Politics & Law* 4(2): 163–80.

Somers, A., and N. Bryant. (1975). Home care: Much needed, much neglected. *Annals of Internal Medicine* 82: 111–12.

Spiegel, A. D. (1983). *Home healthcare: Home birthing to hospice care.* Owings Mills, Md.: National Health Publishing.

Trager, B. (1980). *Home health care and national policy.* New York: Hawthorne Press.

U.S. General Accounting Office. (1982). The elderly should benefit from expanded home health care, but increasing these services will not insure cost reductions (Pub. No. GAO/IPE-83-1). Gaithersburg, Md.: Author.

Vladek, B. (1980). *Unloving care.* New York: Basic Books.

Warhola, C. (1980). *Planning for home health services—A resource handbook* (DHHS Pub. No. [HRA] 80-14017). Washington, D.C.: U.S. Government Printing Office.

Weinstein, S. M. (1987). Home care forum: Cost viewpoints. NITA 10(6): 401–9.

Widmer, G., R. Brill, and A. Schlosser. (1978). Home health care services and cost. *Nursing Outlook,* 26: 488–93.

Williams, S. D. (1987). Promotion... for a home health care agency. *Home Healthcare Nurse* 5(5): 44–45.

Young, S., et al. (1988). Ambulatory AIDS care for those with special needs — children, women, and drug users. *Journal of Ambulatory Care Management* 11(2): 67–80.

FOUR Expanding the Nurse's Influence

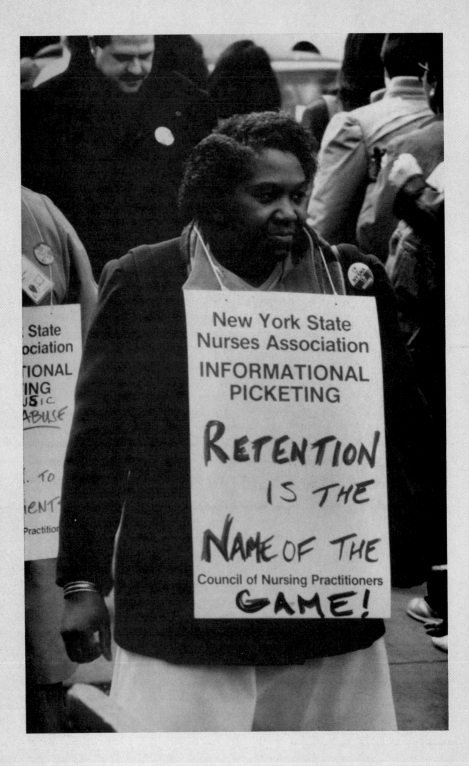

22 Leadership and Managing Change

Leading people to change their beliefs and practices about health lies at the heart of all community health nursing. This aim characterizes work with clients at every level, from individuals to large organizations and communities. At all levels, the ability to influence change requires knowledge and skill in two closely related areas: leadership and management of change.

How do nurses carry out their roles as both leaders and change agents at the community level? With such rapidly expanding opportunities, it is possible to give several examples. One community health nurse becomes a member of the Governor's Commission on the Handicapped. In addition to understanding the entire state as a community and the handicapped as a special population, she urges the commission to formulate new plans for meeting the needs of the handicapped. Another nurse, as a member of a metropolitan health planning board, works to improve health care for a group of Hmong immigrants from Southeast Asia. In a rural community of farms and small towns, another nurse organizes a grass-roots committee concerned about a nearby nuclear generating plant. The committee works to develop an emergency evacuation plan in case of radiation leaks from the plant. All three of these nurses are involved in leadership and change at the community level. They are working to change people's beliefs regarding health and health activities and to involve them in creating organized responses to community problems.

Community health nurses also lead people to change at the organizational level. Let us say that you are a staff nurse in a public health nursing agency. Like the other staff members, you feel overburdened by paperwork. You may feel burned out and lack clear goals for your daily tasks. Setting priorities is difficult. Rather than blaming yourself, you recognize that other staff feel the same way; it is an organizational problem. During a staff meeting, you bring up the problem of job stress and suggest that everyone read an article on the subject to discuss at the next staff meeting. The first discussion is so successful that others follow. At your prompting, a regular staff development meeting evolves with rotating leadership. As the months pass, a new sense of direction emerges among the staff. People feel more competent to cope with job stress, and morale improves. Although you worked informally, you acted as a leader to bring about organizational change. The result not only left individuals feeling better able to cope with their jobs, but also improved the health of the organization.

Community health nurses also seek to influence families to achieve new levels of health. One nurse assists a family in improving its communication; another leads a family through the stress caused by incest and helps its members to change and move to a new level of health. You can act in a leadership capacity with groups, perhaps negotiating a contract with a group to quit smoking or to develop a school program on battered children. The list goes on and on, but in every case the pattern of assuming leadership in order to promote change in health practices is the same. Even with individuals you will seek to influence change. You may negotiate a contract regarding regular exercise with a man recovering from a heart attack. Hardly a day goes by for most community health nurses without deep involvement in leadership and change activities at every level of practice.

Becoming an effective leader and change agent requires specialized knowledge and skills. In this chapter we examine leadership and the management of change. We will see how they are inextricably linked and how community health nurses incorporate them into practice.

LEADERSHIP DEFINED

Many nurses do not see themselves as leaders, nor do they wish to become leaders. All too often, leadership for these nurses has come to mean they must assume a formal position of being in charge. As leaders, they would have to tell other people what to do. Some nurses feel it means being alone at the top of a group or organization, taking all the risks and being held accountable for the outcomes. Many of these conceptions of leadership, however, are based on false premises.

Leadership is *an interpersonal process in which one person influences the activities of another person or group of persons toward accomplishment of a goal in a specific situation* (Hersey and Blanchard, 1988; Moloney, 1979). In its simplest terms, leadership involves setting the pace, going first, and guiding and directing the way people think and act. It is accomplishing goals with and through people (Hersey and Blanchard, 1988). To lead requires interacting with other people to influence them to achieve a goal. Let us look at three major characteristics of leadership implied in this definition.

LEADERSHIP CHARACTERISTICS

First, leadership is *purposeful*: it always has a goal (Adams, 1986). No act of leadership exists without a reason. A mayor wants low-cost housing for the poor; a community nurse wants to see a family change its nutritional habits; a minister wants transportation that is accessible to all the physically handicapped. In each instance, the leader has a purpose and hopes that others will come to share that purpose. A leader will work to achieve goals by making them clear, attainable, specific, and agreeable to the follower constituency.

Second, leadership is *interpersonal*. It is a social exchange, a transaction between the two parties of leader and follower (Nicoll, 1986). These parties share information in a variety of patterns. An authoritarian army general gives direct orders to his military personnel; the president of a garden club makes informal suggestions to club members. In both cases, however, the leader and followers must maintain a relationship that fosters ongoing communication and facilitates the goal-seeking process.

Third, leadership is *influential* (Fritz, 1986). In one small community that existed in a larger city, a nurse received reports that several children had been bitten by rats. A casual survey revealed alleys with piles of garbage and trash that attracted rats. The nurse, as a leader, wanted to influence members of this community to eliminate a public health problem. She could not clean up all the refuse herself, nor would city maintenance crews undertake the responsibility. In order to mobilize the local citizens to achieve this goal, she needed to influence them. She began with the parents of children bitten by rats, influencing them to call their neighbors together. At that meeting, she spoke about the need for eliminating the garbage and trash from alleys. She quietly listened to the discussion and offered suggestions when the group decided to form a committee and hold a clean-up day. As a leader, she offered guidance and direction, thus influencing the ideas and activities of this group of followers.

Leadership, then, in community health means to influence people toward development of an optimally healthy life-style and environment. Any purposeful effort to influence behavior is an example of leadership; thus, every community health nurse can act as a leader (Hersey and Blanchard, 1988). Moreover, according to Moloney (1979), all nurses should exercise leadership. She bases her rationale on the fact that nurses must accept responsibility for revitalizing and upgrading professional nursing practice and for improving health services. She declares: "Accountability for professional practice implies that nurses are functioning as leaders in health care. If nurses are to become accountable for practice, they must broaden their view of what responsible leadership entails" (Moloney, 1979, p. 3). Nurses have many opportunities to exercise leadership. In community health, they may lead citizens; in practice, they may lead clients toward optimal health; as nurse managers, they may lead colleagues to improved practice; and as nurse faculty (Chait, 1988), they may lead their students toward future leadership (Flynn et al., 1987).

LEADERSHIP FUNCTIONS

Leadership functions occur at many levels, each with its own set of activities and sphere of influence. A captain's leadership functions will differ from a corporal's, a governor's from a school board member's, and a corporation president's from an assembly line inspector's. Within community health nursing, the functions of leadership also vary depending upon the nurse's position and work situation. Take, for example, a large community health nursing agency. Listed below are some areas of influence associated with various positions:

Director	Influences organizational policy and decision making
Associate director	Influences management of specific aspects of the organization
Supervisor	Influences structure and process of providing care
Team leader	Influences day-to-day quality of nursing practice
Staff nurse	Influences client health, behavior, and environment

In other settings for community health nursing practice, such as rural or occupational environments, there may be only one nurse present to provide leadership that encompasses many, if not all, of these activities. Beyond the agency itself, the leadership role of each nurse extends to influencing those community attitudes, programs, and environmental factors that affect community health. Each nurse must assess the situation and determine the kind and extent of leadership needed.

What are the functions of leadership in community health nursing? Kouzes and Posner (1987) describe leaders as challenging the process, inspiring a shared vision, enabling others to act, modeling the way, and encouraging the heart. Argyris (1976, p. ix) summarizes several functions: "Leaders... know how to discover the difficult questions, how to create viable problem-solving networks to invent solutions to these questions, and how to generate and channel human energy and commitment to produce the solutions." More specifically, five essential functions are required for effective leadership at any level: (1) the creative function, (2) the initiating function, (3) the risk-taking function, (4) the integrative function, and (5) the instrumental function. These functions do not occur in any particular order; rather, they operate simultaneously throughout the leadership process.

Creative Function

Leaders must be able to envision new and better ways to solve problems. This first step in creativity is then followed by developing methods and activities for carrying out the solutions. This function requires ingenuity, innovation, vision, and a future orientation (Fritz, 1986). For instance, a nurse in a rural agency recognized that the home health aides or homemakers could potentially meet more client needs, find their jobs more fulfilling, and better serve the agency through an expanded role. She revised their job descriptions and instituted an expanded role-training program (Hennes, 1979). The creative leadership function is one that includes generating ideas and developing designs for action. It also involves empowering others to use their own creativity to accomplish goals (Harman, 1986).

Initiating Function

A leader introduces change and sets its process in motion. For a nurse, this function includes convincing clients or followers of the need for change, starting the problem-solving process, and launching the activities needed to carry out the plan. Like all the other leadership functions, it requires decision-making skills. For example, after seeing an increased number of pregnancies, a nurse who works in a high school convinces the girls to start a prenatal counseling group and originates a series of sex education seminars. The initiating function begins the process toward goal accomplishment. It is the stimulus or "push" that starts clients or followers on their course of action (Fritz, 1986).

Risk-Taking Function

Every leader is faced with uncertainty, and to proceed under uncertain conditions is to take risks (Lee, 1987). What nurse, working with a family or group in the community, has not encountered a number of unpredictable variables during the process of planning with clients for health goals? Will this diet control the disease? Will client self-disclosure in this group therapy lead to group acceptance and understanding or to open ridicule and a deteriorated self-image? Will the new drug counseling clinic significantly reduce the problem, or will county funds have been spent needlessly, thus jeopardizing future funding requests? Leaders cannot guarantee outcomes. The leadership process requires careful planning based on all available data and the creation of scenarios in order to predict all possible obstacles and outcomes. It even requires preparation of alternative courses of action, should earlier plans fail. Nevertheless, some variables cannot be predicted beyond a certain point, and leaders must be willing to take chances. They have to be willing to go out on a limb, to expose themselves to possible failure and embarrassment.

Taking chances also means they will expose clients or followers to potential negative outcomes. No leader throughout history has operated without taking risks. Effective leaders, however, take calculated risks (Kouzes and Posner, 1987); they weigh the pros and cons and potential consequences of each action before proceeding. Their concern is to minimize harmful exposure to followers.

Integrative Function

This aspect of the leadership role focuses on strengthening collective ties and uniting clients or followers through a strong sense of purpose. The leader reminds the followers of their goals, encourages pride in their group identity, stabilizes intragroup relations, and mediates interpersonal conflict (Kouzes and Posner, 1987). Community health nurses working with families and groups frequently find members at odds or cross-purposes with one another. Individuals in any group setting tend to have their own hidden agendas and separate needs. One of the nurse leader's jobs is to keep the client group on target by clarifying and reinforcing the goals they have mutually identified. The integrative function requires good interpersonal skills for establishing positive relationships with, as well as between, followers. This function supports the aim of promoting member commitment and cooperation.

Instrumental Function

Leaders must also keep followers moving in the right direction; this is the purpose of the instrumental or facilitative function. Inspired by vision and goals, the leader serves as enabler to move followers to act (Hersey and Blanchard, 1988; Kouzes and Posner, 1987). For nurse leaders, this function involves good communication. They must keep in constant touch with clients or followers, make certain that goals and activities are understood and agreed upon, and encourage both negative and positive feedback. Leaders further stimulate followers to progress toward achievement of goals by reinforcing desired behaviors and by setting the pace themselves. The latter is particularly important for gaining followers' respect and sustained commitment. To set the pace means nurse leaders must demonstrate competence, practice what they preach, and show followers that they believe in them and in what they are asking followers to accomplish.

AREAS OF INFLUENCE

Community health nurses exercise the functions of leadership in ever-widening spheres of influence, as is shown in Figure 22-1. The central aim of this leadership role is to influence community health. The first area of focus is to im-

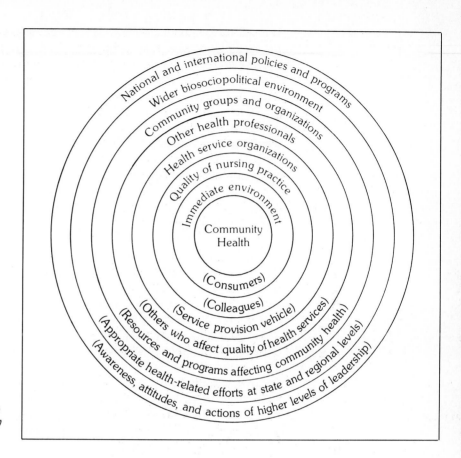

National and international policies and programs
Wider biosociopolitical environment
Community groups and organizations
Other health professionals
Health service organizations
Quality of nursing practice
Immediate environment

Community
Health

(Consumers)

(Colleagues)

(Service provision vehicle)

(Others who affect quality of health services)

(Resources and programs affecting community health)

(Appropriate health-related efforts at state and regional levels)

(Awareness, attitudes, and actions of higher levels of leadership)

Figure 22-1
Areas of potential leadership influence within community health nursing practice.

prove the immediate environment, which includes physical, psychological, social, and spiritual factors, by influencing consumer health-related behavior. Community health nurses exercise leadership when they influence the quality of nursing practice of their co-workers through, for instance, peer consultation and review. They may also influence the service provision vehicle, the agency or organization through which care is offered, by accepting a high-level position or by serving on committees and taking an active part in quality control. Other professionals involved in the health provision system are an additional target of community health nurses' leadership influence. Ongoing communication with colleagues from other disciplines may serve to stimulate these professionals' awareness of health needs and facilitate development of appropriate services. Community health nurses may influence groups and organizations that affect community health, such as clubs, churches, or the legislature, by keeping them informed about health problems and suggesting ways they can improve community health levels. Extending their leadership influence even wider, community health nurses may focus on the wider biosociopolitical environment of the city, county, state, or region (Williams, 1981). For example, a nurse may support anti-smoking programs or campaign for proper disposal of nuclear waste. Finally, community health nursing leadership may extend to influencing national and international policies and programs that affect health, such as those of the World Health Organization. Participating in citizens' lobbies, serving on national committees, or contacting senators and representatives of the U.S. Congress are some of the many possible actions nurses could take. The number of spheres in which the community health nurse exercises a leadership role varies, depending on health needs, the work situation, the nurse's abilities, and available time.

LEADERSHIP STYLES

Some nurses effectively influence people's behavior. Others do not. What explains the difference? What accounts for effective leadership? Some researchers, assuming that certain individuals acquire or are born with leadership qualities, have sought to identify the personality traits of leaders. These efforts have been unsuccessful in establishing any one group of traits that would predict leadership effectiveness (Moloney, 1979).

More recent research has focused on the behavior of leaders during interaction with followers. This approach views leaders' behavior, rather than leaders' personalities, as the chief determinant of leadership effectiveness. From this research, several taxonomies of leadership styles have evolved. We will first consider one that identifies three styles: (1) autocratic leadership, (2) participative leadership, and (3) laissez-faire leadership (Hersey and Blanchard, 1988; Moloney, 1979; Uris, 1964).

Leaders' Behavior

Autocratic Style. The autocratic style is authoritarian. Leaders who adopt this style use their power (usually the power of their position) to influence their followers. The autocratic leader gives orders and expects others to obey without question. This style is generally evident in the military. Suggestions from followers are not, as a rule, invited or accepted. The leader is dominant; the followers have little power or freedom of choice. In times of extreme crisis, an autocratic style may enhance survival. Sometimes a nurse finds that members of a group will expect to be led in an autocratic style. They may see the nurse as the qualified expert among them. Autocratic leadership must be used with caution, and many current organizational structures do not lend themselves to its practice (Kinsman, 1986).

Participative Style. The participative style, a supportive approach, is sometimes called the democratic style. This form of leadership has become increasingly popular in recent years as leaders have sought to involve followers in the decision-making process (Kinsman, 1986). This style tends to promote followers' self-esteem and to increase motivation and productivity (Figure 22-2). Leaders utilizing this style sometimes find it difficult to maintain control and to prevent followers from taking charge while remaining democratic. Some participative leaders permit their followers more freedom and power than others. Generally, however, this leadership style allows followers considerable freedom to make choices (Nicoll, 1986).

Autonomous Style.   The autonomous style means giving followers free rein to pursue goals. The leader maintains a hands-off policy that gives complete freedom of choice to the group members, who set their own objectives, carry out their own activities, and function independently. This style is effective in a group whose members have both the motivation and competence to achieve the goals (Kinsman, 1986). Although someone is formally the leader, this style uses little or no direct influence; rather, the leader sets the overall purpose and encourages follower creativity and innovation.

Task- and Relationship-Oriented Leadership

We discussed earlier the idea that leadership is accomplishing goals with and through people. Consequently, leaders must be concerned with tasks (in order to achieve goals) and with relationships (to show concern for people) (Hersey and Blanchard, 1988). These two dimensions, tasks and relationships, become opposite points of emphasis on a continuum of leader behavior, as is illustrated in Figure 22-3. Research has shown that autocratic leaders tend to be concerned about goals and are task-oriented, whereas participative leaders are concerned about people and emphasize relationships. These two em-

Figure 22-2
As a leader, the nurse seeks to influence clients toward a healthier state. Here the nurse involves a class of senior citizens in a discussion about their health. She uses a participative leadership style.

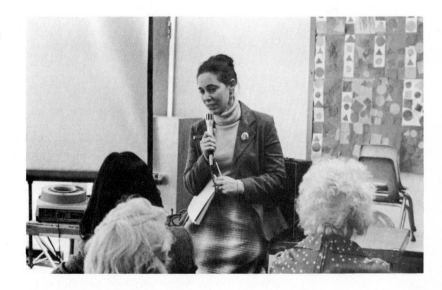

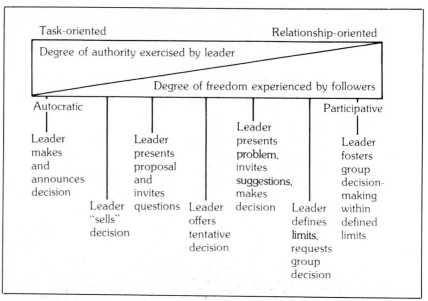

*Figure 22-3
Leadership behavior
continuum.*

phases have led to a new taxonomy of leadership styles as either task-oriented or relationship-oriented (Hersey and Blanchard, 1988).

Leadership behavior research has demonstrated that leadership style has a significant influence on leadership effectiveness. However, since many variables, such as leader personality, follower needs and resources, and the situation, influence effectiveness, no one style can be advocated as best.

Situational-Oriented Leadership

The situational approach to the study of leadership behavior has yielded the most promising results. Based on a recognition that leadership is a relationship between leader, followers, and the situation, it is unrealistic to assume a single, ideal type of leadership behavior. A participative style of leadership used in one organization is not always successful in another similar organization. An integrated style that shows high concern for both tasks and relationships might be appropriate in one setting but not in another. Researchers pursuing the situational approach have concluded that the situation dictates the style of leadership one should use. Because every situation is unique, leadership becomes a dynamic process of adapting one's style to the demands of the situation. Hersey and Blanchard (1988) refer to this process as "adaptive leader behavior." Its implications for community health nursing can be stated thus: the more nurses adapt their style of leadership behavior to meet the particular situation and the needs of clients or followers, the more effective they will be in reaching health-related goals (Bernhard and Walsh, 1981).

The most effective leadership style, then, is an adaptive one. Nurses will need to determine the most appropriate style by assessing the unique qualities of each situation, followers' needs and degree of independence, and their own personalities and abilities (Guidera et al., 1988).

CONDITIONS FOR EFFECTIVE LEADERSHIP

The ultimate test of nurse leadership is in the outcomes. Are goals met? What did the leader accomplish? Reaching a successful outcome involves certain factors. Adherence to these factors will contribute to positive results, but violation of one or more of them will create negative results. They form the conditions necessary for leadership to be effective.

1. Followers must understand the suggestion, advice, or directive in order to make compliance possible (Henry et al., 1987).
2. Followers must be able to carry out the suggestion. They must have or be supplied with the needed resources or abilities (Lee, 1987).
3. The required action must be consistent with the followers' personal values and interests (Fritz, 1986).
4. The required action must be consistent with the followers' collective purposes, values, and norms; that is, followers must be in tune with group or organizational goals (Guidera et al., 1988).

Central and most important to effective leadership is a relationship of trust, respect, and mutual exchange between leader and followers. It is through this transactional relationship that community health nurses can satisfy the conditions for effective leadership and accomplish positive outcomes.

THE NATURE OF CHANGE

"To lead means to effect change" (Moloney, 1979, p. 87). When nurses suggest that postcoronary clients adopt a new, healthier pattern of living, they are asking them to change. Teaching diabetic children how to give themselves insulin is introducing a change. Revising home health aide/homemakers' responsibilities, again, requires that those individuals change. Since community health nursing's responsibility is to accomplish health goals and thus promote change, nurses cannot lead without introducing change. Therefore, it becomes imperative for community health nurses to understand the nature of change, how people respond to it, and how to manage it.

What is change? For some analysts, change means that things are out of balance; they refer to it as an upset in a system's equilibrium (Spradley, 1980; Bennis, Benne, and Chin, 1985). For instance, when the mother in a family becomes ill, that family's normal functioning is thrown off balance. Adjustments are required; new patterns of behavior become necessary. Other observers view change as the process of adopting an innovation (Spradley and McCurdy, 1980). Something different, such as a new diet, is introduced; change occurs when the innovation is accepted, tried, and integrated into daily living. Lippitt (1973, p. 37) defines change as "any planned or unplanned alteration of the status quo in an organism, situation, or process," thus reminding us that change may occur either by design or by default (Rantz et al., 1987). Still others view change in terms of its effect on behavior. They say change is both the altering of a situation and, depending upon how people define the new situation, the way behavior is altered to fit it (Zaltman and Duncan, 1977). We can see that change requires adjustment in thinking and behavior and that people's responses to change vary according to their perceptions of it. Change threatens the security that people feel when following established and familiar patterns (Nordstrom et al., 1987). It generally requires the adoption of new roles. Change is disruptive.

KINDS OF CHANGE

The way people respond to change depends, in part, on the kind of change it is. We can describe the change process as occurring along a continuum between two opposites, evolutionary change and revolutionary change (Gerlach and Hine, 1973).

Evolutionary Change

Evolutionary change tends to be gradual and requires adjustment on an incremental basis. It modifies rather than replaces a current way of operating. Becoming parents, stopping smoking by gradually cutting back on the number of cigarettes smoked each day, and losing weight by eliminating desserts and sweets are examples of evolutionary change. Since it is gradual, this kind of change does not require radical shifts in goals or values; in fact, it may enhance current goals or values (Nordstrom et al., 1987). Less threatening and more readily adopted than revolutionary change, evolutionary change is sometimes considered reform. It resembles variations on a musical theme.

Revolutionary Change

Revolutionary change, in contrast, is more rapid, drastic, and threatening. It may completely upset the balance of the system. It involves different goals and perhaps radically new patterns of behavior (Nordstrom et al., 1987). This kind of change resembles a whole new musical theme. Sudden unemployment, stopping smoking overnight, losing the town's football team in a plane accident, or suddenly removing a child from abusive parents are examples of revolutionary change. In each instance, the people affected have little or no advance warning and time to prepare. High levels of psychic energy and rapid behavior change are required in adapting to revolutionary change; as a result, incapacitation, resistance, or denial of the new situation frequently occurs.

The impact of a proposed change on a system will clearly depend on the degree of the change's evolutionary or revolutionary qualities, a factor to be considered in planning for change. Some situations lend themselves better to one kind of change than the other. A community in need of improved facilities for the handicapped, such as ramps and wider doors, can introduce this change on an evolutionary, incremental basis; whereas a community involved in an unsafe, intolerable, or life-threatening situation, such as a serious epidemic, may require revolutionary change.

STAGES OF CHANGE

The process of change occurs in three stages described by Lewin (cited in Lippitt, Watson, and Westley, 1958; Noone, 1987) as unfreezing, moving, and refreezing.

Unfreezing

Unfreezing, the first stage, occurs when a need for change develops. People are motivated to change either intrinsically or by some external force (Ryan, 1987). During this stage the need for change creates disequilibrium in the system. A system in disequilibrium is more vulnerable to change. People have a sense of dissatisfaction; they feel a void that they would like to fill. Like an amputee eager to use a prosthesis or a community concerned about safe intersections, they are ready for change. Thus, the unfreezing stage involves initiating the change.

Unfreezing may occur spontaneously. A family requests help in solving a problem with alcoholism; a group seeks help in adjusting to retirement. However, the nurse as change agent may need to initiate the unfreezing stage by attempting to motivate clients to see the need for change (Ryan, 1987).

Moving

Moving, the second stage of the change process, occurs when people examine, accept, and actually try out the innovation. For instance, this is the period when participants in a prenatal class are learning exercises or when the elderly in a senior citizens' center are discussing and trying out ways to make their apartments safe from falls. During the moving stage, people experience a series of attitude transformations ranging from early questioning of the innovation's worth to full acceptance and commitment to accomplishing the change. The change agent's role during this stage is to help clients see the value of the change, encourage them to try it out, and assist them in adopting it for use (Cobb-McMahon et al., 1984).

Refreezing

Refreezing, the third and final stage in the change process, occurs when change is established as an accepted and permanent part of the system. The rest of the system has adapted to it. Since it is no longer viewed as disruptive, threatening, or even new, people no longer feel resistant to it. As the change is integrated, the system becomes refrozen and stabilized. We know that refreezing has occurred when weight loss clients, for instance, are regularly following their diets and losing weight, or when senior citizens have installed grab bars in their bathrooms and removed scatter rugs, or when a community has erected stop signs and established crosswalks at dangerous intersections.

Refreezing involves integrating or internalizing the change into the system and then maintaining it. Simply because a change has been accepted and tried does not guarantee that it will last (Spradley, 1980). Often there is a tendency for old patterns and habits to return; consequently, the change agent must take special measures to assure maintenance of the new behavior. We will discuss ways to stabilize change in the next section.

PLANNED CHANGE

Planned change can be defined as a purposeful, designed effort to effect improvement in a system with the assistance of a change agent (Spradley, 1980). Several characteristics in this definition distinguish planned change from unplanned change (Noone, 1987). First, the change is purposeful and intentional; there are specific reasons or goals prompting the change. These goals give the change effort a unifying focus and a specific target. Unplanned change occurs haphazardly, and its outcomes are unpredictable. Second, the change is by design, not by default. Thorough, systematic planning provides structure for the change process, a map to follow toward a planned destination. Third, planned change in community health aims at improvement. That is, it seeks to better the present situation, to promote a higher level of efficiency, satisfaction, or productivity. Just as not all movement is forward, not all change is positive or growth producing. Planned change however, aims to facilitate growth. Finally, the change is accomplished by means of an influencing agent. The change agent serves as a catalyst in developing and carrying out the design; the change agent's role is a leadership role.

PLANNED CHANGE PROCESS

Before initiating planned change, community health nurses need to consider the dynamics of change in the context of system functioning. Any system seeks to achieve and maintain a relative state of equilibrium. It is in the nature of a system to seek this stability in order to maximize its ability to function. Yet the internal and external forces acting upon every system create new needs that, in turn, demand change in order to restore the system to a new level of functioning and equilibrium. For example, toxic fumes emanating from a derailed freight train forced community residents in a southern town to flee. The introduction of this external force upset the community's equilibrium and ability to function. Every effort was made to remove the source of danger and restore the community to normal functioning. The creation of a new need (to eliminate the toxic fumes) led to a change effort (the cleanup process) in order to restore system balance (normal community living). Community health nurses, as change agents, are responsible for seeing that the needs of clients are met through some kind of change and that a new equilibrium is achieved as soon as possible. They can meet clients' needs, effect change successfully, and restore clients to a stable state by conducting planned change.

Planned change involves a systematic sequence of activities that utilizes the nursing process. We shall consider eight basic steps to follow in the successful management of change (Spradley, 1980): (1) recognize symptoms, (2) diagnose need, (3) analyze alternative solutions, (4) select a change, (5) plan the change, (6) implement the change, (7) evaluate the change, and (8) stabilize the change. Figure 22-4 shows how forces acting on a system create a need for change. When we recognize that need, we have begun the change process. This model also illustrates what happens when the nurse fails to respond to the need for change. The need remains and, in fact, may increase. The client system (those involved and affected by the change) and the change agent must work together throughout the entire planned change process. Their respective roles will vary depending upon the situation, but no planned change will be truly effective without recognition and utilization of this helping relationship. The model depicts the client system as variable and vacillating (wavy arrow) because the client system is generally composed of a number of people. It may be an entire community. Thus it will experience many fluctuations in its involvement with the change process. The change agent (straight arrow), as a good leader and manager, analyzes the situation thoroughly, plans carefully, and sets a steady course for effecting the change.

Step 1: Recognize the Symptoms

The first step in managing change is to recognize the symptoms of a need for change. In this step, one should gather and examine the presenting evidence, not diagnose or jump ahead to treatment. For instance, let us say that several clients request help with parenting. Before we can diagnose or plan, we must determine all the indicators of a need. We cannot assume that these clients feel inadequate in the parent role, nor can we assume that they lack information about parenting or are having difficulty with their children. One, all, or perhaps none of these assumptions may be true. Therefore, we first look for

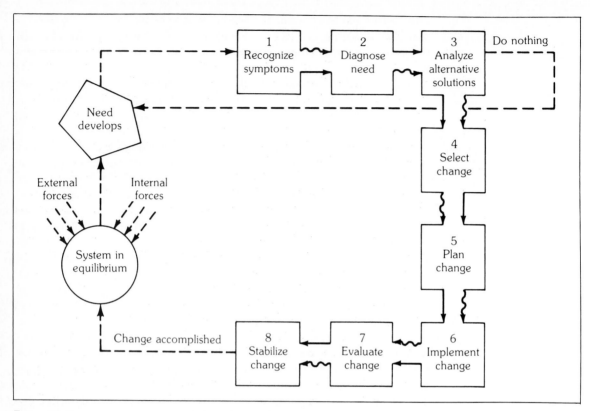

Figure 22-4
Planned change model. The change agent (solid line) and the client system
(wavy line) must work together to effect change.

symptoms and discover that some of the parents have trouble talking to their teenagers, others wonder if their children's behavior is normal, a few question how strictly they should set limits, and still others are not certain about how to handle punishment. These symptoms are pieces of evidence that we will diagnose in the next step. It is an assessment phase. Before moving on, however, we need to ask ourselves as change agents what our motives are for pursuing this change. Inappropriate motives, such as wanting to be needed, can cloud judgment and interfere with effective management of change.

Step 2: Diagnose the Need

Diagnosis means to analyze the symptoms and reach a conclusion about what, if anything, needs changing. First, describe the situation as it is now (the real) and compare it to the way it should be (the ideal). For example, you may notice a great deal of loud arguing and conflict among members of a client family. Although your ideal may be quiet harmony, noisy conflict may be normal, functional behavior for this family. In that case, there is no discrepancy between the real and the ideal and therefore no need for change. If, however, there is a discrepancy between the real and the ideal, then a need exists and a change effort is justified (Hersey and Blanchard, 1988). From speaking with the parents, we recognize that their behavior and concerns indicate a possible lack of information about and confidence in the parenting role. A gap clearly exists between their present and ideal situations; therefore, there is a need.

Next, determine the exact nature and cause of the need. Gathering data by means such as questioning clients, checking the literature, or seeking consultation is important for making a more accurate diagnosis (Porter, 1987). We question the parents in more detail about the difficulties they are having with their children. How do they feel about being parents? What are the most difficult aspects of parenting for them? Have they read any books or used any other resources to help them in their parenting activities? To whom do they talk (if anyone) about parenting problems? When they have a problem handling the raising of their children, how do they usually solve it? We also seek secondary data by checking the literature ourselves to determine the most effective approaches to solving parenting problems. We consult an expert on family life to get ideas about what this group of parents might need, given the symptoms we have seen. We need to come to a conclusion about what specific changes are needed for these parents. Unless the diagnosis is made accurately, the entire change effort may be addressing its attention to the wrong problem. Also, when possible, the client system should help diagnose. We ask the parents to help us determine exactly what it is that they need.

Finally, we must narrow the findings down to a single diagnostic statement that also includes the cause. The parents, we discover after data collection, are insecure in their parenting roles. They believe the insecurity is caused partially by lack of knowledge about how to carry out parental responsibilities. Primarily, however, they are convinced that the cause is lack of a supportive reference group. Most of them live some distance from relatives or no longer maintain close ties with relatives. Our diagnosis for these parents is insecurity in the parenting role. We define the cause to be lack of support as well as some lack of knowledge.

Step 3: Analyze Alternative Solutions

Once we know the diagnosis and its cause, we are ready to identify solutions or various alternative directions to follow. Like the physician who has studied the patient's symptoms and diagnosed the patient as having a duodenal ulcer, we must next decide what general treatment direction to follow. Should it be surgery, diet, medication therapy, or a life-style change approach? At this point the physician does not decide on a specific treatment regimen. That step comes later. Brainstorming is helpful at this point, and the client system should be involved as much as possible in the process. Make a list of all the reasonable broad alternatives, and then analyze them thoroughly to determine the advantages, disadvantages, possible consequences, and risks involved in each. For the parents, we could consider general alternatives such as family counseling, a support group, or education in family life. Each of these alternatives has some advantages and disadvantages toward meeting the parents' need for confidence in their roles.

Next, we analyze each alternative. For example, the counseling solution could provide insight and awareness into family behavior. It would give family members opportunities to express feelings and gain understanding of how other members feel. However, it would not provide a frame of reference that they could use to compare their own parenting behaviors with other acceptable ones, nor would it provide adult peer support for the parents. The consequences of this alternative would most likely be to promote parents' self-understanding and better family communication. Risks would include the possibility that children, especially teenagers, might not be willing to participate and that parents might not gain self-confidence in their roles. We study each alternative to determine its usefulness and feasibility. We also go to the literature again and to other resources, such as consultants, to learn all we can about the best ways to meet the parents' need for change.

Step 4: Select the Change

Having carefully analyzed all the alternatives, we now select the best solution. The parents agree with us that the best solution seems to be a parenting support group. We reexamine the risks involved in the change choice; sometimes a possible course of action may be too costly in time, money, or potential for failure. Also, there may be ways to reduce the risks.

It is important to know what the change is aiming to accomplish; we need a clearly stated goal. For the parenting group, our mutually agreed-upon goal is to provide a supportive, reinforcing climate while increasing members' parenting skills.

Step 5: Plan the Change

This step is at the heart of planned change because it is now that the change agent prepares the design, the blueprint that guides the change action. In steps 1 through 4, data are gathered, a diagnosis made, resources assessed, and a goal established, all preparatory actions for planning the change. The plan tells the change agent and client system how to meet that goal. Preferably they develop the plan together.

We talk with the parents about ways to meet their goal, considering such possibilities as weekly discussion groups on selected topics, monthly meetings with an informed speaker, or reading books and articles on parenting with regular sessions to discuss their application. After analysis and discussion, we decide to meet one evening a month, rotating the location between members' homes. Group sessions will include a variety of approaches: a speaker will be invited every three months; a book or article discussion will be held quarterly; and the remaining meetings will be spent on topics of the group's choice. All sessions will provide opportunities for parents to discuss their concerns or problems. We design this plan around a set of objectives.

The most important activity in planning is to have clear, specific objectives. They should be measurable and, preferably, stated as outcomes. For example, the objective, "By the end of the second session, each parent in the group will have participated in the discussion at least once," is measurable and describes an outcome. Make a list of activities to help you accomplish each objective, and develop a time plan. It is also important to assess the potential costs in terms of time, money, and number of people and materials needed, and to determine the resources available. Design the evaluation plan, and start a list of ways to stabilize (refreeze) the change. During planning, it is useful to perform a force field analysis (Hersey and Blanchard, 1988), a technique developed by Kurt Lewin (1947) for examining all the positive and negative forces in a change situation.

In any situation, there are both driving and restraining forces that influence change. Driving forces push for change. Examples might be clients' desire to be healthier, more productive, or have a safe environment. These are influencing forces in favor of change. Restraining forces, such as apathy, fear of something new, or hostility, work against change, decreasing its possibility. When the strength of the driving forces is equal to the strength of the restraining forces, equilibrium exists. To introduce a change and move the client system to a higher level, that balance must be altered. To do so, the change agent either increases the driving forces, decreases the restraining forces, or both. Force field analysis is a technique that the change agent utilizes to study both sets of forces and to develop strategies to influence them in favor of the change (see Figure 22-5).

The procedure for conducting a force field analysis follows a few simple steps. As change agent, you may conduct it alone, but preferably, you will consult your clients, a change-planning resource group, such as your nursing team, or both. The steps for force field analysis are given below:

1. Brainstorm to produce a list of all driving and restraining forces. (For the parenting group, one driving force is the parents' desire to be better parents; a restraining force might be lack of group agreement on discussion topics.)
2. Estimate the strength of each force.
3. Plot the forces on a chart such as the one shown in Figure 22-5.
4. Note the most important forces; then research and analyze them.
5. List and document possible responses or action steps that might strengthen each important driving force or weaken each important restraining force.

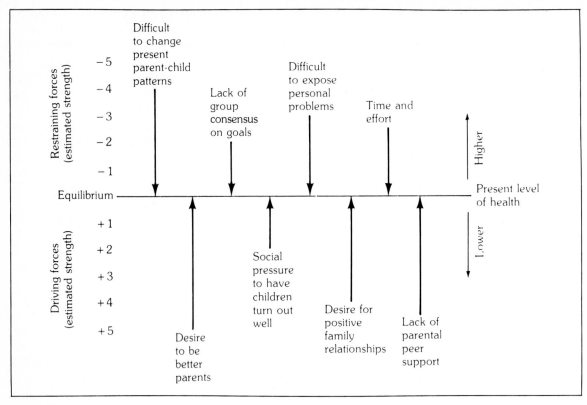

Figure 22-5
Analysis of restraining and driving forces.

Finally, as a consideration in planning the change and in analyzing the driving and restraining forces, study the social network and interaction of the system involved in the change. The change agent needs to be aware of formal and informal leaders, cliques within larger groups, influential persons, the grapevine, and all the other possible social network influences on the change process. For instance, one nurse attempting to change the infant-feeding practices of a young mother failed to consider the strong influence of the grandmother living next door. Another nurse was making no headway with a group of teenage drug addicts until she discovered that their real leader was one of the boys who always sat in the back, not the "captain" appointed by the center director.

Step 6: Implement the Change

The implementation step involves enacting the change plan. Because their objectives and activities have been clearly defined, change agent and client system know exactly what needs to be done and now proceed to do it. The parenting group and their nurse–change agent, for instance, can start the discussion sessions because they know what they want to accomplish and how to go about it. The change plan tells them where they will meet, how often, what they will discuss, and who will be involved. As they move through implementation, they will also know when their objectives have been met and will have a ready-made plan for evaluation and stabilization of the change, once it has been completed.

At the start of implementation, it is important to make certain that all persons concerned are prepared for the change. When working with a family, for example, the nurse may do most of the planning with one or two key members. Do the other family members, who will also be affected by the proposed change, know what to expect? Do they understand the meaning of the change and what will be required of them in adapting to it? An unprepared client system, especially in a large group or organization, may often spell disaster (Kanter, 1985); no matter how well a change effort is planned, people who are unprepared for it may resist it strongly and render it useless.

In some instances, such as introduction of a mass immunization program or a new clinic procedure, it is helpful to do a pilot study. The study is done to try out the change on a small scale, iron out the problems, and revise the change before implementing it into the whole system. One advantage of a pilot study is that it demonstrates to the client system how the change will work on a scale that is small enough not to require any major adaptation or pose any serious threats to present security. It gives people time to adjust their thinking and to discover that the change may not be so bad after all. It is another way of introducing evolutionary change.

Step 7: Evaluate the Change

The success of this step also depends on how well the change is planned. Well-written objectives with specific criteria for their measurement will make the evaluation step much simpler. However, evaluation does not end with saying whether or not the objectives were met. Each objective requires analysis: (1) Was it met? (2) What evidence (documentation) shows that it was met? and (3) Were the best means used to accomplish it, or would some other method have been better? The objective mentioned earlier for the parenting group could be evaluated by saying, yes, it was met. The fact that every person had entered into the discussion by the end of the second session, a point noted by the nurse leader, would be evidence that the objective was met. However, the method used to encourage participation might have been to call on individuals who were not contributing, thus in a sense coercing them into participation. A better method would have been to suggest that some individuals seem more involved than others and that the more active ones might like to solicit ideas from those who had not had an opportunity to speak. Finally, considering the evaluation, the change agent makes needed modifications in the change before stabilization.

Step 8: Stabilize the Change

The final step in the planned change process requires taking measures to reinforce and maintain the change (Figure 22-6). A well-developed change plan includes a design for stabilization. The change agent actively encourages continued use of the innovation by establishing two-way communication; thus any future resistance can be overcome, and the client's full commitment to the change can be maintained (Noone, 1987). Stabilization occurs through soliciting reactions from the client system. Do the clients perceive any potential problems? Do they have doubts? Reinforcing the desired behavior and following up on the change as long as necessary will help assure its permanence. Alcoholics Anonymous, for example, stabilizes the change to non-

Figure 22-6
Positive health behaviors, such as these joggers' regular exercise, must be maintained and reinforced for change to be stabilized and health goals achieved.

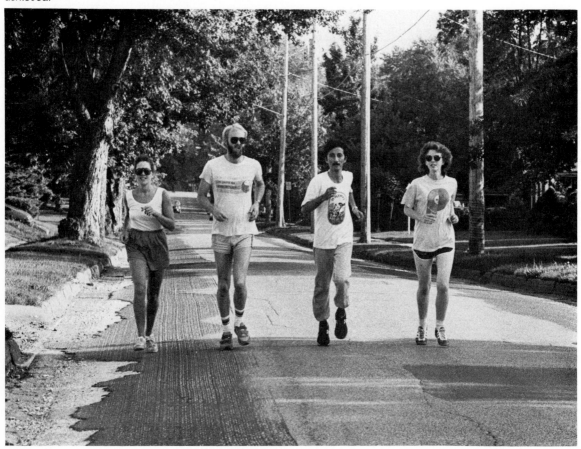

drinking by providing a regular support group that reinforces the nondrinking pattern. The group rewards compliance with praise and replaces drinking with other satisfying experiences, such as social acceptance, to keep the alcoholic from returning to the old behavior. We stabilize our parenting group's changed behavior by calling attention to their increased confidence in their parenting roles and by pointing out the greater number of successes they are having in coping with their children. The group itself decides to give a "Parent of the Month" plaque to the member who demonstrates the most growth in his or her parenting skills. The members also agree to nominate one member as "Parent of the Year" in the community newspaper contest. When stabilization occurs, the system achieves a new equilibrium (see Figure 22-5), and the change agent–client system relationship, at least for this particular change effort, can be terminated.

We have viewed the planned change process primarily in the context of introducing change to smaller aggregates. Community health nurses also utilize these eight steps when managing change at the organization, population group, community, and larger aggregate levels. For example, a nurse may suspect that there is a widespread lack of confidence among young parents. This hypothesis could be tested through an epidemiologic survey to determine parenting needs among the entire community's population of young parents. If symptoms are present (step 1), the nurse, in collaboration with health department personnel or other appropriate professionals, could analyze the symptoms and reach a diagnosis (step 2), perhaps that a large percentage of young parents in the community are lacking in confidence and knowledge of parenting skills. Several approaches to meeting this need could be considered, such as instituting a parenting center in the community with satellite clinics; organizing churches, clubs, or both to sponsor parenting support groups; or working through the community college system to hold workshops and classes on parenting skills (step 3). The most feasible and useful alternative could be selected (step 4), and a parenting program for the community planned (step 5) and implemented (step 6). The nurse, with the other professionals involved, would then evaluate the outcomes (step 7) and make any necessary adjustments in the parenting program before finally stabilizing it (step 8), making certain that this change, undertaken to meet a population group need, remained an established and effectively functioning service.

PLANNED CHANGE STRATEGIES

The literature describes three general change strategies (Bennis, Benne, and Chin, 1985; Haffer, 1986; Zaltman and Duncan, 1977). In any given situation, the change agent may use one or a combination of these strategies to effect a change (Haffer, 1986). They are (1) empirical-rational, (2) normative-reeducative, and (3) power-coercive.

Empirical-Rational

This set of strategies assumes that men and women are rational. When presented with empirical data, people will adopt a new practice because it appears to be in their own best interest. To use this approach, which is common in community health, one simply offers or makes new information available to clients. For instance, most family planning programs use empirical-rational strategies (Fischman, 1973). Clients are given basic information on reproductive anatomy and physiology, and they are told about the benefits of contraception with an explanation of a variety of birth control methods. Health workers hope that once clients have this information, they will adopt some form of birth control. Some clients respond well to this approach, while others do not. The difference lies in client ability and interest in self-help. The nurse–change agent uses empirical-rational strategies with clients who can assume a relatively high degree of responsibility for their own health. In some respects, this set of strategies parallels the participative leadership style, described in Figure 22-2, that fosters maximum client autonomy.

Normative-Reeducative

A second set of change strategies goes beyond merely informing to actively influencing the client system. This approach assumes that attitudes and practices are determined by cultural norms; thus knowledge is necessary but not enough to change behavior (Chin and Benne, 1985). Nurse–change agents who use this set of strategies seek to modify the normative orientations of clients through reeducation (Figure 22-7). They directly influence clients' values, attitudes, skills, and relationships as well as offer new information (Ryan, 1987). This approach attempts to strengthen client self-understanding, self-control, and commitment to new patterns through direct persuasion or manipulation. For example, a health-teaching program that aims to increase safety practices in an industrial setting will, if employing normative-reeducative strategies, not only provide safety information such as posters and warning signs but also use persuasive tactics such as individual rewards for safe practices, division recognition for minimum number of accidents, or discipline for noncompliance. Nurses use normative-reeducative strategies with clients who have a measure of self-care skill but, at the same time, need external assistance to effect lasting behavioral change. This type of client is found in teaching, counseling, and therapy situations.

Power-Coercive

The third set of change strategies uses power to effect change. Change agents may derive power from the *law* (such as health regulations or administrative policies), from *position* (such as political, social, or managerial positions),

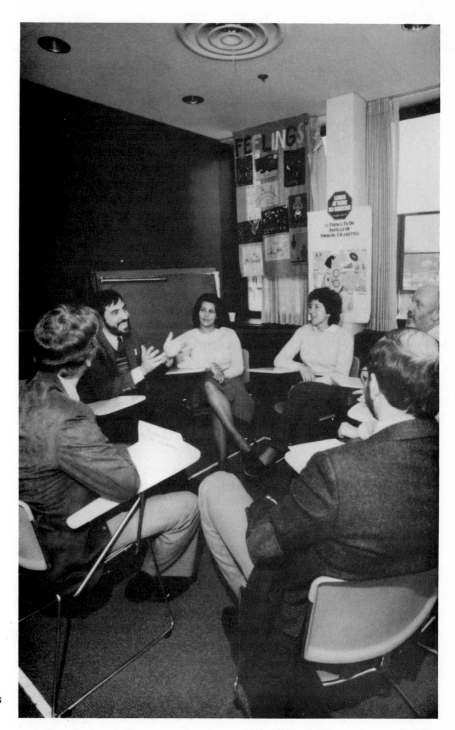

Figure 22-7
*Normative-reeducative
strategies produce
behavioral change by
seeking to influence clients'
values and norms, as in this
"stop smoking" seminar.*

from a *group* (such as a social, work, or professional group), or from *personal power* (such as personal magnetism, competence, or respect of followers) (Gorman et al., 1986). They use this power to coerce change; the result is more or less forced compliance by the client system. Some situations, particularly those that are life-threatening, may require power-coercive strategies. In community health practice, power-coercive strategies may be used with people who cannot help themselves or in situations that threaten the public's health. If officials find a restaurant in violation of health codes, for example, they will most likely require forced compliance or close down the restaurant. Occasionally clients cannot exercise responsibility, perhaps because they are experiencing temporary physical or psychological incapacitation caused, for example, by severe illness or family abuse. In such cases, the nurse may need to use power to effect changes that are in the clients' best interests. Although power-coercive strategies are appropriate in some situations, they should be used with caution because they can rob clients of opportunities to grow in autonomy and capacity for self-care.

Planned change strategies may be combined; for instance, a normative-reeducative approach might have a power backup. We see this combination in programs that, for example, educate and persuade groups of people to be immunized against an impending epidemic or to keep their garbage contained to avoid insect and rodent infestation. Behind this normative-reeducative strategy is an implied power threat of official disapproval, or worse, for noncompliance.

The effectiveness of a change strategy, then, varies with each situation and particularly with the degree of client capacity for self-care. As in the approach to leadership styles discussed earlier in the chapter, the nurse–change agent adapts strategies to fit each change situation.

PRINCIPLES FOR MANAGING CHANGE

Community health nurses introduce change every day that they practice. Every effort to solve a problem, prevent another from occurring, meet a potential community need, or promote optimal client health requires changes. To make these changes truly successful so that desired outcomes are reached, they must be managed well. We shall examine six principles that provide some guidelines for effective management of change.

Involve Persons Affected by the Proposed Change

Persons affected by a proposed change should participate as much as possible in every step of the planned change process (Nicoll, 1986). This involvement is important for several reasons. Collaboration with those who have a vested interest in the change can produce a wealth of ideas and insights that can greatly improve the change plan. Furthermore, such participation can help remove obstacles and reduce resistance. Participation ensures a greater likelihood that the change will be accepted and maintained (Kanter, 1985). One nurse, for instance, when planning for a grandmother's care, involved all the family members, including the grandmother; as a result, she automatically secured their support and cooperation, gained many helpful suggestions that she herself had not considered, and discovered that the grandmother was happier and more responsive to care because the change plan was specifically tailored to her needs.

Be Prepared for Resistance to Change

Because all systems instinctively preserve the status quo, the change agent can expect people to resist change (Fritz, 1986). The homeostatic mechanism operating in any system seeks to maintain equilibrium; change poses a threat to that stability and security. Furthermore, all systems experience inertia; that is, they resist beginning movement. People do not undertake a change until they are convinced of its worth. Resistance may also come from a conflict over goals and methods or from misunderstanding about what the change will mean and require. Involving clients in the planned change process, discussed in the last section, is one way to overcome resistance. Another way is establishing and maintaining open lines of communication in order to make ideas clearly understood and to resolve disagreements quickly. Prepare people thoroughly for the change, provide support and patience during the change process, and encourage response and expression of feelings.

Introduce Change at the Proper Time

The Bible says, that for everything there is a time and a season. Sometimes a change, even a well-designed and much needed one, must be postponed because the present is not the right time to introduce it. The client system may now be experiencing too many other changes to handle the stress of another change. Other projects or activities in which the client system is currently engaged may compete for energy and other resources, depleting those needed to make the proposed change successful. For example, some young mothers, eager to start a book club that focused on discussion of child rearing, had to postpone the project because Christmas was approaching. Shopping, entertaining, and vacations made it impossible to give the kind of time and energy needed to make the book club effective.

Proper timing is as important to a planned change as proper seed planting is to a good harvest. The change idea must be appropriate, the change recipient prepared, the climate right, and the resources available before the change can be fostered to grow into full maturity and usefulness (Cobb-McMahon et al., 1984).

View Change in Terms of Potential Impact on Systems or Subsystems

Every system has many subsystems that are intricately related to and interdependent upon one another. A change in one part of a system affects its other parts, and a change in one system may affect other systems (Chin, 1980). A county community nursing agency made a change in its use of home health aides. Because many homebound clients needed more care than the agency staff could provide, the agency contracted with a private home-care service for extra home health aides. These paraprofessionals worked in the homes of agency clients, supplementing the care given by agency staff. The private company preferred to supervise its own aides, whereas the county agency had a policy of using community health nurses to supervise aides. The county agency was legally responsible and professionally accountable for the quality of care given to clients. The private company wanted to retain control of its workers. The matter was resolved by contracting with another private service. The change, however, had affected the roles of nurses and aides within the system as well as the relationships between the two systems.

This principle reminds the nurse that change does not take place in a vacuum. When workers learn new health and safety practices associated with their jobs, their relationships with each other and with their bosses and their overall productivity in the organization may easily be affected. One must anticipate and prepare for the impact of the proposed change on the clients involved, other persons, departments, organizations, or even geographic areas.

Be Flexible

Unexpected events can occur in every situation. This fifth principle emphasizes two points; first, you need to be able to adapt to unexpected events and make the most of them. Perseverance and flexibility are the marks of a good change manager. One community health nurse had tried unsuccessfully to contact a young mother who was reportedly abusing her two-year-old son. After several phone calls and visits to an empty house, she finally found the mother at home but accompanied by a neighbor who insisted on staying for the entire visit. At first the nurse was angry that the neighbor was interfering with her goal of getting to know the mother. Then she realized that this situation offered an opportunity to learn more about the mother through an acquaintance's eyes and possibly to influence another client as well. She included them both in the discussion, explained what she had to offer in terms of health teaching and support, and eventually won their combined respect and confidence.

The second point to remember about flexibility is that a good change planner anticipates possible blocks or problems by preparing strategies and alternate plans. During step 3 of the planned change process, it is helpful to rank the alternative solutions considered. Then, if the first choice does not work out for some reason, a second alternative is ready to be put into action. Flexibility involves a willingness to consider a variety of options and suggestions from many sources (Haffer, 1986).

Know Yourself

Self-understanding is essential for an effective change agent (Hersey and Blanchard, 1988). As a leader and change agent, how do you define your role? How do others see it? What are your values and motives in relation to each change that you might ask clients to make? What is your personality like and how will it affect the change process? What is your typical leadership style, the one that you most often revert to when not consciously adapting it to the situation? The answers to these questions about yourself will give you much insight into personal behaviors that you may wish to alter in order to be a more effective leader and change agent.

Summary

Community health nurses, at every level of practice, are leaders and change agents. They influence individuals and families to adopt healthier behaviors. They lead groups of people to change their health practices. Formally or informally, they act as leaders to bring about organizational change. At the community level, they are involved in changing people's health beliefs and practices and in promoting organized responses to community health problems.

Leadership is an interpersonal process in which one person influences the activities of another person or group of persons toward accomplishment of a goal in a specific situation. It has three major characteristics. First, it is purposeful; it always has a goal. Second, it is interpersonal; it always involves a social transaction. Third, it means influencing; it always affects other people by altering their beliefs and practices in some manner. Community health nursing leadership aims to influence people toward optimal health as well as upgrade professional nursing practice.

Effective leadership incorporates five essential functions. Exercising the *creative function,* the leader generates ideas and develops innovative plans for action. With the *initiating function,* the leader introduces changes and sets their processes in motion. Good leaders take calculated risks, evidence of the *risk-taking function.* They use the *integrative function* to strengthen the ties among their followers and unite them through a strong sense of purpose. Finally, with the *instrumental function,* effective leaders facilitate the movement of followers in the right direction. Community health nurses utilize these leadership functions in the context of ever-widening spheres of potential influence. They influence consumers; other nurses; health service organizations; other professionals; resources and programs affecting health; and state, regional, national, and even international programs and organizations.

Leadership styles have been studied for many years. The original view that some individuals are born with leadership qualities has been refuted. More recent research supports the fact that leaders' behavior, rather than their personalities, determines their effectiveness. From this research we have drawn three styles of leadership. *Autocratic* leadership is authoritative; orders are given that people are expected to follow. *Participative* leadership is democratic and involves followers in the decision-making process. This style tends to promote followers' self-esteem and to increase their productivity. *Laissez-faire* leadership gives followers complete freedom of choice; they are essentially independent of the leader. Some would argue that this style is not a form of leadership at all.

Leadership encompasses two important dimensions: a concern for accomplishing goals and a concern for relationships with people. The different leadership styles emphasize these dimensions to varying degrees. An autocratic style tends to be task-oriented, while a democratic style tends to be relationship-oriented. Situational leadership integrates both task and relationships by emphasizing one or the other depending upon the situation. This more recent leadership approach has evolved as the most effective because it tailors to each situation the style of leadership one should use.

Change is an outcome of leadership. Our job in community health nursing is to effect change by preventing illness and promoting health. Change, however, is disruptive. Evolutionary change is gradual and requires adjustment on an incremental basis. We introduce this kind of change in many situations. Revolutionary change tends to occur suddenly and is more drastic. It may be necessary to introduce revolutionary change under certain conditions, such as an emergency.

Change occurs in three major stages. First, there is *unfreezing*. It is during this stage that the need for change develops. People become receptive. *Moving*, the second stage, occurs when people accept and try out the innovation. The third stage, *refreezing*, involves maintaining the change as an accepted, established part of the system.

Planned change is a purposeful, designed effort to effect improvement in a system with the assistance of a change agent. It involves a process of eight steps that nurses can follow to manage change:

1. Recognize the symptoms that indicate a need for change.
2. Diagnose the need by analyzing the symptoms and reaching a conclusion about what needs changing.
3. Analyze alternative solutions by first identifying a variety of possible general directions to pursue and then analyzing each of these possibilities in relation to their advantages, disadvantages, and possible outcomes and risks.

4. Select the change alternative that is most feasible and most likely to meet the identified need. Decide on the goal for this change project.
5. Plan the change by developing specific objectives and a set of activities to meet the stated goal. Force field analysis is a useful tool to facilitate change planning.
6. Implement the change by enacting the change plan, making certain that the client system is properly prepared.
7. Evaluate the change, measuring its outcomes and making needed adjustments.
8. Stabilize the change, instituting measures to reinforce and maintain (refreeze) the change.

During planned change, we can use one or a combination of three major strategies. *Empirical-rational* strategies provide basic information and assume that people are rational and will act on this new knowledge because to do so serves their own best interest. *Normative-reeducative* strategies not only give information but also directly influence people to change. *Power-coercive* strategies use power to force change.

Six principles provide community health nurses with guidelines for managing change:

1. Involve the persons affected by the proposed change.
2. Be prepared for resistance to change.
3. Introduce change at the proper time.
4. View any change in terms of its potential impact on systems or subsystems.
5. Be flexible.
6. Know yourself.

Study Questions

You have been asked to chair an ad hoc committee in a community health nursing agency. The committee's task is to plan a health fair for the local community.

1. Discuss how you would exercise each of the five leadership functions as you chaired the planning committee.
2. What would your leadership style be and how would you know whether it was appropriate for this situation?
3. What strategies would you use to ensure that the health fair was viewed by community members as an evolutionary change?
4. Six principles for managing change were presented in this chapter. Briefly discuss how you would use each one as you and your committee developed the health fair.

References

Adams, J. D. (ed.). (1986). *Transforming leadership: From vision to results.* Alexandria, Va.: Miles River Press.

Argyris, C. (1976). *Increasing leadership effectiveness.* New York: Wiley.

Bennis, W. G., K. D. Benne, and R. Chin. (1985). *The planning of change.* 4th ed. New York: Holt, Rinehart and Winston.

Bernhard, L., and M. Walsh. (1981). *Leadership—The key to the professionalization of nursing.* New York: McGraw-Hill.

Chait, R. (1988). What makes a leader in higher education? *Journal of Professional Nursing* 4(3): 223–29.

Chin, R. (1980). The utility of system models and developmental models for practitioners. In J. Riehl and S. Roy (eds.), *Conceptual models for nursing practice.* 2nd ed. New York: Appleton-Century-Crofts.

Chin, R., and D. Benne. (1985). General strategies for effecting changes in human systems. In W. G. Bennis, K. D. Benne, and R. Chin (eds.), *The planning of change.* 4th ed. New York: Holt, Rinehart and Winston.

Cobb-McMahon, B., D. Williams, and J. Davis. (1984). Changing health behavior of community health clients. *Journal of Community Health Nursing* 1(1): 27–31.

Fischman, S. (1973). Change strategies and their application to family planning programs. *American Journal of Nursing* 73: 1771.

Flynn, B., et al. (1987). Preparation of community health nursing leaders for social action. *International Journal of Nursing Studies* 24(3): 239–48.

Fritz, R. (1986). The leader as creator. In J. D. Adams (ed.), *Transforming leadership.* Alexandria, Va.: Miles River Press.

Gerlach, L., and V. Hine. (1973). *Lifeway leap: The dynamics of change in America.* Minneapolis: University of Minnesota Press.

Gorman, S., et al. (1986). Power and effective nursing practice. *Nursing Outlook* 34(3): 129–34.

Guidera, M., et al. (1988). Working with people: In defense of followership. *American Journal of Nursing* 88(7): 1017.

Haffer, A. (1986). Facilitating change: Choosing the appropriate strategy. *Journal of Nursing Administration* 16(4): 18–22.

Harman, W. (1986). Transformed leadership: Two contrasting concepts. In J. D. Adams (ed.), *Transforming leadership.* Alexandria, Va.: Miles River Press.

Hennes, K., Sr. (1979). *Expansion of the aide's role in home care.* Unpublished manuscript. University of Minnesota, Minneapolis.

Henry, B., et al. (1987). Language, leadership, and power . . . research-based theories of language in organizations. *Journal of Nursing Administration* 17(1): 19–25.

Hersey, P., and K. Blanchard. (1988). *Management of organizational behavior: Utilizing human resources.* 5th ed. Englewood Cliffs, N.J.: Prentice-Hall.

Kanter, R. M. (1985). *The change masters.* New York: Simon and Schuster.

Kinsman, F. (1986). Leadership from alongside. In J. D. Adams (ed.), *Transforming leadership.* Alexandria, Va.: Miles River Press.

Kouzes, J., and B. Posner. (1987). *The leadership challenge: How to get extraordinary things done in organizations.* San Francisco: Jossey-Bass Publishers.

Lee, J. L. (1987). Leadership in practice. *Imprint* 34(6): 57–58, 61.

Lewin, K. (1947). Frontiers in group dynamics: Concept, method, and reality in social science; social equilibria and social change. *Human Relations* 1: 5.

Lippitt, G. L. (1973). *Visualizing change: Model building and the change process.* La Jolla, Calif.: University Associates.

Lippitt, R., J. Watson, and B. Westley. (1958). *The dynamics of planned change.* New York: Harcourt, Brace & World.

Moloney, M. (1979). *Leadership in nursing: Theory, strategies, action.* St. Louis: C. V. Mosby.

Nicoll, D. (1986). Leadership and followship. In J. D. Adams (ed.), *Transforming leadership.* Alexandria, Va.: Miles River Press.

Noone, J. (1987). Planned change: Putting theory into practice...utilizing Lippitt's theory. *Clinical Nurse Specialist* 1(1): 25–29.

Nordstrom, R., et al. (1987). Cultural change versus behavioral change. *Health Care Management Review* 12(2): 43–49.

Porter, E. J. (1987). Administrative diagnosis — Implications for the public's health... community nurse-administrators...diagnostic decisions that have preceded service change. *Public Health Nursing* 4(4): 247–56.

Rantz, M., et al. (1987). Change theory: A framework for implementing nursing diagnoses in a long-term-care setting. *Nursing Clinics of North America* 22(4): 887–97.

Ryan, P. (1987). Strategies for motivating life-style change. *Journal of Cardiovascular Nursing* 1(4): 54–66.

Spradley, B. (1980). Managing change creatively. *Journal of Nursing Administration* 10(5): 32–37.

Spradley, J., and D. McCurdy. (1980). *Anthropology: The cultural perspective.* 2nd ed. New York: Wiley.

Uris, A. (1964). *Techniques of leadership.* New York: McGraw-Hill.

Williams, C. A. (1981). Nursing leadership in community health: A neglected issue. In J. McCloskey and H. Grace (eds.), *Current issues in nursing.* Boston: Blackwell Scientific Publications.

Zaltman, G., and R. Duncan. (1977). *Strategies for planned change.* New York: Wiley.

Selected Readings

Adams, J. D. (ed.). (1984). *Transforming work: A collection of organizational transformation readings.* Alexandria, Va.: Miles River Press.

Adams, J. D. (ed.). (1986). *Transforming leadership: From vision to results.* Alexandria, Va.: Miles River Press.

Aspree, E. S. (1975). The process of change. *Supervisor Nurse* 6(10): 5–24.

Bennis, W. G., K. D. Benne, and R. Chin. (eds.). (1985). *The planning of change.* 4th ed. New York: Holt, Rinehart and Winston.

Bernhard, L., and M. Walsh. (1981). *Leadership — The key to the professionalization of nursing.* New York: McGraw-Hill.

Brooten, D., L. Hayman, and M. Naylor. (1978). Leadership for change: A guide for the frustrated nurse. *American Journal of Nursing* 78: 1526–29.

Brooten, D., L. Hayman, and M. Naylor. (1978). *Leadership for change: A guide for the frustrated nurse.* Philadelphia: J. B. Lippincott.

Burns, J. M. (1978). *Leadership.* New York: Harper & Row.

Castledine, G. (1985). Change: Crucial to the future of nursing practice. *Nursing Practice* 1(2): 76–79.

Chait, R. (1988). What makes a leader in higher education? *Journal of Professional Nursing* 4(3): 223–29.

Chin, R., and D. Benne. (1985). General strategies for effecting changes in human systems. In W. G. Bennis, K. D. Benne, and R. Chin (eds.), *The planning of change* 4th ed. New York: Holt, Rinehart and Winston.

Cobb-McMahon, B., D. Williams, and J. Davis. (1984). Changing health behavior of community health clients. *Journal of Community Health Nursing* 1(1): 27–31.

Conway, M. E. (1978). Clinical research: Instrument for change. *Journal of Nursing Administration* 8(12): 27–32.

Council of Community Health Nurses. (1986). *Community-based nursing services: Innovative models.* ANA Publication No. CH-13: 1–91.

Deal, J. (1977). The timing of change. *Supervising Nurse* 8(9): 73–79.

Flynn, B., et al. (1987). Preparation of community health nursing leaders for social action. *International Journal of Nursing Studies* 24(3): 239–48.

Fritz, R. (1986). The leader as creator. In J. D. Adams (ed.), *Transforming leadership.* Alexandria, Va.: Miles River Press.

Gorman, S., et al. (1986). Power and effective nursing practice. *Nursing Outlook* 34(3): 129–34.

Grissum, M. (1976). How you can become a risk taker and a role breaker. *Nursing '76* 6(11): 89–98.

Guest, R., P. Hersey, and K. Blanchard. (1977). *Organizational change through effective leadership.* Englewood Cliffs, N.J.: Prentice-Hall.

Guidera, M., et al. (1988). Working with people: In defense of followership. *American Journal of Nursing* 88(7): 1017.

Haffer, A. (1986). Facilitating change: Choosing the appropriate strategy. *Journal of Nursing Administration* 16(4): 18–22.

Harman, W. (1986). Transformed leadership: Two contrasting concepts. In J. D. Adams (ed.), *Transforming leadership.* Alexandria, Va.: Miles River Press.

Harvey, E. B. (1988). Change. *Kansas Nurse* 63(4): 6–7.

Hein, E. and M. J. Nicholson. (1982). *Contemporary leadership behavior: Selected readings.* Boston: Little, Brown.

Henry, B., et al. (1987). Language, leadership, and power... research-based theories of language in organizations. *Journal of Nursing Administration* 17(1): 19–25.

Hersey, P., and K. Blanchard. (1988). *Management of organizational behavior: Utilizing human resources* 5th ed. Englewood Cliffs, N.J.: Prentice-Hall.

Horsley, J. A. (1986). Factors associated with innovation in nursing practice. *Family and Community Health* 9(1): 1–11.

Kanter, R. M. (1985). *The change masters.* New York: Simon and Schuster.

Kinsman, F. (1986). Leadership from alongside. In J. D. Adams (ed.), *Transforming Leadership.* Alexandria, Va.: Miles River Press.

Kouzes, J., and B. Posner. (1987). *The leadership challenge: How to get extraordinary things done in organizations.* San Francisco: Jossey-Bass Publishers.

Lancaster, J. (1980). An ecological orientation toward change: Considerations for leadership in nursing. *Image* 3(4): 12–15.

Lebsack, C. (1986). Dealing with leadership changes. *Nursing Success Today* 3(12): 32–36.

Lee, J. L. (1987). Leadership in practice. *Imprint* 34(6): 57–58, 61.

Levy, J. A. (1987). Women's leadership status in the American Public Health Association. *American Journal of Public Health* 77(12): 1537–38.

Lippitt, G. L. (1973). *Visualizing change: Model building and the change process.* La Jolla, Calif.: University Associates.

Lippitt, R., J. Watson, and B. Westley. (1958). *The dynamics of planned change.* New York: Harcourt, Brace & World.

McCloskey, J. C., et al. (1987). Leadership in nursing. *Annual Review of Nursing Research* 5: 177–202.

McNally, J. M. (1986). Live as on a mountain — Leadership, the great potential. *Journal of Professional Nursing* 2(6): 380–90.

Moloney, M. (1979). *Leadership in nursing: Theories, strategies, action.* St. Louis: C. V. Mosby.

Muller, H. J., et al. (1988). Women in power: New leadership in health industry. *Health Care for Women International* 9(2): 63–82.

Nicoll, D. (1986). Leadership and followship. In J. D. Adams (ed.), *Transforming leadership.* Alexandria, Va.: Miles River Press.

Noone, J. (1987). Planned change: Putting theory into practice . . . utilizing Lippitt's theory. *Clinical Nurse Specialist* 1(1): 25–29.

Nordstrom, R., et al. (1987). Cultural change versus behavioral change. *Health Care Management Review* 12(2): 43–49.

Olson, J. K., et al. (1988). Learning planned change: A practicum for RN students. *Journal of Nursing Education* 27(4): 178–80.

Porter, E. J. (1987). Administrative diagnosis — Implications for the public's health . . . community nurse-administrators . . . diagnostic decisions that have preceded service change. *Public Health Nursing* 4(4): 247–56.

Powers, D. M. (1986). A new style of nursing leadership. *Canadian Nurse* 82(10): 18–19.

Rantz, M., et al. (1987). Change theory: A framework for implementing nursing diagnoses in a long-term-care setting. *Nursing Clinics of North America* 22(4): 887–97.

Rodgers, J. (1973). Theoretical considerations involved in the process of change. *Nursing Forum* 12: 161–74.

Rogers, E. (1983). *Diffusion of innovations.* 3rd ed. New York: Free Press.

Rothman, J., J. Erlich, and J. Teresa. (1981). *Changing organizations and community programs.* Beverly Hills, Calif.: Sage Publications.

Rothman, J. (1974). *Planning and organizing for social change: Action principles from social science research.* New York: Columbia University Press.

Rubin, I., M. Plovnich, and F. Fry. (1974). Initiating planned change in health care systems. *Journal of Applied Behavioral Science* 10: 107–24.

Ryan, P. (1987). Strategies for motivating life-style change. *Journal of Cardiovascular Nursing* 1(4): 54–66.

Sanders, I. T. (1975). Professional roles in planned change. In R. M. Kramer and H. Specht (eds.), *Readings in community organization practice.* 2nd ed. Englewood Cliffs, N.J.: Prentice-Hall.

Schaller, L. E. (1972). *The change agent: The strategy of innovative leadership.* Nashville, Tenn.: Abingdon.

Spickerman, S., et al. (1988). Use of learning modules to teach nursing leadership concepts. *Journal of Nursing Education* 27(2): 78–82.

Spradley, B. (1980). Managing change creatively. *Journal of Nursing Administration* 10(5): 32–37.

Tough, A. (1985). How adults learn and change. *Diabetes Education* 11: 21–25.

Wakefield-Fisher, M. (1986). Women in administration. *Nursing Success Today* 3(3): 3–8.

Watzlawick, P., J. Weaklund, and R. Fisch. (1974). *Change: Principles of problem formation and problem resolution.* New York: Norton.

Williams, C. A. (1981). Nursing leadership in community health: A neglected issue. In J. McCloskey and H. Grace (eds.), *Current issues in nursing.* Boston: Blackwell Scientific Publications.

Wright, S. G. (1985). Change in nursing: Application of change theory to practice . . . joint appointments. *Nursing Practice* 1(2): 85–91.

Zaltman, G., and R. Duncan. (1977). *Strategies for planned change.* New York: Wiley.

Zimmerman, B. M. (1979). Changes of the second order. *Nursing Outlook* 27: 199–201.

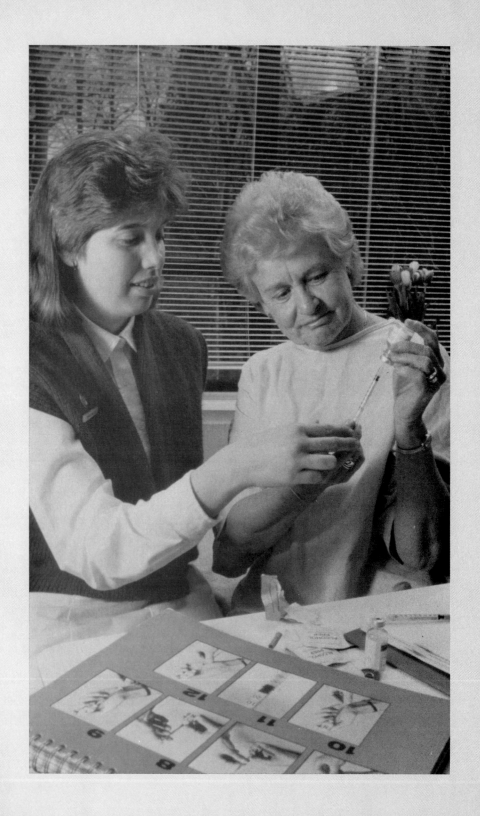

23 Quality Assurance in Community Health Nursing

Pamela J. Thul-Immler

In an era of cost concerns, it is easy to overlook quality. How do we ensure that clients receive high-quality care? For instance, when we design a plan of care for Mrs. Dimitre, who needs post-CVA rehabilitation, how can we be certain that she receives good care? How do we ensure high-quality teaching and learning in the prenatal classes given at our neighborhood center? To assure quality in our practice as community health nurses we need to be familiar with quality assurance and know how to design and implement it in our day-to-day work.

This chapter is intended to introduce the reader to the use of quality assurance in health care, and particularly in community health nursing. Quality assurance is a rapidly growing field, with its own terminology, technology, and applications. At the end of this chapter we include a glossary of terms frequently used in quality assurance.

DEFINITION OF QUALITY ASSURANCE

Quality assurance is a form of health care evaluation. It seeks to assure that sufficient health care services are provided in a timely manner and that the services provided have a high likelihood of improving the health and the perception of health of the recipient(s) of care. (Blum, 1981; Hyman, 1982). These goals are met through a three-pronged process:

1. *Quality assessment* to determine whether the services provided are of high quality.
2. *Problem identification* to locate any specific deficiencies or opportunities to improve the care provided.
3. *Corrective action* to resolve known problems and improve care (JCAHO, 1988; Lalonde, 1987; MDH, 1980).

Many organizations view quality assurance processes as tools that facilitate ongoing self-evaluation and improvement. For-profit industries consider quality control programs essential to their profitability. It is easiest to talk about quality control measures in product-oriented industries, such as the fast-food industry, that have used these processes for decades. In these industries, when a product has been developed, field-tested, and perfected for marketing, it is up to the company's managers to assure that the product is of uniform quality and equally satisfies customers wherever it is sold. The company institutes tight controls on purchasing of ingredients, preparation, handling, and presentation of its product. All of these measures are designed to bring back satisfied customers.

Do we in the health care field know what our customers want, need, and like? Can we identify satisfied consumers of health care services? Often the answer to these questions is no. This leaves us in a situation of not really knowing how to target our services.

We are not naïvely suggesting that studying and instituting tight controls on how specific community health nursing services are delivered will result in satisfied clients or healthier clients. The effects and benefits of health care services are the result of multiple factors; formal health care is only one (Januska, Engle, and Wood, 1976). We are suggesting, however, that it makes sense to make the best use of nursing time and other resources to serve those who will benefit most or who are at greatest risk for illness, injury, or death. When we can demonstrate that various nursing interventions are effective, highly satisfactory, and cost efficient within a given group, these interventions should be consistently chosen over interventions that do not withstand such tests (Palmer, 1983).

Community health nursing deals with individuals, families, and other subgroups within larger populations. Whether in a public health agency, community clinic, health department, school, or other setting, our unique population-focused role carries with it the challenge of sorting out top-priority health care needs from the many competing client needs (White, 1982).

We all know that there are many arenas in community health where the current system of services falls short of effectively meeting the needs of large segments of the population. We frequently see preventable injuries, illnesses, and deaths caused by accidents, chemical abuse, sexually transmitted diseases, domestic violence, and suicide. Deficiencies in health services also appear in the way we manage the needs of those with existing problems, such as adolescent parents, handicapped children, frail elderly, and those entrenched in cycles of poverty and illness.

New and innovative public health programs arise out of the realization by public health practitioners that time-honored methods of addressing such problems may have little current impact on their incidence or prevalence in the specific population at risk. New strategies must be found. Such realizations come out of self-reflection on public health services (Figure 23-1) and, in turn, this reflection requires objective data about those services. The pro-

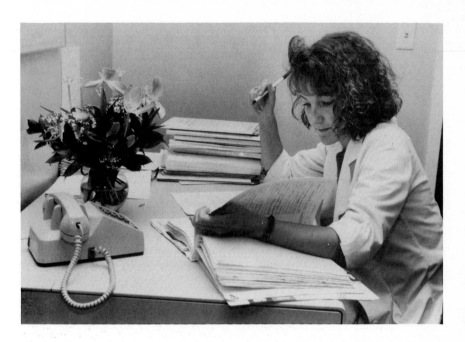

Figure 23-1
Quality assurance efforts
begin with self-reflection
on health service delivery.

cess of quality assurance provides a framework for collecting and evaluating data on an ongoing basis (Januska, Engle, and Wood, 1976).

QUALITY ASSURANCE IN COMMUNITY HEALTH NURSING

Irene, an experienced community health nurse, was preparing to orient a new nurse at her agency. While reviewing the maternal-child health (MCH) component of her job, Irene reflected, "We've always provided MCH services, and I believe we do it well. I know that I am careful in my assessments and the plans that I develop when working with mothers and children. These plans are usually received favorably by my clients, and the results are good for the most part. But do other nurses cover the same issues when they assess and teach? Do I cover all of the important issues with each family? Do we agree as a team of public health nurses what the critical issues are and how to deal with them? Do we know what our clients think about the care they receive?"

Irene began to realize that she didn't have a clear picture of what should be expected of the new nurse in her care of MCH and other clients. She suggested that a group of the experienced nurses at her agency work together to develop some basic guidelines for MCH care that could be used to orient new staff and to evaluate the quality of services provided.

Quality assurance is important to community health work because when we attempt to influence the health of individuals or populations, the limited resources available must be put to the most effective use (Brook and Lohr, 1981). We provide many services to individuals, and we also develop wide-reaching services, such as immunization programs to prevent outbreaks of certain illnesses in the community at large.

It is critical for community health nurses to be able to evaluate the quality of their own nursing process, since this is the area of nursing that is most under the control of nurses (Phaneuf, 1976). By contrast, the structures through which care is given and the particular client outcomes frequently are not as easy for nurses to control. An example is the thrust in the health industry over the last decade to contain costs. Limited health care dollars pose a potent stimulus for change in the delivery of health care services. This trend raises the question of whether we are to be concerned primarily with serving the needs of clients, providers, or purchasers of care such as insurers and employers. It is critical that professions such as nursing be able to define appropriate or inappropriate care and know what constitutes underservice (Harris, Peters, and Yuan, 1987).

While nurses who deliver care directly to clients are not managers as such, quality assurance is largely a "management" activity. Though community health nurses may not be responsible for a staff or agency budget and functioning, they are responsible for managing a caseload of clients with needs of varying degrees of urgency. They must provide priority services within allowable resources that will promote the highest possible level of personal and group functioning and health. Thus, any activities the community health nurse engages in to assure these ends can be called quality assurance activities (Davidson, 1978; O'Grady, 1986).

Some quality assurance activities for community health nurses include prioritizing care needs for a caseload of clients for the day, seeking supervision with skills development or with a difficult case, systematizing charting so that needed documentation is efficiently completed (e.g., using flow sheets to chart MCH visits), proposing better ways to organize care of chronically ill clients, or establishing new agency procedures. All of these actions demonstrate that nurses are reflecting on their work and looking for ways to improve care. Staff meetings and case conferences are common settings for nurses to bring the lessons of their practice to the larger group for examination and potential adoption.

It is the role of nursing administration to develop a formalized quality assurance program for reviewing organizational structure, processes of delivering nursing care, and outcomes of that care. These formal evaluations include nursing peer review audits, client satisfaction assessments, review of agency policies and procedures, analysis of demographic information, and the like (Berman, 1988).

Nurses who are new to formal quality assurance activities need to have positive first experiences with it. We who are trained to provide direct care often view auditing and evaluation as a waste of time that takes us away from the work for which we're best suited. What we miss in this argument is that direct service providers are the best judges of care problems and their potential solutions. It is critical, then, that quality assurance reviews focus on issues relevant to staff concerns and be structured so that they can be accomplished quickly and with minimal effort. The clearer, more concise, and less time-consuming the actual evaluation process is, the more likely staff will be willing to participate (Orlikoff and Snow, 1984). If those who provide health services have an opportunity to examine the care they provide in a systematic manner, they can and will generate useful ideas for improving that care and identifying care issues sooner. They are in the best position to design more efficient and effective services for a widening circle of target populations (Flynn and Ray, 1979).

DIMENSIONS OF QUALITY HEALTH CARE

A major goal of community health nursing is to provide high-quality care to clients. To strive for quality care and then to evaluate it requires a measurable definition of the concept of quality. We can draw from the work of the National Association of Community Health Centers (NACHC), who define a quality community health program as providing

> "...health care that effectively betters the health status and satisfaction of the population within the resources that the individual and society make available for that care" (Benson, 1985; p. 1)

This definition acknowledges that health care resources are limited and that the priorities placed on health by consumers vary.

To further our understanding of quality health care, the NACHC has proposed five dimensions of quality that they believe to be essential in the development and maintenance of quality community health programs. We have added a sixth.

A quality program:

1. addresses all of the interrelated health needs of a whole person or community (*comprehensiveness*);
2. will demonstrate that it can and does affect in a positive manner the health status of not only the individual but also the population (*effectiveness*);
3. can demonstrate a high degree of satisfaction among recipients, not only to services, but also to their resulting health status (*acceptability*);
4. can demonstrate that its services are readily accessible to its population on a timely basis despite the financial, cultural, emotional, and geographic barriers that may be intervening (*accessibility*);

5. will demonstrate that it consistently makes the best use of available resources (*efficiency*) (Benson, 1985);
6. can demonstrate that the system and its providers use the best available knowledge and judgment to contribute to the health and satisfaction of clients (*provider competence*) (Palmer, 1983).

The six dimensions outlined provide a framework for evaluating the quality of health care service delivery. Consider how the six dimensions might be used. A nurse concerned about the care of adolescent mothers might ask, in relation to the first dimension, "Are we looking at all the health care needs of our typical teen mothers?" Second and third, "Are these young mothers actually functioning at a higher level as a result of our care and do we know that they are satisfied with our care?" Fourth, "Do we connect with these women during their first trimester and find ways to effectively interact with them to meet their needs throughout their pregnancy and postpartum period?" Fifth, "Are the services provided consistent with the specific mothers' needs or too generalized to make efficient use of available funds?" Finally, "Are we nurses using the most current information and resources to serve these women?" Such questions provide the basis for studying each dimension of quality. Later in this chapter we will discuss the process of quality assurance in greater depth.

HISTORICAL PERSPECTIVES

Let us examine nursing's evolution as a self-regulating profession from three perspectives: (1) clinical competence of nurses, (2) organizational competence, and (3) nursing care review processes.

CLINICAL COMPETENCE OF NURSES

The move to assure quality in health care has its roots in the professions of medicine and nursing. Both physicians and nurses as young professional groups in the mid-1800s assumed responsibility for maintaining standards within their disciplines for the services that each provided. This role began with assuring minimum levels of education and later included guarding clinical competence via licensure and clinical certification (Nutting and Dock, 1907).

Nursing education began with a few intuitive, service-minded people who applied practical knowledge in the care of the ill. Today it includes standardized basic and advanced educational systems. Throughout early efforts to build consistency into nursing education, the goal was always to prepare nurses with sufficient experience and academic work to meet the needs of typical patients of the day. Thus, over time educational standards necessarily have changed. Various accrediting organizations arose in the early 1900s to oversee and stimulate nursing schools to stay abreast with changes in health care. Today's National League for Nursing (NLN) is one such agency (NLN, 1960).

Prior to the Depression nursing licensure was already required in most states as an effort to further ensure safe practice (Goodrich, 1912). Each state legislature controlled the state's nursing practice act to ensure that minimum standards of education, practice, and expertise were maintained. Today many states require continuing education units (CEUs) as part of their qualifications for nursing license renewal. The American Nurses Association (ANA) and other professional organizations provide clinical certification for nurses in more than 20 different clinical specialities including community health nursing (ANA, 1982). Certification exams and ongoing CEU requirements provide additional means for achieving and maintaining high-level nursing skills.

ORGANIZATIONAL COMPETENCE

As health care organizations have developed and diversified, many methods for managing large staffs, multiple departments, and missions have emerged. Organizational structures and methods were designed to promote effective operations of hospitals and other health care organizations. The many responsibilities that health care agencies have to their clients, staffs, boards of directors, and funders complicate their functioning and sometimes compromise care.

Institutional attention to quality-of-care issues began to be seen in the 1940s and '50s when it became clear that organizations delivering health care services must govern those services to achieve both the organization's goals and the health care goals of their consumers (Bull, 1985). External certification and accreditation processes began at about the same time. These processes validated organizations' ability to provide adequate service. Accrediting bodies, such as the Joint Commission on Accreditation of Hospitals (commonly referred to as the Joint Commission) examine all types of health care organizations to aid them in attending to all facets of their operations, thus promoting an effective balance in priorities. Throughout the 1970s and '80s, the Joint Commission, a voluntary accrediting body, and the Professional Review Organizations, which in 1972 began certifying all organizations receiving Medicare/Medicaid dollars, both shifted their primary emphasis to the impact of organizational functioning on quality of care. They began to consider the effects of such factors as staff recruitment, organizational structure, management effectiveness, billing practices, and planning on quality. Both bodies continue to require evidence of effective quality assurance programs in all agencies that they certify. These accrediting bodies focused most of their attention on hospitals during the '70s. In the '80s the attention shifted to include ambulatory care, long-term care, and home health care. This shift occurred for many reasons, but the high costs of care and competition for health care dollars were leading reasons for such agencies to seek accreditation (Werner, 1985).

Involvement of the federal government in regulating the delivery of health care services increased after the passage of Medicare in 1965. Equal access to health services was the primary emphasis of public health care initiatives in the 1960s. Attention to rising health care costs was the work of the 1970s. In the '80s the questions of quality of care and cost effectiveness of care were issues across the nation. Thus, quality assurance began to play a specific protective function to prevent an erosion of minimal standards of care (Rinke, 1987; Brook and Lohr, 1981).

Numerous requirements for internal health care reviews now affect nursing. How nurses review client care is sometimes left up to the agency (as with Professional Review Organizations), giving them great flexibility in determining what aspects of care to study. Other types of review do not allow for such individuality. For instance, the audits required by the Federal Bureau of Community Health Services, which funds many community clinics nationwide, require that evaluation focus on five specific aspects of clinic and nursing care. The five evaluation foci are (1) immunization of children, (2) family planning education of adolescents, (3) abnormal Pap smear follow-up, (4) adult hypertension follow-up, and (5) childhood anemia screening.

Initiatives for quality review are already arising from health insurers, state Medicaid programs and professional organizations. This trend is expected to continue through the 1990s (Palmer, 1983; Gallant and Meisenheimer, 1985).

NURSING CARE REVIEW PROCESSES

Formal quality assurance activities in the health care field began in earnest in the early 1970s. Nursing's quality assurance efforts generally pre-dated those of other health care fields and included initial standard setting, formal auditing, and peer review methods developed and used during the 1950s and '60s (Phaneuf, 1976; Bull, 1987).

Patient care and nursing care reviews form the basis of quality assurance, providing specific patient care data for problem identification. The value of reflecting back on one's efforts became very evident in Florence Nightingale's work during the Crimean War. Though appropriate care for that era was being provided to injured soldiers, unexpected deaths occurred at alarming rates. It was through Florence Nightingale's rigorous review of the soldiers' care (Who was dying? How was dying patients' care different from that of similar patients who survived?) that she discovered a contributing problem. An infested air vent located near the bed where most of the men died was one source for the men's lethal acquired infections. In this case an inadequate part of the health care structure was compromising the overall quality of care. Florence Nightingale was the first person to set standards for nursing. She conducted systematic statistical record keeping as early as 1860 (Kopf, 1978).

The development of the nursing process after World War II formalized the notion of evaluation as a necessary part of the thinking process of all nursing practice. Record keeping was incorporated into evaluation more than a decade later when the problem-oriented medical record was implemented across the country, thus routinizing evaluative documentation in nursing records (National League for Nursing, 1974b). This was significant to quality assurance because it made the nurses' internal problem-solving process available to outsiders for evaluation. Thus the quality assurance tools that began to be developed for nursing during the '50s could be used to assess nurses' decision-making activities.

Froebe and Bain stated in the mid-1970s that " . . . the profession of nursing, large both numerically and operationally, should not await the implementation of outside surveillance before instituting a systematic method of quality assurance evaluation" (Froebe and Bain, 1976, p. vii).

Over the past 35 years nursing has developed more formalized nursing care review models and implemented them throughout the profession. The American Nurses Association has contributed to formal quality assurance evaluative processes through development of models, quality of care review guidelines, and nursing care standards, including those for community health nursing. Nursing has adapted and applied these models, guidelines, and standards in many inpatient, ambulatory care, and community nursing settings (American Nurses Association, 1973-1988).

In its 1988 Peer Review Guidelines the American Nurses Association proposed that nurses bear primary responsibility and accountability for the quality of nursing care their clients receive. ANA went on to say that "Standards of nursing practice provide a means for measuring the quality of nursing care a client receives. Each nurse is responsible for interpreting and implementing the standards of nursing practice. Likewise, each nurse must participate with other nurses in the decision-making process for evaluating nursing care. This process is peer review" (ANA, 1988, p. 3).

MODELS FOR QUALITY ASSURANCE

To better conceptualize the quality assurance process, let us first turn to a tested model. The American Nurses Association provided a quality assurance model in 1974 that remains true to the process of quality assurance as it is practiced today (ANA, 1975). Once a quality assurance committee or nursing peer-review group has been established to deal with quality assurance issues, the major steps in the process are as outlined below.

1. *Identify values.*
   There needs to be consensus within the practice group or organization as to the values underlying its area of practice. These values should be consistent with the organization's philosophy and the standards

and ethics of the professional practice group. A community health nursing agency, for example, must determine when the common good takes priority over individual rights (Westfall, 1987).

2. *Identify standards and criteria.*

   Specific structure, process, and outcome standards relevant to the setting should be identified. These should reflect both the values identified above and the entire scope of practice of the group or organization. (We will discuss this step in more detail later when we describe conducting a quality assurance study.) Related measurable criteria should then be developed to elaborate on the standards and to be used as the basis for judging nursing practice decisions. It is important for the whole group of peers or a representative group to be involved in this step of the process (JCAHO, 1988).

3. *Collect data.*

   Methods for collecting both descriptive and quantitative data are needed to determine the degree to which standards and criteria have been met. This step should be planned before actual data collection is done. Methods may include record audits, retrieval of statistical information already collected, or client surveys.

4. *Analyze and interpret data.*

   The reviewers analyze the data collected in light of the agreed-upon standards and criteria and make judgments about strengths, deficiencies, or problems related to quality. Particular areas that reviewers should consider in this stage are appropriateness of nursing decisions and the timeliness, efficiency, and effectiveness of nursing care.

5. *Identify courses of action.*

   The reviewers identify suitable courses of action to reward strengths, correct deficiencies, solve problems, and prevent future problems.

6. *Choose actions.*

   The reviewers, depending on their role in the organization, will either make recommendations to administrative and peer groups or select appropriate courses of action themselves.

7. *Take action.*

   If empowered to do so, the reviewers implement the action(s) chosen. Otherwise, the reviewers should receive reports of follow-up on their recommendation from those who have taken the actions. In either case, the results of recommended actions should be reevaluated at a specified future date by the same review group (ANA, 1988; JCAHO, 1988; Ingram and Harmon, 1987).

These seven steps are often depicted in a circular model to emphasize the feedback nature of the process (see Figure 23-2). Information that is gained by studying given aspects of nursing care is fed back into the system over and over again. Each decision about how care is to be provided or changed is then based on solid information gained from studying clients actually being served and the nurses providing services (Schmele, 1987).

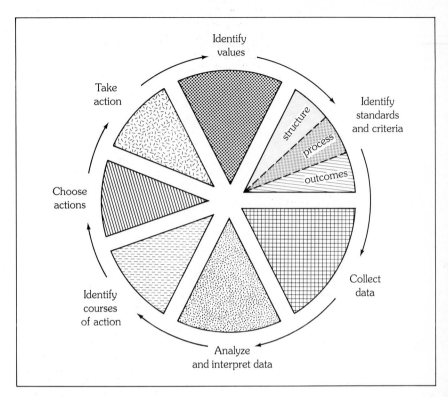

Figure 23-2
ANA quality assurance model (adapted from N. Lang, A Model for Quality Assurance in Nursing, *1974, as reprinted in* A Plan for Implementation of Standards of Nursing Practice, ANA, *1975, p. 15).*

To take the ANA model one step further, we can add an upward dimension to the feedback loop. Consider the process of quality assurance as a dynamic, upwardly spiralling feedback loop of information and care decisions that enables nurses and organizations alike to identify specific ways to improve the quality of care they provide and ensure that those improvements are effective and sustained.

The model in Figure 23-3 displays this idea in graphic form. The right pole of the model represents the continuum of clients' health needs and personal health actions taken to meet those needs. The left pole depicts the points of contact between the health care system and clients. The quality assessment activities that nurses use to look at their clients and the nursing care provided is reflected in the spirals' movement from pole to pole. Each occasion of quality assessment leads to revision of nursing care or plans and the implementation of changes. Any changes will again be assessed at a future date as part of the ongoing review process.

As the spiralling process repeats itself over and over, the quality of care should improve, and the effects of that care on clients' health status will move clients upward along the continuum towards optimum health. For example, clients are better equipped to make healthy dietary decisions if they are supported and educated effectively by nurses. Thus it behooves nurses

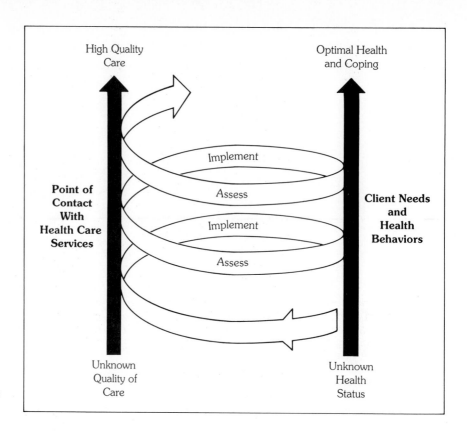

Figure 23-3
Upwardly spiralling quality
assurance feedback loop.

to ascertain that their care is effective and that they are open to quality assurance recommendations for increasing effectiveness.

This model makes two basic assumptions: first, that specific nursing activities are known to maintain and promote health, and second, that positive results are brought about by positive interventions.

Again referring to the model in Figure 23-3, one notices the physical space between the two poles in which the spiral moves. This distance allows nurses to step back from the everyday demands of direct client care to look more critically at that care and the desired outcomes. More specifically, stepping back from the process prompts us to do the following things:

1. Identify and prioritize the health problems and needs of the populations that we serve.
2. Determine the systems, nursing actions, or outcomes in terms of client behaviors that we strive to facilitate.
3. Examine the success or failure of our efforts with a specific group.
4. Adjust nursing care, systems, or client goals as needed.
5. Plan for future quality assessments.

QUALITY ASSURANCE VERSUS PROGRAM EVALUATION

The process of reflecting on one's nursing practice as a guide for change shares some similarities with program evaluation, although the two differ in some important respects. When we talk about program evaluation we refer to examining a specific component or nursing program within a larger organization. Most organizations, including nursing agencies, encompass a number of programs. For example, the health promotion activities within a local community health nursing agency may include well-child services, nutritional counseling, blood pressure screening, and other services (Bower, Linc, and Denega, 1988).

Evaluation in this context sets out to answer the following question: "Did this program achieve the goals and objectives set forth for it?" When we plan programs we ideally develop specific goals identifying who the program is supposed to serve and what services will be provided over what period of time and with what resources. We then develop objectives that describe how to accomplish the goals in measurable terms (Lieske, 1985).

The basic question of quality assurance, "Did the nursing care provided meet the desired standards for quality and did it result in the desired outcomes for the clients served?" is not answered when doing program evaluation unless such a question is specifically built into the goals of the program being evaluated. We recommend incorporating quality-focused objectives into the planning of any service-related programs. Then quality issues are dealt with routinely within all organizational program evaluations.

Quality assurance activities seek to ask the above question about all important aspects of a community health nursing agency's programming on a continuous basis (Berman, 1988). Granted, a specific program such as health screening of the elderly may be the focus for quality assurance review at one point in time, but that review fits into the whole fabric of a system-wide effort to assure that the elements of quality care are present.

COMMUNITY HEALTH NURSING AGENCIES AND QUALITY ASSURANCE

Quality assurance programs in community health agencies are typically fragmented (Ingram and Harmon, 1987). Monitoring of specific aspects of care is often done in response to funders' requirements for periodic progress reports rather than as part of a larger program (Januska, Engle, and Wood, 1976).

Quality assurance programs within community health nursing agencies may take a number of forms, depending on the values of the organization's leadership, the time resources available, and the staff's experience in research and quality assurance work. Some small agencies that provide home health care services are able to do only the auditing and clinical reporting required by Medicare or other funders. Larger agencies are more likely to incorporate additional voluntary types of quality assessment and review into their programs, due in part to the greater potential that larger staffs may have quality assurance experience and sufficient supervisory personnel to initiate, coordinate, and implement actual studies. Ideally, a comprehensive community health nursing quality assurance program will address in some fashion all of the important agency services to assure formal or informal review of those services for quality and efficiency (Januska, Engle, and Wood, 1976; Kerfoot and Watson, 1985).

Peer review committees are the basic working unit for accomplishing specific studies in quality assurance. A quality assurance committee is by definition made up of staff representing all of the important program components within an agency and often includes concerned community members as well (American Nurses Association, 1988; Ortega and Agbayani, 1987; Lang, 1976). Agency board members also can provide valuable perspective and expertise. In a small agency a quality assurance committee may include the entire staff: the director, community health nurses, nutritionist, and other support staff such as physical and occupational therapists and clerical workers. A quality assurance committee in a larger agency may be composed of a nursing representative or supervisor from each field team and representatives of specialized programs such as maternal and child health, home health care, or services for disabled children. While the community health nursing director may sit on the committee, it is important to distinguish the role of the quality assurance committee as separate from that of administration.

A quality assurance committee performs the following tasks:

1. Identifies those areas of care where practice patterns indicate that more knowledge is needed by staff. Updated information on AIDS might be an example.
2. Determines the strengths and weaknesses of nursing care. Perhaps the staff provides positive support for AIDS clients but gives partially inaccurate information on AIDS prevention.
3. Evaluates the quality and quantity of nursing care being provided. The committee might examine the accuracy and amount of community teaching given on AIDS.
4. Provides data to utilize as the basis for recommendations for new or revised policies. For example, the agency might use data on the number of nursing care plans demonstrating inadequate AIDS background to institute a policy of periodic mandatory staff education on AIDS.

Thus, a quality assurance committee identifies topics and groups for study, plans and implements studies, assesses the results, and makes recommendations to administration for problem resolution (ANA, 1988; Ingram and Harmon, 1987).

Administration, on the other hand, should support the evaluative work of the committee, solicit its recommendations, and respond effectively (Berman, 1988). Examples of effective responses on the part of administration include providing leadership in planning staff education programs, providing nursing supervision of staff, and assuming major responsibility in developing policies and procedures (MDH, 1980).

PLANNING A QUALITY ASSURANCE STUDY

Quality assurance is a group of evaluative processes, both formal and informal, that seek to answer the question, "Is care effective and acceptable to those served?" An integrated quality assurance program includes review of several interconnected aspects of care: the *structure* of the health care agency or delivery system, the *process* of provision of care, the *outcomes* of care relative to health status of care recipients, and the *impact* of that care on the larger system in which recipients' health is embedded (Blum, 1981).

In *structural* evaluation one assumes that using better qualified staff, improved physical facilities and an effective administration will result in delivery of high-quality care. The organization's management, facilities, and staff competence are the focus of standards and evaluation. In *process* evaluation the activity of the health professionals involved is assessed. The assumption is that specific nursing activities are known to be related to positive client outcomes and that these activities maintain and promote health. *Outcome* appraisal examines the final consequences of the service and assumes that good results are the result of good care. *Impact* evaluation goes beyond outcome to explore the consequences on the target population, both anticipated and unanticipated, of health professionals' actions taken to reach a goal (Davidson, 1978; Blum, 1981; Lalonde, 1987; Rinke, 1987; Berman, 1988).

In spite of the recommendation that all aspects of care be evaluated, until recently community health nursing has evaluated primarily structure and process aspects of care (Harris, Peters, and Yuan, 1987). This situation is understandable for several reasons. Government and other regulatory bodies have had reporting requirements that used only structural and process standards. These have comprised the bulk of quality assurance monitoring done by many agencies. Also, development and field testing of outcome standards is a complex task requiring much skill, time, and focused commitment by personnel. Resource limitations have precluded large-scale efforts to branch out into the outcome arena for most individual agencies. Finally, the reliability of using outcomes as the primary measure of quality care is limited in that clients may have bad outcomes despite receiving good care. Many factors other than specific health interventions can and do influence outcomes (Donabedian, 1969).

The quality assurance process is similar to the nursing process. Routine, disciplined use of the nursing process can be an informal method for assuring quality of care. In formal client care reviews the nurse collects relevant objective and subjective data about a given group of clients from whatever data sources are relevant (chart notes, statistical data, or surveys) and seeks to make a diagnosis or to identify client care problems. Those areas of care identified as questionable in terms of consistency of care or outcome will then be studied in more detail. Once the problem has been studied and understood, then corrective actions can be proposed, implemented, and reviewed for their effectiveness at a later date. This more formalized process truly mirrors the nursing process and can be readily learned and used effectively by nurses.

A number of quality assurance initiatives have been published nationally in recent years as resources for public health agencies, home health care agencies, and ambulatory care services. Examples include *Outcome Criteria for Preventive Services and Home Health Care* by the Public Health Nursing Section of the Minnesota Department of Health (MDH, 1986); *Model Standards for Community Health Programs,* whose second draft was published in 1985 as a collaborative project by the American Public Health Association, the Department of Health and Human Services, and others as a framework for developing community standards; and most recently, *Outcome Measures in Home Care* by Rinke et al., which presents a sampling of efforts nationally "to develop and measure outcome indicators for community-based nursing services" (Rinke et al., 1987, p. viii). Some reliable and valid measurement scales are also beginning to emerge and are applicable to CHN practice. Examples include the *General Symptom Distress Scale,* a client distress rating tool (Lalonde, 1987); a scale that relates nursing diagnosis to cost of care delivered in home care settings (Harris, Peters, and Yuan, 1987); and the *Slater Scale,* which measures nursing competencies in client care (Hough and Schmele, 1987).

CONDUCTING A QUALITY ASSURANCE STUDY

In order to carry out a useful and effective quality assurance study it is important to follow a logical sequence of actions. We will base our sequence on the models discussed earlier. The reader is reminded that quality assurance studies are planned and carried out by a designated committee or peer group who have been given the charge of examining specific health care services for quality-of-care issues. Figure 23-4 provides a summary of the steps to be taken in conducting a quality assurance study.

TOPIC IDENTIFICATION

How does a quality assurance committee select topics or problems worthy of study? This can be done in several ways:

1. Select from the most common types of nursing services provided by the organization.

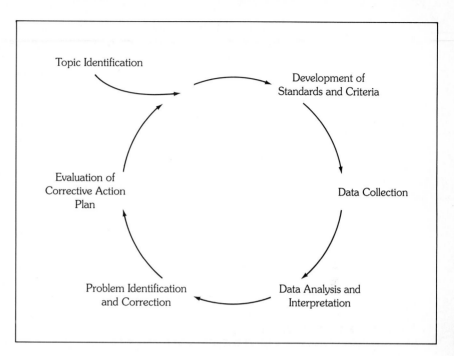

Figure 23-4
Steps of a quality assurance study (adapted from Lang, 1974; American Nurses Association, 1975; Davidson, 1977; Palmer, 1983).

2. Select from the highest-risk populations that are being served in which nursing intervention can significantly improve the health status of the client.
3. Select from obvious incidents reported by staff and clients.
4. Detect problems by scanning client care data in specific program areas (Palmer, 1983; Kerfoot and Watson, 1985; MDH, 1986).

Nursing services used most frequently, such as well-child care, self-care education with chronically ill adults, or various screening programs, are excellent topics with which to begin study. Generally these services involve all of the nursing staff and consume a significant amount of nursing care time.

Focusing on commonly served high-risk groups presents an opportunity to optimize care delivery as well as to benefit high-risk clients. Children living in neighborhoods with high lead toxicity rates from leaded paint in older homes stand to benefit tremendously by a consistently implemented lead screening, treatment, and advocacy program. Without study such a program would not be certain to achieve its goals of decreasing lead toxicity among area children.

Incidents of poor client outcome are important topics for further study. Many clinics routinely review records of deceased or hospitalized clients to assess whether any aspect of the clinic's care might have prevented these occurrences. For instance, a case in which a child has shown repeated high serum lead levels and requires hospitalization for chelation could stimulate the clinic's examination of the adequacy of parent education on environmental sources of lead. The clinic could also explore the effectiveness of its advocacy with the city lead abatement staff to assure needed repairs in leaded homes and the removal of families to safe housing while repairs are being made.

A final means for selecting quality review topics is to scan various types of client care data. Data sources that suggest a need for review might include statistical reports that tabulate the types and amounts of services provided over time, records of clients who heavily utilize agency services, and closed records. Many community clinics, home health programs, and community health nursing agencies already do periodic record reviews that can be very useful in identifying quality of care problems for further study. An example might be quarterly monitoring of the level of childhood immunization among all children served by an agency.

Quality review topic selection may be influenced by several of the above considerations. For instance, a local community health nursing agency decided to study care of infants in its area. Based on routine birth certificate review the agency attempted nursing visits with all mothers and infants in the first three months of life in the entire county. This represented both a large proportion of the nurses' caseloads and also an ill-defined area of nursing practice.

DEVELOPMENT OF STANDARDS AND CRITERIA

Having selected a topic or problem for review, a quality assurance review committee must next clearly articulate standards and criteria against which to measure the actual care provided. Clinical *standards* are defined as desired goals for health care activities that can be used to evaluate care on one of three levels: structure, process, or outcome of care. *Criteria,* on the other hand, are specific, measurable indicators that standards or goals have been achieved (Beckman, 1987).

Standards are expressed as statements of who is responsible for what behavior and the desired frequency of the behavior, as in "a teenage client chooses her/his own specific birth control method in 100 percent of cases" or "the nurse assesses all pregnant clients for risk of physical abuse."

Criteria state more specifically what can be observed about the behavior of the client or nurse that gives evidence that the standard is being met. One often needs more than a single criterion to substantiate a given standard. Several criteria substantiate the teen client's choice of birth control method: "the client (1) states goal or intent for birth control, (2) can describe alternate methods of contraception, and (3) states chosen method." Only one criterion may be necessary for assessment of abuse in pregnancy: "the primary nurse documents the use of pregnancy abuse risk scale to assess for physical violence with each pregnant client by the second visit."

Numerous authors speak to the process of standard and criteria development (Davidson, 1978; American Nurses Association and Sutherland Learning Associates, 1982; Palmer, 1983; Beckman, 1987; Rinke, 1987; O'Leary, 1988). Formal standards of care and practice are available for many nursing care areas. These have been developed on the national level by groups of professional peers. Examples include ANA standards for community health, maternal-child, home health nursing and others (ANA, 1973–1986); American Public Health Association (APHA) model standards for community preventive health services (APHA, 1985); the American Academy of Pediatrics and the Federal Maternal-Child Health Program standards for pediatric public health. To date, no comprehensive standards for community health nursing programs have been developed (Ingram and Harmon, 1987).

The Public Health Nursing Section of the Minnesota Department of Health (MDH) has outlined a method for developing outcome criteria that clearly illustrates this process (see Table 23-1). It is applicable to CHN agencies as well as other community agencies and ambulatory centers. According to the MDH method, criteria development consists of five steps once a topic area has been identified (MDH, 1986). These steps are described below and summarized in Table 23-1.

1. *Define a population.*

   Once one has chosen a topic, it is critical to specifically define those who will be considered in an audit. This is important for two reasons. First, the types of clients being reviewed must be familiar to the nurses for the review to be meaningful and valid. Second, it would be impossible to select cases for audit without clear guidelines for who will be included or excluded. Useful characteristics to include in defining the population are age, sex, relationship, and health status. Thus, Table 23-1 shows that children of both sexes who are from 0 to 3 months old and live in one- and two-parent families will be reviewed and standards set for their care.

2. *Identify typical problems and needs.*

   This step enables nurses who are familiar with the population to gain a holistic view of the group before choosing areas that may benefit from nursing intervention. Returning to Table 23-1, we see that growth and development, preventive health care, and adequate familial support and income are clearly part of the constellation of infant needs.

3. *Select priority problems.*

   This step follows and determines the decisions for nursing intervention. The number of priority problems should be limited to enable realistic handling of them by the peer group. Only two priority needs were chosen in the case of the infant group since these are the ones most likely to be influenced by nursing care.

4. *Establish desired outcomes.*

   Outcomes are the expected end results or expected changes in the client population's health status resulting from nursing care received (MDH, 1986, p. 15). As shown in Table 23-1, we expect that children will demonstrate normal growth and development patterns by eating appropriate foods and attaining weight and height levels consistent with their ages.

5. *List criteria to measure the outcomes.*
Criteria state more specifically what can be observed about the behavior of clients to give evidence that the outcome is being achieved. Sometimes several criteria may be needed to substantiate a given outcome. Use verbs to clearly describe client behavior; this helps reviewers to recognize when the desired behavior has been demonstrated. The statements "children eat..." and "children demonstrate normal weight..." from our example show how verbs describe client behavior.

Some practical guidelines for writing criteria include: keep criteria simple, include only the most essential items, limit the number of criteria, specify achievement rather than intention, and be sure content is up-to-date and relevant to the setting (Palmer, 1983; O'Leary, 1988).

Many authors recommend that if criteria are developed by people other than the entire professional clinical staff to whom they will be applied, a ratification process should be undertaken before actual peer review is started. This process can simply mean sending the criteria to a vote of the entire professional staff and adjusting criteria by consensus. In other circumstances it may involve a more complicated review for clinical accuracy and validation of the criteria as quality indicators. A major benefit of the ratification process is the

Table 23-1
Outcome Criteria Development

Steps	Illustrations
1. Define a population.	Infants between 0 and 3 months old in one- and two-parent families (both male and female).
2. Identify typical problems and needs of clients in population.	Children need stimulation and support for growth and development. Children need well-child health care. Parents need to adjust to their new responsibilities and to utilize support systems. Parents need adequate income to support family.
3. Select priority problems amenable to nursing intervention.	First two needs in item 2 above.
4. Establish desired or expected client outcomes (*). 5. List observable criteria to measure outcomes (–).	*Children attain normal growth and development. –Children eat foods as appropriate to age. –Children demonstrate normal weight and height on growth charts. –Children demonstrate 50% of behaviors on bonding scale. *Children receive regular well-child care. –Children are up to date on immunizations per health department guidelines or specific recommendations. –Children see doctor according to schedule set by doctor or EPSDT guidelines.

Source: Adapted from printed materials of the Section for Public Health Nursing of the Minnesota Department of Health, Minneapolis, 1986.

opportunity to enlist the support of the clinical staff in principle and practice of quality assurance reviews (Phaneuf, 1976; Davidson, 1978; MDH, 1980).

Standards and criteria should be used with caution. They are not intended as whips to keep service providers in line. Rather, they should serve as firm but gentle reminders of our quality concerns and of the ways we can improve our practice. Many factors influence whether people's health has been favorably affected by nursing or other professional intervention. These factors need to be considered when peer review committees apply quality standards and criteria.

In general, we recommend that each case reviewed should meet the screening criteria. If a case does not meet a given criterion, that case should be subjected to more detailed review by a peer. Such detailed review can often uncover the other unique factors impinging on the health status of the client in question. Often such factors as marital problems, unemployment, or chemical dependency are more powerful influences on client decision-making than is nursing care. Detailed peer review may reveal these variables or identify service delivery problems that influence outcomes, such as documentation backlogs, referral breakdowns, and inadequate staff performance (Davidson, 1977).

DATA COLLECTION

To plan a study or audit that will accurately evaluate whether predetermined standards and criteria for quality nursing care have been met, a quality assurance committee must ask a number of questions:

1. Is the information needed to make a judgment about a specific aspect of nursing care available in the present system?
2. How would that information be obtained most efficiently? Namely, what records or other data sources are needed, and who can accurately and objectively assess the records for the presence or absence of criteria?
3. How many cases need to be reviewed to give a representative picture of the specific aspect of care being evaluated? How will those cases be identified?
4. What specific steps must each reviewer go through to adequately assess a case?
5. What kind of secondary review should be done on those cases that do not meet the criteria? (Palmer, 1983)

In carefully answering each of these questions, the committee can design a detailed data collection plan that is objective and efficient. The care review plan in Table 23-2 addresses these questions.

While developing criteria, the committee needs to identify whether substantiating data for each nursing activity and client outcome was actually available in the current system of record keeping. If the current system could

Table 23-2
Well-Child Care Review Plan for 0- to 3-Month-Old Infants

Criteria and standards: Previously established by nursing quality assurance committee (see Table 23-1, items 4 and 5).

Data sources needed: Infant/family record—specifically, narrative notes, and education and screening flow sheets.

Persons responsible for review: All community health nurses currently on quality assurance committee.

Sample selection: The records staff randomly selects 10% or 20 cases (whichever is greater) from all of the 0- to 3-month-old infants who received nursing care during the months of January through March, 1989. Both open and closed cases at the time of the review are included.

Data retrieval procedure: Reviewers examine each assigned chart comparing the nursing visit documentation to the list of expected nursing activities and infant outcomes (criteria) on the audit sheet. They note the presence or absence of each criterion on the audit form for each infant. They also note any exceptions to a given criterion before assessing its presence or absence on the audit form.

Cases are excluded from the audit if:
—an RN did not visit the family
—the infant did not meet the age or visit criteria.

Secondary review: Done by the entire committee on any case that the RN reviewer determines is deficient in an important aspect of care.

not provide such information, then it may be necessary to develop new procedures and documentation such as flow sheets or case data bases before actual case reviews can be done. The plan then identifies specific data sources to be used for a given review in order to facilitate data retrieval.

In some organizations non-clinical personnel, such as records and secretarial staff, do the actual record reviews. In others, the clinical staff or peer review committee members do the reviews (Davidson, 1978; Kline, Tracy, and Howell, 1980; Palmer, 1983; Rinke, 1987). Philosophical differences between quality assurance professionals account for this apparent paradox. One can design a study so that nonprofessional, less costly staff can objectively and accurately abstract useful data for quality-of-care issues. The same study can use professional clinical staff for analysis and interpretation of that data as the most efficient and effective use of their clinical expertise (Davidson, 1978). Proponents of having professionals review individual cases argue that there are clinical judgments that need to be made while assessing for quality of care since there are many intervening variables that may influence care decisions. No less important are the additional issues that a clinician may identify as a result of reviewing a group of cases (Smeltzer, Hinshaw, and Feltman, 1987). This is an ideal way to identify other areas of care that need attention, as in the case of nurses dealing with mothers of young infants. While the care of infants may be appropriately addressed, the mothers' needs for family planning information might have been overlooked. Since it may be unrealistic to review all infant cases for quality of care, the quality assurance committee would seek to select a smaller group or sample of cases to be representative of all infants receiving nursing services in a given time period. It is generally accepted that a sample of 20 randomly selected cases will provide useful information. If the population to be sampled numbers more than 200, some sources recommend that the sample include more than 20 cases.

The timing of the review can be done in different ways. In many community health nursing agencies cases are opened and closed within a brief time period, while others remain open for years. *Concurrent* nursing care review is concerned with the identification of nursing care priorities and the provision of optimal nursing care while the patient is still receiving services. *Retrospective* review examines documented care already given (Figure 23-5). Its purpose is to identify deficiencies in the organization and administration of nursing care, to correct such deficiencies through education and administrative change, and to periodically assess performance to assure that improvements are maintained (Davidson, 1978). In our example the review is retrospective in that it examines care already received and infant outcomes noted during a particular time period (January through March, 1989) to identify patterns of nursing care and variations in care.

The actual procedure for data retrieval and documentation varies from audit to audit, but it should be stated specifically so that each reviewer assesses each case the same way. This enhances the objectivity, accuracy, and reliability of the results, and these factors will be important for later decision making. Excluded cases and exceptions to each criteria need to be noted so that the final combined results of the study describe the quality and outcomes of nursing care among the specified group of young infants.

Secondary record review by nursing peers of those children who did not receive the recommended care or whose health outcomes were compromised provides an opportunity for in-depth assessment of care. This can benefit the

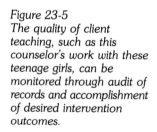

Figure 23-5
The quality of client teaching, such as this counselor's work with these teenage girls, can be monitored through audit of records and accomplishment of desired intervention outcomes.

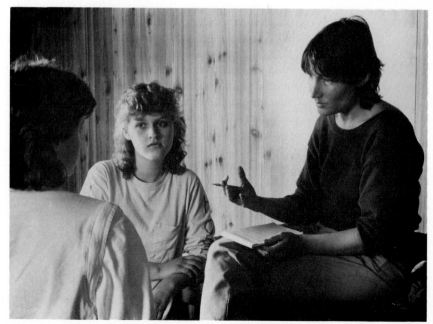

recipients and providers of care if quality-of-care problems actually exist. We will discuss this topic further in the next section.

DATA ANALYSIS AND INTERPRETATION

After auditing an individual record, the reviewer determines whether the care meets the standards or is deficient in some way, then summarizes the entire group of records. The summary consists of adding up the number of cases fulfilling each criterion and computing their percentage of the total sample. For example, the reviewer can calculate the proportion of infants who met half of the items on the maternal bonding scale after two visits. This report gives an overview of how the documented care compares with preestablished outcomes for the desired group (Driever, 1988).

The reviewer then presents this summary to the quality assurance committee for data analysis along with the records of cases not meeting the specific criterion. These nursing peers review the specific cases first. They use their judgment upon review of the data available in each record to determine if not meeting the criterion is clinically justified in any of the cases. If the group members decide that failure to meet a criterion represents a deficiency in care, they then make an effort to describe and understand the problem and its possible causes (MDH, 1980). The quality assurance committee applies the same analysis to the audit summary, looking for strengths and weaknesses in practice across all records. The group then determines and recommends what type of corrective action will remove the cause of an identified problem, who is to implement the action, and when the action is to be taken. They may recommend that the problem be taken back to the entire staff for brainstorming to identify resolution ideas (JCAHO, 1988). For example, if all of the charts are found to be deficient in the same area, such as anticipatory guidance on safety concerns, this could be a clue that the nurses need additional education in this area or that their caseload exceeds the capabilities of the nurses to provide minimum expected preventive education. Once the cause is determined to be a staffing issue the quality assurance committee makes its recommendation to the director to reassess the nursing caseload requirements by the end of the following quarter and implement appropriate changes to give nurses adequate time to address critical education issues (Wilbert, 1985; Mottet, 1987).

PROBLEM IDENTIFICATION AND CORRECTION

Once the peer review group has analyzed the study findings and identified strengths, weaknesses, and opportunities to improve nursing care, their next job is to identify the interventions that are likely to result in improved care and/or client outcome. The types of corrective action needed will vary with the circumstances. If a system problem is interfering with care, a new or revised policy or procedure may be sufficient to address the problem. For example, a lengthy infant safety assessment tool may be prohibitive for use by nurses in a 30-minute infant visit and thus needs to be modified to guarantee nursing safety assessment.

Education needs are frequently identified as part of an initial corrective action plan. Many administrators and quality assurance professionals alike agree that education and a shared understanding of problem situations often result in improved care and outcomes (Davidson, 1978; Wilbert, 1985). In general, nurses and other providers of care desire to provide high-quality services (Figure 23-6). Given adequate resources, including sufficient time, information, and support, good care is the norm. There are occasions where quality-of-care problems result from individual providers' performance. The peer group makes recommendations for counseling or another type of personnel intervention by the individual's supervisor.

Whether the quality assurance committee actually implements the corrective action plan or simply submits recommendations for such plans to administration depends on the authority vested in the committee. Whichever the case, the plans should clearly state what is to be done, when, and by whom. These recommendations should be included as the completion of the audit analysis and interpretation (Lieske, 1985b).

EVALUATION OF CORRECTIVE ACTION PLAN

The feedback loop of the quality assurance cycle is closed with an evaluation of the corrective action plan. This evaluation determines the effectiveness of a given set of interventions in improving the quality of a specific nursing care component. This is done by reauditing the specific problem areas at a pre-

Figure 23-6
Quality care is more likely to occur when staff have been thoroughly trained and oriented to the setting and to clients' needs. Here a nurse conducts a class for nurses' aides.

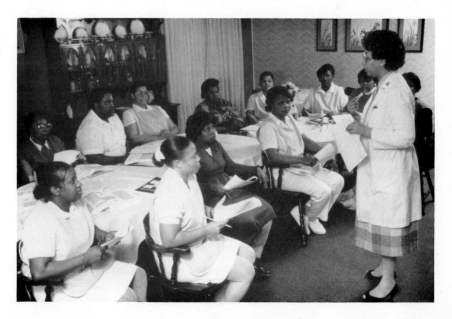

determined time following implementation of the action plan. Such an audit is often built into a larger study. It can also be completed in an abbreviated form using the steps already described, but with only the "problem" criteria being examined. In our example, the quality assurance committee repeats the same infant care audit for subsequent quarters of the year. They focus their analysis on the quality and quantity of documented infant safety assessments. This review gives evidence to the effectiveness of the staffing changes that were implemented (Wilbert, 1985; JCAHO, 1988).

If the problem persists in follow-up audits, then the review committee renews its efforts to understand the problem and to recommend appropriate action(s). The priority of the problem needs to be considered at this point. In our example, assuring infant safety in the home is certainly a priority. The nursing staff's allegiance to a specific assessment tool or procedure may need to be questioned as a priority if this remains the obstacle to adequate and timely assessment. Thus, the nurses must explore other options for assessing safety that take less time to implement and require less time for staff orientation, but are effective and achievable in each infant case. If a new tool is adopted, the quality assurance committee must alter the audit criteria to reflect this. This ensures evaluation of the new procedure or tool in future audits. The feedback loop repeats itself over and over again until the problem no longer exists.

Summary

Quality assurance is a set of systematic evaluation processes. It seeks to assure that sufficient health care services are provided in a timely manner and that those services provided have a high likelihood of producing a positive effect on the health and perception of health of those being served.

In this chapter we have emphasized the importance of quality assurance for community health nursing as a means for defining and assuring appropriateness and adequacy of nursing care. The changing health care climate necessitates that such definitions come from within the profession of nursing; otherwise, they will be imposed from forces outside of nursing, namely insurers and other purchasers of health care.

Over time the practice of peer review has become more specific as standards of practice and client care have been refined and new methodologies have been validated. Whether quality assurance is practiced formally or informally, any time practicing nurses monitor, assess, and make judgments about the quality and appropriateness of care as measured against professional standards, then the interests of clients are being served.

Study Questions

1. Name the six descriptors (dimensions) of a quality community health program discussed early in the chapter. Taking an existing program in your community, evaluate its quality based on these dimensions.

2. Using the American Nurses Association's quality assurance model, describe the steps for establishing a quality assurance program in a community family planning agency.
3. Select a community program about which you have some knowledge. Identify one topic for quality assurance study and develop one or more standards and criteria against which to measure the actual service provided.

Glossary of Terms

Audit: An organized effort whereby practicing professionals monitor, assess, and make judgments about the quality and appropriateness of nursing care provided by peers as measured against professional standards of practice.

Concurrent review: A quality assessment process that looks at specific elements of care while the care is in progress. Open audits, joint home visits by a nurse and her supervisor, and care conferences are examples.

Criteria: Predetermined, measurable indicators that a given standard of care has been met. Criteria state specifically what can be observed about the behavior of the client or nurse to give evidence that the standard is being met.

Peer review committee: The basic working unit of any quality assurance program. For community health nursing, it is composed of registered nurses actively engaged in the practice of nursing who have knowledge of and experience providing nursing care with the client group being studied.

Professional Review Organizations (PRO): Organizations of physicians mandated to monitor the necessity, appropriateness and quality of health services financed by federal funds. PROs have focused on hospitals until recently. Currently Medicare-certified home health agencies and HMOs caring for the elderly are beginning to prepare for review by PROs. It is expected that some Medicaid-funded programs will be reviewed by PROs in the foreseeable future.

Quality: The degree to which services provided are properly matched to the needs of the population, are technically correct, and achieve beneficial impact.

Quality assurance: A three-phase process that involves (1) comparison of a health care situation against preestablished criteria believed to represent quality care; (2) identification of care strengths, deficiencies, and opportunities to improve; and (3) introduction of changes in the health care system based on information supplied in the first two phases.

Quality assurance package or program: The grouping of tools that comprise an evaluation system within an organization. This concept is based on the premise that an organization undertakes many activities that contribute to the assurance of quality and that these must be organized in such a way as to include all important program components.

Retrospective review: A quality assessment process that looks at patterns of care over a specified period of time in the past. Examples include closed record audits and statistical review of trends in services provided.

Standards of care: The desired goals for health care activities that can be used to plan and evaluate care. Standards are developed for several levels of care: the structure, process, outcome, and impact of care. They are expressed as statements of who is responsible for what behavior and the desired frequency of that behavior.

Utilization review: A process that seeks to eliminate the overuse of health care services and thus decrease payments for those services. This is done via examination of client data to ensure that any given client requires the specific service in a given setting at a given time.

References

American Nurses Association (ANA). (1973). *Standards: Maternal-child health nursing practice.* Kansas City, Mo.: Author.

American Nurses Association. (1974). *Standards: Community health nursing practice.* Kansas City, Mo.: Author.

American Nurses Association. (1975). *A plan for implementation of standards of nursing practice.* Kansas City, Mo.: Author.

American Nurses Association. (1976a). *Guidelines for review of nursing care at the local level.* Kansas City, Mo.: Author.

American Nurses Association. (1976b). *Quality assurance workbook.* Kansas City, Mo.: Author.

American Nurses Association. (1982). *Credentialing in nursing: Contemporary developments and trends.* Kansas City, Mo.: Author.

American Nurses Association. (1986). *Standards of home health nursing practice.* Kansas City, Mo.: Author.

American Nurses Association. (1988). *Peer review guidelines.* Kansas City, Mo.: Author.

American Nurses Association and Sutherland Learning Associates. (1982). *Nursing quality assurance management/learning system.* Kansas City, Mo.: Author.

American Public Health Association. (1985). *Model standards: A guide for community preventive health services.* (2nd ed.). Washington, D.C.: Author.

Beckman, J. S. (1987). What is a standard of practice? *Journal of Nursing Quality Assurance* 1(2): 1–6.

Benson, D. S. (1985). *Position paper on quality health care.* Unpublished paper submitted to Clinical Directors Subcommittee of the National Association of Community Health Centers.

Berman, S. (1988). Quality assurance in ambulatory health care. *Quality Review Bulletin* 13(1): 18–21.

Blum, H. L. (1981). *Planning for health: Generics for the eighties.* (2nd ed). New York: Human Sciences Press.

Bower, D., L. Linc, and D. Denega. (1988). *Evaluation instruments in nursing.* (Pub. No. 15-2178). New York: National League for Nursing.

Brook, R. H., and K. N. Lohr. (1981). Quality of care assessment: Its role in the 1980s. *American Journal of Public Health* 71(7): 681–82.

Bull, M. J. (1985). Quality assurance: Its origins, transformations, and prospects. In C. G. Meisenheimer, *Quality assurance: A complete guide to effective programs.* Rockville, Md.: Aspen Systems.

Davidson, S. V. (1977). *Nursing care evaluation: Concurrent and retrospective review criteria.* St. Louis: C. V. Mosby.

Davidson, S. V. (1978). Community nursing care evaluation. In B. W. Spradley (ed.), *Readings in community health nursing.* Boston: Little, Brown.

Donabedian, A. (1969). Medical care appraisal: Quality and utilization. In American Public Health Association, *Guide to medical care administration.* New York: Author.

Driever, M. J. (1988). Interpretation: A critical component of the quality assurance process. *Journal of Nursing Quality Assurance* 2(2): 55–58.

Flynn, B. C., and D. W. Ray. (1979). Quality assurance in community health nursing. *Nursing Outlook* 27: 650–53.

Froebe, D. J., and T. Bain. (1976). *Quality assurance programs and controls in nursing.* St. Louis: C. V. Mosby.

Gallant, B. and C. G. Meisenheimer. (1985). The future of quality. In C. G. Meisenheimer, *Quality assurance: A complete guide to effective programs.* Rockville, Md.: Aspen Systems.

Goodrich, A. (1912). A general presentation of the statutory requirements of the different states. *American Journal of Nursing* 12: 100–105.

Harris, M. D., D. A. Peters, and J. Yuan. (1987). Relating quality and cost in a home health care agency. *Quality Review Bulletin* 13(5): 175–81.

Hough, B. L., and J. A. Schmele. (1987). The Slater scale: A viable method for monitoring nursing care quality in home health. *Journal of Nursing Quality Assurance* 1(3): 28–38.

Hyman, H. H. (1982). *Health planning: A systematic approach.* (2nd ed.). Rockville, Md.: Aspen Systems.

Ingram, H. H., and L. Harmon. (1987). Quality assurance in a public health agency. *Quarterly Review Bulletin* 12(11): 372–76.

Januska, C., J. Engle, and J. Wood. (1976). *Status of quality assurance in public health nursing.* Washington, D.C.: American Public Health Association, Public Health Nursing Section.

Joint Commission on Accreditation of Healthcare Organizations (JCAHO). (1988). *Ambulatory health care standards manual.* Chicago: Author.

Kerfoot, K. M., and M. Watson. (1985). Research-based quality assurance: The key to excellence in nursing. In J. C. McClosky and G. H. Kennedy (eds.), *Current issues in nursing.* 2nd ed. Boston: Blackwell Scientific Publications.

Kline, M. M., M. L. Tracy, and S. D. Howell. (1980). Quality assurance in public health. *Nursing and Health Care* 4: 192–96.

Kopf, E. W. (1978). Florence Nightingale as statistician. *Journal of Research in Nursing and Health* 1(3): 93–102.

Lalonde, B. (1987). The general symptom distress scale: A home care outcome measure. *Quality Review Bulletin* 12(7): 242–50.

Lang, N. (1976). Issues in quality assurance. In American Nurses Association, *Issues in Evaluation Research.* Kansas City, Mo.: Author.

Lieske, A. M. (1985a). Quality assurance and research. In C. G. Meisenheimer, *Quality assurance: A complete guide to effective programs.* Rockville, Md.: Aspen Systems.

Lieske, A. M. (1985b). Reporting mechanisms. In C. G. Meisenheimer, *Quality assurance: A complete guide to effective programs.* Rockville, Md.: Aspen Systems.

Minnesota Department of Health (MDH), Section of Public Health Nursing. (1980). *Outcome auditing: One component of a quality assurance program.* Rev. ed. Minneapolis: Author.

Mottet, E. A. (1987). Monitoring is only the beginning: Critical element is the plan for action. *Journal of Nursing Quality Assurance* 1(3): 23–27.

National League for Nursing. (1960). *Accreditation of educational programs in nursing conducted by hospitals.* New York: Author.

National League for Nursing. (1974a). *Community health services in the health care delivery system.* (Pub. no. 21-1524). New York: Author.

National League for Nursing. (1974b). *The problem-oriented system: A multidisciplinary approach.* (Pub. no. 20-1546). New York: Author.

Nutting, M. A., and L. L. Dock. (1907). *A history of nursing.* New York: G. P. Putnam's Sons.

O'Grady, T. P. (1986). *Creative nursing administration: Participative management into the 21st century.* Rockville, Md.: Aspen Systems.

O'Leary, D. S. (1988). The need for clinical standards of care. *Quality Review Bulletin* 13(2): 31–32.

Orlikoff, J. E., and A. Snow. (1984). *Assessing quality circles in health care settings: a guide for management.* Chicago: American Hospital Publishing, Inc.

Ortega, T. S., and F. P. Agbayani. (1987). Compliance with standards of nursing practice: Use of a peer review system. *Journal of Nursing Quality Assurance* 1(2): 39–65.

Palmer, R. H. (1983). *Ambulatory health care evaluation: Principles and practice.* Chicago: American Hospital Association.

Phaneuf, M. C. (1976). *The nursing audit: Self-regulation in nursing practice.* 2nd ed. New York: Appleton-Century-Crofts.

Rinke, L. T. and A. A. Wilson (eds.). (1987). *Outcome measures in home care: Research* (vol. 1) and *Service* (vol. 2). New York: National League for Nursing.

Schmele, J. A. (1987). A method to implement nursing standards in home care. *Journal of Nursing Quality Assurance* 1(2): 43–52.

Smeltzer, C. A., A. S. Hinshaw, and B. Feltman. (1987). The benefits of staff nurse involvement in monitoring the quality of patient care. *Journal of Nursing Quality Assurance* 1(3): 1–7.

Werner, J. (1985). PSROs and hospital accreditation. In J. C. McCloskey and C. H. Kennedy (eds.), *Current issues in nursing.* 2nd ed. Boston: Blackwell Scientific Publications.

Westfall, U. E. (1987). Standards of practice: Nursing values made visible. *Journal of Nursing Quality Assurance* 1(2): 21–30.

White, M. S. (1982). Construct for public health nursing. *Nursing Outlook* 30: 527–30.

Wilbert, C. C. (1985). Selecting topics/methodologies. In C. G. Meisenheimer, *Quality assurance: A complete guide to effective programs.* Rockville, Md.: Aspen Systems.

Selected Readings

American Nurses Association. (1973). *Quality assurance for nursing care.* Kansas City, Mo.: Author.

American Public Health Association. (1982). Definition and role of public health nurses in delivery of health care (Policy Statement No. 8132). *American Journal of Public Health* 72: 210–12.

Barkauskas, V. H. (1983). Effectiveness of public health nurses' home visits to primiparous mothers and their infants. *American Journal of Public Health* 73: 573–80.

Bussmann, J. W., and S. V. Davidson. (1981). *PSRO: The promise, perspective and potential.* Menlo Park: Addison-Wesley.

Davidson, S. V. (1976). *PSRO utilization and audit in patient care.* St. Louis: C. V. Mosby.

Decker, F., L. Stevens, M. Vancini, and L. Wedeking. (1979). Using patient outcomes to evaluate community health nursing. *Nursing Outlook* 27: 278–82.

Joint Commission for Accreditation of Hospitals. (1986). *Monitoring and evaluation in nursing services.* Chicago: Author.

Journal of Nursing Quality Assurance. (1986). Balancing quality and cost, 1(1), entire issue.

Lewis, E. M. (1985). Administrative support. In C. G. Meisenheimer, *Quality assurance: A complete guide to effective programs.* Rockville, Md.: Aspen Systems.

Litwack, L., L. Linc, and D. Bower. (1985). *Evaluation in nursing: Principles and practice.* (Pub. No. 15-1976). New York: National League for Nursing.

Milio, N. (1975). Values, social class and community health services. In A. Cox and A. Mead (eds.), *A sociology of medical practice.* London: Macmillan.

Minnesota Department of Health, Section of Public Health Nursing. (1986). *Outcome criteria for preventive services and home health care.* Rev. ed. Minneapolis: Author.

Mowry, M. M., and R. A. Korpman. (1986). *Managing health care costs, quality and technology.* Rockville, Md.: Aspen Systems.

National League for Nursing. (1980). Criteria for documentation to measure the quality of care in the home health agency. (Pub. No. 21-1306). In National League for Nursing, American Public Health Association, Accreditation of Home Health Agencies and Community Nursing Services, *Criteria and standards manual.* New York: Author.

Nightingale, F. (1860). *Notes on nursing: What it is and what it is not.* New York: D. A. Appleton.

Rezler, A. G., and B. J. Stevens. (1978). *The nurse evaluator in education and service.* New York: McGraw-Hill.

Schmele, J. A. (1985). A method for evaluating nursing practice in a community setting. *Quality Review Bulletin* 11(4): 115–22.

Schroeder, P. S., and R. M. Marbusch. (1984). *Nursing quality assurance: A unit-based approach.* Rockville, Md.: Aspen Systems.

Smith-Marker, C. G. (1988). Practical tools for quality assurance: Criteria development sheet and data retrieval form. *Journal of Nursing Quality Assurance* 2(2): 43–54.

United States Department of Health and Human Services, Public Health Service, Health Services Administration. (1982). *Instruction manual for bureau of community health services common reporting requirements.* Rockville, Md.: Author.

Wandelt, M. A., and D. S. Stewart. (1975). *Slater nursing competencies rating scale.* New York: Appleton-Century-Crofts.

Weed, L. (1970). *Medical records: Medical education and patient care.* Chicago: Year Book Medical Publishers.

While, A. (ed.). (1986). *Research in preventive community nursing care: Fifteen studies in health visiting.* (Wiley Series, vol. 4) Great Britain: John Wiley and Sons.

Whittaker, A., and L. McCanless. (1988). Nursing peer review: Monitoring the appropriateness and outcome of nursing care. *Journal of Nursing Quality Assurance* 2(2): 24–31.

Wyszewianski, L., J. R. C. Wheeler, and A. Donabedian. (1982). Market-oriented cost containment strategies and quality of care. *Milbank Memorial Fund Quarterly/ Health & Science* 60(4): 518–50.

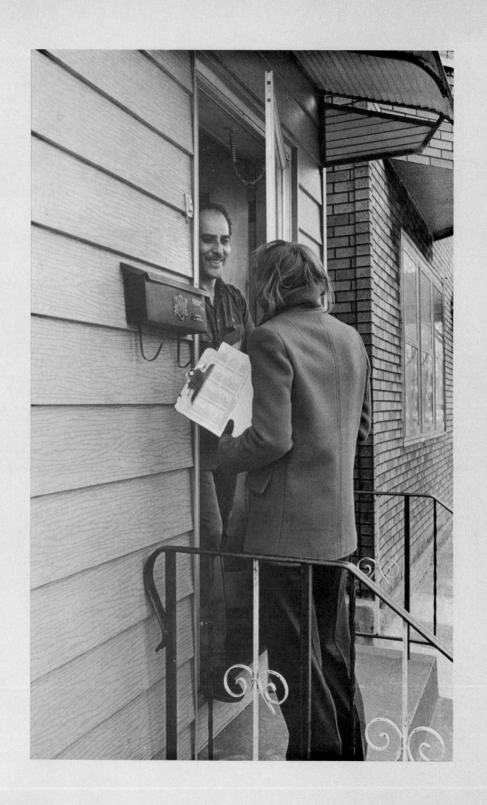

24 Research in Community Health Nursing

Dorothy Brockopp

We can view the nature of clinical practice in community health nursing and therefore the focus for research activities from two vantage points. One view is that community health nursing is nursing practice that occurs outside of an institution and within the community. The direct care provided by the nurse is emphasized and the issues of health maintenance, continuity of care, and disease prevention are in the forefront of practice (deTornyay, 1980). Another view of community health nursing, endorsed in this text, identifies the community itself rather than an individual as the client. This approach to nursing practice requires the community health nurse to identify the boundaries of a given community (boundaries may be based on location or special interests) and develop an understanding of the population within the boundaries. In addition, the nurse may identify a community in terms of its location. Data can then be gathered on the characteristics of the population within the specified boundaries. The nurse may identify subgroups as being at risk for particular health problems, such as individuals who might develop AIDS, teenagers likely to become pregnant, and children at risk for malnutrition. If the community is the client, knowledge regarding all relevant health concerns or potential concerns is necessary for the provision of effective clinical services (Williams, 1988).

Whether the approach to the clinical practice of the community health nurse is described as service provided for individuals and groups within the community, or as practice that focuses on the community as a client, the underlying framework for conducting research remains the same. The community health nurse alone, or in collaboration with colleagues, (1) identifies an area of interest, (2) specifies a research question or statement, (3) reviews the literature, (4) selects a conceptual model, (5) chooses a research design, (6) collects and analyzes data, (7) interprets the results, and (8) communicates the findings. These eight steps make up the research process. Regardless of the focus, conducting research provides an exciting opportunity for community health nurses to examine questions of interest, design effective research projects, and add their findings to a body of nursing knowledge and thereby promote the level of health of at-risk populations.

In this chapter we review the framework for conducting research within the context of community health nursing. Published examples of community health nursing research, as well as ideas generated from clinical practice, are presented within each step of the process.

IDENTIFYING THE AREA OF INTEREST

The unique focus of community health nursing influences the selection of an area of interest. The community health nurse researcher functions within a context that emphasizes disease prevention, wellness, and the active involvement of clients in their care (Figure 24-1). Clients' physical and social environments, as well as their biopsychosocial and spiritual domains, are of major concern. Community health nurses think in terms of the broader community and therefore their research efforts are developed with the needs of the community in mind.

Examples of areas of interest within the community health context include terminal illness among the poor (McGrath, 1986), self-help groups for family-member caregivers of elderly clients (Pesznecker and Zahlis, 1986), funding home care as a means of containing health care costs (Knollmueller, 1984), and self-care activities of clients with breast cancer (Dodd, 1984). In each instance a group within the community has been identified as having particular health care needs. In addition, the likelihood exists that if these needs are not met, the community as a whole could suffer.

The indigent who are terminally ill are at risk of dying without adequate emotional and perhaps physical support. Families who take care of elderly ill individuals may feel considerable stress from the demands created by their situation. The cost of health care is an overriding concern for many groups within society. Various subpopulations within the community would suffer should the cost of providing care escalate beyond society's ability to pay. Individuals diagnosed with breast cancer are vulnerable to a variety of emotional and physiological side effects of their disease.

The impact of these problems on the community is obvious. When the health care needs of the dying, the elderly, and disease-specific groups are not met, the quality of life experienced by the entire community may be at risk. Selecting an area to investigate that can facilitate an improvement in health status for a particular group enhances the existence of the individuals within the group as well as that of the larger community.

A discussion of research interests within community health raises the question, "What is the difference between a research study and an epidemiologic study?" Epidemiology specifically studies the health and illness states of populations. It is a type of research. Community health nursing research

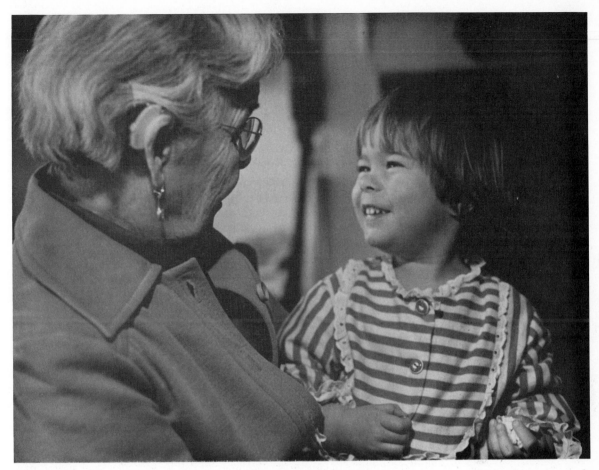

Figure 24-1
The needs of the elderly are an important subject for research. Community
health nurses are particularly interested in identifying health-promoting
activities, such as this joyful visit between grandmother and granddaughter.

may include conducting epidemiologic investigations, and in Chapter 9 we
examine this process in detail. However, a community health research focus
may be broader, extending to questions other than those solely addressed by
epidemiology. These questions are examined in the next section.

SPECIFYING A RESEARCH QUESTION

The area of interest selected for investigation may evolve out of clinical practice or articles in journals, newspapers, or books. For example, newspaper
articles on AIDS may prompt community health nurses to look at the impact

of the disease on their communities. Experiences within clinical practice may motivate nurses to investigate health care administrative issues, environmental concerns such as air quality, or the effectiveness of immunization programs.

After selecting an area of interest, the researcher must next narrow the topic and formulate a specific research question or statement. A carefully formulated research question or statement facilitates the effective completion of a project. For example, the question, "What do women know about early detection of breast cancer?" provides little direction in relation to the remaining steps in the research process. The question, "What is the status of women's knowledge regarding the American Cancer Society's seven recommendations for breast cancer screening?" posed by Fox et al. (1987) gives more specific focus and direction to the research project. The latter question ties knowledge to specific recommendations that form a basis for measurement. Specifying a clear research question provides direction for the investigator and enables the reader to understand the study. Increasingly, nurses are seeking funding for their research, and it is important for them to clearly specify what they want to examine. Funding agencies carefully scrutinize research proposals for their feasibility, value, and use of appropriate methods.

When several community health nurse researchers selected as their area of interest the impact of cancer diagnosis on their community, a number of specific questions surfaced. Questions they addressed included, "What are the cognitive, emotional, and physical needs perceived as important by family members of cancer patients during three phases of illness?" (Tringali, 1985), "Have men in a demographically at-risk population been exposed to the concepts of testicular cancer and testicular self-examination?" (Blesch, 1986), and "What are the cancer-prevention learning needs of parents and their 6th-, 7th-, and 8th-grade children?" (Krohner, McBurney, and Wadelin, 1988).

Each research question identifies the population to be addressed, i.e., family members of cancer patients, men at risk for testicular cancer, and parents and their 6th-, 7th-, and 8th-grade children. In addition, each question describes what is to be measured, i.e., cognitive, emotional, and physical needs, concepts of testicular cancer and testicular self-examination, and cancer prevention learning needs. The specificity of the question assists the reader to understand clearly the focus of the research and also provides direction for investigators.

Taking the group of individuals diagnosed with cancer in any given community, one can focus on many areas of research interest and formulate great numbers of specific questions. What preventive measures might address such areas as nutrition, pollution, and stress? Possible targets for investigation include health maintenance and promotion, educational needs of cancer survivors, and vocational concerns of individuals diagnosed with cancer. The community health nurse's interest in the active involvement of clients in their care could also be explored with this cancer population. How effective are various preventive activities, such as self-examination? What problems surround maintenance activities, such as self-administration of medications?

The formulation of a specific research question or statement generally occurs over time. The initial wording of a question or statement may change considerably as investigators learn more about their topic and work to narrow the field of study. An initial attempt may be refined several times before the final product is achieved.

REVIEWING THE LITERATURE

Community health nurse investigators, having chosen an area of interest for a research project and begun to specify the problem, need to develop an understanding of the previous research in that area. They may have chosen their area of interest as a result of reading a number of studies or because of their clinical experience. In either case, they need to further develop their ideas by reviewing available literature (Figure 24-2).

Reviewing the literature, and thereby developing an in-depth understanding of the topic under consideration, ensures that the research project extends prior knowledge and has a firm theoretical base. Advantages to the investigators include the ability to provide justification for their proposed project and to facilitate the development of their research design. Much can be learned regarding methodology from reading studies already completed.

For example, a study conducted by Whall et al. (1985) was designed to examine a specific problem among the chronically mentally ill who reside in the community. They designed their study to test the feasibility of using non-licensed psychiatric aftercare personnel to monitor clients for symptoms of tardive dyskinesia(TD). Tardive dyskinesia is a syndrome that is characterized by involuntary, repetitive movements of various body parts (tongue, lips, face, extremities) and is associated with prolonged use of medications prescribed in the treatment of mental illness.

The review of the literature reported in this study covers a number of important points. The definition of the syndrome, its accepted association with specific medications, hypotheses regarding the physiology of TD, diagnosis, prevalence rate, possible predisposition, and treatment are described within the context of prior research. Early detection is seen as important to effective treatment, and therefore questions (for research investigation) regarding the monitoring of these clients for symptoms flow from the literature reviewed. Because the individuals live in residential homes, health care professionals cannot monitor these clients on a continuous basis for possible symptoms—thus the interest in training home personnel.

The authors of this article have obviously conducted an in-depth review of the literature. This kind of comprehensive review helps to ensure that the investigators have the basic knowledge necessary to design a successful project. In addition to being comprehensive, the review needs to cover all recent works (from the past five years) and should include any major contributions to the field, regardless of their date of origin.

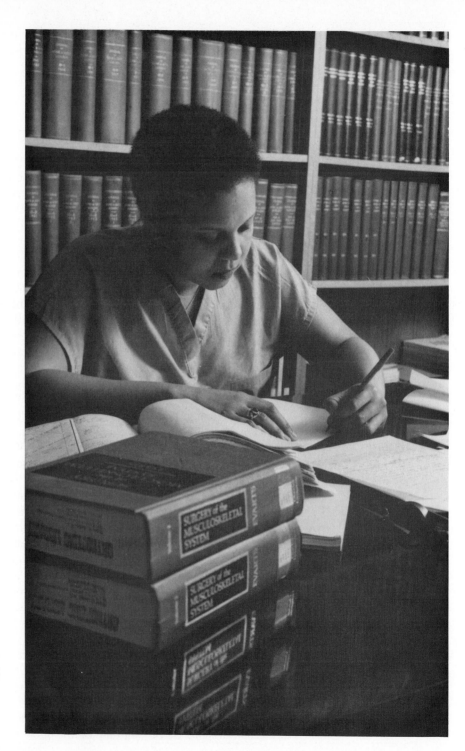

Figure 24-2
After choosing an area
of interest for community
health research, the nurse
must develop the idea
further by reviewing
available literature on
the subject.

SELECTING A CONCEPTUAL MODEL

A conceptual model for a given research topic clarifies the focus of study and helps make sense of the findings. The conceptual context enables investigators to approach the same topic from different perspectives. For example, investigators who attempt to examine the effects of chronic back pain on absenteeism from work may view pain from a physiological perspective or a psychological perspective, or they may use a model that incorporates both psychological and physiological concepts. The perspective or model from which investigators develop their research idea can influence the definitions of their major concerns, the design of their project, and eventually their results.

For example, Morgan and Borden (1985) studied the interaction between public health nurses and perinatal clients during home visits. They chose a symbolic interaction model originated by Mead (1934) to describe their view of interaction. Interaction was seen as a means by which individuals organize and interpret various symbols in their environment. They assessed both verbal and nonverbal behaviors. Another group of investigators could approach the same issue — the interaction of public health nurses and perinatal clients — from a different perspective. They could use a model that emphasized the importance of touch in nurse-client interactions, thereby changing what was measured as well as the results of the study.

CHOOSING A RESEARCH DESIGN

The design of a research project represents the overall plan for carrying out the study. This overall plan guides the conduct of the study and, depending on its effectiveness, can influence investigators' confidence in their results. The major purpose in selecting a particular design is to try to control as much as possible those factors that are not included in the study but can influence the results.

Complete descriptions of various research designs, specific methodologies, and sample selection are available in basic nursing research texts. For the purposes of this chapter, we have identified a few important considerations underlying design selection. Two major categories in terms of design are experimental versus nonexperimental. A requirement of experimental designs is that the investigators "do something" and then measure the consequences of the activity. For example, Lancaster et al. (1986) designed a project to measure the effects of three different approaches used to assist individuals to stop smoking. These three approaches constituted the "doing something" of the experimental design. The effects of these approaches were then measured.

Community health nurses could evaluate the effects of interventions designed to encourage a variety of health-promoting behaviors. Such interventions might include educational programs that would support home-care activities, assist teenage mothers to care for their children, and enhance compliance to medical regimens. In each of these instances an activity is designed, carried out, and its effectiveness measured.

Another important distinction exists within the experimental category of research. There are true experiments and quasi-experiments. The true experiment is characterized by "doing something" (manipulating one of the variables), assigning subjects to groups in a specific manner (randomization), and by comparing one group of subjects who experience the manipulation to another group that does not (the use of a control group). The quasi-experimental design lacks either the randomization of subjects or the formation of a control group. Community health nurses conduct quasi-experiments more often than true experiments because it is often difficult (sometimes impossible) to provide a treatment for only one-half of a group and/or to randomize subjects. An important ethical consideration is to protect human rights while conducting research. Nurses must inform subjects of the research protocol and obtain their consent to participate.

Community health nurses frequently use nonexperimental research designs. Examples of this approach could include examining the relationship between sex and smoking behaviors among adolescents, describing the emotional needs of families of clients with AIDS, or determining the attitudes of parents in a given community toward sex education in the schools. In each of these instances the focus of the research would be on the relationships observed or the description of what exists.

Nonexperimental designs are often the precursors of experiments. For example, King and Winett (1986) designed a study to describe the levels and sources of stress among working women. They compared career women (university faculty and non-academic professionals) and working women (clerical workers, office personnel). In this study a description of the levels and sources of stress found in these two groups permitted the investigators to make suggestions regarding appropriate interventions for dealing with stress. Others could then design experimental or quasi-experimental studies to test the effect of the intervention.

COLLECTING AND ANALYZING DATA

The value of the data collected in a given research project largely depends on the care taken to apply and measure the concepts (variables) of concern. For example, investigators examining the attitudes of hypertensive men toward a specific weight-loss program would need to define what is meant by attitudes, how attitudes are measured, who a hypertensive man is, and how blood pressure levels, age, ethnic backgrounds, and the like are used to define this population. If considerable attention is not paid to clearly defining the variables involved in the study and to the accurate measurement of those variables, the results of the study may have little meaning.

Similarly, the accuracy of the measuring instrument used can affect the value of the results of a study. Some evidence that an instrument measures what it is supposed to measure (validity) and is consistent in its measurement of a given concept within a particular population (reliability) is necessary to ensure meaningful results. Instruments may be designed by the investigators, or pre-tested instruments may be used.

Dawkins et al. (1988) examined health orientations, beliefs, and use of health services among minority, high-risk expectant mothers. They developed their own instruments and pre-tested them in a pilot study. De Von and Powers (1984) examined the health beliefs and psychosocial adjustment to illness among clients with hypertension. They used instruments to measure compliance and psychosocial adjustment to illness that had been designed and tested by other investigators. Both approaches to measuring the variables of interest are acceptable; however, using available instruments of known reliability and validity saves considerable time. Unfortunately, within the area of nursing research, instruments appropriate to the measurement of nursing concepts often are unavailable.

The actual collection of data can involve methods of self-reporting, observation, physiological assessment, or document analysis (Figure 24-3). For example, investigators examining the stress level of the caregiver when a family member chooses to die at home might (1) design or use an existing paper-and-pencil questionnaire or interview schedule (self-report), (2) outline a schema for observing caregivers as they function in the home (observation), (3) measure various physiological indicators of stress (physiological assess-

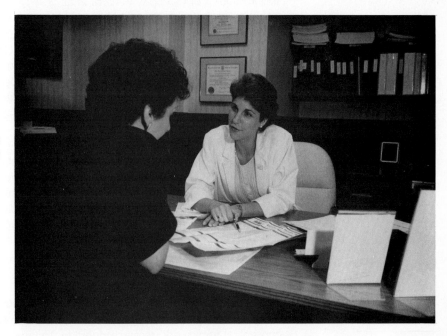

Figure 24-3
Gathering data on issues related to preventing illness is an important feature of community health nursing research. Here, an HMO nurse collects information from a client. HMOs maintain a broad data base on healthy clients, and such information can be useful in research related to illness prevention.

ment), or (4) analyze the diaries kept by caregivers in an attempt to identify their levels of stress (document analysis). In most instances the nature of the data to be collected dictates the best method of collection. One or more methods will be more appropriate, given the topic of concern.

Once collected, data must be analyzed so that meaningful interpretation can be made. Statistical procedures simply reduce great amounts of information to smaller chunks that can be easily interpreted. When deciding on an appropriate statistical procedure, it is helpful to consider the two major categories of statistical analysis: descriptive and inferential statistics.

Descriptive statistics do what the title suggests. They describe in an organized fashion the data collected. Calculating the average number or mean of a particular set of occurrences or its frequency are two examples of descriptive statistics. Rudman and Steinhardt (1988) in their study on fitness in the workplace reported the percentages of employees who would be willing to pay to participate in a health and fitness program. Fox et al. (1987), in their study on the status of women's knowledge regarding breast cancer screening, reported that 58 percent of the women had accurate information regarding the correct age for a baseline mammogram, 46 percent understood the recommendation regarding the frequency of mammograms between 40 and 49, and only 34 percent knew that women over 50 should have annual mammograms. These investigators used a statistical procedure designed to describe the data they collected.

Inferential statistics are used to imply that relationships seen in the group of individuals studied (sample) are likely to exist in the larger group of concern (population). For example, Ventura et al. (1984) were interested in whether or not an intervention designed to improve foot-care habits, reduce smoking, and increase exercise would reduce the number of peripheral-vascular-disease-related illnesses within this particular population. One group of clients experienced the intervention, and the other group did not. Using inferential statistical procedures, researchers found a difference between the groups in terms of their exercise levels. The groups of clients who experienced the intervention were more likely to maintain their usual exercise behaviors or to increase them than were subjects in the control group.

The specific descriptive and inferential techniques used to analyze data can be found in a variety of basic research and statistics texts. Regardless of the procedure used, descriptive techniques provide an overall picture of results. Inferential techniques permit investigators to identify the likelihood that the relationship(s) found are real and that they can be replicated with other samples taken from the same population.

INTERPRETING RESULTS

The explanation of the findings of a study flows from the previously formulated research plan. Findings need to make sense in relation to the identified conceptual framework, research question, literature review, and methodology.

When findings support the directions developed in the research plan, their interpretation is relatively straightforward. For example, a group of community health nurse investigators might design a study to determine the effect of parenting classes on the self-esteem of single welfare mothers between the ages of 21 and 35. They could use Coopersmith's (1967) ideas on self-esteem as their conceptual model, hypothesize that self-esteem will improve as a result of the classes, and design an experiment to test their idea. If self-esteem does in fact increase, their finding flows logically from their framework.

If the findings do not support the hypothesis of the study, investigators question various aspects of the research in order to develop an explanation. In this instance a number of questions could be posed. Coopersmith related feelings of success in an endeavor to self-esteem. Can that position be inaccurate? Could the parenting classes have been ineffective? Perhaps they did not enhance feelings of success. Were there problems with the methodology used — perhaps too few subjects, or intervening occurrences that affected the results? All of these questions and more could be considered in an attempt to explain the results.

If the study is descriptive in nature, i.e., one that was designed to describe particular characteristics of a population, the direction of the findings is not a concern. A detailed, accurate report of the results and their implications is appropriate. Given either an experimental or descriptive design, the importance of accuracy cannot be overemphasized. Leaps of faith when reporting the results of a study are not desirable unless labeled as such. One could not conclude, for example, from the study on the parenting classes that these classes develop expert parenting skills, given that parenting skills were not assessed.

A valuable contribution can be made to the advancement of nursing knowledge when investigators use their results to make suggestions for future research. The investigators' knowledge of a particular area and their experience in conducting a specific study give them an excellent background for identifying future research possibilities.

COMMUNICATING FINDINGS

Community health nurse investigators may want or be required to communicate their findings in a variety of ways. There is little purpose in conducting research if the results are not communicated in some fashion to interested colleagues (Figure 24-4). Detailed reports may be required by funding agencies. Papers may be accepted for presentation at conferences. Articles may be written for nursing journals. In each case guidelines are available to assist researchers to appropriately communicate their results.

In terms of both journals and conferences, community health nurses can select on the basis of their specialty or the specific area under investigation. For example, a study examining risk factors associated with cancer might be accepted for publication in *Public Health Nursing* or in the *Oncology Nursing Forum*. Similarly, presentations at conferences can be selected in relation to

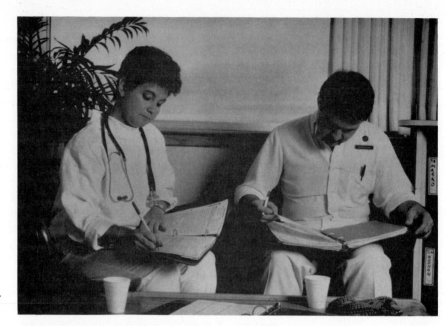

Figure 24-4
Community health nurses
may collaborate with
physicians to study health
problems. Here the nurse
(on the right) and the doctor
discuss client records.

the specialty area or the topic of concern. Community health nurses also have a responsibility to evaluate existing research reports. To do so builds a knowledge base for enhancing clinical practice and generates new questions for further research.

Summary

Involvement in community health nursing research can be an exciting opportunity to enhance a variety of skills and add to a body of nursing knowledge. It also provides community health nurses with an opportunity to promote health and prevent illness among at-risk populations. The basic research process includes the following eight steps: (1) identify an area of interest, (2) specify a research question or statement, (3) review the literature, (4) select a conceptual framework, (5) choose a research design, (6) collect and analyze data, (7) interpret the results, and (8) communicate the findings. While the process is the same regardless of nursing specialty, community health nurses have a unique opportunity to expand nursing knowledge in relation to the structure and functioning of communities. The steps described in this chapter provide an overview for nurses interested in applying the research process to community health issues.

Study Questions

1. You notice a group of small children playing in a vacant, unfenced lot bordered by a busy street. List three research questions you might consider using to study the situation.

2. You want to determine whether a group of sexually active teenagers who are at risk of AIDS would be receptive to an educational program on AIDS. Describe a conceptual framework you might use in your study and defend your choice.

3. Assume you have just completed a study on the effectiveness of a series of birth control classes in three high schools. Your results show a reduction in the number of pregnancies over last year. Name three nursing journals to which you might submit an article on your study findings. Get the name and address of the journal's editor and obtain the journal's instructions for publication.

References

Blesch, K. S. (1986). Health beliefs about testicular cancer and self-examination among professional men. *Oncology Nursing Forum* 13(1): 29–33.

Coopersmith, S. (1967). *The antecedents of self-esteem.* San Francisco: W. H. Freeman & Company.

Dawkins, C., N. Ervin, L. Weissfield, and A. Yan. (1988). Health orientation, beliefs, and use of health services among minority, high-risk expectant mothers. *Public Health Nursing* 5(1): 7–11.

deTornyay, R. (1980). Public health nursing: The nurse's role in community-based practice. *Ann. Rev. Public Health* 1: 83–94.

DeVon, H. A., and M. J. Powers. (1984). Health beliefs, adjustment to illness, and control of hypertension. *Research in Nursing and Health* 7(1): 10–16.

Dodd, M. (1984). Self-care for patients with breast cancer to prevent side effects of chemotherapy: A concern for public health nursing. *Public Health Nursing* 4: 202–9.

Fox, S., D. Klos, C. Tsou, and J. Baum. (1987). Breast cancer screening recommendations: Current status of women's knowledge. *Family and Community Health* 10(3): 39–50.

King, A., and R. Winett. (1986). Tailoring stress-reduction strategies to populations at risk: Comparisons between women from dual-career and dual-worker families. *Family and Community Health* 9(3): 42–50.

Knollmueller, R. (1984). Funding home care in a climate of cost containment. *Public Health Nursing* 1(1): 16–22.

Krohner, K. M., B. H. McBurney, and J. W. Wadelin. (1988). Assessing cancer prevention learning needs of parents and their 6th-, 7th-, and 8th-grade children. *Oncology Nursing Forum* 15(1): 59–64.

Lancaster, J., K. Ellison, G. Myers, and J. Van Matre. (1986). Evaluation of freedom from smoking among Alabama residents. *Family and Community Health* 8(4): 36–47.

McGrath, B. B. (1986). The social networks of terminally ill skid road residents: An analysis. *Public Health Nursing* 3(3): 192–205.

Mead, G. H. (1934). *Mind, self, and society.* Chicago: University of Chicago Press.

Morgan, B., and M. Borden. (1985). Nurse-patient interaction in the home setting. *Public Health Nursing* 2(3): 159–67.

Pesznecker, B., and E. Zahlis. (1986). Establishing mutual-help groups for family-member caregivers: A new role for community health nurses. *Public Health Nursing* 3(1): 29–37.

Rudman, W., and M. Steinhardt. (1988). Fitness in the workplace. The effects of a corporate health and fitness program on work culture. *Health Values: Achieving High-Level Wellness* 12(2): 4–17.

Tringali, C. A. (1985). The needs of family members of cancer patients. *Oncology Nursing Forum* 13(4): 65–70.

Ventura, M., D. Young, M. Feldman, P. Pastore, S. Pikula, and M. Yates. (1983). Effectiveness of health promotion interventions. *Nursing Research* 33(3): 162–67.

Whall, A., V. Engle, J. Floyd, and J. Agers. (1985). Monitoring for tardive dyskinesia: A community-based approach. *Public Health Nursing* 2(3): 168–77.

Williams, C. (1988). Population-focused practice: The basis of specialization in public health nursing. In M. Stanhope and J. Lancaster (eds.), *Community health nursing process and practice for promoting health.* St. Louis: Mosby.

Selected Readings

Amos, L. K. (1985). Influencing the future of nursing research through power and politics. *Community Nursing Research* (Fall) 18: 1–14.

Arnold, J. M., et al. (1986). Belief systems which influence research in nursing: Implications for preparing future investigators. *Journal of Nursing Education* 25(8): 325–27.

Brett, J. (1987). Use of nursing practice research findings. *Nursing Research* 36(6): 344–49.

Brockopp, D., and M. Hastings-Tolsma. (1988). *Fundamentals of nursing research,* Boston: Little, Brown.

Brunt, J. H. (1985). Nursing research and philosophy: A delicate balance. *Nursing Forum* 22(1): 19–21.

Carper, B. (1978). Fundamental patterns of knowing in nursing. *Advances in Nursing Science* 1(1)(Oct.): 13–23.

Carr, A. M. (1988). Development of public health nursing literature. *Public Health Nursing* 5(2): 81–85.

Closs, J. (1987). Research issues: Biological science and nurses. *Senior Nurse* 7(5): 45.

Crane, J. (1985). Using research in practice: Research utilization—nursing models. *Western Journal of Nursing Research* 7(4): 494–97.

Davis, A. J. (1987). Ethical issues in nursing research . . . . international nursing research. *Western Journal of Nursing Research* 9(3): 400–402.

Diekelmann, N. (1986). Why research in nursing education? *Nurse Educator* 11(1): 4–5.

Duffy, M. (1985). A research appraisal checklist for evaluating nursing research reports. *Nursing and Health Care* 6(10)(Dec.) 538–47.

Duffy, M. (1986). Qualitative research: An approach whose time has come. *Nursing and Health Care* 7(5): 237–39.

Duffy, M. (1988). Health promotion in the family: Current findings and directives for nursing research. *Journal of Advanced Nursing* 13(1): 109–17.

Fontes, H. (1986). Stratifying research curricula—The logical next step. *Nursing and Health Care* 7(6): 293–95.

Gortner, S. (1983). The history and philosophy of nursing science and research. *Advances in Nursing Science* 5(2)(Jan.): 1–8.

Hashings-Tolsma, M. T., et al. (1986). Stimulating research: A sensory model. *Western Journal of Nursing Research* 8(2): 197–205.

Hinshaw, A. S. (1988). Using research to shape health policy. *Nursing Outlook* 36(1): 21–24.

Hodson, K. E. (1986). Research in nursing education and practice: The ecological methods perspective. *Western Journal of Nursing Research* 8(1): 33–48.

Hollander, R. B., et al. (1986). Health education research in the workplace. *Health Education* 17(3): 34–37.

Keane, A., et al. (1986). Industry and nursing research: A compatible couple? *Nursing Economics* 4(3): 128–30.

Larson, E. (1986). Guidelines for collaborative research with industry. *Nursing Economics* 4(3): 131–33.

Lindaman, C. (1984). Dissemination of nursing research. *Image: The Journal of Nursing Scholarship* 16(2)(Spring): 57–58.

Martin, K. (1988). Research in home care. *Nursing Clinics of North America* 23(2): 373–85.

McKechnie, M., et al. (1985). Developing research skills in occupational health nursing: Where to begin? *Occupational Health Nursing* 33(10): 515–16.

Morris, J. M. (1985). Descriptive study of the practice of community health nurses with infants at risk for developmental disabilities. *Journal of Community Health Nursing* 2(1): 53–60.

Myers, A. H., et al. (1987). Smoking behavior among participants in the Nurses' Health Study. *American Journal of Public Health* 77(5): 628–30.

Oda, D., J. Fine, and D. Heilbron. (1986). Impact and cost of public health nurse telephone follow-up of school dental referrals. *American Journal of Public Health* 76(11): 1348–49.

Rogers, B. (1985). Developing research skills in occupational health nursing: Where to begin? *Occupational Health Nursing* 33(10)(Oct.): 515–16.

Roncoll, M., et al. (1988). Nursing research: What it costs and who will pay. *Nursing and Health Care* 9(2): 76–80.

Ross, F. (1985). Uneasy bedfellows... district nursing and research. *Nursing Times* 81(44): 38–39.

Smith, M., and P. Horns. (1987). The future for research. *Nursing and Health Care* (Jan.): 22–25.

Sorofman, B. (1986). Research in cultural diversity: Defining diversity. *Western Journal of Nursing Research* 8(1): 121–23.

Stern, P. N., et al. (1985). Using grounded theory methodology to study women's culturally based decisions about health. *Health Care Women International* 6(1): 1–24.

Swanson, E., and J. McCloskey. (1986). Publishing opportunities for nurses. *Nursing Outlook* 34(5)(Sept.–Oct.): 227–35.

Wilson, H. (1987). *Introducing research in nursing.* Menlo Park, Calif.: Addison-Wesley.

Windsor, R. A., et al. (1986). Guidelines and methodological standards for smoking cessation intervention research among pregnant women: Improving the science and art. *Health Education Quarterly* 13(2): 131–61.

Young-Graham, K. (1986). Research cuts breed new challenges for public health nursing. *Public Health Nursing* 3(2): 69–70.

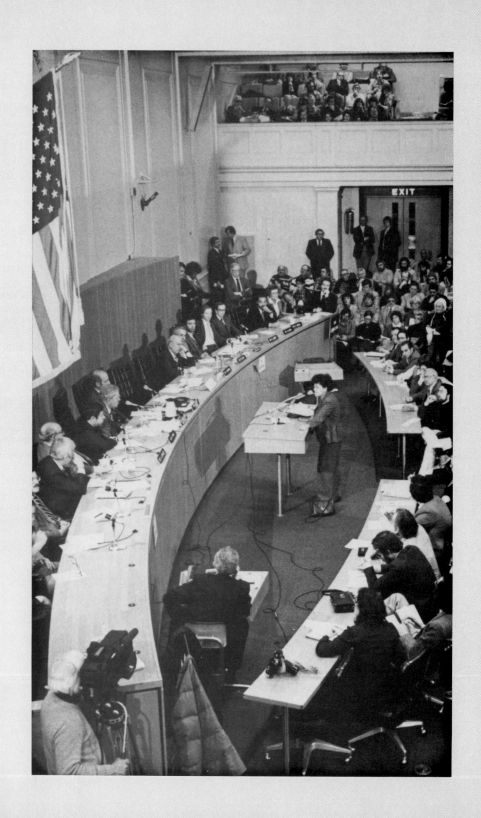

25 Political Involvement and Community Health Advocacy

Terry W. Miller

Community health nursing has undergone many changes since its inception in the late 1880s, and so has health policy. Historically, and dangerously, nurses have placed blind trust in other health care providers, such as physicians, insurance companies, and politicians, to develop, regulate, and finance the U.S. health care system. Behind all legislation and health care regulation are power struggles. The outcomes determine the availability and quality of all social services. To a great extent, health policy and nursing practice rest upon legislative action at the state and federal levels. Many people, even a health care bill's originator, are unaware of a bill's total impact on health care. In other words, the intent of a policy is not always its actual outcome. Consultation with nurses and other important implementers of the policy may not be considered. Clearly, nurses need to develop an operational knowledge of health policy and political process in order to protect individuals, families, communities, and nursing practice.

In this chapter we will examine health policy and the political process as they relate to community health nursing. The aim is not to isolate or differentiate community health nursing from other health professions or even other nursing specialties. The purpose is to emphasize the need for community health nurses to understand their role and power in providing an essential influence and unique perspective in health care.

WHAT IS POLICY?

Many definitions of social or public policy have been proposed in recent years as the study of policy has become a more formalized and highly funded academic field. Many of the most respected universities in the country support schools of public affairs. Nursing's representation in such schools has been minimal. These schools arose out of need and demonstrate the relevancy, as well as the complexity, of understanding policy and political process today.

Basically, policy is what an institution, organization, agency, or government chooses to do or not to do. Policy can (and should) be written, formally, but many policies are unwritten, unclear, or "hidden" to prevent public or legal review. Either way, policy includes all actions of an institution, organization, agency, or government. Government policy, whether the government is local, state, or federal, is public policy (Dye, 1978).

More specifically, health policy pertains to the deliberative allocations of resources to health care. Resources include people, facilities, time, and money. To see health policy only from an economic perspective is a mistake. Not to consider the costs of health care is a greater mistake, as the outcry of the public, followed by politicians, demonstrates. Policy usually begins as health laws but may be secondary to other types of legislation. For instance, military policy on nuclear defense affects health policy, whether intentionally or not. Since resources are limited, distribution in one area affects or determines the availability of resources in another area.

Most policies are created to express the collective interests and beliefs of the social system or institution that generates them. Unfortunately, many people within a social system or institution allow others to determine policy for them instead of with them (Litman and Robins, 1984). Community health nurses' primary mission is to promote and preserve the health of aggregates or populations. In order to fulfill this mission, nurses should be policymakers, as well as policy followers (Courtney, 1987). Even within the profession, some nurses lack the vision to promote community health. They define the client as an individual patient and nothing more.

Various health policies can be categorized by their social impact or outcomes. *Distributive* health policies promote nongovernmental activities thought to be beneficial to society as a whole. Title VIII, the Nurse Training Act, of the Public Health Service Act is such a distributive policy. It establishes a federal subsidy for nursing education. *Redistributive* health policy changes the allocation of resources from one group to usually a broader or different group. Medicare illustrates this type of redistributive policy. *Competitive* regulation through health policy limits or structures the provision of health services by designating who can deliver them. Nurse licensure is a form of such regulation at state level. Protective regulation sets conditions under which various private activities can be undertaken. Although professional licensure is most commonly identified by professions as first and foremost protecting the public, such policy is competitive regulation in terms of its social impact. Professional standards review organizations or certificates of need are more clearly defined as protective regulation.

Health policy comes from many sources. On the surface it appears to emanate from the government, but in reality, policymakers take their cues from many sources. Community health nurses should be one of the major sources of influence (Courtney, 1987), even though many strong and well-organized forces resist nursing's direct involvement in the politics and policy-making of health care.

POLICY SYSTEMS AND POLICY ANALYSIS

All people are political creatures in the sense that they live within the context of many political systems. The more obvious political systems are the state and federal governments. The political system within a community may be less formalized or apparent but also has a profound influence on the collective health and well-being of community residents.

Political systems, such as city and county governments, are interrelated and complex, and they generate policies. Therefore, they are also policy systems. A community health nurse needs a simple policy analysis framework for determining the intentions and possible capacity of political and policy systems. This framework allows the nurse to protect herself and, most important, to protect the client, whether it be a community or individual.

Policy analysis is the systematic identification of causes or consequences of policy and the factors that influence it (Litman and Robins, 1984). Often nurses confuse policy advocacy with policy analysis. This mistake can be detrimental in community health nursing. Policy advocacy is subjective; policy analysis should be objective. What is most important is that policy analysis should come before policy advocacy.

Nurses can take several approaches when looking at a policy, such as mandatory preschool immunizations, that affects the health of a community or target population. They can look at the reasons for policy formulation, the groups of people affected by the policy, or the policy's possible long-range consequences. Focusing on the policy's consequences makes the policy an independent variable and the social, economic, or political conditions in the community dependent variables. This impact approach to policy analysis produces two general questions to be answered: (1) Who benefits from this policy? and (2) Who loses from this policy? Whether or not the policy should be advocated by the community as a whole depends upon the degree to which the policy benefits the community without being detrimental to individuals or the country.

Figure 25-1 provides a simple model for studying health policy. If nurses know something about the forces shaping health policy and the policy process, then they are in a better position to influence policy outcomes. The model identifies four major stages in the policy process: formulation, adoption, implementation, and evaluation. Policy formulation has to do with identifying goals, problems, and potential solutions. Policy adoption refers to the authorized selection and specification of means to achieve goals, resolve problems, or both. Implementation follows adoption and occurs when the policy is put to use. Policy evaluation means comparing policy outcomes or effects with the intended or desired effects.

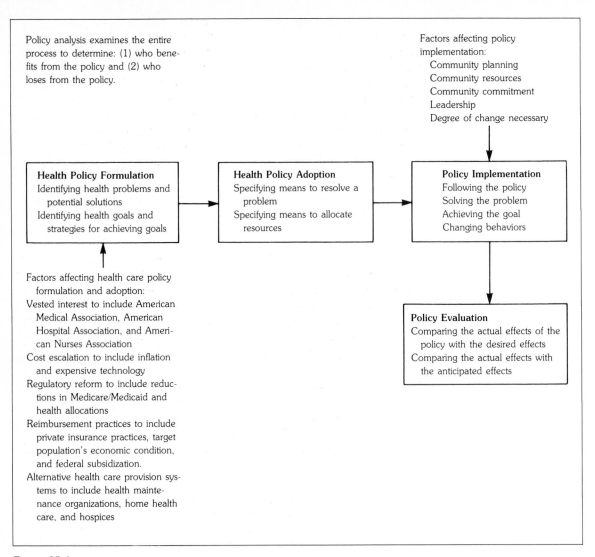

Policy analysis examines the entire process to determine: (1) who benefits from the policy and (2) who loses from the policy.

Factors affecting policy implementation:
 Community planning
 Community resources
 Community commitment
 Leadership
 Degree of change necessary

Health Policy Formulation
Identifying health problems and potential solutions
Identifying health goals and strategies for achieving goals

Health Policy Adoption
Specifying means to resolve a problem
Specifying means to allocate resources

Policy Implementation
Following the policy
Solving the problem
Achieving the goal
Changing behaviors

Factors affecting health care policy formulation and adoption:
Vested interest to include American Medical Association, American Hospital Association, and American Nurses Association
Cost escalation to include inflation and expensive technology
Regulatory reform to include reductions in Medicare/Medicaid and health allocations
Reimbursement practices to include private insurance practices, target population's economic condition, and federal subsidization.
Alternative health care provision systems to include health maintenance organizations, home health care, and hospices

Policy Evaluation
Comparing the actual effects of the policy with the desired effects
Comparing the actual effects with the anticipated effects

Figure 25-1
Policy analysis model.

Policy Formulation and Adoption

Health policy formulation is the stage at which a policy is conceptualized and ultimately defined. It is approached in at least two ways. Most commonly, a health problem is identified, such as the increased infant mortality rate associated with teenage pregnancy. Health policy is developed to correct the particular health problem. Another approach to policy formulation emphasizes health planning more than corrective actions, at least initially. Health goals and strategies for achieving the goals are identified. In this more proactive approach, resources may be created as well as allocated for health services. Whereas both approaches to policy formulation may lead to the solution of a health problem, the goal-oriented approach is less reactive in that it does not require problem identification before the making of health policy.

The social and political conditions that affect policy formulation are limitless, but public need and public demand should be the strongest influences (Hancock et al., 1985). Health care providers can stimulate a community to identify its health needs and demand health policies to fufill its needs. During this process the community health nurse recognizes that each community is unique, with its own mix of health services and public expectations.

Today there are increasing demands for better quality health services, better access to health services, better cost control of health services, and more health services. Expensive technologies, consumer naïveté, and reimbursement procedures that reward inefficiency while disassociating care from actual costs, hinder the fulfillment of these demands. Americans have grown to believe that health care is a basic human right, and nursing has supported this belief. But Americans are no longer capable nor willing to pay for the present system with its rapidly escalating costs. Indeed, health care is undergoing a metamorphosis.

What should be the role of community health nurses in policy formulation? All professions face the continuing problem of making their knowledge useful to society (Dye, 1978). Community health nursing, as does all of nursing, faces the challenge of determining its appropriate relationship with the government. In this determination there are certain requirements to be met.

Community health nurses are community advocates. Their role is to increase the community's health awareness and to support the community's decisions regarding health policies (Courtney, 1987). This recognition of a community's rights in determining its health policies inherently involves conflict. Nurses as decision makers are often under pressure to define specific goals, delegate or implement actions to achieve these goals, and even to establish controls to see that a community moves toward these goals. Sometimes specific health goals prove elusive or they have no validity save that they are agreed upon. One thing is certain: the goals, constraints, and consequences of actions are seldom known precisely at a community level.

Policy Implementation

Implementation of health policy occurs when an individual, group, or community puts the policy into use. It involves overt behavior changes as the policy is put into nursing practice. The degree and extent of compliance with a policy is the most direct measure of the policy's implementation (Sabatier and Mazmanian, 1981). Non-compliance refers to conscious or unconscious refusal to follow the policy directives. Community health nurses have always been health policy implementers and, recently, evaluators, regardless of whether or not these roles were consciously chosen.

Implementation of health policy is an essential part of effective, comprehensive client care for many documentable reasons. It should now be apparent that policies come in many forms and may have statutory or nonstatutory origins. Nurses are most cognizant of the latter in the form of procedure manuals and institutional guidelines. Communities are most aware of policies that limit or restructure their activities and growth, such as curfews and zoning regulations.

Once a health policy is written and adopted, its successful implementation depends heavily upon the manipulation of many variables. For example, the implementation of day-care standards depends, in part, on how they are interpreted and what resources are available to enforce them. The community health nurse as an implementer assesses the capacity of the community to formulate and define strategies that will enhance the community's compliance with the policy. This phase of policy analysis does not focus on the merits or shortcomings of the policy as is done in policy formulation, adoption, and evaluation.

Policy Evaluation

Comparing what a health policy does with what it is supposed to do is evaluation. Evaluation of a policy should result in continuance of the policy in its original form, revision or modification of the policy, or termination of the policy. Laws and policies are created to express the collective and powerful interests of the political system that generated them (Litman and Robins, 1984). The need for a particular health policy may be temporary, but a policy is difficult to change once adopted and implemented. Once a policy system is in operation, vested interests evolve as a result and become political influences. These vested interests under the guise of jobs, positions, titles, and wealth are perceptibly jeopardized by any change in the health policy that helped create them. Hence, tradition or old policies tend to prevail.

Regardless of the factors that affect policy evaluation, continual comparison of what a community believes about and wants in health care with what it is getting is necessary. As community advocates, nurses have a responsibility to increase community awareness of health issues. They help the community make sure that its health needs are met through productive, desirable health policies.

Perhaps the major premise that should underlie policy evaluation is that the goal of health policy is to design a system whereby health services are equitably distributed and appropriate care is given to the right people at a reasonable cost (Donley, 1982). This premise leads to the following basic criteria for evaluation:

1. Are the health services appropriate?
2. Are the health services accessible?
3. Are the health services comprehensive?
4. Is there continuity of care?
5. Is the quality of the services adequate?

6. Is the efficiency of the services adequate?
7. Is there an ongoing evaluation of the services?
8. Is appropriate action taken based on the findings of the evaluation?

DETERMINING A COMMUNITY'S HEALTH POLICY NEEDS

It is essential that the community health nurse take an active role in determining a community's health policy needs. The nurse serves as a facilitator in assessing the community's unique health care needs in relation to its existing health care policies. Legislation and policy must be reviewed from the community's viewpoint, as opposed to an individual's viewpoint (Williams, 1983). Both public health efforts and community health systems are confronted with conflicting interests when individual rights interfere with aggregate rights. However, the community health nurse's primary mission is to promote and preserve the health of populations or aggregates for the benefit of the entire community.

To identify the health policy needs of a community requires an ongoing comprehensive assessment of the community, or what some policy analysts call a "community diagnosis." In Chapter 13 we identified the dimensions or variables of a community that are important in making a community assessment. Public opinion polls sometimes provide data for policy formulation but should be examined carefully to avoid biased research design. Two polls on smoking, one in Michigan and the other in Los Angeles, were countered when flawed design influenced by tobacco interests was discovered (Perlstadt and Holmes, 1987).

STEPS IN COMMUNITY ORGANIZATION FOR POLITICAL ACTION

Organizing a particular community for political action involves taking the following steps:

1. *As the community health nurse, identify yourself as a potential community organizer.* In this beginning step, nurses must perform a self-assessment in terms of what they have to offer the community.
2. *Identify problems, concerns, and issues.* This information should come from the community's perspective, not merely that of individuals. Such information may be obtained directly by conducting a survey in the community and indirectly by looking at vital statistics, voting practices, and the life-style of the community.
3. *Assess the physical community.* Physical environment can have a significant influence on a community. Characteristics of the setting in which a population lives set the stage for particular health problems

and practices. Information about the physical environment can be obtained from a variety of resources (*see* Chapter 13).

4. *Assess community strengths, resources, and interests.* This information is an important indicator of the community's health potential and ability to organize for political action. In this step, the nurse identifies community skills and assesses community strengths and limitations.

5. *Assess political influences in the community.* Each community has its own power base and political structure. The community health nurse must understand that power is an essential and primary concept inherent to all political and policy systems (Kalisch and Kalisch, 1982). Power is perceived as a limited entity and therefore is not given freely, even when "deserved" or "earned." Historically, the four most powerful health interest groups have been physicians, hospitals, insurance companies, and the drug industry (Lee, Estes, and Ramsey, 1984). Gaining knowledge of community political systems enables the nurse to identify key people and operations that are essential to the successful implementation of health goals. The community health perspective has a political advantage in terms of votes if the community is clearly defined and can be unified on a particular health issue.

6. *Evaluate alternative courses of action.* Community decision making is facilitated when the community is well informed. The nurse can play an important role in the decision-making process by helping to identify possible outcomes and alternative courses of action to meet health goals. Each community, as well as each individual, is different in its perspective of a situation. Decision making will be influenced by the impact the decision can have on the social systems of the community.

7. *Redefine objectives, priorities, and the community health nurse's goals.* After a careful assessment of the community's needs, the community health nurse must compare the relationship between existing programs and policies as they relate to the defined needs and goals. If an incongruent relationship does exist, plans must be made to redefine and reshape existing and future policy directions.

8. *Develop a plan of action.* Planning for an entire community requires the nurse to collaborate with other professionals and representatives of the community's social systems (Figure 25-2). Each member of the planning team is considered an equal resource, and each member's input is vital to the successful implementation of the plan.

9. *Implement the plan.* Implementation of a plan requires several important considerations: involvement by representatives of the population to be affected, proper timing, and preparedness.

10. *Evaluate the outcome of the planned action.* Evaluation of a plan or program requires analyzing the observed outcomes based on the specific goals, objectives, and criteria that were adopted. Evaluation should be a continuous process that guides decision making for the future.

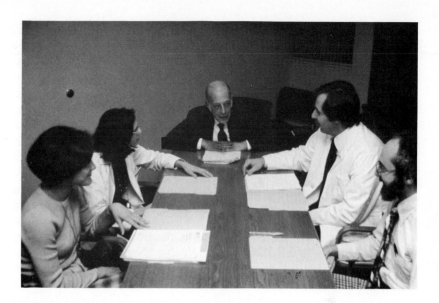

Figure 25-2
This group of professionals is meeting to accomplish a health planning task.

THE LEGISLATIVE PROCESS AND INFLUENCING LEGISLATION

Theoretically, at the local level health policies are guidelines for the implementation of health laws. A community's policy system exerts its control in distributing its health resources through its health policies. Sometimes nurses and clients come to think of policies as statutes and therefore as difficult to change as law. In reality, community health policies are often an interpretation of health laws and at best serve as a strategy for implementing health laws, whether they be state or federal.

The nurse's role as an indirect care provider includes active involvement in the community's political arena (Bagwell and Clements, 1985). Nurses particularly have a responsibility to generate new ways of providing health care and to modify or improve existing health care (Kalisch and Kalisch, 1982). In order to influence and initiate changes in the health care system, the nurse needs to know about the legislative process. The nurse also needs to know how to influence the passage of legislation or modify existing legislation (Williams, 1983). These skills are essential for all professional nurses because they are major ways that nurses can provide leadership in the improvement of health care.

HOW A BILL BECOMES LAW

In the United States, all nurses have opportunities to provide input on the initiation, formulation, and revision of legislation at the local, state, and federal levels. Proposed drafts of bills originate from many places because the sources of legislative ideas are relatively unlimited. An idea may be forwarded to a legislator by individuals, groups, government agencies, or other interested parties. The process can be initiated when a concerned citizen or group writes or talks to a legislator.

The legislative process is well defined and governed by rules at all levels of government (U.S. House of Representatives, 1981). The process is similar at the state and federal levels, with the exception of some minor peculiarities. Public libraries have copies of a state's legislative process, or the nurse may write to the state's printing office for information.

There is a requirement that certain types of federal bills be started in the House of Representatives, as opposed to the Senate. This may not be true at the state level, depending upon the particular state's constitution. Once a senator or representative is found who is willing to author a bill, discussion takes place about what current law needs changing or what needs to be added to existing laws. When authoring a bill, a senator or representative consults with a legislative council. This council consists of legal specialists who assist legislators with the drafting of bills. The drafted bill is returned to its originator in the form of an "author copy." Content is carefully reviewed to ascertain that the bill does in fact state what it was intended to state.

A bill can be introduced at any time while the House is in session as long as the sponsoring representative has endorsed the bill and placed the proposal in the House's hopper. The procedure is more formal for the Senate, and any senator can postpone a bill by raising objections to it. All sponsored bills are assigned a legislative number and referred to committee. Currently there are 20 standing committees of the Senate, 27 standing committees of the House of Representatives, and 4 joint committees. Most standing committees have two or more subcommittees.

Formal statements and details pertaining to each bill are published in the *Congressional Record* and printed for distribution. At the federal level, a bill may be considered at any time during the two-year life of that Congress.

The chairperson of the committee to which a bill has been referred must submit the bill to the appropriate subcommittee within a specified time period, usually two weeks. The exception is when the majority of the committee members of the majority party vote to have the bill considered by full committee. Traditionally, many committees and subcommittees have held to a policy that any member who insists on a committee hearing on a particular bill should have it. Standing committees must have regular meetings at least once per month, and the chairperson may call additional meetings.

The legislators appointed to a committee conduct the hearing on a bill. At the federal level a bill may have no hearings or several hearings at one time in different committees. At the federal level, the author of a bill is seldom a member of the committee hearing the bill, while at the state level, the bill's author may have privileges not available to other legislators or the audience.

The committee chairperson selects individuals to present testimony first at hearings. Individuals or representatives of groups who have requested to speak about the bill may or may not be called for testimony. It is a frustrating political reality that one may go to committee hearings planning to speak or expecting to hear witnesses, only to find that the voting action was determined before the meeting. Astute individuals and groups not only monitor legislation but also tactfully lobby legislators before committee and subcommittee hearings.

After studying a bill and possibly hearing testimony, a committee may approve a bill in its original form and forward it. More commonly, the bill is revised and then forwarded or set aside. If a committee votes to pass a bill, a committee report is written that includes the bill's purpose, scope, and the reasons for the committee's approval. Containing a section-by-section analysis of the bill, the report is one of the most valuable sources of information regarding policy formulation and adoption.

Amendments to state bills and federal bills are handled differently. At the state level, the original bill retains its assigned number throughout the legislative process regardless of amendments. At the federal level, amending occurs in "mark-up" sessions. A new bill is printed and reintroduced with a new number following each mark-up session. Obviously, it is more difficult to follow a bill through the federal process. Also, it should be noted that more than 25,000 bills and joint resolutions are introduced in the average two-year U.S. Congress. Less than 10 percent of these are enacted as laws (U.S. House of Representatives, 1981).

In summary, there are three types of recommendations the committee can make. First, *due pass* means the committee approves the bill and is ready to forward it. Second, *due pass with amendments* means the committee has revised the bill. Third, the committee may refer the bill to another committee. If the bill is set aside by any committee it will eventually die; therefore, committees constitute veto points for bills.

Following committee action, the bill goes on the calendar and awaits being read before the originating house. The house considers the bill, and at this point its author states reasons why the bill is needed and responds to questions. Only legislators of the house may speak at the floor vote. The house may pass the bill or defeat the bill at the third reading. If the author knows in advance that there are not enough votes for the bill's passage, he or she will take action to delay the vote. At this point considerable compromise, negotiating, trade-offs and other strategies come into play. Success greatly depends upon the author's power base and political maneuvering.

If a bill passes the first house, it is forwarded to the second house. For example, if a bill passes the Senate, it then goes to the House of Representatives. It enters as a new bill with an introduction and first reading. In the second house the bill will again be assigned to committee. The committee will recommend due pass, due pass as amended, or amend and rerefer. Following this committee's actions, the bill has a second reading on the floor of the second house. The third reading results in a floor vote. If there are any changes in the bill by the second house, it is returned to the originating house for concurrence. When significant differences prevent concurrence, the bill is referred to a conference committee consisting of members from both houses.

The conference committee action is a very important step to which the public has no access. This committee determines which version of the bill, or a compromise of the bill, will go forward in the conference report. After adoption by both houses, the bill is enrolled and goes to the president.

The president has three options; he may sign, hold, or veto the bill. Signing the bill causes it to become law. Holding the bill without signing it causes the bill to become law after a delay of ten days if Congress is still in session. Vetoing the bill sends it back to Congress with the president's objections attached. Congress can override this veto by a two-thirds majority vote in both houses, and if the veto is overridden, the bill becomes law despite the president's objections.

Figure 25-3 outlines the process by which a bill becomes law. The fact remains that statutory law is only the beginning. The legislature enacts statutory law that enables a government agency to administer that law by means of regulation. Law is measured only in court. There are few laws other than criminal law by which one may be cited for noncompliance without going through a report mechanism. The government agency administers the law through regulation. In the case of registered nurses, it is the Board of Registered Nursing that administers laws relating to nursing education, licensure, and practice, most often called the Nurse Practice Act. That is the group accountable for disciplining registered nurses who do not meet the law.

A POLITICAL STRATEGY

Community health nursing must be clearly defined as having a necessary and integral role with clear-cut responsibilities in the health care system (Young, 1981). The role must be understood and appreciated by the public and legislators. The "selling" or marketing of the role can begin at the community or grass-roots level but must also occur at the state and national levels. Ideas of opposition groups or interest groups with conflicting goals must be met with constructive criticism and compromise. During this process of defining and marketing nursing, nurses should present a positive and unified image to the public, the legislators, and opposition groups (McCloskey and Grace, 1981). Nursing, like all other professions, has internal struggles and disagreements, but politically successful professions avoid public disclosure of internal discontent. Nursing holds a great deal of power, but that power remains unexerted (Gorman and Clark, 1986). A change in image is coming. Nurses outnumber all other health care providers and are as well educated as most. They have enhanced the health care system throughout all its struggles. Nurses need to improve their individual and collective self-concept. They must assist each other in achieving the highest possible levels of maturity, education, public service, and professionalism (Henderson, 1981; Young, 1981). Again, the focus should be on construction and growth.

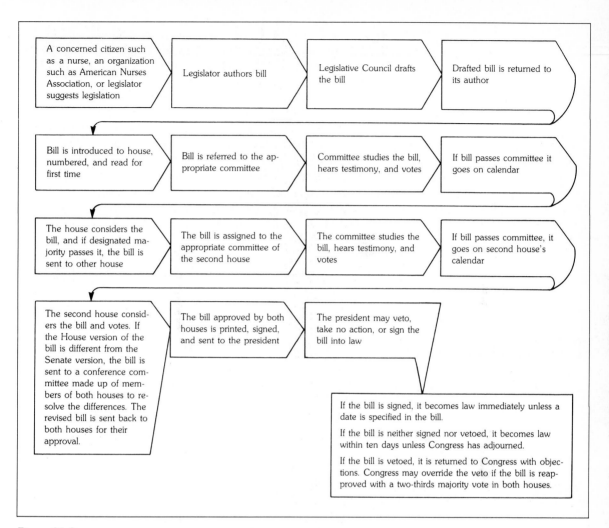

Figure 25-3
This flow chart diagrams the legislative process
through which a bill becomes a federal law.

Nurses must give each other credit for their accomplishments. Community health as a movement was created by nurses, yet others are ready to take the credit. Many leaders in nursing have received little recognition by nurses themselves. People in other fields who have done less and even borrowed heavily from nursing's ideas and practices have received tremendous recognition because they sell their accomplishments and have their colleagues' respect. Nurses must learn to support and assist one another. They must learn to be personally and politically assertive (McCloskey and Grace, 1981).

Policy research has shown that economic resources continue to be the major determinant of public policy, although the attitudes of political leaders appear to be increasingly important (Dye, 1978). The fact that the bulk of federal law presently originates in the executive branch of the government supports this conclusion. A great deal of emphasis has been placed on pluralistic political variables such as voter participation, party competition, and majority party control.

A greater financial base for promoting nursing will have to be established. Remarkably, while nurses willingly give their services and energy, they hesitate to share their money. As with any investment, nurses must first put money into the investment before expecting any returns. Also, it must be recognized there is an inherent risk to be taken before any short-term or, more importantly, long-term gains can be expected. That is, gains for clients and for the profession as a whole have been minimized because of nursing's present stage of political development. Once the profession assumes the authority, autonomy, and recognition it deserves, individual nurses will have the economic freedom to achieve their personal goals.

INDIVIDUAL GUIDELINES FOR POLITICAL INVOLVEMENT

Three major goals should be accomplished by the nurse as an individual in the political arena. They are generating support, creating legitimacy, and resolving conflicts (Monsama, 1979; Archer and Goehner, 1982). These goals are fulfilled when the community health nurse follows certain guidelines.

Generating Support

1. Present yourself well by promoting a positive and professional image. Dress and act accordingly.
2. Communicate your ideas effectively. Be knowledgeable, prepared, and state your position well. Use clear, concise, and understandable terms.
3. Learn the importance of socialization skills. Being a legislator is a 24-hour-a-day position. Invite a legislator to a social event at which a subject can be discussed in a relaxed manner.
4. Get yourself known. Network both within and outside the profession.
5. Recognize your skills to initiate, organize, and participate as well as use nursing process. Apply these skills to the political process.
6. Know your representatives at the local, state, and federal levels. Know allies in legislation. Keep in touch with them and keep them informed of health issues and their potential impact.
7. Make a concerted effort to influence a legislator to take a particular position on prospective legislation. Become involved in lobbying, writing, and presenting testimony when legislators hold hearings on prospective legislation.
8. Support a candidate's campaign by donating money or by volunteering time and energy. Campaign for candidates who support nursing and community health, provided the rest of their political platform is agreeable.

9. Join a political action committee (PAC). PACs are formed to permit a group to endorse and financially back up candidates who will support the group's position on issues.

Creating Legitimacy

1. Keep abreast of current issues in health care and nursing. Share your information with your colleagues.
2. Register to vote. Encourage others to do so. Hold a voters' registration drive. Be sure to vote and communicate with legislators when a health issue surfaces.
3. Belong and become involved in professional nursing organizations such as the American Nurses Association and the National League for Nursing, and outside professional organizations, such as the American Public Health Association and the American Hospital Association.
4. Become involved on committees and boards within your agency and community, such as boards of directors, state boards of registered nursing, health planning boards and committees, city planning boards, and the League of Women Voters.
5. Run for office. Start by running for an office at the local level, or, if you are known in your community, consider state or national office. Nurses need representation from nurses in the governmental system at all levels.
6. Become knowledgeable of the political process. Become familiar with committees handling health care legislation.

Resolving Conflict

1. Plan your strategies well. Be able and willing to negotiate and compromise, or you may lose the enire battle. However, do not sell out your profession to meet the goals of other professions.
2. Be proactive rather than reactive on health issues whenever possible. It gives you time to anticipate, accumulate resources, and more freedom to negotiate — all for better control.
3. Communicate with tact and respect. Each person has a right to his or her own beliefs. Avoid insults and overly aggressive behavior. Balance cooperation, collaboration, strength, and assertiveness.
4. Put politics into perspective. Every political position has pros and cons. Weigh each carefully and avoid tunnel vision.

COMMUNICATING WITH PUBLIC OFFICIALS

One form of political participation is communicating with legislators. The purpose of this contact is to sway the public official's views toward or against a specific bill or political position. The nurse can influence a legislator's opinion by means of oral and written communication through telephone calls, personal visits, telegrams, mailgrams, and letters. To be effective as a private citizen or as a member of a group, the nurse needs to know the process and appropriateness of each type of communication.

Written Communication

Legislators are more likely to be influenced by letters that express personal opinion and provide useful data than by form letters or mass telegrams. Form communications are tallied by a secretary or administrative assistant, but personal communication often reaches legislators directly. A considerable amount of data convincingly presented is necessary to change a legislator's opinion.

Effective communication persuades with facts, logic, and brevity. It requires the nurse to be well prepared. In writing a public official, the following points should be considered:

1. A neat, clear handwritten letter is acceptable, although a typewritten letter is preferable. Always address the letter appropriately with name and address on the letter and envelope.

President	The President
	The White House
	Washington, D.C. 20500
	My dear Mr. President:
	Most respectfully yours,

U.S. Senator	The Honorable Terry Miller
	Senate Office Building
	Washington, D.C. 20510
	My dear Senator Miller:
	Yours very truly,

U.S. Congressperson	The Honorable Terry Miller
	House Office Building
	Washington, D.C. 20515
	My dear Mr. or Ms. Miller:
	Yours very truly,

Governor	The Governor:
	State Capitol
	City, State Zip
	Dear Governor:
	Respectfully yours,

Mayor or City   Mayor Terry Miller (or) Councilperson
   Councilperson   Terry Miller
                              City Hall
                              City, State Zip

                              Dear Mayor Miller: (or) Dear Mr. or Ms.
                                Miller:
                                      Yours very truly,

2. When a bill is in committee, correspond with all members of the committee. The content of the letter may be the same, but each letter should be individually typed or handwritten.
3. There are no extra points for length, so plan the wording of your letter to make points concisely. The following is a content outline of what is appropriate to include in the correspondence:
   (a) One sentence that clearly states the issue
   (b) One sentence that clearly states your individual or group position
   (c) A statement that delineates the status of the proposed legislation (for example, where it is in the legislative process and what appears to be its disposition)
   (d) A list of the reasons to support or oppose the pending legislation
      (1) Financial
      (2) Groups adversely affected
      (3) Weaknesses of opposing view
      (4) Specific benefits that override weaknesses of your view, benefits of the opposing view, or both
   (e) Specific data that support these reasons
      (1) Dollar amounts
      (2) Number of groups affected and their names
      (3) Numbers within those groups
      (4) Delineation of processes, systems, equipment, and loopholes that have adverse or positive effects
   (f) A clear, concise statement of the action that you want the legislator to take on the piece of legislation: vote for or against the legislation; meet with you or your organization; ask for additional information; convey contents of letter to interested, influential persons; provide you with those persons' names and titles so that you can contact them, or other similar action.

Personal Visits

An amazing number of bills are enacted with no input from constituents. Lobbyists exert great influence, as do other legislative colleagues and persons who use the physical proximity of sitting close to a legislator or the persuasive tactic of trading favors to sway legislators' decisions.

Personal visits by nurses to their legislators can have a profound impact. Many legislators welcome additional expert information and respect the professional commitment involved in making the visit. Because legislators are very busy, with as little as three to five minutes for an interview, the nurse will make the visit more profitable by sending a briefing sheet or letter prior to the meeting. Discussion with a legislator's staff members can also be worthwhile. These individuals do the legislator's background research and help to develop the positions and language contained in the bills. Staff members are often more knowledgeable than the legislator about the issues and have more time to discuss them.

Community health nurses, as advocates for a health issue, must know the opposition's arguments and be prepared to counter them. The prepared nurse will communicate far more effectively with the legislator and his or her staff.

ATTENDING HEARINGS

Community health nurses attending a legislative hearing can have considerable impact on a pending bill or proposed regulation (Bagwell and Clements, 1985). Singly or as an organized group, the nurses' physical presence communicates to legislators that they are concerned, informed, and ready to take action. Again, nurses need to be prepared in advance of the hearing. Resources, such as a government relations committee or the state nurses' association, can provide useful information on the issues surrounding the bill. Other existing communication networks, such as nurses involved in political action committees, can provide additional information.

PROVIDING TESTIMONY

Once a community health nurse is versed in the particular topic of a bill, he or she may want to provide testimony (Figure 25-4). Testimony may be given verbally at the time of a hearing, or it may be written in advance. What should be included in it differs little from what should be included in a letter, with the exception of supportive materials, such as actual research or survey data.

Party has significant impact on the conduct of legislative business. Legislators have a party or partisan affiliation, and the numbers of any given party in one of the houses make a considerable difference in the conducting of business. At times votes follow party lines and platforms rather than respond to the information provided at the hearing or through letters. For this reason an organized lobbying group can be one helpful means to facilitate change.

All the standing committees of the legislature use the hearing process to discuss bills. During a hearing, amendments are introduced and discussed, and it is the hearing process that government agencies use to discuss proposed regulations. Legislative protocol favors the bill's author and the committee chairperson. They have more rights and privileges for the conduct of business.

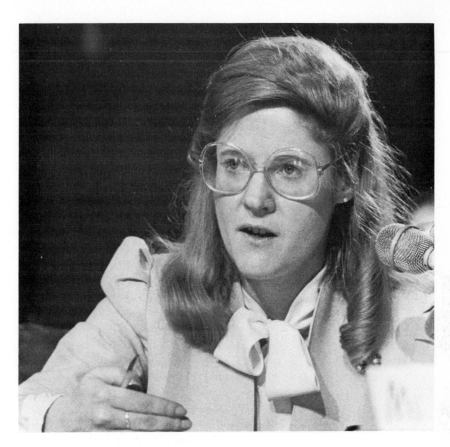

Figure 25-4
Advance preparation
enables the nurse to
communicate clearly and
convincingly, as this nurse
does while testifying before
a legislative committee.

If you as a community health nurse are in support of a bill and wish to testify, contact the author. If you are opposed to a bill and wish to testify, notify the author and the chairperson. Organized groups with registered lobbyists are most familiar with the process and may provide the best entrée to providing testimony. Remember, votes are counted by the author before a committee meets, and if the number is not sufficient for a due pass, there are many ways to keep the house from taking an official vote.

RESOURCES

The following is a brief compilation of resources covering some major facets of the policy studies area. There is no pretense that it is comprehensive. The chief objective is to provide directions in which political contacts and knowledge can be developed by the community health nurse.

A full-time clearinghouse with an extensive full-time staff would be required to review all the government publications in circulation. The nurse has to focus her or his reading and depend upon professional and political organizations and current nursing literature for guidance. The office of the *Federal Register* is responsible for the publication of laws, presidential documents, and the *United States Government Organization Manual.* Each act of Congress and public laws are accumulated for each congressional session in the *United States Statutes at Large.* Five times each week the *Federal Register* lists the regulations of government agencies, notices, executive orders, and presidential proclamations having general applicability and legal effect at the time. The annually updated *Code of Federal Regulations* lists all government regulations currently in effect. Presidential materials such as speeches and messages are available in the *Weekly Compilation of Presidential Documents.* Both the U.S. Senate and the U.S. House of Representatives keep a journal of their proceedings, but neither includes debates. The *Congressional Record* contains a complete record of everything said on the floor of both houses. It is printed bimonthly by the U.S. Government Printing Office and available by writing the Superintendent of Documents, U.S. Government Printing Office, Washington, D.C. 20402. Health statistics may be obtained from the National Center for Health Statistics, Hyattsville, Maryland 20872.

Just as there is an overwhelming number of federal publications, there is an overwhelming number of national, state, and local organizations. The *Encyclopedia of Associations,* published annually, is a comprehensive source of detailed information concerning nonprofit American organizations. The inclusion of for-profit groups in the list suggests that they are voluntary or not primarily for the purpose of profit generation. Citizen action groups, projects, and programs are also included. It is available in libraries and through the Gale Research Company in Detroit, Michigan.

Organizations politically significant to community health nurses are numerous. A listing of some of them at the national level is included at the end of this chapter.

The very diversity of policy articles requires a variety of journals. There are currently several publications that include articles and research directly related to health and health care from a policy analysis perspective. In the United States, the oldest of these journals is probably *Public Policy.* It offers detailed, theory-based case studies. Some other journals are *Policy Sciences, Policy Studies Journal,* and *Policy Analysis.*

An excellent resource specifically for nursing is the American Nurses Association Government Relations Division, which publishes *From the Washington Office.* This bulletin gives overviews of federal policy and laws, the voting records of legislators, and the action needed for nursing at the national level. The address of the division is 1030 15th Street, NW, Washington, D.C. 20005.

CONCLUSION

It is logical to anticipate that the 1990s will be characterized by increasing regulations regarding the costs, quantity, and quality of health care (Litman and Robins, 1984). Hence, the community health nurse must set forth an analysis framework that realistically assesses the capacity of a policy system to formulate, define, and implement health laws. Understanding the economic structure of a policy system or a community is integral to understanding its limits. More essentially, the economic structure reveals what motivates the policy system. Although the nurse knows a well-planned community program based on disease prevention and health promotion is more cost-effective than a disease treatment program, many policymakers do not. The experience of Santa Clara County's public health nurses' successful reversal of budget cuts gives testimony to this fact (Couser et al., 1986).

A community's health is strongly affected by many forces outside it. Funding limitations and reimbursement policies from third-party payers often dictate how nurses spend their time. Diagnosis-related groupings have undergone rapid growth as a significant financial base of health care agencies. The home health care boom has forced public health agencies to compete with private institutions. Social security benefits have undergone new restrictions. A nurse's evaluation of a law or policy in relation to a community should identify these external forces and their impact on the population.

The role of government in the organization, provision, and subsidization of health care has evolved from that of a protector of public health and provider of limited services to that of a policy setter and major underwriter of the entire health care system. Nurses must be politically active, because, as Litman and Robins (1984) point out, he who pays the piper calls the tune.

Both nurses and communities have a common goal, and that is the best possible health care for all. Nurses and communities can formulate, implement, and evaluate health policies to achieve this goal. Nurses cannot solve problems by blaming others nor by waiting passively for others to solve a community's health problems. Communities are learning what they want at the same time that they are learning how to get it.

Understanding politics and the policy-making process requires an integration of the findings and insights of many disparate studies into a reasonably comprehensive and verifiable framework. This framework can serve as a guide for future research and lead to a theory of policy process for nursing practice. The research information will make health policy formulation and implementation more cost-effective and community-oriented.

Summary

Community health nurses need to understand and become involved in the development of health policy and in the political process to protect the public's health. Furthermore, nurses need to exercise decision-making power in the political arena to enhance their own professional image and practice.

Social policy is what an institution, organization, agency, or government chooses to do or not to do. It may be written or unwritten. Health policy refers to the choices made regarding distribution of resources — people, facilities, time, and money — to health care. Policies ideally reflect the collective interests and beliefs of the group affected by them. However, in many instances a few individuals determine policy for the rest of the group. If community health nurses are to fulfill their mission of promoting, protecting, and preserving the health of aggregates, they must become policy makers as well as policy implementers.

Political systems, such as city government, generate policies and thus are policy systems. To determine the intentions of political systems, the nurse needs a framework for objective policy analysis, in contrast to the subjective activity of policy advocacy. One such framework for studying health policy involves analyzing the four stages of the policy process. Policy formulation includes identifying goals, problems, and potential solutions. Policy adoption refers to authorizing the selection and specification of the means to achieve the goals, resolving the problems, or both. Policy implementation is putting the policy to use. Policy evaluation means comparing policy outcomes with intended effects.

Legislation and policy related to community health must be analyzed from an aggregate perspective. Therefore, the community health nurse benefits from being able to diagnose the community and from assuming an active role in community organization. Steps in community organization for political action include: (1) identify oneself as a community organizer, (2) identify problems, (3) assess the physical community, (4) assess community resources and interests, (5) assess community politics, (6) evaluate alternative actions, (7) redefine objectives and priorities, (8) develop a plan, (9) implement the plan, and (10) evaluate the outcomes.

Community health policies are guidelines for implementing health laws. As such, they are subject to interpretation and change. Community health nurses can influence the development of policies as well as laws by learning about the legislative process and becoming appropriately involved.

A bill becomes law by going through various stages at any of which nurses can have input. These stages are governed by rules at all levels of government. Each bill undergoes a prescribed series of reviews before passage or rejection. Information about the process and the content of bills is available to nurses from several sources.

A political strategy available to community health nurses is to define and market nursing to the public and to legislators. Prerequisite to this is nursing's need to be internally supportive and reinforcing (in every way, including financially) in order to present a strong, unified front and have an impact on the health care system.

The politically involved nurse aims to accomplish the three goals of generating support, creating legitimacy, and resolving conflicts. The nurse can influence legislation by communicating with public officials through letters or phone calls, by personally visiting legislators, by attending hearings, and by providing testimony.

Many resources exist to assist the nurse with political contacts and information. Community health nurses must recognize societal changes and their potential impact on community health, and become active in the political process.

Study Questions

Select one bill related to health currently (or recently) under consideration by your state legislature.

1. Describe the bill and the issues involved in it.
2. Who is sponsoring it and why?
3. Who is opposing it and why?
4. Who will it affect, if passed, and in what ways will it affect them?
5. Discuss what you, as a community health nurse, could do to be involved in this bill.
6. Write a letter to your legislator regarding this bill (or some other health issue of concern to you).

Organizations Politically Significant to Community Health Nurses

American Academy of Nurses
c/o American Nurses Association
2420 Pershing Road
Kansas City, MO 64108

American Association of Nursing Service Administrators
840 North Lake Shore Drive
Chicago, IL 60611

American Association of Occupational Health Nurses
3500 Piedmont
Suite 400
Atlanta, GA 30305
Publications include *AAOH Newsletter* and *Occupational Health Nursing*

American Civil Liberties Union
132 W. 43rd Street
New York, NY 10036
Publications include the newsletter *Civil Liberties Alert*

American College of Nurse Midwives
1522 K Street, NW
Suite 1120
Washington, DC 20005
Publications include *Journal of Nurse Wifery* and the newsletter *Quickening*

American Indian Nurses Association
P.O. Box 1588
Norman, OK 73071
Publications include the *Newsletter of the AINA*

American Nurses Association
2420 Pershing Road
Kansas City, MO 64108
Publications include the *American Journal of Nursing* and *The American Nurse*

American Public Health Association
1015 15th Street, NW
Washington, DC 20005
Publications include the *American Journal of Public Health, The Nation's Health,* and *Washington Newsletter*

Association of Rehabilitation Nurses
2506 Gross Point Road
Evanston, IL 60201
Publications include *Rehabilitation Nurses*

Association of State Democratic Chairs
1625 Massachusetts Avenue, NW
Washington, DC 20036

Chamber of Commerce of the United States
Public Affairs Department
1615 H Street, NW
Washington, DC 20006
Publications include *Elections Guide* and *They Grade the Congress*

International Council of Nurses
Box 42
1211 Geneva, Switzerland

League of Women Voters
1730 M Street, NW
Washington, DC 20005

National Association of Hispanic Nurses
12400 7th Avenue, NW
Seattle, WA 98177

National Association of School Nurses
7395 South Kramer Street
Englewood, CO 80112
Publications include *School Nurse*

National Black Nurses Association, Inc.
P.O. Box 1835B
Boston, MA 02118

National League for Nursing
10 Columbus Circle
New York, NY 10019
More significant policy publications include *Public Policy Bulletin* and *Nursing Health Care*

National Organization for Women
425 13th Street, NW
Suite 1048
Washington, DC 20004

National Student Nurse Association
10 Columbus Circle
New York, NY 10019
Publications include *Imprint*

National Women's Political Caucus
1411 15th Street, NW
Suite 1110
Washington, DC 20005
Publications include *Women's Political Times*

Nurses' Coalition for Action in Politics
1030 15th Street, NW
Suite 408
Washington, DC 20005

Public Citizen
P.O. Box 19404
Washington, DC 20036

Republican National Committee
310 First Street, SE
Washington, DC 20003

References

Archer, S. E., and P. A. Goehner. (1982). *Nurses: A political force.* Monterey, Calif.: Wadsworth Health Sciences Division.

Bagwell, M., and D. Clements. (1985). *A political handbook for health professionals.* Boston: Little, Brown.

Courtney, R. (1987). Community practice: Nursing influence on policy formulation. *Nursing Outlook* 35(4): 170–73.

Couser, S., G. Daly, J. Grisham, and B. Rieder. (1986). Health in the balance. *Nursing Outlook* 34(1): 25–27.

Donley, R. (1982). Nursing and the politics of health. In N. L. Chaska (ed.), *The nursing profession: A time to speak* (pp. 844–57). New York: McGraw-Hill.

Dye, T. R. (1978). *Policy analysis: What governments do, why they do it, and what difference it makes.* Tuscaloosa, Ala.: University of Alabama.

Gorman, S., and N. Clark. (1986). Power and effective nursing practice. *Nursing Outlook* 34(1): 129.

Hancock, T., et al. (1985). Beyond health care: Proceedings of a conference on healthy public policy. *Canadian Journal of Public Health* 76(3)(Suppl. 1): 99–104.

Henderson, G. (1981). Nurses as risk takers. In J. McCloskey and H. Grace (eds.), *Current issues in nursing.* Boston: Blackwell Scientific Publications.

Kalisch, B. J., and P. A. Kalisch. (1982). *Politics of nursing,* Philadelphia: J. B. Lippincott.

Lee, P. R., C. L. Estes, and N. Ramsey. (1984). *The nation's health.* 2nd ed. San Francisco: Boyd and Fraser.

Litman, T. J., and L. S. Robins. (1984). *Health politics and policy.* New York: Wiley.

McCloskey, J., and H. Grace. (1981). Nurses must be personally and politically assertive. In J. McCloskey and H. Grace (eds.), *Current issues in nursing.* Boston: Blackwell Scientific Publications.

Monsama, S. V. (1979). *American politics: A systems approach.* New York: Holt, Rinehart and Winston.

Perlstadt, H., and R. Holmes. (1987). The role of public opinion polling in health legislation. *American Journal of Public Health* 77(5): 612–14.

Sabatier, P., and D. Mazmanian. (1981). *Effective policy implementation.* Lexington, Mass.: Lexington Books.

U.S. House of Representatives. (1981). *Our American government: What is it? How does it function? 150 questions and answers* (House Document No. 96-351). Washington, D.C.: U.S. Government Printing Office.

Williams, C. A. (1983). Making things happen: Community health nursing and the policy arena. *Nursing Outlook* 31: 225–28.

Young, W. B. (1981). Political action for professionalization. In J. McCloskey and H. Grace (eds.), *Current issues in nursing.* Boston: Blackwell Scientific Publications.

Selected Readings

Aiken, L. H. (ed.). (1982). *Nursing in the 1980's: Crises, opportunities, challenges.* Philadelphia: J. B. Lippincott.

American Nurses Association. (1980). *Nursing: A social policy statement.* (ANA Pub. NP-63 35M). Kansas City, Mo.: Author.

Anderson, E., and J. McFarlane. (1988). *The community as client: Application of the nursing process.* Philadelphia: J. B. Lippincott.

Archer, S. E., and P. A. Goehner. (1982). *Nurses: A political force.* Monterey, Calif.: Wadsworth Health Sciences Division.

Bagwell, M. (1980). Motivating nurses to be politically aware. *Nursing Leadership* 3(4): 4–6.

Bagwell, M. and D. Clements. (1985). *A political handbook for health professionals.* Boston: Little, Brown.

Baker, N., and C. Hart. (1981). Nurses in action. *Nursing and Health Care* 2(3): 130–32.

Berg, M., B. Taylor, L. Edwards, and E. Y. Hakanson. (1979). Prenatal care for pregnant adolescents in a public high school. *Journal of School Health* 49(1): 32–35.

Binder, J. (1983). Toward a policy perspective for nursing. *Nursing Economics* 1(1): 47–50.

Booth, R. Z. (1983). Power: A negative or positive force in relationships? *Nursing Administration Quarterly* 7(4): 10–20.

Braden, C. J., and N. L. Hervan. (1976). *Community health: A systems approach.* New York: Appleton-Century-Crofts.

Brower, T. H. (1982). Advocacy: What it is. *Journal of Gerontological Nursing* 8(3): 141–43.

Brown, B. J. (1981). Reviewing the past and current status of nursing's role in influencing governmental policy for research and training in nursing. In J. McCloskey and H. Grace (eds.), *Current issues in nursing.* Boston: Blackwell Scientific Publications.

Courtney, R. (1987). Community practice: nursing influence on policy formulation. *Nursing Outlook* 35(4): 170–73.

Couser, S., G. Daly, J. Grisham, and B. Rieder. (1986). Health in the balance. *Nursing Outlook* 34(1): 25–27.

Davis, A. J., and M. A. Aroskar. (1978). *Ethical dilemmas and nursing practice.* New York: Appleton-Century-Crofts.

de Kieffer, D. (1981). *How to lobby Congress.* New York: Dodd, Mead.

DelBueno, D. J. (1986). Power and politics in organizations. *Nursing Outlook* 34: 124.

Donley, R. (1982). Nursing and the politics of health. In N. L. Chaska (ed.), *The nursing profession: A time to speak* (pp. 844–57). New York: McGraw-Hill.

Dye, T. R. (1978). *Policy analysis: What governments do, why they do it, and what difference it makes.* Tuscaloosa, Ala.: University of Alabama.

Ellis, J. R., and C. L. Hartley. (1984). *Nursing in today's world: Challenges, issues, and trends.* Philadelphia: J. B. Lippincott.

Fisher, F. (ed.). (1980). *Politics, values, and public policy: The problem of methodology.* Boulder, Colo.: Westview Press.

Goodwin, R. (1982). *Political theory and public policy.* Chicago: The University of Chicago Press.

Gorman, S., and N. Clark. (1986). Power and effective nursing practice. *Nursing Outlook* 34(1): 129.

Hagberg, J. (1984). *Real power.* Minneapolis: Winston Press.

Hambrick, R., Jr. (1980). A guide for the analysis of policy arguments. In F. Fisher (ed.), *Politics, values, and public policy: The problem of methodology.* Boulder, Colo.: Westview Press.

Hancock, T., et al. (1985). Beyond health care: Proceedings of a conference on healthy public policy. *Canadian Journal of Public Health* 76(3)(Suppl. 1): 99–104.

Hein, E. C., and M. J. Nicholson. (1982). *Contemporary leadership behavior: Selected readings.* Boston: Little, Brown.

Henderson, G. (1981). Nurses as risk takers. In J. McCloskey and H. Grace (eds.), *Current issues in nursing.* Boston: Blackwell Scientific Publications.

Jenkins, W. I. (1978). *Policy analysis: A political and organizational perspective.* New York: St. Martin's Press.

Kalisch, B. J., and P. A. Kalisch. (1982). *Politics of nursing.* Philadelphia: J. B. Lippincott.

Lamar, E. K. (1985). Communicating personal power through nonverbal behavior. *Journal of Nursing Administration* 15(1): 41–44.

Lee, P. R., C. L. Estes, and N. B. Ramsey. (1984). *The nation's health.* 2nd ed. San Francisco: Boyd and Fraser.

Levine, M. (1981). Conditions contributing to effective implementation and their limits. In J. Crecine (ed.), *Research in public policy analysis and management.* Greenwich, Conn.: Jai Press.

Lindel, A. R. (1988). Power and politics: Tools for survival. *Nurse Educator* 4(3): 223–29.

Litman, T. J., and L. S. Robins. (1984). *Health politics and policy.* New York: Wiley.

Maraldo, P. J. (1982). Politics: A very human matter. *American Journal of Nursing* 82(7): 1104–5.

McCloskey, J., and H. Grace. (1981). Nurses must be personally and politically assertive. In J. McCloskey and H. Grace (eds.), *Current issues in nursing.* Boston: Blackwell Scientific Publications.

McLaughlin, M. (1976). Implementation as mutual adaptation. In W. Williams and R. Elmore (eds.), *Social program implementation* (pp. 167–80). New York: Academic Press.

Monsama, S. V. (1979). *American politics: A systems approach.* New York: Holt, Rinehart and Winston.

Moore, E., and D. Oakley. (1983). Nurses, political participation, and attitudes toward reform in the health care system. *Nursing and Health Care* 4(9): 504–6.

Nakamura, R., and F. Smallwood. (1980). *The politics of policy implementation.* New York: St. Martin's Press.

National League for Nursing. (1979). *The emergence of nursing as a political force* (NLN Pub. No. 41-1760). New York: Author.

National League for Nursing. (1982). Political action committees (PACs). *Public Policy Bulletin* 1(4).

National League for Nursing. (1982). Reimbursement for nurses in the primary care arena: A cost savings for health care. *Public Policy Bulletin* 1(5).

Perlstadt, H., and R. Holmes. (1987). The role of public opinion polling in health legislation. *American Journal of Public Health* 77(5): 612–4.

Puetz, B. E. (1984). Networking. *Public Health Nursing* 1(3): 174–77.

Raven, B. H., and R. W. Haley. (1980). Social influence in a medical context. *Policy Studies Review Annual* 4: 626–48.

Sabatier, P., and D. Mazmanian. (1980). The implementation of public policy: A framework for analysis. *Policy Studies Review Annual* 4: 181–203.

Sabatier, P., and D. Mazmanian. (1981). *Effective policy implementation.* Lexington, Mass: Lexington Books.

Somers, A. R. (1983). Competition or regulation — or both. *CHA Insight* 7(19).

Somers, A. R. (1983). New marching order for health care. *CHA Insight* 7(18).

Stevens, K. R. (ed.). (1983). *Power and influence: A source book for nurses.* New York: Wiley.

Thompson, T. (1980). An ordinal evaluation of the consumer participation process in community health programs. *Nursing Research* 29: 50–54.

U.S. House of Representatives. (1981). *How our laws are made* (House Document No. 97-120). Washington, D.C.: U.S. Government Printing Office.

U.S. House of Representatives. (1981). *Our American government: What is it? How does it function? 150 questions and answers* (House Document No. 96-351). Washington, D.C.: U.S. Government Printing Office.

Van Meter, D., and C. Van Horn. (1975). The policy implementation process: A conceptual framework. *Administration and Society* 6(4): 85–89.

Williams, F. C., and C. A. Williams. (1972). Ethical issues in health care policy. In Miller and Flynn (eds.), *Current perspectives in nursing,* pp. 121–32. St. Louis: C. V. Mosby.

Williams, C. A. (1983). Making things happen: Community health nursing and the policy arena. *Nursing Outlook* 31: 225–28.

Young, W. B. (1981). Political action for professionalization. In J. McCloskey and H. Grace (eds.), *Current issues in nursing.* Boston: Blackwell Scientific Publications.

Zaretsky, H. W. (1983). Planning for competition. *CHA Insight* 7(10), special issue.

Credits

The author and publisher would like to thank the following sources for granting permission to use their material:

Figure 1-2 (p. 9): From *Health Is a Community Affair,* Harvard University Press, 1967. Reprinted by permission of the publisher.

Table 2-1 (p. 34): From A.P.H.A. Position Paper in *American Journal of Public Health,* 65, 189–192, 1975. Reprinted by permission.

Figures 2-4 and 2-5 (pp. 38-39): Reproduced by permission from *Public Health Administration and Practice,* 8th ed., by J. J. Hanlon and G. E. Pickett. St. Louis, 1984, Times Mirror/Mosby College Publishing.

Figure 2-7 (p. 50): From Gibson, R. M., Levit, K. R., Lazenby, H., and Waldo, D. R.: National Health Expenditures, *Health Care Financing Review,* Vol. 6, No. 2. HCFA Pub. No. 03195. Office of Research and Demonstrations, Health Care Financing Administration. Washington. U.S. Government Printing Office, Dec. 1984.

Figure 3-2 (p. 70): From "Construct for Public Health Nursing" by Marla Salmon White in *Nursing Outlook,* November/December 1982. Copyright © 1982 by American Journal of Nursing Company. Reprinted by permission.

Table 4-3 (p. 123): Adapted from E. M. Duvall and B. Miller, *Marriage and Family Development,* 6th edition. 1985. Reprinted by permission of Harper & Row Publishing Company.

Tables 4-4 and 4-5 (pp. 124 and 125): From *The Family Life Cycle,* edited by Elizabeth A. Carter and Monica McGoldrick. Copyright © 1980 by Gardner Press, Inc., New York. Reprinted by permission of the publisher.

List on p. 153: From "Transcultural Nursing" by Anita J. Gagnon in *Nursing and Health Care,* March 1983, p. 130. Copyright © 1983 by Technomic Publishing Company, Inc. Reprinted by permission of the National League for Nursing.

List on pp. 170–71: From "The Use of Values Clarification in Nursing Practice" by Diane B. Uustal in *Continuing Education in Nursing,* May–June 1977. Copyright © 1977 by Charles B. Slack, Inc. Reprinted by permission.

Figures 6-4, 6-5, 6-6 (pp. 171–72): From "Values Clarification in Nursing: Application to Practice" by Diane B. Uustal in *American Journal of Nursing,* December 1978, Vol. 78, No. 12. Copyright © 1978 by American Journal of Nursing Company. Reprinted by permission.

List at top of p. 175: From "Ethics as a Component of the Curriculum" by Theresa Stanley in *Nursing and Health Care,* September 1980. Copyright © 1980 by Technomic Publishing Company, Inc. Reprinted by permission.

List on pp. 175–76: From *Ethics in Nursing* by Joyce B. Thompson and Henry O. Thompson. Reprinted by permission of the authors.

Figure 6-7 (p. 176): From "A Proposed Model for Critical Ethical Analysis" by Leah Curtin in *Nursing Forum* 17, 1978. Reprinted by permission.

Figure 9-4 (p. 245): From *Primer of Epidemiology* by G. D. Friedman. Reprinted by permission of McGraw-Hill Publishing Company.

Figure 9-5 (p. 254): From "Patterns of Reported Rape" by J. Sanford et al. in *American Journal of Public Health,* May 1979, p. 483. Copyright © 1979 by the American Public Health Association, Inc. Reprinted by permission.

Figure 9-6 (p. 262): From "A Cluster of Unexplained Deaths in a Nursing Home in Florida" by J. Sachs et al. in *American Journal of Public Health,* July 1988, p. 807. Copyright © 1988 by the American Public Health Association, Inc. Reprinted by permission.

Figure 9-7 (p. 263): From "Childhood Injury Deaths: A National Analysis" by A. Waller et al. in *American Journal of Public Health,* March 1989. Copyright © 1989 by the American Public Health Association, Inc. Reprinted by permission.

List on p. 287: From M. Sloan and B. T. Schommer, "The Process of Contracting in Community Nursing" in *Readings in Community Health Nursing,* Third Edition. (Boston: Little, Brown and Company, 1986), pp. 244–45.

Figure 11-1 (p. 307) and list on p. 311: From Malcolm S. Knowles, *The Modern Practice of Adult Education: From Pedagogy to Andragogy,* copyright © 1980, pp. 43–44, 57–58. Adapted by permission of Prentice-Hall, Inc., Englewood Cliffs, New Jersey.

List on p. 327: From G. Caplan, *Principles of Preventive Psychiatry* (New York: Basic Books, 1964).

Table 12-2 (p. 338): From "Crisis and Motivation: A Theoretical Model" by Stephen L. Fink in *Archives of Physical Medicine and Rehabilitation,* 48: 592, 1966. Copyright © 1966 by the American Congress of Rehabilitation Medicine. Reprinted by permission.

Figure 12-4 (p. 341): From "Crisis Transition Sequence" by Ralph G. Hirschowitz in *Levinson Letter.*

List on pp. 382–83: From *Community Health Analysis* by G. E. Alan Dever. Copyright © 1980 by Aspen Systems Corporation. Reprinted by permission of Aspen Publishers, Inc.

Lists on pp. 414–15: From E. Sampson and M. Marthas, *Group Process for the Health Professions* (New York: John Wiley & Sons, 1981).

Figures 15-5 and 15-6 (pp. 451 and 452): From Adele Holman, *Family Assessment,* pp. 64–65, 70. Copyright © 1983 by Sage Publications, Inc. Reprinted by permission of Sage Publications, Inc.

Table 17-1 (p. 503): "Childhood Immunization Schedule." Reprinted by permission of the American Academy of Pediatrics.

Poem on p. 522: "A Prayer/Pledge of Responsibility for Children" by Ina J. Hughes in *What Every American Should by Asking Political Leaders in 1988.* Reprinted by permission of the author.

List on pp. 540–41: From "Surveillance of Occupational Illness and Injury" by E. Baker, J. Melius, and J. Millar in *Journal of Public Health Policy,* Summer 1988. Copyright © 1988 by the Journal of Public Health Policy, Inc. Reprinted by permission.

Tables 19-1 and 19-2 (pp. 574 and 580): From *Introduction to Environmental Health,* edited by Daniel S. Blumenthal. Copyright © 1985 by Springer Publishing Company, Inc., New York, New York 10012. Reprinted by permission.

Figures 19-3 and 19-5 (pp. 576 and 583): From P. W. Purdom, *Environmental Health* (New York: Academic Press, 1980).

Figure 21-6 (p. 641): "Home Care Bill of Rights." Reprinted by permission of Ramsey County Public Health Nursing Service.

Figure 22-3 (p. 662): Adapted from P. Hersey and K. Blanchard, *Management of Organizational Behavior: Utilizing Human Resources,* Third Edition (1977). Reprinted by permission of Prentice-Hall Publishing Company.

Figure 23-2 (p. 699): Adapted from "A Model for Quality Assurance in Nursing" by Norma Lang, 1974. Reprinted with permission from *A Plan for Implementation of the Standards of Nursing Practice,* p. 15. Copyright © 1975 by the American Nurses Association, Kansas City, MO.

Table 23-1 (p. 707): "Outcome Criteria Development." Reprinted by permission of Ramsey County Public Health Nursing Service.

Photo Credits

Unless otherwise credited, all photographs are the property of Scott, Foresman and Company. *Chapter 1 Opener (p. 2):* Spencer Grant/Leo de Wys. *Figure 1-4 (p. 11):* Lori Bennett. *Figure 1-7 (p. 19):* From M. Blackwell, *Care of the Mentally Retarded.* Boston: Little, Brown, 1979. *Chapter 2 Opener (p. 26):* Nancy Lutz/The Picture Cube. *Figure 2-1 (p. 30):* Paul Conklin. *Figure 2-6 (p. 41):* WHO Photo. *Figure 2-8 (p. 52):* Courtesy of the Harvard Community Health Plan, Boston. *Figure 2-9 (p. 55):* Frank Siteman/The Picture Cube. *Chapter 3 Opener (p. 64):* Susan Van Etten/The Picture Cube. *Figure 3-3 (p. 75):* Courtesy of the Visiting Nurses' Association Collection, Boston. *Figure 3-4 (p. 77):* Courtesy of the Visiting Nurses' Association Collection, Boston. *Figure 3-6 (p. 88):* Lori Bennett. *Figure 3-7 (p. 91):* Billy E. Barnes/Stock Boston. *Chapter 4 Opener (p. 98):* Michael Weisbrot and Family. *Figure 4-1 (p. 102):* Richard Hutchings. *Figure 4-2 (p. 106):* Myrleen Ferguson/Photo Edit. *Figure 4-3 (p. 111):* Ulrike Welsch. *Figure 4-4 (p. 113):* Edward Slaman. *Figure 4-5 (p. 116):* Edward Slaman. *Figure 4-6 (p. 117):* From C. Schuster and S. Ashburn, *The Process of Human Development: A Holistic Approach.* Boston: Little, Brown, 1980. *Chapter 5 Opener (p. 130):* Ulrike Welsch. *Figure 5-3 (p. 136):* Lori Bennett. *Figure 5-4 (p. 138):* Courtesy of the Mount Vernon News. *Figure 5-5 (p. 141):* Burk Uzzle/Magnum Photos. *Figure 5-6 (p. 145):* Michael Weisbrot and Family. *Figure 5-7 (p. 148):* Charles Kennard/Stock Boston. *Figure 5-8 (p. 150):* Mimi Forsyth/Monkmeyer Press Photo Service. *Chapter 6 Opener (p. 162):* Joel Gordon Photography. *Figure 6-1 (p. 165):* Richard Hutchings. *Figure 6-3 (p. 170):* Edward Slaman. *Chapter 7 Opener (p. 190):* David E. Kennedy/TexaStock. *Figure 7-1 (p. 194):* From M. Blackwell, *Care of the Mentally Retarded.* Boston: Little, Brown, 1979. *Figure 7-2 (p. 198):* From M. Blackwell, *Care of the Mentally Retarded.* Boston: Little, Brown, 1979. *Figure 7-3 (p. 199):* Courtesy of the Harvard Community Health Plan, Boston. *Figure 7-4 (p. 203):* David Powers/Stock Boston. *Chapter 8 Opener (p. 212):* © 1982 Joel Gordon Photography. *Figure 8-2 (p. 217):* Courtesy of the Mount Vernon News. *Figure 8-5 (p. 229):* Courtesy of Beth Israel Hospital, Boston. *Chapter 9 Opener (p. 236):* Larry Mulvehill/Photo Researchers. *Figure 9-1 (p. 238):* Wallowitch. *Chapter 10 Opener (p. 272):* Hazel Hankin/Stock Boston. *Figure 10-1 (p. 281):* Courtesy of the Harvard Community Health Plan, Boston. *Figure 10-2 (p. 285):* Courtesy of the Harvard Community Health Plan, Boston. *Figure 11-2 (p. 308):* From C. Schuster and S. Ashburn, *The Process of Human Development: A Holistic Approach.* Boston: Little, Brown, 1980. Photo by Glenn Jackson. *Figure 11-3 (p. 312):* SIU/Custom Medical. *Figure 11-4 (p. 319):* Courtesy of Beth Israel Hospital, Boston. Photograph by Michael Lutch. *Chapter 12 Opener (p. 324):* El Paso Times. *Figure 12-1 (p. 331):* Courtesy of the Mount Vernon News. *Figure 12-2 (p. 333):* Ted Carland/ Courtesy The American Red Cross. *Figure 12-3 (p. 338):* Paul Conklin. *Figure 12-5 (p. 343):* Courtesy of the Mount Vernon News. *Figure 13-2 (p. 367):* Photograph by Robert Isaacs for Time Inc. *Figure 13-3 (p. 368):* Copyrighted Chicago Tribune Company, all rights reserved. *Figure 13-6 (p. 378):* Bob Daemmrich/Stock Boston. *Figure 13-7 (p. 386):* David R. Frazier Photolibrary. *Chapter 14 Opener (p. 392):* Tom Pantages. *Figure 14-1 (p. 395):* Paul Conklin. *Figure 14-2 (p. 397):* Courtesy of Beth Israel Hospital, Boston. Photograph by Michael Lutch. *Figure 14-4 (p. 402):* Courtesy of Beth Israel Hospital, Boston. *Figure 14-5 (p. 424):* Courtesy of the Mount Vernon News. *Chapter 15 Opener (p. 434):* Spencer Grant/Marilyn Gartman Agency. *Figure 15-1 (p. 442):* Karin Rosenthal/Stock Boston. *Figure 15-2 (p. 444):* Michael Grecco/Stock Boston. *Figure 15-3 (p. 446):* Jeffry W. Myers/Stock Boston. *Figure 15-4 (p. 447):* Sarah Putnam/The Picture Cube. *Chapter 16 Opener (p. 470):* Bryce Flynn/Stock Boston. *Figure 16-1 (p. 473):* David Witbeck/The Picture Cube. *Figure 16-2 (p. 475):* George W. Gardner/ The Image Works. *Figure 16-4 (p. 482):* Michael McGovern/The Picture Cube. *Figure 16-5 (p. 484):* Lori Bennett. *Chapter 17 Opener (p. 492):* Michael D. Sullivan/TexaStock. *Figure 17-1 (p. 495):* Lori Bennett. *Figure 17-2 (p. 503):* Paul Conklin. *Figure 17-3 (p. 506):* Nick de Gregory/ Leo de Wys. *Figure 17-4 (p. 508):* Andrew Brilliant/Carol Palmer. *Figure 17-5 (p. 511):* Edward Slaman. *Figure 17-6 (p. 515):* Courtesy of LaEsperanza Development Center, San Mateo, Ca. *Figure 17-7 (p. 516):* © Diana O. Rasche. *Chapter 18 Opener (p. 528):* Mark Chester/Leo de Wys. *Figure 18-1 (p. 533):* Photograph by Marilee Caliendo. *Figure 18-2 (p. 539):* Michael O'Brien. *Figure 18-3 (p. 545):* Photograph by Denny Lorentzen from *Newsletter,* National Swedish Board of Occupational Safety & Health, January 1981. *Figure 18-4 (p. 547):* Courtesy of the Harvard Community Health Plan, Boston. *Chapter 19 Opener (p. 562):* Lisa Law/The Image Works. *Figure 19-1 (p. 564):* John Colwell/Grant Heilman Photography. *Figure 19-2 (p. 572):* Michael D. Sullivan/TexaStock. *Figure 19-4 (p. 578):* Joe Travers/Gamma-Liaison. *Figure 19-5 (p. 582):* Ellis Herwig/The Picture Cube. *Figure 19-7 (p. 586):* © 1989 Nelson/ Custom Medical Stock Photo. All Rights Reserved. *Figure 19-8 (p. 589):* Dion Ogust/The Image Works. *Chapter 20 Opener (p. 596):* Suzanne Murphy. *Figure 20-1 (p. 600):* Nita Winter/The Image Works. *Figure 20-2 (p. 602):* Paul Conklin. *Figure 20-3 (p. 606):* © 1979 David Franklin for Time Inc. *Figure 20-4 (p. 607):* Lori Bennett. *Figure 20-5 (p. 610):* Fred Broadwell. *Figure 20-6 (p. 615):* Anna Kaufman Moon/Stock Boston. *Chapter 21 Opener (p. 624):* Alan Carey/The Image Works. *Figure 21-1 (p. 630):* David Schaefer. *Figure 21-2 (p. 632):* Paul Conklin. *Figure 21-3 (p. 633):* Paul Conklin. *Figure 21-5 (p. 640):* Paul Conklin. *Chapter 22 Opener (p. 652):* John Griffin/The Image Works. *Figure 22-2 (p. 661):* Courtesy of Beth Israel Hospital, Boston. *Figure 22-6 (p. 674):* David Conklin. *Figure 22-7 (p. 677):* Jacqueline Durand. *Chapter 23 Opener (p. 688):* Shelly R. Harrison/Decisive Moments. *Figure 23-1 (p. 691):* Lori Bennett. *Figure 23-5 (p. 711):* John Maher/The Picture Cube. *Figure 23-6 (p. 713):* Miro Vintoniv/Stock Boston. *Figure 24-1 (p. 723):* Joel Gordon Photography. *Figure 24-2 (p. 726):* Shelly R. Harrison/Decisive Moments. *Figure 24-3 (p. 728):* Alan Carey/The Image Works. *Figure 24-4 (p. 731):* Shelly R. Harrison/Decisive Moments. *Chapter 25 Opener (p. 736):* Sandra Johnson/The Picture Cube. *Figure 25-2 (p. 745):* Courtesy of the Harvard Community Health Plan, Boston. *Figure 25-4 (p. 755):* Copyright © 1983 *The American Nurse.* Reprinted with permission.

Index